Veterinary Vaccines

Veterinary Vaccines: Principles and Applications

Published by

The Food and Agriculture Organization of the United Nations

and

John Wiley & Sons Limited

Edited by

Samia Metwally
Senior Animal Health Officer
Animal Production and Health Division
Food and Agriculture Organization of the United Nations

Gerrit Viljoen
Section Head, Animal Production and Health
Joint FAO/IAEA Center
International Atomic Energy Agency

Ahmed El Idrissi
Former, Senior Animal Health Officer
Animal Production and Health Division
Food and Agriculture Organization of the United Nations

Food and Agriculture Organization of the United Nations

WILEY Blackwell

This edition first published 2021

The Food and Agriculture Organization (FAO) is a specialized agency of the United Nations that leads international efforts to defeat hunger. Our goal is to achieve food security for all and make sure that people have regular access to enough high-quality food to lead active, healthy lives. With over 194 member states, FAO works in over 130 countries worldwide. We believe that everyone can play a part in ending hunger.

Registered Office
John Wiley & Sons, Inc., 111 River Street, Hoboken, NJ 07030, USA
John Wiley & Sons Ltd, The Atrium, Southern Gate, Chichester, West Sussex, PO19 8SQ, UK

Editorial Office
9600 Garsington Road, Oxford, OX4 2DQ, UK

For details of our global editorial offices, customer services, and more information about Wiley products visit us at www.wiley.com.

Wiley also publishes its books in a variety of electronic formats and by print-on-demand. Some content that appears in standard print versions of this book may not be available in other formats.

Library of Congress Cataloging-in-Publication Data

Names: Metwally, Samia, editor. | Viljoen, Gerrit J., editor. | El Idrissi, Ahmed, editor.
Title: Veterinary vaccines : principles and applications / edited by Samia Metwally, Gerrit Viljoen, Ahmed El Idrissi.
Other titles: Veterinary vaccines (Metwally)
Description: Hoboken, NJ : Wiley-Blackwell, 2021. | Includes bibliographical references and index. | Description based on print version record and CIP data provided by publisher; resource not viewed.
Identifiers: LCCN 2020029897 (print) | LCCN 2020029898 (ebook) | ISBN 9781119506270 (epub) | ISBN 9781119506263 (adobe pdf) | ISBN 9781119505952 (hardback) | ISBN 9781119505952q(hardback) | ISBN 9781119506263q(adobe pdf) | ISBN 9781119506270q(epub)
Subjects: | MESH: Vaccines | Vaccination–veterinary | Livestock | Poultry | Animal Diseases–prevention & control
Classification: LCC SF918.V32 (ebook) | LCC SF918.V32 (print) | NLM SF 918.V32 | DDC 636.089/5372–dc23
LC record available at https://lccn.loc.gov/2020029897
LC record available at https://lccn.loc.gov/2020029898

Cover Design: Wiley
Cover Images: United States Department of Agriculture, public domain

Set in 9.5/12.5pt STIXTwoText by SPi Global, Chennai, India

Printed in Singapore
M089438_260321

Contents

List of Contributors

Alexandra Adams BSc, PhD
Professor of Aquatic Immunology and Diagnostics
Institute of Aquaculture, School of Natural Sciences
University of Stirling
Stirling, Scotland, UK

William Amanfu DCM, MS
International Veterinary Consultant
Formerly Animal Health Officer
FAO/UN
Rome, Italy

John Atkinson BSc Hons
Technical Manager, Ruminants
MSD Animal Health
Milton Keynes
Buckinghamshire, UK

Paul Barnett CBiol MRSB PhD
Biologicals Assessor
Veterinary Medicines Directorate
Addlestone, Surrey, UK

Carrie Batten Dr PhD
Head of Vascular Research Laboratory
The Pirbright Institute
Woking, Surrey, UK

Imane Belkourati DVM
Head of Quality Assurance
MCI Santé Animale
Mohammedia, Morocco

Abdelali Benkirane DVM, PhD
Full Professor
Microbiology, Immunology and Contagious
Diseases Unit, Department of Pathology
and Veterinary Public Health
Institut Agronomique et Vétérinaire Hassan II
Rabat, Morocco

José Maria Blasco PhD
Ad Honorem Researcher
Animal Health Department IA2 CITA
Universidad de Zaragoza
Zaragoza, Spain

Michèle Bouloy
Head of Research Unit "Molecular Genetics of Bunyavirus"
Department of Virology
Institut Pasteur
Paris, France

Zineb Boumart PhD
Research and Development Coordinator
MCI Santé Animale
Mohammedia, Morocco

Ian Brown MIBiol PhD
Head of Virology Department
Director of OIE/FAO International Reference
Laboratory for Avian Influenza and Newcastle Disease
Animal and Plant Health Agency
Addlestone, Surrey, UK

Emanuele Campese MSc
Researcher
Italian Reference Centre for Anthrax
Istituto Zooprofilattico Sperimentale
della Puglia e della Basilicata
Foggia, Italy

Peter Cargill BVM, CertPMP, MRCVS
Director
Wyatt Poultry Veterinary Services
Hereford, UK

Bryan Charleston BVM, MSc, PhD, MRCVS
Director
The Pirbright Institute
Pirbright, Surrey, UK

Adela Chavez PhD
Postdoctoral Researcher
CIRAD, UMR ASTRE
Petit-Bourg
Guadeloupe, French West Indies
CIRAD INRA, ASTRE
University of Montpellier
Montpellier, France

Karin Darpel VetMed, MRCVS, PhD
Head of Orbivirus Research
The Pirbright Institute
Woking, Surrey, UK

Klaus Depner DVM
Senior Scientific Officer
FAO Reference Centre for Classical Swine Fever
Friedrich-Loeffler-Institut
Greifswald, Germany

Adama Diallo DVM, PhD
Adviser to the Director
ISRA/LNERV
Dakar Hann, Senegal
UMR CIRAD-INRA ASTRE
Montpellier
France

Klaas Dietze DVM
Senior Scientific Officer
FAO Reference Centre for Classical Swine Fever
Friedrich-Loeffler-Institut
Greifswald, Germany

Meritxell Donadeu DVM, MSc
Visiting Research Fellow
Faculty of Veterinary and Agricultural Sciences
Veterinary Clinical Centre
The University of Melbourne
Werribee, Australia

Adelia Donatiello MSc
Researcher
Italian Reference Centre for Anthrax
Istituto Zooprofilattico Sperimentale della Puglia e della Basilicata
Foggia, Italy

Baptiste Dungu DVM, PhD
CEO
Onderstepoort Biological Products SOC Ltd
Onderstepoort, South Africa

Mehdi El Harrak DVM, PhD
R&D Director
MCI Santé Animale
Mohammedia, Morocco

Monique Eloit DVM
Director General
World Organization of Animal Health (OIE)
Paris, France

Lawrence Elsken BS, DVM
Vice President of Global Development
EDGE Veterinary Vaccines Consulting Group, LLC
Ames, Iowa, USA

Fatima Fakri DVM, PhD
Head of In Vitro Quality Control
MCI Santé Animale
Mohammedia, Morocco

Marisa Farber PhD
Researcher
INTA, CONICET, Instituto de Biotecnología
Buenos Aires, Argentina

Antonio Fasanella DVM, PhD
Director of the National Reference Center for Anthrax and General Director
Italian Reference Centre for Anthrax
Istituto Zooprofilattico Sperimentale della Puglia e della Basilicata
Foggia, Italy

Patricia Foley DVM, PhD
Risk Manager
Policy, Evaluation, and Licensing
Center for Veterinary Biologics
USDA APHIS
Ames, Iowa, USA

Alf-Eckbert Füssel DVM
Deputy Head
Animal Health and Welfare Unit
European Commission
Brussels, Belgium

Antonio Garmendia MSc, PhD
Professor of the Department of Pathobiology and Veterinary Science
University of Connecticut
Storrs, Connecticut, USA

Giuliano Garofolo DVM
Researcher
Reference Laboratory for Brucellosis
Istituto Zooprofilattico Sperimentale
dell'Abruzzo e del Molise
Teramo, Italy

Donna Gatewood DVM, MS
President and Chief Operating Officer
EDGE Veterinary Vaccines Consulting Group, LLC
Ames, Iowa, USA

Mohamed Gharbi DVM, MSc, PhD
Professor
Laboratoire de Parasitologie, Ecole
Nationale de Médecine Vétérinaire de Sidi Thabet
University of Manouba
Sidi Thabet, Tunisia

Carol Gibbs PhD
Senior Staff Microbiologist
Policy, Evaluation, and Licensing
Center for Veterinary Biologics
USDA APHIS
Ames, Iowa, USA

Amanda Gibson BSc(Hons), PhD
Immunologist
Department of Pathology and Pathogen Biology
The Royal Veterinary College
Hatfield, Hertfordshire, UK

Amy Gill DVM, PhD
Senior Staff Veterinarian
Policy, Evaluation, and Licensing
Center for Veterinary Biologics
USDA APHIS
Ames, Iowa, USA

Jihane Hamdi *DVM, PhD Student*
Vaccine Production Team
MCI Santé Animale
Mohammedia, Morocco

Ahmed El Idrissi DVM, PhD
Formerly Senior Animal Health Officer
Animal Production and Health Division
Food and Agriculture Organization of the United Nations
Rome, Italy

Richard Hill Jr DVM, MS
USDA – Retired

Philippe Holzmuller Eng. PhD, HDR
CIRAD INRA, ASTRE
University of Montpellier
Montpellier, France

Pascal Hudelet DVM
Head
Veterinary Public Health Technical Services
Merial, France

April Johnson DVM, MPH, PhD
Veterinary Medical Officer, USDA APHIS
Veterinary Services, Field Operations
Alabama, USA

Alasdair King BVMS
Director of Intergovernmental Veterinary Health
Merck Animal Health
Madison, New Jersey, USA

Babett Kobe
Scientific Assistant and Assessor
Veterinary Division
Paul Ehrlich Institut
Langen, Germany

Charles Lamien MSc, PhD
Technical Officer
Animal Health, Animal Production and
Health Laboratory, Joint FAO/IAEA
Division of Nuclear Techniques
in Food and Agriculture, Department of
Nuclear Sciences and Applications
International Atomic Energy Agency
Vienna, Austria

Marie-Frédérique Le Potier PhD
Head of the Swine Virology and Immunology Unit
ANSES – Laboratoire de Ploufragan/Plouzané
National Reference Laboratory
for Classical Swine Fever
Ploufragan, France

Alessio Lorusso DVM, PhD
Veterinary Medical Officer
Virology Unit
Istituto Zooprofilattico Sperimentale
Dell'Abruzzo E Molise
Teramo, Italy

Nicholas Lyons MA, VetMB, MSc, PhD, DipECBHM, MRCVS
Research Fellow
The Pirbright Institute
Pirbright, Surrey, UK

James MacLachlan BVSc, PhD
Distinguished Professor
School of Veterinary Medicine
University of California, Davis
Davis, California, USA

Isabel Marcelino PhD
CIRAD, UMR ASTRE
Petit-Bourg
Guadeloupe, French West Indies
CIRAD INRA, ASTRE
University of Montpellier
Montpellier, France

Dominique Martinez PhD
CIRAD, UMR ASTRE
Petit-Bourg
Guadeloupe, French West Indies

Samia Metwally DVM, PhD
Senior Animal Health Officer
Animal Production and Health Division
Food and Agriculture Organization of the United Nations
Rome, Italy

Maria Montoya PhD
Centro de Investigaciones Biológicas (CIB-CSIC)
Madrid, Spain

Edgardo Moreno PhD
Research Leader – Immunology Laboratory
Programa de Investigación en Enfermedades Tropicales
Escuela de Medicina Veterinaria
Universidad Nacional
Heredia
Instituto Clodomiro Picado
Universidad de Costa Rica
San José, Costa Rica

Ignacio Moriyón PhD
Professor
Instituto de Saludad Tropical y Departamento de Microbiología y Parasitología
Universidad de Navarra
Pamplona, Spain

Douglas Murtle BS
Senior Biologics Specialist
USDA-APHIS-VS-DB-Center for Veterinary Biologics
Ames, Iowa, USA

Waithaka Mwangi PhD
Associate Professor
Vaccine and Adjuvant Development Program
Department of Diagnostic Medicine/Pathobiology (DMP)
College of Veterinary Medicine
Kansas State University
Manhattan, Kansas, USA

Ivancho Naletoski DVM, PhD
Animal Production and Health Section
Joint FAO/IAEA Division of Nuclear Techniques in Food and Agriculture Department of Nuclear Sciences and Applications
International Atomic Energy Agency
Vienna, Austria

Nick Nwankpa DVM, MSC, PhD
Director
African Union Pan African Veterinary Vaccine Centre
Debre-Zeit, Ethiopia

Mark Pagala BS
Assistant Director
Microbiology
USDA-APHIS-VS-DB-Center for Veterinary Biologics
Ames, Iowa, USA

David Paton MA, VetMB, PhD
Veterinary Adviser
The Pirbright Institute
Woking, Surrey, UK

Anton Pernthaner DVM, Habil
Senior Scientist
Hopkirk Research Institute
Palmerston North, New Zealand

Rabindra Prasad Singh PhD
Head of the Division of Biological Products
ICAR – Indian Veterinary Research Institute
Bareilly
Uttar Pradesh, India

Monica Reising PhD
Senior Staff Statistician
USDA APHIS
Ames, Iowa, USA

Gourapura Renukaradhya DVM, MS, PhD
Associate Professor
Food Animal Health Research Program, OARDC
Veterinary Preventive Medicine
The Ohio State University
Wooster, Ohio, USA

James Roth DVM, PhD
Distinguished Professor
Director of the Center for Food Security and Public Health
Department of Veterinary Microbiology and Preventive Medicine
College of Veterinary Medicine, Iowa State University
Ames, Iowa, USA

Charles Rupprecht VMD, MS, PhD
CEO
LYSSA LLC
Atlanta, Georgia, USA

Matthew Sandbulte PhD
Scientist
Center for Food Security and Public Health
Department of Veterinary Microbiology and Preventive Medicine
Iowa State University
Ames, Iowa, USA

Giovanni Savini DVM, PhD
Scientific Director
Istituto Zooprofilattico Sperimentale
Dell'Abruzzo E Molise
Teramo, Italy

Melisse Schilling DVM
Senior Staff Veterinarian
Policy, Evaluation, and Licensing
Center for Veterinary Biologics
USDA APHIS
Ames, Iowa, USA

Renee Schnurr BSc
Section Leader
Inspection and Compliance
USDA-APHIS-VS-DB-Center for Veterinary Biologics
Ames, Iowa, USA

David Siev DVM, MS
Policy, Evaluation, and Licensing
Center for Veterinary Biologics
USDA APHIS
Ames, Iowa, USA

Heather Simpson PhD
Professor Emeritus
Institute of Veterinary, Animal and Biological Sciences
Massey University
Palmerston North, New Zealand

Leslie Sims BVSc(Hons), MANZCVS
Director
Asia Pacific Veterinary Information Services
Montmorency, Australia

Rohana Subasinghe BSc, MSc, PhD
Managing Director
FUTUREFISH Pvt. Ltd.
Rajagiriya, Sri Lanka

David Swayne DVM, MSc, PhD
Center Director
Southeast Poultry Research Laboratory
Agricultural Research Service
US Department of Agriculture
Athens, Georgia, USA

Elma Tchilian PhD
Group Leader
Swine Influenza Immunology, Livestock Viral Diseases
The Pirbright Institute
Pirbright, Surrey, UK

François Thiaucourt PhD
Head of Bacteriology Team
UMR, CIRAD-INRA, ASTRE
Montpellier, France

Karim Tounkara DVM, PhD
OIE Regional Representation for Africa
Bamako, Mali

Eeva Tuppurainen DVM, MSc, PhD, MRCVS
Senior Scientist
Friedrich-Loeffler-Institut
Greifswald, Germany

Saleh Umair DVM, M.Phil, PhD
Scientist
Hopkirk Research Institute
Palmerston North, New Zealand

Hermann Unger DVM
Animal Production and Health Section
Joint FAO/IAEA Division of Nuclear
Techniques in Food and Agriculture,
Department of Nuclear Sciences
and Applications
International Atomic Energy Agency
Vienna, Austria

Nathalie Vachiéry PhD
Unit Director
CIRAD, UMR ASTRE
Petit-Bourg
Guadeloupe, French West Indies
CIRAD INRA, ASTRE
University of Montpellier
Montpellier, France

Thierry van den Berg
Operational Director Viral Diseases
Veterinary and Agrochemical Research Centre
Brussels, Belgium

Piet van Rijn PhD
Professor
Department of Virology
Central Veterinary of Wageningen University
Research Center (CVI)
Lelystad, The Netherlands

Gerrit Viljoen DSc
Section Head
Animal Production and Health Section
Joint FAO/IAEA Division of Nuclear Techniques
in Food and Agriculture Department of Nuclear
Sciences and Applications
International Atomic Energy Agency
Vienna, Austria

Veronika von Messling DVM
Director
Veterinary Medicine Division
Paul Ehrlich Institut
Langen, Germany

Dirk Werling Dr, VetMed, PhD
Professor and Chair of Molecular Immunology
Department of Pathology and Pathogen Biology
The Royal Veterinary College
Hatfield, Hertfordshire, UK

Esther Werner
Deputy Head of Veterinary Division and Head
of Section "Assessment of Immunological
Veterinary Medicinal Products"
Paul Ehrlich Institut
Langen, Germany

Viskam Wijewardana BVSc, PhD
Animal Health Officer
Animal Production and Health Section
Joint FAO/IAEA Division of Nuclear Techniques
in Food and Agriculture Department of Nuclear
Sciences and Applications
International Atomic Energy Agency
Vienna, Austria

Ralph Woodland BSc, PhD
Retired (Previously Senior Biologicals Assessor)
Veterinary Medicines Directorate
Addlestone, Surrey, UK

Teresa Yeary PhD
Biologics Specialist
Inspection and Compliance
USDA-APHIS-VS-DB-Center for Veterinary Biologics
Ames, Iowa, USA

Stéphan Zientara DVM PhD HDR
Director
ANSES Laboratoire de Santé Animale
Maisons-Alfort, France

Foreword

For centuries, vaccinating animals has been the most cost-effective and sustainable measure to prevent and control infectious emerging and reemerging diseases. A prominent example of the merit of vaccination practices in eliminating major infectious animal epizootics is that of rinderpest, which was declared to have been eradicated in 2011. Veterinary vaccines can also help protect the health of people from zoonotic diseases.

The proper use of a quality and effective vaccine provides significant benefits to stakeholders and food security, from the reduction in livestock mortality, increased milk production, savings by reducing antibiotic and acaricide treatments, and alleviating the impact of antimicrobial resistance. The effects of livestock vaccination provide a positive impact on rural, livestock-dependent families, contributing to reducing poverty at the household level and in turn help us achieve the core mandate of the Food and Agriculture Organization of the United Nations and many of the Sustainable Development Goals.

The increase in global investment in livestock and its products signifies the demand for the development of new vaccines and vaccine production in accordance with international standards, effective vaccination strategies and their application. The need for advanced knowledge among vaccine producers, users and decision makers led to the publication of this comprehensive book addressing the principles and applications of veterinary vaccines for livestock.

This is the first book that provides a thorough review on a wide variety of topics regarding the role of veterinary vaccines, vaccine international standards, immune response, current and novel vaccines, production and quality control and more importantly a comprehensive review of vaccines for 13 high impact transboundary and zoonotic diseases. The book encompasses 29 chapters written by 97 leading experts, spanning 51 academic institutions, private and public sectors and regional and international organizations.

What I found impressive about this book is the high level of technical and practical information and guidelines it contains. I am confident that it will be valuable to a wide audience, including government authorities, decision makers, field veterinarians, livestock keepers, scientific community, vaccine producers and veterinary students.

I wish to thank the editors, authors, and their institutions for bringing together the first edition of this Veterinary Vaccines book in celebration of the 75th anniversary of the Food and Agriculture Organization of United Nations (FAO). A highly relevant publication that enhances the knowledge on vaccine principles and its applications to protect animal and public health and secure safe animal food for future generations.

Dr QU Dongyu

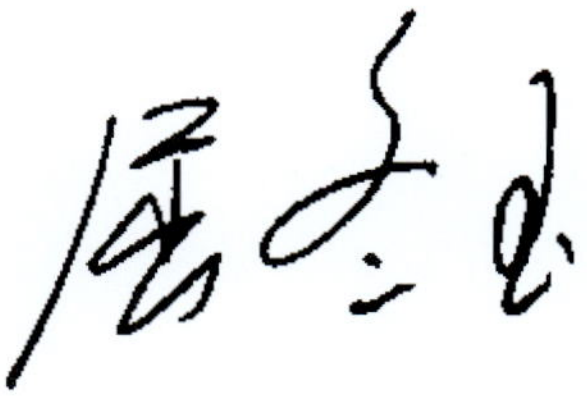

Director-General
Food and Agriculture Organization of
the United Nations (FAO)

Acknowledgments

There are many people, institutions, public and private sectors, and organizations that we would like to thank for their invaluable contributions. The contributions of all the authors and co-authors are greatly appreciated in order to produce their chapters.

We acknowledge the key role played by Drs Paul Barnett (The Pirbright Institute) and Akiko Kamata (FAO) in assisting the Editors in the design of the outline of book, and Dr David Paton (The Pirbright Institute) in the technical editing of the chapters. We are especially grateful to Dr Juan Lubroth, the former Chief Veterinary Officer of FAO, for his inspiration and support in the production of the book. Our thanks to Dr Berhe Tekola, Director of Animal Production and Health Division of FAO, for continued support.

Our profound appreciation is given to Ms Beate Werner for her invaluable assistance in liaising with the authors for the completion of the chapters and in selection of the publisher. Special appreciations to Dr Shija Jacob (FAO) in taking the key role in coordinating the submission of the final chapters to the publisher. Special thanks to Mr Paul Howard (FAO), Claudia Ciarlantini (FAO), Ms Cecilia Murguia (FAO) for their invaluable support throughout the production of the book.

We are particularly grateful for the financial support received from GALVmed that was kindly arranged for us by Drs Baptiste Dungu (former Senior R&D Director) and Jeremy Salt (Senior R&D Director).

Our most heartfelt thanks are due to our families for their help, forbearance, and understanding.

The Editors
Samia Metwally
Gerrit Viljoen
Ahmed El Idrissi

Introduction

First Edition

Over the past 200 years, following Louis Pasteur's first vaccine experiments, veterinary vaccines have played a central role in protecting animal and public health enabling efficient production of food animals, which is of significant importance to communities that rely on livestock to meet their nutritional and economic needs. Vaccines are now available for a range of important viral, bacterial, and parasitic diseases that have a major economic and public health impact.

Current veterinary vaccines based on inactivated and conventionally attenuated pathogens have illustrated good outcomes in the control of various types of animal diseases and therefore contribute significantly to animal welfare and safe food. However, vaccines also have their limitations, necessitating the application of different technologies to overcome the drawbacks and ensure the availability of safer and more efficacious vaccines. Improved understanding of the immunogenic and protective antigens of pathogens coupled with the advent in molecular genetics has opened the way for new generation vaccines. They afford numerous advantages over conventional vaccines, including ease of production, immunogenicity, and safety.

Manufacturing quality assured veterinary vaccines, whether conventional or new generation, and making them available on a large scale, requires the use of complex production methods, stringent quality control at every stage of the process, licensing regulations, and reliable distribution channels that ensure the products are potent and effective at their point of use. Reliable vaccine production and commercialization at affordable prices is the cornerstone of developing appropriate vaccination policies and strategies for prevalent animal diseases. This book primarily addresses the aforementioned aspects and provides vaccine users and stakeholders with concise, authoritative, and readily available information on vaccinology and vaccine immune response in animal populations.

Section I of this book is devoted to the importance of veterinary vaccines for animal health, animal welfare, and public health. Authors provide an overview of the benefits and challenges of vaccines for livestock species in the context of the growing human population, the global demand for meat, eggs, and dairy products, the rising standards of living in developing countries, and the changes in animal husbandry. This perspective is completed by a comprehensive technical review of the principles of vaccinology and immune response, vaccination strategies, implementation, and monitoring.

The following section provides an update on the current and future vaccines available for diseases caused by virus, bacteria, protozoans, rickettsia, and parasites in terrestrial and aquatic animals. The authors highlight the features of each vaccine category, challenges, research gaps, and technical options for the development of new generation vaccines and their possible impact on the design and modulation of novel vaccines or new approaches for their administration.

Section III of the book is dedicated to all aspects of vaccine production, quality control, licensing, and accessibility. It provides detailed schemes of in-process and final product quality control and testing to ensure the consistency of the vaccine quality. Aspects of external assessment, registration of veterinary vaccines, vaccine accessibility, and commercialization are also addressed. This section covers a comprehensive review of vaccine strategic reserves, or banks, as an adjunct to the control of important veterinary diseases.

The final section of the book provides a full review on vaccines and vaccination against selected high impact animal and zoonotic diseases. For each of the 13 diseases or group of pathogens addressed in this section, the book examines historical and current trends for immunization practices, the type of vaccines commercially available and those under development, practical recommendations and guidance on vaccination strategies, vaccine specifications, factors affecting vaccine efficacy and safety, and monitoring vaccine effectiveness after vaccination campaigns.

We believe that this first edition will be invaluable and instrumental to the scientific community, vaccine producers, stakeholders, field veterinarians, veterinary authorities, and veterinary students.

Although every effort was made to complete this book in as short a time as possible, it proved to be a more formidable and daunting task than anticipated, which took seven years from inception to publication. We sincerely hope that this book will help promote not only vaccine production and access to quality assured vaccines but also the control of infectious animal and zoonotic diseases so is the health of people and their livestock.

The Editors

Section I

Importance of Veterinary Vaccines

1

The Role of Veterinary Vaccines in Livestock Production, Animal Health, and Public Health

James Roth and Matthew Sandbulte

Department of Veterinary Microbiology and Preventive Medicine, Center for Food Security and Public Health, College of Veterinary Medicine, Iowa State University, Ames, Iowa, USA

1.1 Introduction: The Need for Veterinary Vaccines

The growing human population and rising standards of living in developing countries add to the global demand for meat, eggs, and dairy products. Changes in animal agriculture in recent decades include larger and denser populations of livestock species. Infectious diseases that degrade the health and productivity of livestock herds can be economically devastating and destabilize food supplies. Zoonotic transmission of infectious organisms from food-producing animals to humans is a significant threat to public health. There is an array of strategies used to control infectious diseases of livestock species, including facility sanitation, isolation or culling of infected animals, selection of disease-resistant genetic stock, treatment with antibiotics, and vaccination.

Vaccines are biological products designed to induce immune responses specific to pathogenic microorganisms, in order to prevent or reduce infectious diseases. Veterinary vaccines are a cost-effective method to prevent animal disease, enhance the efficiency of food production, and reduce or prevent transmission of zoonotic and food-borne infections to people. Safe and effective animal vaccines have become essential to modern society. The cost of producing enough animal protein to feed the 7 billion people on Earth would be dramatically higher without vaccines to prevent epizootics in food-producing animals. The lack of vaccines would leave farmers, communities, and countries more vulnerable to economically devastating livestock diseases. Zoonotic diseases such as brucellosis and leptospirosis would be much more prevalent in humans without effective vaccines for use in animals.

Rinderpest is a powerful example of how livestock vaccination, combined with other control measures, can dramatically improve animal health and human well-being. Rinderpest is an acute, highly contagious, viral disease of cattle, domesticated buffalo, and some species of wildlife. In 1889, cattle shipped from India carried the rinderpest virus to Africa, causing an epidemic that established the virus on the continent. Initially, approximately 90% of the cattle in sub-Saharan Africa died as well as many sheep and goats. The loss of draft animals, domestic livestock, and wildlife resulted in mass starvation, killing a third of the human population in Ethiopia and two-thirds of the Maasai people of Tanzania. The reduced number of grazing animals allowed thickets to form in grasslands. These thickets served as breeding grounds for tsetse flies, the vector for trypanosomes, resulting in an outbreak of trypanosomiasis (African sleeping sickness) in humans. This rinderpest epidemic is considered by some to have been the most catastrophic natural disaster ever to affect Africa. The Global Rinderpest Eradication Programme was a large-scale international collaboration involving vaccination, local and international trade restrictions, and surveillance. In 2011, rinderpest infection was declared to be eradicated from the world's livestock and wildlife, marking one of veterinary medicine's greatest achievements (OIE 2011).

Continuing improvement and increased use of livestock vaccines will promote the health and welfare of animals, promote efficient food production, reduce economic losses to producers, and reduce the dangers of zoonotic diseases. For animal vaccines to make a significant impact on animal and public health, they must be widely used, which means they must be affordable. This chapter provides an overview of the benefits and challenges of vaccines for livestock species.

Veterinary Vaccines: Principles and Applications, First Edition. Edited by Samia Metwally, Gerrit Viljoen, and Ahmed El Idrissi.

1.2 Diversity of Veterinary Vaccines

Because a variety of livestock and poultry species are raised around the world and each species is susceptible to an array of bacterial, viral, and parasitic infectious agents, it is not surprising that many diverse vaccines are produced in the world. Livestock vaccines are developed and licensed for a variety of purposes, which are sometimes different from the purposes of human vaccines. Examples would be food safety vaccines to reduce the shedding of *Salmonella* by poultry and *Escherichia coli* 0157/H7 by cattle. Livestock vaccines are primarily used to improve the efficiency of production of food animals. The cost of the vaccine is an important consideration as to whether the vaccine will be used. It must contribute to profitability for the producer in the long run to be widely accepted. Vaccination against zoonotic diseases also can be used to reduce or eliminate the risk of human infection (e.g. rabies, brucellosis). Wildlife vaccines are generally used for zoonotic diseases (e.g. oral bait vaccines for rabies), or in some cases in conjunction with disease control programs in domestic species (e.g. brucellosis vaccine for bison and elk, oral bait vaccines for classic swine fever in feral swine).

Today, in the USA alone, there are about 1280 active licenses for nonautogenous veterinary vaccine products, including vaccines that consist of viruses, bacterins, bacterial extracts, toxoids, and many combinations (USDA-APHIS 2014). Licensed animal vaccines are available for some diseases where vaccines are not available for analogous human diseases, such as brucellosis and bovine respiratory syncytial virus in cattle, and *Mycoplasma hyopneumoniae* in swine. Veterinary vaccines have a distinct advantage in that they can be developed and licensed much more quickly and at much less cost than human vaccines. The ability to conduct safety and efficacy studies, including vaccination/challenge experiments, in the target species greatly facilitates licensing of veterinary vaccines. Liability issues associated with adverse reactions are much less restrictive for manufacturers of veterinary vaccines than for manufacturers of human vaccines. In addition, veterinary vaccines produced in developing countries may undergo less rigorous approval processes than in developed countries.

The equine West Nile virus vaccine is an example of how an animal vaccine can be developed and licensed quickly to meet an emergency situation (Brown et al. 2016). The West Nile virus was discovered in the USA in August 1999. The veterinary vaccine industry, working in cooperation with the US Department of Agriculture (USDA) Center for Veterinary Biologics, quickly developed an effective vaccine to prevent the disease in horses. By August 2001, an equine vaccine for West Nile virus was conditionally licensed by the USDA. West Nile virus vaccine is now considered one of the core equine vaccines in the USA (American Association of Equine Practitioners – Vaccination guidelines). The vaccine has also been used off label to protect some endangered birds, such as California condors (Chang et al. 2007). Porcine circovirus 2 vaccines (Chae 2012) and influenza pandemic H1N1 vaccines (AVMA 2010) for swine are additional examples of newly emerging diseases for which veterinary vaccines were developed and licensed quickly.

1.3 Vaccines and Food Production

Veterinary vaccines are used in livestock to maintain animal health and improve overall production. More efficient animal production and better access to high-quality protein are essential to feed the growing population. According to the United Nations Department of Economic and Social Affairs Population Division, the world population was approximately 7 billion in 2014, and is estimated to increase to just over 8 billion in 2025 and to reach 9.1 billion people in 2050 (Figure 1.1). The United Nations Food and Agriculture Organization (FAO) estimates that 805 million people were undernourished in 2014 (FAO, IFAD, and WFP 2014). There were dramatic increases in world meat and egg production between 1962 and 2006 (Figure 1.2). The FAO projected that feeding a world population of 9.1 billion people will require overall food production to increase by 60% between 2007 and 2050 (FAO 2009; Alexandratos and Bruinsma 2012). The global demand for beef, pork, poultry, and other animal protein sources will increase sharply by the year 2050 (Figure 1.2). Vaccines that preserve animal health and improve production will be important components in meeting this need.

The economic structures of livestock husbandry are unique in the developing world, where many livestock and poultry are raised in small household settings. Even when licensed vaccines are commercially available for livestock pathogens of concern in a region or country, many producers cannot afford to use them. Reliable statistics on the use of livestock vaccines across the developing world are very scarce. A survey performed in Tanzania in 2008–2009 provided useful socioeconomic data on household livestock keeping in a sub-Saharan African context. A majority of rural households in Tanzania reported livestock-related income. Approximately 60% of households reported the presence of livestock disease in their herd/flock during the year of the survey. Only about 29% of households reported any use of vaccination in their animals. It could be inferred that the small livestock holders in Tanzania have

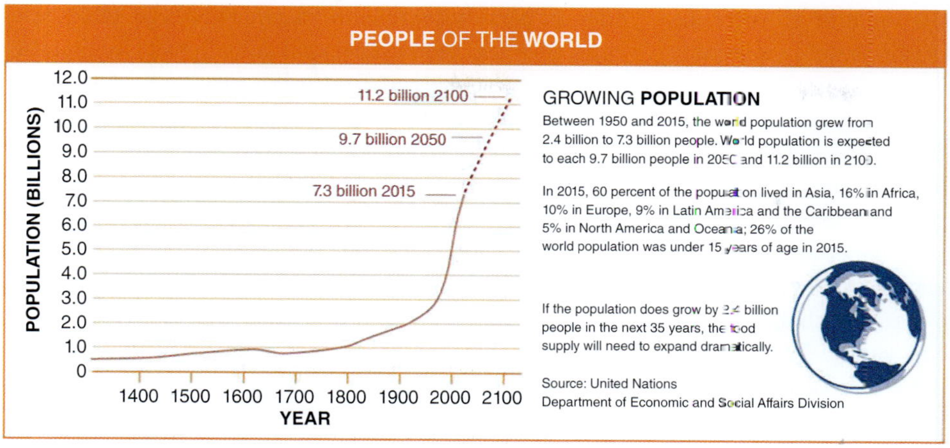

Figure 1.1 Global population growth in recent centuries, projected through 2100. Source: Reprinted with permission from Roth et al. (2016).

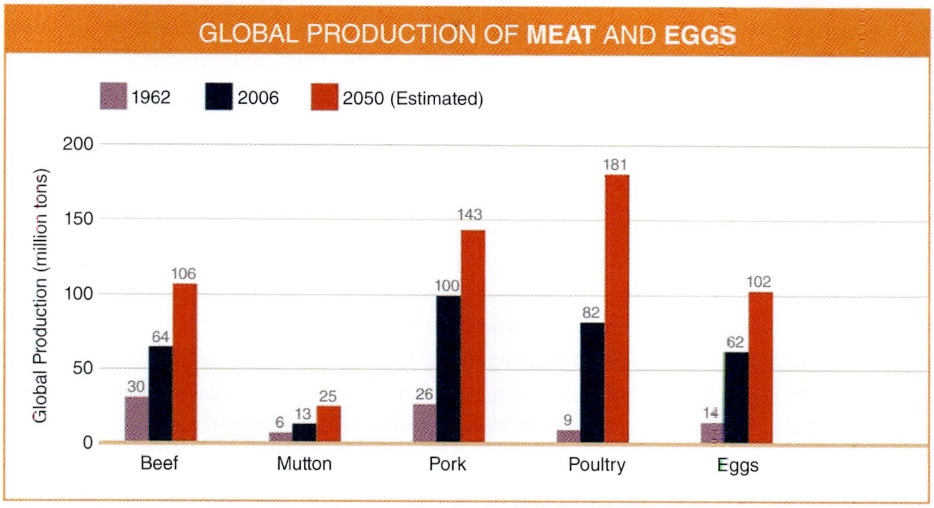

Figure 1.2 Global production of meat and eggs. Between 1962 and 2006 the production of major classes of animal-derived food increased by twofold or greater. Production of these food sources is projected to increase substantially again over the first half of the twenty-first century. Similar growth is reported for milk production, except on a larger scale: 344M tons in 1962, 664M tons in 2006, 1077M tons projected in 2050. Vaccines and other methods of controlling infectious diseases in livestock and poultry help to maximize food production. Source: Data from Table 4.18 of Alexandratos and Bruinsma (2012).

insufficient access to effective vaccines either due to cost or lack of availability, and the same is likely true in many other countries (Covarrubias et al. 2012).

Foot and mouth disease (FMD) virus is a tremendous burden to meat and dairy production in many parts of the world, especially developing countries. It is estimated that 2% of cattle in the world are infected with FMD virus in a year (Knight-Jones and Rushton 2013). The direct production losses from FMD – the majority of which are borne by China, India, and Africa – are estimated at roughly US$ 7.6 billion per year (Knight-Jones and Rushton 2013). Losses include not only diminished animal weight gain and milk production, but also loss of traction power when draft animals are infected. There are also indirect economic costs, such as restrictions to livestock export. In countries where FMD virus is endemic, vaccination has an important role in protecting cattle, pigs, and buffalo, thus reducing the economic impact of the disease. It is estimated that the world's livestock are immunized with 2.35 billion doses of FMD vaccine annually (Knight-Jones and Rushton 2013). The positive impact of FMD vaccination in endemic countries would be greater if vaccine doses were less expensive and induced longer-lasting immunity (Kitching et al. 2007). Even countries recognized as FMD free, which often cease vaccination, have an economic burden from the virus. They must maintain costly preventive measures and prepare resources to respond in the event of an outbreak emergency, such as vaccine banks (discussed in a section below).

Antibiotics are widely used to control bacterial pathogens of livestock and to promote efficient food production. However, there are increasing concerns related to antibiotic resistance associated with the extensive use of antibiotics in veterinary and human medicine (Dibner and Richards 2005). Producers may choose either vaccines or antibiotics to control some diseases based on cost, if both options are available. For example, swine ileitis caused by *Lawsonia intracellularis* can be controlled by either vaccination or antibiotics, along with good management practices. Swine producers will use the approved control method that is most cost effective. If regulatory requirements for a biologics company to obtain and maintain a license to produce the vaccine were to increase beyond what is essential, then the cost of the vaccine would increase and producers would opt to use less vaccine and more antibiotics. Affordable and available vaccines reduce reliance on antibiotics for animal health.

1.4 Vaccines for Control of Zoonotic Diseases

Vaccines to control zoonotic diseases in food animals, companion animals, and even wildlife have had a major impact on reducing the incidence of zoonotic diseases in people. Some examples of veterinary vaccines for zoonotic diseases that have been, or could be, used to control infections in animals, thereby reducing transmission of the infectious agent to people, include rabies, brucellosis, leptospirosis, influenza, Rift Valley fever, nipah, hendra, Japanese encephalitis, and Q fever. Without rabies vaccines, it is unlikely that families would be willing to keep cats and dogs as pets. Recombinant vaccinia-vectored rabies vaccines have also been used successfully in baits for oral vaccination campaigns to reduce the incidence of rabies in wild animals (Pastoret and Brochier 1996). Vaccines for brucellosis were instrumental in the *Brucella abortus* eradication program in the USA. Many countries continue to have severe problems with brucellosis in cattle, small ruminants, and people due to a lack of available *Brucella* vaccines for animals (FAO 2010). An additional concern related to *Brucella* vaccines is that they are live vaccines which can infect and cause symptoms in people (Ashford et al. 2004). New-generation safer vaccines for brucellosis are needed.

Similarly, vaccinating livestock against various *Leptospira* serovars can reduce the incidence of human leptospirosis, which in severe cases can cause miscarriage or death. The tapeworm parasite *Taenia solium*, which is transmitted between pigs and humans, is a major cause of adult-onset epilepsy in developing countries (Spickler 2005). In recent field trials, an experimental *T. solium* vaccine administered to scavenging pigs protected them against transmission of the parasite (Jayashi et al. 2012). These promising results suggest that pig vaccination could become an effective way to break the cycle of *T. solium* transmission to people in the developing world.

Emerging and exotic animal diseases are a growing threat to human and animal health and jeopardize food security (Figure 1.3). Increases in human and animal populations, with accompanying environmental degradation, global warming, spread of arthropod vectors, and globalized trade and travel, enhance opportunities for transfer of pathogens within and between species. The resulting diseases pose enormous challenges now and for the future.

In most of the world, increased demand for animal protein has resulted in intensified commercial food animal production and/or expanded "backyard" production.

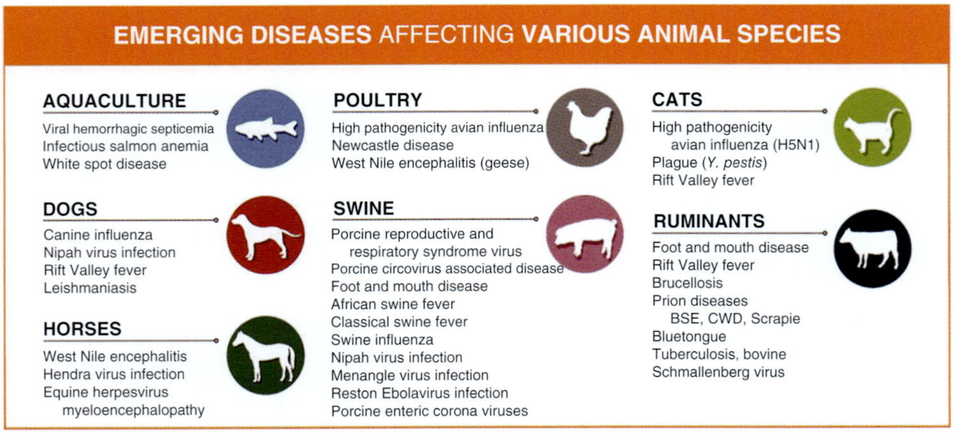

Figure 1.3 Emerging diseases affecting various animal species. Source: Reprinted with permission from Roth et al. (2016).

Both types of production present unique challenges for disease emergence and control. Large commercial operations with high concentrations of animals produce high-quality protein for human consumption at reduced costs. These operations typically have some degree of biosecurity, vaccination programs, and veterinary care. However, the high concentration of animals may facilitate the emergence of pathogens due to extensive replication in large numbers of animals, enhancing the potential for mutation and adaptation to the species. They also present concerns regarding animal welfare and environmental preservation. "Backyard" production of poultry, pigs, and small ruminants can efficiently use household waste for feed and can be an important supplement to dietary protein and income. However, the close interaction with humans, especially children, presents an increased risk of zoonotic disease transfer (e.g. avian influenza and *Brucella melitensis*). "Backyard" animal production rarely has biosecurity or adequate vaccination. Emerging zoonotic diseases of both food and companion animals are a major threat to public health. It is inevitable that the world will continue to experience emerging disease outbreaks in the coming decades. Rapid development of animal vaccines can play a key role in controlling emerging diseases.

There are several examples of vaccines successfully developed against emerging equine viruses, including Venezuelan equine encephalitis, West Nile, and hendra (Broder et al. 2013; Bowen et al. 2014). Vaccination against these agents lowers the risk of zoonotic infections. Several countries have used vaccines, together with other eradication measures, to control high pathogenicity avian influenza virus (H5N1) in poultry. From 2002 to 2010, it is reported that many billions of doses were administered to poultry, mostly in China (Chapter 18) (Swayne 2012). This practice is considered to have reduced disease and mortality in chicken flocks, while also reducing the number of human infections, which have very high fatality rates. Rift Valley fever virus, a devastating pathogen of ruminants and a virulent zoonotic agent, is seen as a prime target for animal vaccine development (Monath 2013). Continued development of more cost-efficient, safe, and effective vaccines against zoonotic agents will foster improvement of human health, animal health, and food security.

1.5 Vaccines to Improve Food Safety

Recently, vaccines have been developed to reduce the shedding of organisms that cause food-borne diseases in people. Vaccines are available for *E. coli* O157:H7 in cattle and *Salmonella enterica*, serovars *enteritidis* and *typhimurium*, in chickens. These vaccines typically do not improve the health of the vaccinated animal, but reduce the intestinal colonization and shedding of pathogens that may contaminate animal products for human consumption (Thomson et al. 2009; Desin et al. 2013). The severity of the *S. enteritidis* outbreak in people in the USA in 2010 due to consumption of contaminated eggs (Cima 2010) could have been reduced or prevented if the associated chickens had received an *S. enteritidis* vaccine. Numerous other microorganisms, common in livestock, cause food-borne disease outbreaks in people, so there may be future opportunities to broaden the use of livestock vaccines for food safety purposes.

1.6 Vaccine Banks

In countries where a particular animal infectious disease does not exist – either due to eradication or because it was never endemic to the region – vaccination against the agent will usually not be practiced. When there is no market for vaccines, the biologics companies do not have an incentive to develop, license, and manufacture them. However, there is often a continuing risk that the agent will be (re)introduced. This requires readiness to respond quickly to control an outbreak, especially because herd immunity to the agent no longer exists.

In the USA, the Department of Agriculture and the Department of Homeland Security have recognized the need to have approved vaccines for important animal diseases that are not currently present within the country's borders. US animal agriculture is highly vulnerable to the introduction of foreign diseases, most notably FMD. A Homeland Security Presidential Directive mandated the establishment of a National Veterinary Stockpile (NVS), a national repository that can deploy within 24 hours "sufficient amounts of animal vaccine, antiviral, or therapeutic products to appropriately respond to the most damaging animal diseases affecting human health and the economy" (Bush 2004). Although the USA is a partner in the North American FMD Vaccine Bank, the present supply is not sufficient to meet the needs of an FMD outbreak. European Union states, Japan, Australia, and New Zealand also maintain FMD vaccine banks (Hagerman et al. 2012). The World Organization for Animal Health has established vaccine banks for avian influenza, FMD, and peste des petits ruminants (PPR) and has shipped doses to many countries in the developing world.

Vaccine banks or stockpiles are expensive to establish and maintain, so robust funding is required. Also, establishing an emergency plan for vaccination against an emerging or foreign animal disease can be complicated from the regulatory standpoint. In some cases, a disease-free country does not issue a regular vaccine license, but issues a conditional license for use in the event of an outbreak. Safety and efficacy criteria for conditional licensure may be different from criteria for a vaccine used against endemic diseases. A functional program of foreign animal disease preparedness requires cooperation among veterinary and public health agencies, regulators, and vaccine manufacturers.

1.7 Successes and Challenges

As discussed above, one of the greatest successes in the use of vaccination to control an animal disease was the global eradication of rinderpest virus. This was achieved using the Plowright vaccine, a conventional live attenuated virus that was generated by serial passages of a virulent rinderpest strain in primary calf kidney cells (Plowright 1984). Other striking examples of vaccine successes and challenges can be seen in some important swine viruses. Aujeszky's disease virus (also called pseudorabies virus) has been successfully eradicated from swine herds in numerous countries, including the USA. An important innovation aiding that success was vaccines with glycoprotein gene deletions (Mengeling et al. 1997; Pensaert et al. 2004). These deletions allow diagnostic tests that differentiate between infected and vaccinated animals (the DIVA strategy). With these tools, it is possible to conduct screening and selective culling in the eradication campaigns, without forgoing the use of immunization to protect herds.

After its discovery in the late 1990s, the porcine circovirus 2 (PCV2) was found to be widespread in major swine-producing countries. It was etiologically linked to postweaning multisystemic wasting syndrome and other clinical syndromes with great economic impact. Subunit and inactivated virus vaccines for PCV2 were developed commercially, became widely adopted, and led to significant improvements in swine health and productivity (Beach and Meng 2012).

On the other hand, efforts to produce effective vaccines against porcine reproductive and respiratory syndrome virus (PRRSV) and influenza A viruses of swine (IAV-S) have been less successful. These economically important viruses have been identified for many years, but current vaccines do not provide reliable control of infection and disease. A major hurdle in both cases is the antigenic variability of the viruses. One concept for improved vaccines against antigenically variable viruses like PRRSV and IAV-S is to identify epitopes that are highly conserved across the various strains. Vaccines that target the conserved epitopes would have the potential to supply broad cross-protection (Khanna et al. 2014). Utilizing new adjuvants, vaccine vectors, delivery mechanisms, or rationally designed live attenuated viruses might also lead to more effective vaccines against these viruses.

Across the spectrum of livestock infectious diseases, there are many with no proven vaccines and others with inadequate vaccine options. Live and killed Newcastle disease virus vaccines are used extensively in some endemic countries, yet frequent outbreaks continue, possibly because genetic mutations in the pathogenic strains allow them to evade the immunity induced by the vaccines (Ashraf and Shah 2014). A live *Mycoplasma mycoides* subsp. *mycoides* vaccine against contagious bovine pleuropneumonia has existed in Africa for half a century, but problems with its efficacy and duration of immunity have been recognized (Jores et al. 2013). Improvements in vaccine technologies, such as adjuvants and recombinant vectors, can potentially aid the development of vaccines against many pathogens. However, one of the disadvantages faced in veterinary vaccine development is that the potential financial returns are much less than for human vaccines. Veterinary vaccines have lower sales prices and smaller potential market value. Consequently, there is a lower investment in research and development for animal vaccines compared to human vaccines, although the range of hosts and pathogens is greater.

1.8 Policies on Use of Vaccines in Disease Control Programs

In some situations, infectious disease agents pose a threat to animal health, human health, food security, or economic stability, but producers do not have the ability or strong incentive to pay for vaccination. Such situations may include endemic diseases in developing countries, zoonotic and food-borne diseases that do not cause serious sickness in livestock, and emerging or exotic diseases that have a small probability of spreading to the given region. For disease control and eradication programs, it is often necessary for governments or other entities to provide financial support. An example would be the current interest in eradication of PPR. Regardless of how the expense is met, a low cost per unit of vaccine is critical to achieving widespread vaccination of the susceptible livestock.

1.9 Summary

The consequences of livestock and poultry infectious diseases are felt throughout the world, regardless of wealth or veterinary medical infrastructure. When livestock diseases are not controlled effectively, global food production is diminished and public health is often put at risk. This explains the vital importance of vaccines for food-producing animals. The fact that so many people depend on livestock and poultry for their livelihoods and as a source of food limits policy options, complicates local and global trade decisions, and raises political sensitivities. It is inevitable that the world will continue to experience the emergence of new human and animal diseases in the coming decades. This challenge requires that veterinary, medical, and public health communities work together locally and internationally. Affordable, safe, and effective livestock vaccines will continue to be an important tool to protect human health, animal health, food safety, and food security.

Acknowledgments

Portions of this chapter were adapted from a 2011 review article authored by James Roth (Roth 2011).

References

Alexandratos, N.B.J. and Bruinsma, J. (2012). World Agriculture Towards 2030/2050: The 2012 Revision. ESA Working Paper No. 12-03. Food and Agriculture Organization of the United Nations. www.fao.org/docrep/016/ap106e/ap106e.pdf

Ashford, D.A., di Pietra, J., Lingappa, J. et al. (2004). Adverse events in humans associated with accidental exposure to the livestock brucellosis vaccine RB51. *Vaccine* 22 (25–26): 3435–3439.

Ashraf, A. and Shah, M.S. (2014). Newcastle disease: present status and future challenges for developing countries. *Afr. J. Micriobiol. Res.* 8 (5): 411–416.

AVMA. (2010). Swine-use H1N1 vaccine approved under conditional license. JAVMANews. www.avma.org/javma-news/2010-01-15/swine-use-h1n1-vaccine-approved-under-conditional-license

Beach, N.M. and Meng, X.J. (2012). Efficacy and future prospects of commercially available and experimental vaccines against porcine circovirus type 2 (PCV2). *Virus Res.* 164 (1–2): 33–42.

Bowen, R.A., Bosco-Lauth, A., Syvrud, K. et al. (2014). Protection of horses from West Nile virus Lineage 2 challenge following immunization with a whole, inactivated WNV lineage 1 vaccine. *Vaccine* 32 (42): 5455–5459.

Broder, C.C., Xu, K., Nikolov, D.B. et al. (2013). A treatment for and vaccine against the deadly Hendra and Nipah viruses. *Antiviral Res.* 100 (1): 8–13.

Brown, G.B., Spickler, A.R., Galyon, J., and Roth, J.S. (2016). Descriptions of incursions of foreign, transboundary and emerging animal diseases. In: *Transboundary and Emerging Diseases of Animals* (eds. A.R. Spickler, J.A. Roth, J. Galyon and G.B. Brown), 96–100. Ames: Center for Food Security and Public Health, Iowa State University.

Bush, G.W. (2004). Homeland Security Presidential Directive 9: Defense of United States Agriculture and Food. United States Department of Homeland Security. www.gpo.gov/fdsys/pkg/PPP-2004-book1/pdf/PPP-2004-book1-doc-pg173.pdf

Chae, C. (2012). Commercial porcine circovirus type 2 vaccines: efficacy and clinical application. *Vet. J.* 194 (2): 151–157.

Chang, G.J., Davis, B.S., Stringfield, C., and Lutz, C. (2007). Prospective immunization of the endangered California condor (*Gymnogyps californianus*) protects this species from lethal West Nile virus infection. *Vaccine* 25 (12): 2325–2330.

Cima, G. (2010). Vaccine use up since Salmonella outbreak. *J. Am. Vet. Med. Assoc.* 237 (12): 1356–1357.

Covarrubias, K., Longin, N., and Zezza, A. (2012). Livestock and livelihoods in rural Tanzania: a descriptive analysis of the 2009 National Panel Survey. World Bank Open Knowledge Repository, Washington DC. https://openknowledge.worldbank.org/bitstream/handle/10986/17885/866280WP0Live00Box385181B00PUBLIC0.pdf?sequence=1&isAllowed=y

Desin, T.S., Köster, W., and Potter, A.A. (2013). Salmonella vaccines in poultry: past, present and future. *Expert Rev. Vaccines* 12 (1): 87–96.

Dibner, J.J. and Richards, J.D. (2005). Antibiotic growth promoters in agriculture: history and mode of action. *Poult. Sci.* 84 (4): 634–643.

FAO. (2009). High Level Expert Forum – How to Feed the World in 2050. FAO, Rome. www.fao.org/fileadmin/templates/wsfs/docs/Issues_papers/HLEF2050_Global_Agriculture.pdf

FAO. (2010). *Brucella melitensis* in Eurasia and the Middle East. FAO Animal Production and Health Proceedings No. 10. FAO, Rome. www.fao.org/docrep/012/i1402e/i1402e00.pdf

FAO, IFAD, and WFP. (2014). The State of Food Insecurity in the World 2014. Strengthening the enabling environment for food security and nutrition. FAO, Rome. https://sustainabledevelopment.un.org/content/documents/1717The%20State%20of%20Food%20Insecurity%20in%20the%20World%202014.pdf

Hagerman, A.D.M., McCarl, B.A., Carpenter, T.E. et al. (2012). Emergency vaccination to control foot-and-mouth disease: implications of its inclusion as a U.S. policy option. *Appl. Econ. Perspect. Policy* 34 (1): 119–146.

Jayashi, C.M., Kyngdon, C.T., Gauci, C.G. et al. (2012). Successful immunization of naturally reared pigs against porcine cysticercosis with a recombinant oncosphere antigen vaccine. *Vet. Parasitol.* 188 (3–4): 261–267.

Jores, J., Mariner, J.C., and Naessen, J. (2013). Development of an improved vaccine for contagious bovine pleuropneumonia: an African perspective on challenges and proposed actions. *Vet. Res.* 44 (1): 122.

Khanna, M., Sharma, S., Kumar, B., and Rajput, R. (2014). Protective immunity based on the conserved hemagglutinin stalk domain and its prospects for universal influenza vaccine development. *BioMed. Res. Int.* 2014: 546274.

Kitching, P., Hammond, J., Jeggo, M. et al. (2007). Global FMD control – is it an option? *Vaccine* 25 (30): 5660–5664.

Knight-Jones, T.J. and Rushton, J. (2013). The economic impacts of foot and mouth disease – what are they, how big are they and where do they occur? *Prev. Vet. Med.* 112 (3–4): 161–173.

Mengeling, W.L., Brockmeier, S.L., Lager, K.M., and Vorwald, A.C. (1997). The role of biotechnologically engineered vaccines and diagnostics in pseudorabies (Aujeszky's disease) eradication strategies. *Vet Microbiol* 55 (1–4): 49–60.

Monath, T.P. (2013). Vaccines against diseases transmitted from animals to humans: a one health paradigm. *Vaccine* 31 (46): 5321–5338.

OIE. (2011). Final Report of the 79th General Session. OIE, Paris. www.oie.int/doc/ged/D11931.PDF

Pastoret, P.P. and Brochier, B. (1996). The development and use of a vaccinia-rabies recombinant oral vaccine for the control of wildlife rabies; a link between Jenner and Pasteur. *Epidemiol. Infect.* 116 (3): 235–240.

Pensaert, M., Labarque, G., Favoreel, H., and Nauwynck, H. (2004). Aujeszky's disease vaccination and differentiation of vaccinated from infected pigs. *Dev. Biol.* 119: 243–254.

Plowright, W. (1984). The duration of immunity in cattle following inoculation of rinderpest cell culture vaccine. *J. Hyg.* 92 (3): 285–296.

Roth, J.A. (2011). Veterinary vaccines and their importance to animal health and public health. *Procedia Vaccinol.* 5: 127–136.

Roth, J.A., Galyon, J., and Brown, G.B. (2016). Causes and consequences of transboundary and emerging diseases of animals: role of the veterinarian. In: *Transboundary and Emerging Diseases of Animals* (eds. A.R. Spickler, J.A. Roth, J. Galyon and G.B. Brown), 14–27. Ames: Center for Food Security and Public Health, Iowa State University.

Spickler, A.R. (2005). Taenia Infections. Ames: Center for Food Security and Public Health, Iowa State University. www.cfsph.iastate.edu/DiseaseInfo/factsheets.php

Swayne, D.E. (2012). The role of vaccines and vaccination in high pathogenicity avian influenza control and eradication. *Expert Rev. Vaccines* 11 (8): 877–880.

Thomson, D.U., Loneragan, G.H., Thornton, A.B. et al. (2009). Use of a siderophore receptor and porin proteins-based vaccine to control the burden of *Escherichia coli* O157:H7 in feedlot cattle. *Foodborne Pathog. Dis.* 6 (7): 871–877.

USDA-APHIS. (2014). Current Veterinary Biologics Product Catalogue. www.aphis.usda.gov/animal_health /vet_biologics/publications/currentprodcodebook.pdf

2

Principles of Vaccinology and Vaccine Immune Response

María Montoya[1] and Elma Tchilian[2]

[1] *Centro de Investigaciones Biológicas (CIB-CSIC), Madrid, Spain*
[2] *Swine Influenza Immunology, Livestock Viral Diseases, The Pirbright Institute, Woking, Surrey, UK*

2.1 Introduction

Edward Jenner recognized that dairymaids who frequently contracted cowpox were often immune to smallpox, which led him to use cowpox to inoculate people against smallpox. Jenner named the process *vaccination* (derived from the Latin word *vacca*, "cow") and Pasteur in his honor extended the term to the stimulation of protection to other infectious agents. Vaccination eventually resulted in the complete eradication of smallpox in humans and rinderpest in cattle, and is one of the most effective medical interventions ever introduced.

The aim of vaccination is to induce a long-lasting protective immune response to an infectious pathogen or toxic moiety from a pathogen, using a nonvirulent or nontoxic antigen preparation. As a result, in the event of an actual encounter with the infectious agent or toxin, the host is either completely protected against harm or is able to mount a very rapid and potent secondary immune response to reduce the harm, rather than a slow and less effective primary response. In this chapter, we will review how the adaptive immune response protects against the attack of pathogens, describing the major types of lymphocytes, B and T cells, and the different forms of immune protection they provide. We will discuss how best to deliver vaccines using adjuvants and delivery platforms, how to differentiate vaccinated from infected animals, how to assess protection after vaccination, and the features of active, passive, and herd immunity.

2.2 The Concept of Immune Conversion

The immune system protects the organism from attack by pathogens. It is composed of many cell types, the majority of which are organized into separate lymphoid tissues and organs. Because pathogens can attack at many different sites of the body, molecules and cells of the immune system circulate in the blood as well as residing in the tissues so that a rapid response can be made. The innate system is the first line of defense against infection. It works rapidly, giving rise to acute inflammatory responses, and has some specificity for microbes but no memory. Some of the most important cells in the innate system are phagocytes that can ingest microbes and kill them.

In contrast, the second line of defense, the adaptive immune response, takes longer to develop, is highly specific, and responds more quickly to a microbe that it has encountered previously ("memory"). The adaptive immune system starts acting even as the innate immune system is dealing with the invading microbe, and especially if it is unable to contain it.

Innate and adaptive immunity work together. For example, the phagocytic cells produce important cytokines that help induce the adaptive immune response. Cytotoxic T cells kill virus infected cells, but these have to be cleared from the body by phagocytic cells. Complement components of the innate system can be activated directly by microbes, but they can also be activated by antibodies, molecules of the adaptive immune system.

The adaptive immune system contains two major types of lymphocytes: thymus-derived (T) and bone marrow-derived (B) lymphocytes. T cells mature under the influence of the thymus and on stimulation with antigen, give rise to cellular immunity. B cells mature mainly in the bone marrow and mediate humoral immunity, which involves soluble molecules – antibodies (immunoglobulins, Ig). Both T and B cells have randomly generated receptors so that each cell is specific for a different foreign substance (antigen). When an antigen is introduced into the body,

Veterinary Vaccines: Principles and Applications, First Edition. Edited by Samia Metwally, Gerrit Viljoen, and Ahmed El Idrissi.

lymphocytes with receptors for this antigen encounter and bind it, proliferate, and give rise to clones of cells specific to the antigen. These cells or their products specifically interact with the antigen to neutralize or eliminate it.

Antibodies are key effectors of adaptive immunity. In addition to proliferation after encountering with antigen, B cells undergo somatic mutation, giving rise to high-affinity antibodies, as well as Ig class switching to produce antibody molecules with different effector functions (IgG, IgA, and IgE). Thus, for both B and T cells, immunological memory consists of increased numbers of cells with specificity for the antigen. T memory cells have a range of different effector functions while memory B cells produce high-affinity antibodies, also with different effector functions.

While the immunoglobulin (IgM and IgD) receptors on B cells can interact directly with antigen in solution, T cells require peptide moieties from processed protein antigens to be presented in the context of major histocompatibility complex (MHC) molecules. Antigen processing and presentation is typically performed by specialized antigen-presenting dendritic cells. It is important for vaccines to induce the type of immunity able to neutralize the pathogen: antibody (B cell) and/or cell-mediated (or T cell) immunity.

2.2.1 Antibodies

Antibodies, either produced as result of immunization or passively administered to the host, are often very effective in preventing infection. Antibodies can prevent the pathogen from entering the host's tissues and cells (neutralization) and can mediate killing of the pathogen (phagocytosis or cytotoxicity) (Figure 2.1a). The ability of the antibody to neutralize and promote cytotoxicity depends on its avidity, isotype, subclass, and ability to fix complement and recruit phagocytic cells. Antibodies may also prevent damaging effects on cells by neutralizing toxins such as those produced by the *Giardia* parasite and *Diphtheria* and *Clostridium* species of bacteria. IgG antibodies are primarily effective in the blood and tissues whereas IgA plays an important role at mucosal surfaces, where it helps prevent viral or bacterial access to the mucosal lining cells (Loehr et al. 2001; Sedgmen et al. 2004; Meeusen et al. 2007).

There are two components of antibody memory. First, preexisting antibodies are readily available and able to bind the infectious agent at the time of infection, avoiding the need for the host's immune system to respond. Specific antibody can be maintained at a relatively high level for many years, probably produced mainly by long-lived plasma B cells in the bone marrow. The second component of antibody memory is memory B cells, which may also be crucial for vaccine-mediated protection. In this case, contact with the pathogen stimulates antigen-specific memory B cells, induced by the vaccine, to proliferate and differentiate to short-lived plasmablasts, which rapidly produce large amounts of antibody. Contact of memory B cells with antigen is also important in boosting long-lived plasma cell numbers and maintaining serum antibody concentrations for the next encounter with the pathogen.

Immune responses to infectious agents usually produce antibodies directed at multiple epitopes but only some of these confer protection. The specificity of antibodies is influenced not only by the repertoire of B cells but also by the specificity of T cells. Linked recognition, in which antigen-specific B and T cells provide mutually activating signals, leads to affinity maturation and Ig isotype switching, which is often required for efficient pathogen neutralization. This process requires that B cells present an appropriate peptide epitope for T cells and typically, the T cell epitope is contained within the region of a protein recognized by the B cell.

Sometimes, however, immunization may have unpredicted, pathological consequences. The formalin-inactivated respiratory syncytial virus (RSV) vaccine provides an example of vaccine-enhanced disease, which is thought to be due to production of low-avidity, poorly neutralizing antibodies that are not protective. In addition, immune complexes and complement activation contribute to pathology as well as an inappropriate, Th2-biased immune response (Acosta et al. 2015). Another example of the pathological consequences of inappropriate immunization, although with a different mechanism, is vaccine-associated enhanced respiratory disease (VAERD). This has been observed in pigs when heterologous influenza A virus infection occurs after vaccination with mismatched whole inactivated vaccine (Gauger et al. 2011). VAERD is associated with the presence of high-titer cross-reacting antibodies targeting the conserved stem domain of the viral hemagglutinin molecule (Khurana et al. 2013). This phenomenon is relevant to the current field situation in the USA where inactivated vaccines are used, which are frequently mismatched to the circulating swine viruses.

2.2.2 Cell-Mediated Immune Protection

Cell-mediated immunity is mediated by T lymphocytes, which can recruit and activate other cell populations, including macrophages, neutrophils, and natural killer (NK) cells by releasing cytokines, as well as directly killing infected cells. Two major classes of T cells can be distinguished by their expression of the surface co-receptor molecules CD4 and CD8. CD4 cells recognize peptide epitopes displayed on MHC class II molecules and mainly produce cytokines that activate other cells, including B cells (helper function).

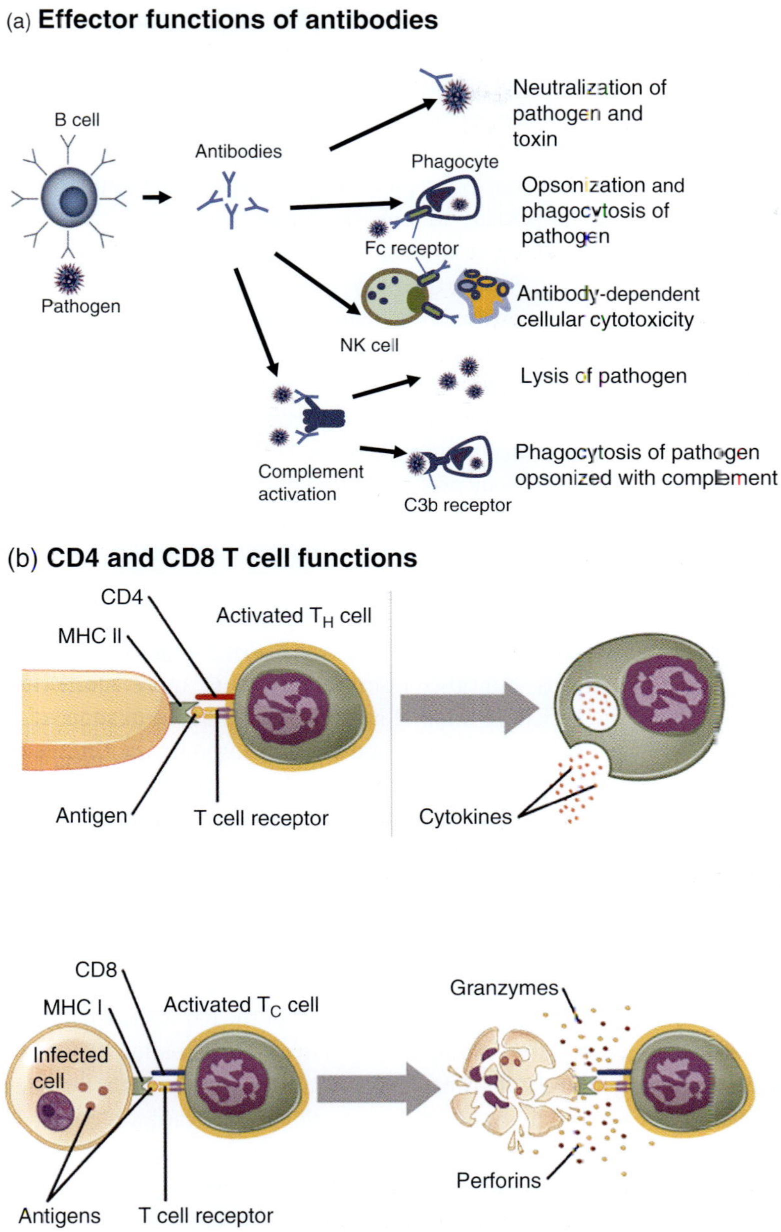

Figure 2.1 Effector functions of antibodies and T cells. (a) Effector functions of antibodies and the cells which mediate them. Fc and complement receptors play a major role in recruiting cells of the innate immune system. (b) Antigen peptides presented on MHC class II recruits CD4 T cells, which in turn produce cytokines which activate other cells. Peptides presented on MHC class I by infected cells activate CD8 T cells which lyse the infected cells but also produce cytokines.

CD8 T cells recognize peptides displayed by MHC class I molecules and, as well as releasing cytokines, can directly kill infected target cells (Figure 2.1b). While antibodies play a major role in combating extracellular infections and may neutralize viruses, cell-mediated immunity is essential for eradicating many viral infections as well as certain bacterial, fungal, and protozoal intracellular infections, for example bovine tuberculosis.

T cells that have encountered antigen and responded (memory and activated cells) can be distinguished from those that have not (naïve cells) by the surface molecules they express. Until recently, it was assumed that T cell memory existed in two compartments, defined in a pivotal study by Lanzavecchia and colleagues (Sallusto et al. 1999). Central memory cells (T_{CM}) are identified by expression of lymph node homing molecules and are found mainly in blood and lymph nodes. Like naïve cells, they recirculate through secondary lymphoid organs, are able to synthesize interleukin (IL)-2 and respond to antigen contact in lymph nodes by proliferation and differentiation to effector cells.

Effector memory T cells (T_{EM}) are defined in blood by the absence of lymph node homing molecules and are able to enter inflammatory sites in nonlymphoid tissues, where they can respond immediately to pathogen-infected cells. T_{EM} maintain heightened effector-like functions such as cytolytic activity of CD8 T cells or production of cytokines by CD4 and CD8 T cells.

However, more recently, a third memory T cell population has been identified: the tissue resident memory T cells (T_{RM}). T_{RM} are largely sessile and do not circulate. Recent studies have revealed that at least in some circumstances, T_{RM} are more effective at protecting nonlymphoid tissues from pathogens than migratory T_{CM} and T_{EM} (Park and Kupper 2015; Mueller and Mackay 2016) and that their abundance has been grossly underestimated (Steinert et al. 2015). These studies suggest that it will be necessary to establish memory T cells in tissues if rapid T cell-mediated control of infection is the goal, as may be the case for diseases such as influenza and tuberculosis. Most studies of T_{RM} so far have been performed in mice, but veterinary species provide unique opportunities to assess T_{RM} in large animals in the context of vaccination and infection.

2.3 Use of Adjuvants

Adjuvants are substances incorporated into or injected simultaneously with antigen that stimulate enhanced, longer-lived immune responses (derived from the Latin *adiuvare*, "to help"). The use of adjuvants in veterinary vaccines is less regulated than in human vaccines and a large number are currently used in veterinary vaccines, which in many cases are not fully specified in product descriptions because of commercial sensitivity. Most adjuvants are used within inactivated or subunit vaccines due to their low immunogenic profile. On the other hand, live-attenuated vaccines rarely require adjuvants because they usually elicit strong immune responses. By using adjuvants in the vaccine formulation, the challenges of reduced immunogenicity of inactivated and subunit vaccines can be overcome while maintaining the high safety profile of the vaccine. Several adjuvants are under development with a view to eliciting similar immune responses to live-attenuated vaccines.

Generally speaking, two types of action have been described for adjuvants: immunostimulation and depot effects (Table 2.1) (reviewed in Gerdts 2015). Immunostimulation results from the activity of molecules, which directly enhance immune responses. The majority of immunostimulants target pattern recognition receptors (PRRs), which are molecules expressed by lymphoid cells that recognize pathogen-associated molecular patterns (PAMPS) that are not present on mammalian cells. PRRs include toll-like receptors (TLRs), lectins and cytoplasmic nucleotide-binding oligomerization domain-like receptors (NLRs), and retinoic acid inducible gene I-like receptors (RLRs). The interaction of PAMPS with PRRs in antigen-presenting cells, particularly dendritic cells that are crucial for processing and presenting antigen to T cells in primary immune responses, is critical for initiating and amplifying immune responses and many newer adjuvants target these receptors.

Immunostimulants include TLR agonists such as bacterial flagellins, lipoplysaccharides (LPS) and CpG oligodeoxynucleotides (CpGODN). Synthetic oligonucleotides containing unmethylated CpG motifs are powerful immunostimulants, acting through TLR9. Different families of CpGODN can preferentially stimulate different cells – B cells, NK, dendritic cells (DC) or CD8 cells involved in immune responses. Cytokines can also amplify immune responses.

Depot effects of adjuvants prevent antigen dispersal and promote slow release. Depot vehicles can deliver not only antigens but also immunostimulants more effectively. They include mineral salts such as alum, emulsions such as Freund's adjuvant, liposomes, virosomes, and immune-stimulating complexes (ISCOMs). In reality, many adjuvants combine both immunostimulation and antigen depot effects to varying degrees (see Table 2.1).

Alum was introduced in the 1920s for vaccines against diphtheria and tetanus toxoid, and is widely used in veterinary vaccine formulations. Antigens are absorbed onto particles of aluminum salts and the adjuvant activity is ascribed to both the depot effect of the particles and immunostimulation due to induction of inflammation. Water-in-oil emulsions were first introduced as adjuvants by Jules Freund in the 1930s. Like alum, this adjuvant was designed to release antigen over an extended period at the injection site, acting as an antigen depot. Complete Freund's adjuvant consists of a water-in-paraffin oil emulsion and inactivated mycobacteria, which provide the immunostimulant; the incomplete form lacks mycobacteria. Freund's adjuvant is still used when a strong adjuvant is needed and inflammation is not an important drawback (Spickler and Roth 2003).

The montanides are similar to incomplete Freund's adjuvant but are biodegradable and have been used in veterinary vaccines (e.g. foot and mouth disease [FMD] virus, rotavirus, coronavirus, hemorrhagic septicemia). Ribi, a commonly used formulation for experimental work, combines a water-in-oil emulsion incorporating monophosphoryl lipid A (MLA) and mycobacterial trehalose dimycolate (TDM). MLA is a derivative of one of the most potent stimulators of antigen-presenting cells, namely lipid A from gram-negative bacterial LPS.

Table 2.1 Most commonly used adjuvants, their mode of action, and advantages versus disadvantages are shown with some examples and references.

Type of adjuvant	Ascribed mode of action	Advantages/disadvantages	Examples	References
Mineral salts	DE by retaining Ag IS by inducing cell injury resulting in danger signals that induce inflammation	Th2 inducer (Ab-mediated protection) Used for extracellular pathogens	Alum (aluminum potassium sulfate) Alhydrogel (aluminum hydroxide) Adju-Plus (aluminum phosphate) Imject Alum (aluminum hydroxide and magnesium hydroxide)	De Gregorio et al. (2008), Marrack et al. (2009), McKee et al. (2009)
Oil-in-water/ water-in-oil emulsions	DE at the injection site with slow release of Ag IS by inducing inflammation	Slow release of Ags for a prolonged period of time	MF59 Ribi Montanide adjuvants (Seppic) Incomplete Freund's adjuvant Emulsigen-D (MVP Technologies)	Galliher-Beckley et al. (2015), Lai et al. (2015), Shah et al. (2015)
Saponins	NU	Powerful inducers of both T cell and humoral immune responses	Quil-A (InvivoGen) ISCOMS, ISCOMATRIX (CSL) QS-21 (Cambridge Biotech Corp.)	Morein et al. (1984), Sanders et al. (2005), Drane et al. (2007), Sun et al. (2009), de Costa et al. (2011), Morelli et al. (2012)
Toll-like receptors (TLR) ligands	IS by activation of signaling pathways (induction of proinflammatory cytokines)	Powerful inducers of immune responses Toxicity	LPS PolyI:C CpG ODN	Mutwiri et al. (2003), Nichani et al. (2004), Dar et al. (2010)
Particles	Ag delivery	Delivering the vaccine antigens directly to antigen-presenting cells (mucosal and systemic)	Poly-(DL-lactide-coglycolide) Polyphosphazenes	Mutwiri et al. (2005), Eng et al. (2010a,b), Shah et al. (2014)

(Continued)

Table 2.1 (Continued)

Type of adjuvant	Ascribed mode of action	Advantages/disadvantages	Examples	References
Liposomes, VLP, and virosomes	Ag delivery and IS	Previous knowledge of protective Ag	Monophosphoryl lipid A (MLA)	Alving et al. (2012), Crisci et al. (2012), Korsholm et al. (2012), Gerdts et al. (2013), Schwendener (2014)
		Stability	CAF01	
			Cationic liposome–DNA complexes (CLDCs)	
			Listeriolysin O	
			Calicivirus-like particles	
Combinations	DE and IS as they contain 2–3 individual adjuvant components, often at a lower dose or formulated into smaller particles	Synergistic effect that may exceed the sum of the individual effects	MF59™ (Novartis Inc.)	Mutwiri et al. (2007, 2011), Garlapati et al. (2010), Skibinski et al. (2011), Dar et al. (2012), Auray et al. (2013)
		Cost-effective	AS03™ (Glaxo Smith Kline Inc.)	
		Easy to formulate	IC31™ (Valneva Inc.)	
		Systemic and mucosal administration		

Ab, antibody; Ag, antigen; DE, depot effect; IS, immunostimulation; NU, not understood; VLP, virus-like particles.

Recently, particle-based adjuvants have been extensively studied, in the form of both nanoparticles and microparticles. They offer the advantage of delivering the vaccine antigens directly to antigen-presenting cells, since antigen-presenting cells preferentially take up particulate antigen. Also, particulate vaccine formulations offer the advantage of delivering the vaccine to the mucosal surfaces, including oral and nasal routes of delivery (Mutwiri et al. 2005).

Particulate antigens elicit much better immune responses than soluble proteins. Liposomes, virosomes, and virus-like particles (VLP) have been used to present monomeric antigens in multimeric form to take advantage of this. Similarly, ISCOMs trap antigens in cage-like structures with saponins. Quil-A adjuvant is used in a wide variety of veterinary vaccines, and contains the water-extractable fraction of saponins from the South American tree, *Quillaja saponiara Molina*. Saponins induce strong responses to T cell-dependent and -independent antigens as well as strong CD8 responses.

Most pathogens gain entry into the body via mucosal surfaces and the induction of immune responses at these surfaces can be crucial in providing the best protection against disease (Sedgmen et al. 2004). However, immunizing via mucosal surfaces is particularly challenging, as the induction of excessive inflammation in the intestine or respiratory tract can cause serious side effects. Nevertheless, some of the adjuvants described above can be used as intestinal mucosal adjuvants, with certain molecules being particularly effective, most notably cholera toxin, *E. coli* heat-stable enterotoxin and *Pertussis* toxin, which augments the expression of the co-stimulatory molecules CD86 on B cells and CD28 on T cells and increases interferon (IFN)-γ production. However, fewer safe adjuvants for respiratory use are available.

2.4 Passive Immunity, Induced Immunity, and Individual/Herd Protection

2.4.1 Passive Immunity

Passive immunity can be acquired by the administration of antibodies, usually IgG, either intravenously or intramuscularly. Immune sera are derived from individuals who have high antibody titers to particular microbes and can thus provide rapid protection against infections such as rabies or those caused by *Clostridium* species. The administered antibodies are catabolized and must be administered frequently to maintain a protective titer. However, with the repeated administration of antibodies, antibodies to the infused immunoglobulin may be induced, leading to immune complex formation and serum sickness. In veterinary medicine, antibody administration is primarily used for companion animals, but reduction in the cost of recombinant (monoclonal) antibodies will make passive immunotherapy increasingly feasible.

During pregnancy, maternal antibodies are transferred across the placenta to the fetus, providing passive immunity that protects the newborn during the first months of life. Such passively transferred antibodies can, in some instances, also be a disadvantage as the presence of maternal antibody in the newborn may inhibit effective immunization. Thus, immunization against some antigens must be delayed until the titer of the maternal antibodies has decayed. In contrast, newborn piglets and ruminants for example do not have maternal antibodies at birth as these proteins cannot cross the placenta in these species and although newborns are able to mount immune responses, their immune system is underdeveloped at birth, and less able to respond to pathogens and vaccines for the first few weeks. Therefore, a common strategy for piglets in the USA, for example to control influenza virus infection, is to vaccinate the sows, which then transfer this protection to their piglets in colostrum. As the maternal antibodies decay, however, the piglets become susceptible to infection. In the offspring of vaccinated sows, the antibodies persist up to 14–16 weeks, while they often disappear around 6 weeks in piglets born to exposed but unvaccinated sows (Sandbulte et al. 2015).

2.4.2 Induced Immunity

Induced immunity refers to any intervention whereby an immune response is induced in a given organism. Induced responses are stimulated by administration of vaccines containing microbial products with or without adjuvants in order to obtain long-term immunological protection against the pathogen. The nature of the induced response is determined by the vaccine formulation, dose, frequency, and route of administration.

Vaccine-induced protection is affected by age, nutrition, physiological state, underlying infections, and other factors. Commensal microbial communities (microbiota) colonize barrier surfaces of the skin, vagina, and upper respiratory and gastrointestinal tracts of all mammals and consist of bacteria, fungi, and protozoa. Studies using gnotobiotic (germ-free), antibiotic-treated or selectively colonized mice have demonstrated that signals from commensal bacteria can influence immune cell development, susceptibility to disease and vaccine-induced protection. With aging, T cell function is reduced and the affinity of antibodies and response to vaccination become diminished. Therefore, multiple factors affect immune function, and determine the longevity of the response to immunization and the morbidity or mortality should infection supervene.

2.4.3 Herd Immunity

Herd immunity results from vaccination of a significant proportion of the group, which not only protects those individuals but also reduces pathogen exposure and disease incidence in those not vaccinated. This indirect vaccine effect is due to reduction of pathogen load and transmission within the group as a whole. Thus, herd immunity refers to a particular threshold proportion of immune individuals that should lead to a decline in incidence of infection. This threshold directly depends on the basic reproduction rate (R_0) as the number of secondary infections produced by a typical case of an infection in a population that is entirely susceptible. For example, influenza infection commonly exhibits an R_0 of 2–4 and requires vaccination of 50–75% of the population to achieve the herd immunity threshold (White and Vynnycky 2010).

Although herd effects may be considered, the outcome measure for human vaccine evaluation is typically the status of the individual. In contrast, in veterinary medicine, herd immunity is more commonly assessed and much more important, as disease management is often at group level and concerns control of spread between herds, rather than spread within already infected herds (Knight-Jones et al. 2014).

2.5 Vaccine Delivery Systems

There are two major routes of administration: systemic and mucosal (Table 2.2). The majority of vaccines in veterinary practice are delivered via needle injection by systemic (parenteral) immunization usually carried out by administering the vaccine intradermally, subcutaneously, or intramuscularly. This approach works when a relatively small number of animals require vaccination and for diseases in which systemic immunity, principally antibody-mediated protective immunity, is important.

Nonetheless, as most infectious agents gain entry to the body through mucosal surfaces, mucosal immunity is critical for protection and recently it has also become clear that the most effective means of inducing this form of immunity is by targeting vaccines to the mucosa, rather than systemically (Beverley et al. 2014). This is because this route is most effective in generating mucosal T_{RM}. Immunization via the respiratory tract is highly protective experimentally against several pulmonary diseases in livestock, including bovine tuberculosis, respiratory syncytial virus in cattle, African swine fever, and porcine reproductive and respiratory syndrome virus. For example, targeting Bacillus Calmette-Guerin (BCG) or adenoviral vectors expressing tuberculosis antigens to the respiratory tract is a more effective way to induce protection in mice (Forbes et al. 2008), guinea pigs, cattle (Dean et al. 2015) and nonhuman primates (Jeyanathan et al. 2015) than parenteral immunization. Similarly, intranasal administration of a

Table 2.2 Vaccine delivery systems.

Type of delivery	Administration	Advantages/disadvantages
Parenteral	Intradermal Subcutaneous Intramuscular	Systemic immunity (generally Ab mediated) Good for a small number of animals
Mucosal	Intranasal	Local immunity Prevent infection at the entry point Induce potent mucosal immunity
In ovo	To eggs	Reproducible and reliable Generates systemic immunity in the adult animal Can be applied to a large number of eggs
Oral	In water	Ease of administration Lack of stress Ag has to be mass-produced inexpensively Applicable to animals of all sizes Lack of dose control Ag need to be protected against degradation
Oral	In a bait (for wild animals)	The Ag has to be mass-produced inexpensively Ag has to be robust and stable Vaccine preparation should be compatible with bait delivery systems

Ab, antibody; Ag, antigen.

recombinant chimpanzee adenovirus expressing respiratory syncytial virus F, N, and M2-1 proteins is highly protective in calves (Taylor et al. 2015) and intranasal administration of killed porcine reproductive and respiratory syndrome virus vaccine antigens entrapped within nanoparticles induces strong cross-protective immunity against heterologous challenge in pigs (Binjawadagi et al. 2014).

In cattle and pets, several vaccines are delivered by the intranasal route using mucosal atomization devices: NOBIVAC KC, a vaccine for *Bordetella bronchiseptica* and canine parainfluenza virus in dogs; TRACHERINE, a vaccine for infectious bovine rhinotracheitis (IBR) virus in cattle; and Rispoval RS + PI3 against bovine parainfluenza and bovine RSV.

In poultry, vaccine delivery systems include needle inoculation using wing web vaccination or *in ovo* injection. *In ovo* vaccination has been rapidly adopted as the method of choice for immunizing chickens against Marek's disease and other poultry diseases in many countries because it is reproducible, reliable, generates systemic immunity in the adult animal and can be rapidly applied to large numbers of eggs (Ricks et al. 1999). In recent years, the search for alternative methods of vaccine delivery not requiring a needle and syringe has been accelerated by the need for ease and speed of delivery, improved safety and compliance, decreased costs, and reduction of side effects associated with injection. For example, alternatives to injection in poultry include the incorporation of vaccines into drinking water, eye drops, aerosols, and sprays such as those used in avian influenza control programs (Swayne 2009). Other delivery methods are also being investigated, like a gene gun in the case of DNA vaccine delivery, but these new technologies have not yet advanced to the stage of routine use in livestock (Huang et al. 2006; Loudon et al. 2010).

In fish, needle injection has been used with all its associated problems but needle-free routes, such as dispersing vaccines in the water or food, are being explored. The oral route is attractive for its ease of administration of antigens, lack of stress, and because it is applicable to fish of all sizes. It may also be used for oral boosting during grow-out periods in cages or ponds. However, so far, few commercial vaccines are available due to lack of efficacy and challenges associated with production of large quantities of antigens. Antigens also need to be protected against degradation before they reach the sites where immune induction occurs. Currently, encapsulation techniques are being explored in the quest to protect antigens against digestive degradation, as well as to target them for appropriate immune induction in the host (Mutoloki et al. 2015).

Vaccination of wild animals poses additional problems, both in delivery of the vaccine and maintaining its stability in the environment. For practical reasons, oral delivery is the most likely route of choice for wildlife vaccine development and this method has proved successful, for example, against rabies. The first field trials using a recombinant vaccinia virus rabies vaccine targeting foxes and deployed in bait were initiated in Europe late in the 1980s and continued into the early 1990s. Oral rabies vaccination programs have also been implemented in the USA and southern Canada principally targeting raccoons and coyotes in the former and red foxes in the latter, as the major wildlife reservoirs. As in Europe, wide-scale oral rabies vaccination has been successful in reducing the incidence of rabies among target species.

The main limitation to oral vaccination efficacy for wild animals lies within the immunogen itself as it has to be mass-produced inexpensively, while maintaining safety and efficacy. Vaccine immunogens must also be robust, stable, and compatible with bait delivery systems. In addition, the vaccine vehicle must deliver sufficient quantities of the immunogen to induction sites in order to stimulate a protective immune response. Technologies used include development of biocompatible encapsulation materials for the immunogen. Alternatively, the form of the immunogen itself can be modified to suit the delivery conditions. One example is the use of lyophilized preparations of attenuated or gene-mutated/avirulent variants of the rabies virus for vaccination of Arctic foxes in polar environments. This avoids the loss of efficacy of the more widely used recombinant vaccinia virus that occurs in sub-zero temperatures (reviewed in Cross et al. 2007).

2.6 Assessing Protection Delivered Through Vaccination – Mode and Level of Protection

The efficacy of new vaccines is evaluated by potency tests in which the relevant species of animal is vaccinated and then challenged with the target live pathogen. The percentage of animals that survive or show reduced disease symptoms/pathogen replication following challenge is compared with nonvaccinated controls. Effective vaccines should protect 80–100% of animals, at least from serious disease. The potential benefits of an effective vaccine (e.g. promotion of health and well-being, and protection from illness and its physical, psychological, and socioeconomic consequences) must be considered against the risk of adverse events following immunization. Less effective vaccines may be acceptable if they are safe and economical and nothing better is available.

Vaccination is a powerful tool for the control of infectious diseases; however, its efficacy in disease prevention depends on implementing correct strategies, for example targeted vaccination of animals at high risk or mass vaccination of all animals, as well as the level of vaccination and herd immunity (as described above). Cost is an important constraint in farming.

A central target of vaccine research is to identify vaccine-induced immune responses that correlate with protection from infection or disease. According to the Food and Drug Administration of the USA, a correlate of protection is a laboratory parameter that is associated with protection from the occurrence of clinical disease as shown after sufficient and controlled trials (FDA 1997). Such immune correlates of protection (iCOP) can then be used to predict the protective efficacy of a vaccine in a new setting, when vaccine efficacy is not directly observed, for example across vaccine lots, different populations, or in different species. If the predictions are reliable, then use of iCOP provides an efficient way to guide the development, evaluation, and utilization of vaccines. However, empirically validating iCOP may be challenging and it is still unresolved for many diseases (Table 2.3).

Both cell-mediated and humoral immune parameters have been investigated as potential iCOP, reflecting the type of immunological response that is required for protective efficacy against the relevant pathogen (see Figure 2.1) (Thakur et al. 2012). While the majority of vaccines have been developed empirically with little understanding of the underlying mechanism of action, their success most often relates to induction of strong humoral immune responses. However, protection against most intracellular infections requires a cell-mediated immune response (e.g. *Salmonella* infection, tuberculosis, *Chlamydia*, or Apicomplexan parasites) and others are only resolved if both forms of protection are present (Tham and Studdert 1987; Scott and Geissinger 1999; McVey and Shi 2010). The mechanisms of vaccine-induced protection may also vary widely between different pathogens, in different species, according to the dose of pathogen to which the individual is exposed, and different routes of exposure (Meeusen et al. 2007). These problems make it difficult to identify iCOP that can be used with confidence for diseases other than those in which antibody is the dominant protective mechanism (see Table 2.3). Despite the importance of identifying iCOP, there are few methods for predicting protective immunity (Thakur et al. 2012). It is also worth noting that although iCOP correlate with protection, they may not measure the key mechanisms of protection. Protection depends on preexisting neutralizing antibodies and/or preactivated T cells at the time of infection, as documented by the importance of maternal antibodies around birth for survival of the offspring. However, detection of activated T cells or neutralizing antibodies does not necessarily indicate protection.

Table 2.3 Main gaps in our knowledge.

- Identifying immune correlates of protection after vaccination for each disease
- How best to administer vaccines to induce tissue resident memory T cells (T_{RM}) and determine the duration of T_{RM} induced protection
- How best to induce long-term memory in veterinary species and the mechanisms involved
- New and effective adjuvants and delivery systems, particularly for mucosal use
- How to predict adverse effects of vaccines
- How to induce cross-reactive immunity to different serotypes/genotypes of a pathogen
- How to develop vaccines for complex pathogens or chronic infections

It is important to consider whether vaccination can prevent infection completely or prevent disease symptoms only. In the latter case, the host does not suffer from disease but the pathogen continues to circulate in the herd under immune pressure. This may induce genetic change leading to emergence of new strains with higher pathogenic potential. A good example is the use of commercial Marek's disease vaccines that protect with great efficacy against the development of the disease but do not prevent infection or transmission. In the years following the introduction of Marek's disease vaccine, strains of increased virulence have been isolated from vaccine breakdowns, suggesting that the use of increasingly potent vaccine regimens could be driving Marek's disease virus to evolve to increasing virulence (Davison and Nair 2005).

2.7 Benefits of Using DIVA Vaccines

In situations such as that described above for Marek's disease virus, where virus may continue to circulate in spite of vaccination, better control of disease can be achieved if a test is available to differentiate between infected and vaccinated animals (DIVA test). DIVA tests detect immunity to one or more proteins in the wild-type microorganism that are not present in the vaccine, either serologically or using assays for cell-mediated immunity. Therefore, naturally infected animals can be detected in a vaccinated population and measures taken to prevent further pathogen transmission. During the global eradication of rinderpest virus, a safe and effective live attenuated vaccine and a suitable companion diagnostic test were implemented. Unfortunately, those diagnostic tests did not follow the DIVA concept. While the vaccine was successfully applied across much of the developing world to protect livestock against rinderpest virus, the serological response to vaccination did not differ from that seen following natural infection with field isolates of rinderpest virus. Therefore, serosurveillance tests were not able to differentiate between naturally infected and vaccinated animals. This delayed recognition of countries as being free from rinderpest virus as serological naivety in cattle populations had to be demonstrated for several years following the cessation of vaccination (Buczkowski et al. 2012).

DIVA vaccines and their companion tests are now available for several diseases including IBR, pseudorabies, classic swine fever (CSF), and FMD. DIVA vaccines were first used for the eradication of pseudorabies (Aujeszky's disease) in pigs. The vaccines are based on recombinant deletion mutants lacking the gE envelope glycoprotein and thymidine kinase genes. The accompanying tests score pigs as seropositive for gE antibodies. DIVA vaccines against IBR of cattle, caused by the bovine herpesvirus 1 (BHV-1), work on a similar principle. Currently available FMD vaccines can be prepared from purified and chemically inactivated whole virus particles. The nonstructural proteins (NSPs) are separated from the virus particles so that serological assays detecting antibodies against NSP are indicators of infection. For CSF, a baculovirus-expressed recombinant E2-subunit vaccine is on the market. The surface glycoprotein E2 is the most antigenic protein of CSF virus and elicits a neutralizing antibody response, which can protect pigs against CSF. For DIVA purposes, enzyme-linked immunosorbent assays (ELISAs) were developed which detect antibodies against the viral envelope glycoprotein Erns. In another example, an inactivated heterologous vaccine was used in order to control a low-pathogenic avian influenza infection (H7N1) in Italy in 1999–2000. The vaccine virus contained the same hemagglutinin subtype (H7) as the wild-type virus but a different neuraminidase (N3). The companion test, an indirect immunofluorescence assay, detected antibodies against N1 (reviewed in Pasick 2004). A similar strategy is used in other countries like China and the USA.

Emergency vaccination using DIVA vaccines could be an important control tool for disease outbreaks in densely populated livestock areas. DIVA vaccination might also limit the number of culled animals in the process of disease eradication (e.g. in a FMD epidemic), thereby enhancing public acceptance of disease control measures and limiting economic damage. Therefore, the DIVA concept is recommended for inclusion in any new vaccine development.

2.8 Summary

One of the greatest triumphs of human and veterinary medicine has been the ability to harness immune mechanisms through vaccination to protect against a wide range of diseases. In recent years, vaccine development has used the tools of modern molecular biology and genomics to characterize the molecules of the immune system, identify target antigens of pathogens, develop recombinant vectors to deliver antigens, and map the exact specificity of immune responses. However, despite these significant achievements, we still face many gaps in our knowledge and challenges (see Table 2.3)

References

Acosta, P.L., Caballero, M.T., and Polack, F.P. (2015). Brief history and characterization of enhanced respiratory syncytial virus disease. *Clin. Vaccine Immunol.* 23 (3): 189–195.

Alving, C.R., Rao, M., Steers, N.J. et al. (2012). Liposomes containing lipid A: an effective, safe, generic adjuvant system for synthetic vaccines. *Expert Rev. Vaccines* 11 (6): 733–744.

Auray, G., Facci, M.R., van Kessel, J. et al. (2013). Porcine neonatal blood dendritic cells, but not monocytes, are more responsive to TLRs stimulation than their adult counterparts. *PLoS One* 8 (5): e59629.

Beverley, P.C., Sridhar, S., Lalvani, A., and Tchilian, E.Z. (2014). Harnessing local and systemic immunity for vaccines against tuberculosis. *Mucosal Immunol.* 7 (1): 20–26.

Binjawadagi, B., Dwivedi, V., Manickam, C. et al. (2014). An innovative approach to induce cross-protective immunity against porcine reproductive and respiratory syndrome virus in the lungs of pigs through adjuvanted nanotechnology-based vaccination. *Int. J. Nanomed.* 9: 1519–1535.

Buczkowski, H., Parida, S., Bailey, D. et al. (2012). A novel approach to generating morbillivirus vaccines: negatively marking the rinderpest vaccine. *Vaccine* 30 (11): 1927–1935.

Crisci, E., Fraile, L., Moreno, N. et al. (2012). Chimeric calicivirus-like particles elicit specific immune responses in pigs. *Vaccine* 30 (14): 2427–2439.

Cross, M.L., Buddle, B.M., and Aldwell, F.E. (2007). The potential of oral vaccines for disease control in wildlife species. *Vet. J.* 174 (3): 472–480.

Dar, A., Nichani, A., Lai, K. et al. (2010). All three classes of CpG ODNs up-regulate IP-10 gene in pigs. *Res. Vet. Sci.* 88 (2): 242–250.

Dar, A., Lai, K., Dent, D. et al. (2012). Administration of poly[di(sodium carboxylatoethylphenoxy)]phosphazene

(PCEP) as adjuvant activated mixed Th1/Th2 immune responses in pigs. *Vet. Immunol. Immunopathol.* 146 (3–4): 289–295.

Davison, F. and Nair, V. (2005). Use of Marek's disease vaccines: could they be driving the virus to increasing virulence? *Expert Rev. Vaccines* 4 (1): 77–88.

De Costa, F., Yendo, A.C., Fleck, J.D. et al. (2011). Immunoadjuvant and anti-inflammatory plant saponins: characteristics and biotechnological approaches towards sustainable production. *Mini-Rev. Med. Chem.* 11 (10): 857–880.

De Gregorio, E., Tritto, E., and Rappuoli, R. (2008). Alum adjuvanticity: unraveling a century old mystery. *Eur. J. Immunol.* 38 (8): 2068–2071.

Dean, G.S., Clifford, D., Whelan, A.O. et al. (2015). Protection induced by simultaneous subcutaneous and endobronchial vaccination with BCG/BCG and BCG/adenovirus expressing antigen 85A against *Mycobacterium bovis* in cattle. *PLoS One* 10 (11): e0142270.

Drane, D., Gittleson, C., Boyle, J., and Maraskovsky, E. (2007). ISCOMATRIX adjuvant for prophylactic and therapeutic vaccines. *Expert Rev. Vaccines* 6 (5): 761–772.

Eng, N.F., Garlapati, S., Gerdts, V. et al. (2010a). PCEP enhances IgA mucosal immune responses in mice following different immunization routes with influenza virus antigens. *J. Immune Based Ther. Vaccines* 8: 4.

Eng, N.F., Garlapati, S., Gerdts, V. et al. (2010b). The potential of polyphosphazenes for delivery of vaccine antigens and immunotherapeutic agents. *Curr. Drug Delivery* 7 (1): 13–20.

FDA. (1997). Guidance for industry: for the evaluation of combination vaccines for preventable diseases: production, testing and clinical studies. US Department of Health and Human Services Food and Drug Administration Center for Biologics Evaluation and Research. Report No. 97N-0029. www.fda.gov/downloads/BiologicsBloodVaccines/GuidanceComplianceRegulatoryInformation/Guidances/Vaccines/UCM175909.pdf

Forbes, E.K., Sander, C., Ronan, E.O. et al. (2008). Multifunctional, high-level cytokine-producing Th1 cells in the lung, but not spleen, correlate with protection against *Mycobacterium tuberculosis* aerosol challenge in mice. *J. Immunol.* 181 (7): 4955–4964.

Galliher-Beckley, A., Pappan, L.K., Madera, R. et al. (2015). Characterization of a novel oil-in-water emulsion adjuvant for swine influenza virus and *Mycoplasma hyopneumoniae* vaccines. *Vaccine* 33 (25): 2903–2908.

Garlapati, S., Eng, N.F., Wilson, H.L. et al. (2010). PCPP (poly[di(carboxylatophenoxy)-phosphazene]) microparticles co-encapsulating ovalbumin and CpG oligo-deoxynucleotides are potent enhancers of antigen specific Th1 immune responses in mice. *Vaccine* 28 (52): 8306–8314.

Gauger, P.C., Vincent, A.L., Loving, C.L. et al. (2011). Enhanced pneumonia and disease in pigs vaccinated with an inactivated human-like (delta-cluster) H1N2 vaccine and challenged with pandemic 2009 H1N1 influenza virus. *Vaccine* 29 (15): 2712–2719.

Gerdts, V. (2015). Adjuvants for veterinary vaccines – types and modes of action. *Berl. Munch. Tierarztl. Wochenschr.* 128 (11–12): 456–463.

Gerdts, V., Mutwiri, G., Richards, J. et al. (2013). Carrier molecules for use in veterinary vaccines. *Vaccine* 31 (4): 596–602.

Huang, Y., Babiuk, L.A., and van Drunen Littel-van den Hurk, S. (2006). The cell-mediated immune response induced by plasmid encoding bovine herpesvirus 1 glycoprotein B is enhanced by plasmid encoding IL-12 when delivered intramuscularly or by gene gun, but not after intradermal injection. *Vaccine* 24 (25): 5349–5359.

Jeyanathan, M., Shao, Z., Yu, X. et al. (2015). AdHu5Ag85A respiratory mucosal boost immunization enhances protection against pulmonary tuberculosis in BCG-primed non-human primates. *PLoS One* 10 (8): e0135009.

Khurana, S., Loving, C.L., Manischewitz, J. et al. (2013). Vaccine-induced anti-HA2 antibodies promote virus fusion and enhance influenza virus respiratory disease. *Sci. Transl. Med.* 5 (200): 200ra114.

Knight-Jones, T.J., Edmond, K., Gubbins, S., and Paton, D.J. (2014). Veterinary and human vaccine evaluation methods. *Proc. R. Soc. B* 281 (1784): 20132839.

Korsholm, K.S., Andersen, P.L., and Christensen, D. (2012). Cationic liposomal vaccine adjuvants in animal challenge models: overview and current clinical status. *Expert Rev. Vaccines* 11 (5): 561–577.

Lai, C.H., Tang, N., Jan, J.T. et al. (2015). Use of recombinant flagellin in oil-in-water emulsions enhances hemagglutinin-specific mucosal IgA production and IL-17 secreting T cells against H5N1 avian influenza virus infection. *Vaccine* 33 (35): 4321–4329.

Loehr, B.I., Rankin, R., Pontarollo, R. et al. (2001). Suppository-mediated DNA immunization induces mucosal immunity against bovine herpesvirus-1 in cattle. *Virology* 289 (2): 327–333.

Loudon, P.T., Yager, E.J., Lynch, D.T. et al. (2010). GM-CSF increases mucosal and systemic immunogenicity of an H1N1 influenza DNA vaccine administered into the epidermis of non-human primates. *PLoS One* 5 (6): e11021.

Marrack, P., McKee, A.S., and Munks, M.W. (2009). Towards an understanding of the adjuvant action of aluminium. *Nat. Rev. Immunol.* 9 (4): 287–293.

McKee, A.S., Munks, M.W., MacLeod, M.K. et al. (2009). Alum induces innate immune responses through macrophage and mast cell sensors, but these sensors are not required for alum to act as an adjuvant for specific immunity. *J. Immunol.* 183 (7): 4403–4414.

McVey, S. and Shi, J. (2010). Vaccines in veterinary medicine: a brief review of history and technology. *Vet. Clin. N. Am.-Small.* 40 (3): 381–392.

Meeusen, E.N., Walker, J., Peters, A. et al. (2007). Current status of veterinary vaccines. *Clin. Microbiol. Rev.* 20 (3): 489–510.

Morein, B., Sundquist, B., Hoglund, S. et al. (1984). Iscom, a novel structure for antigenic presentation of membrane proteins from enveloped viruses. *Nature* 308 (5958): 457–460.

Morelli, A.B., Becher, D., Koernig, S. et al. (2012). ISCOMATRIX: a novel adjuvant for use in prophylactic and therapeutic vaccines against infectious diseases. *J. Med. Microbiol.* 61 (Pt 7): 935–943.

Mueller, S.N. and Mackay, L.K. (2016). Tissue-resident memory T cells: local specialists in immune defence. *Nat. Rev. Immunol.* 16 (2): 79–89.

Mutoloki, S., Munang'andu, H.M., and Evensen, O. (2015). Oral vaccination of fish – antigen preparations, uptake, and immune induction. *Front. Immunol.* 6: 519.

Mutwiri, G., Pontarollo, R., Babiuk, S. et al. (2003). Biological activity of immunostimulatory CpG DNA motifs in domestic animals. *Vet. Immunol. Immunopathol.* 91 (2): 89–103.

Mutwiri, G., Bowersock, T.L., and Babiuk, L.A. (2005). Microparticles for oral delivery of vaccines. *Expert Opin. Drug Delivery* 2 (5): 791–806.

Mutwiri, G., Gerdts, V., Lopez, M., and Babiuk, L.A. (2007). Innate immunity and new adjuvants. *Rev. Sci. Tech.* 26 (1): 147–156.

Mutwiri, G., Gerdts, V., van Drunen Littel-van den Hurk, S. et al. (2011). Combination adjuvants: the next generation of adjuvants? *Expert Rev. Vaccines* 10 (1): 95–107.

Nichani, A.K., Mena, A., Popowych, Y. et al. (2004). In vivo immunostimulatory effects of CpG oligodeoxynucleotide in cattle and sheep. *Vet. Immunol. Immunopathol.* 98 (1–2): 17–29.

Park, C.O. and Kupper, T.S. (2015). The emerging role of resident memory T cells in protective immunity and inflammatory disease. *Nat. Med.* 21 (7): 688–697.

Pasick, J. (2004). Application of DIVA vaccines and their companion diagnostic tests to foreign animal disease eradication. *Anim. Health Res. Rev.* 5 (2): 257–262.

Ricks, C.A., Avakian, A., Bryan, T. et al. (1999). In ovo vaccination technology. *Adv. Vet. Med.* 41: 495–515.

Sallusto, F., Lenig, D., Forster, R. et al. (1999). Two subsets of memory T lymphocytes with distinct homing potentials and effector functions. *Nature* 401 (6754): 708–712.

Sandbulte, M.R., Spickler, A.R., Zaabel, P.K., and Roth, J.A. (2015). Optimal use of vaccines for control of influenza a virus in swine. *Vaccines (Basel)* 3 (1): 22–73.

Sanders, M.T., Brown, L.E., Deliyannis, G., and Pearse, M.J. (2005). ISCOM-based vaccines: the second decade. *Immunol. Cell Biol.* 83 (2): 119–128.

Schwendener, R.A. (2014). Liposomes as vaccine delivery systems: a review of the recent advances. *Ther. Adv. Vaccines* 2 (6): 159–182.

Scott, F.W. and Geissinger, C.M. (1999). Long-term immunity in cats vaccinated with an inactivated trivalent vaccine. *Am. J. Vet. Res.* 60 (5): 652–658.

Sedgmen, B.J., Meeusen, E.N., and Lofthouse, S.A. (2004). Alternative routes of mucosal immunization in large animals. *Immunol. Cell Biol.* 82 (1): 10–16.

Shah, R.R., O'Hagan, D.T., Amiji, M.M., and Brito, L.A. (2014). The impact of size on particulate vaccine adjuvants. *Nanomedicine (Lond)* 9 (17): 2671–2681.

Shah, R.R., Dodd, S., Schaefer, M. et al. (2015). The development of self-emulsifying oil-in-water emulsion adjuvant and an evaluation of the impact of droplet size on performance. *J. Pharm. Sci.* 104 (4): 1352–1361.

Skibinski, D.A., Baudner, B.C., Singh, M., and O'Hagan, D.T. (2011). Combination vaccines. *J. Global Infect. Dis.* 3 (1): 63–72.

Spickler, A.R. and Roth, J.A. (2003). Adjuvants in veterinary vaccines: modes of action and adverse effects. *J. Vet. Intern. Med.* 17 (3): 273–281.

Steinert, E.M., Schenkel, J.M., Fraser, K.A. et al. (2015). Quantifying memory CD8 T cells reveals regionalization of immunosurveillance. *Cell* 161 (4): 737–749.

Sun, H.X., Xie, Y., and Ye, Y.P. (2009). Advances in saponin-based adjuvants. *Vaccine* 27 (12): 1787–1796.

Swayne, D.E. (2009). Avian influenza vaccines and therapies for poultry. *Comp. Immunol. Microbiol. Infect. Dis.* 32 (4): 351–363.

Taylor, G., Thom, M., Capone, S. et al. (2015). Efficacy of a virus-vectored vaccine against human and bovine respiratory syncytial virus infections. *Sci. Transl. Med.* 7 (300): 300ra127.

Thakur, A., Pedersen, L.E., and Jungersen, G. (2012). Immune markers and correlates of protection for vaccine induced immune responses. *Vaccine* 30 (33): 4907–4920.

Tham, K.M. and Studdert, M.J. (1987). Antibody and cell-mediated immune responses to feline calicivirus following inactivated vaccine and challenge. *Zentralbl Veterinarmed B* 34 (9): 640–654.

White, R.G. and Vynnycky, E.V. (2010). *An Introduction to Infectious Disease Modelling*. Oxford: Oxford University Press.

3

Role of Regional and International Organizations in Vaccine International Standards

Karim Tounkara[1], Nick Nwankpa[2], Lawrence Elsken[3], and Monique Eloit[4]

[1] OIE Regional Representation for Africa, Bamako, Mali
[2] Department of Rural Economy and Agriculture, African Union Commission, African Union Pan African Veterinary Vaccine Centre (AU-PANVAC), Debre-Zeit, Ethiopia
[3] EDGE Veterinary Vaccines Consulting Group, LLC, Ames, Iowa, USA
[4] World Organization for Animal Health (OIE), Paris, France

3.1 Introduction

The production of vaccine – a biological product – provides a great opportunity for variability, which should be controlled to the greatest extent possible, to ensure the purity, safety, potency, and efficacy of the vaccine and the batch-to-batch uniformity independently of the place of its production. In this process, standardization of vaccine production is vital. Several key international and regional organizations play major roles in the global standardization and harmonization of vaccine production and use, through the production of standards in the form of guides, manuals, and monographs. Some of these standards include the World Organization for Animal Health (OIE) manual of diagnostic tests and vaccines for terrestrial animals; the European Pharmacopoeia (EP) monographs on vaccines and other immunological human medicinal products; the International Cooperation on Harmonization of Technical Requirements for Registration of Veterinary Products (VICH) monographs; and the United States Department of Agriculture Animal, Plant Health Inspection Service (USDA-APHIS), Veterinary Biologics regulations and guidance.

3.2 The Need for International Vaccine Standardization

As a rule, a vaccine should not be used if the national quality control authority does not approve its use. These control authorities should strive to establish control standards and procedures that ensure a finished product of the highest quality possible. Each country has a range of veterinary legislation, aimed at regulating the control, sale, and use of veterinary medicinal products. These legislations stipulate the minimum requirements for quality, which usually require testing by a laboratory under state supervision.

In developed countries, quality control and biological standardization have always been a prerogative of the state, and quality standards have been developed at a national, regional, or international level. Until recently, these were relatively new notions in developing countries. Although most African countries have, in recent years, adopted veterinary medicinal products legislation, very few of them offer an effective regulatory system for licensing and/or monitoring the quality of biological products, such as vaccines, to ensure that only those that are pure, safe, and potent are used in animal disease control programs. In many cases, veterinary biological products are licensed according to the "dossier" submitted by the supplier and not according to laboratory or field data.

The reality of the globalization of trade and the introduction of technical barriers to trade dictates that harmonization and standardization of requirements for veterinary vaccines must be instituted at regional and international levels in order to safeguard the economic, environmental, and social welfare of the planet.

Recent scientific and technical developments have led to a rapid expansion in the number and complexity of biologicals, with new products, including vaccines and new biotechnologies, posing new challenges for standardization.

Veterinary Vaccines: Principles and Applications, First Edition. Edited by Samia Metwally, Gerrit Viljoen, and Ahmed El Idrissi.

3.3 Key International and Regional Organizations and Their Functions

3.3.1 International Vaccine Standardization Organizations

The key international organizations responsible for addressing the issue of veterinary vaccine standardization are the OIE, the Food and Agriculture Organization of the United Nations (FAO), the Global Alliance for Livestock Veterinary Medicines (GALVmed) and the Health for Animals (formerly International Federation for Animal Health) (Blancou and Truszczynski 1995) (Figure 3.1). The World Health Organization (WHO) is not directly involved in standardizing or testing vaccines for veterinary use but some approaches used for human vaccines may be similar and it has an interest in pathogens which are transmissible to human beings (e.g. zoonoses, toxins in food).

3.3.1.1 World Organization for Animal Health

The Office International des Epizooties (OIE) was created through the international agreement signed on January 25, 1924, in Paris by 28 countries. In May 2003, the OIE became the World Organization for Animal Health, but kept its

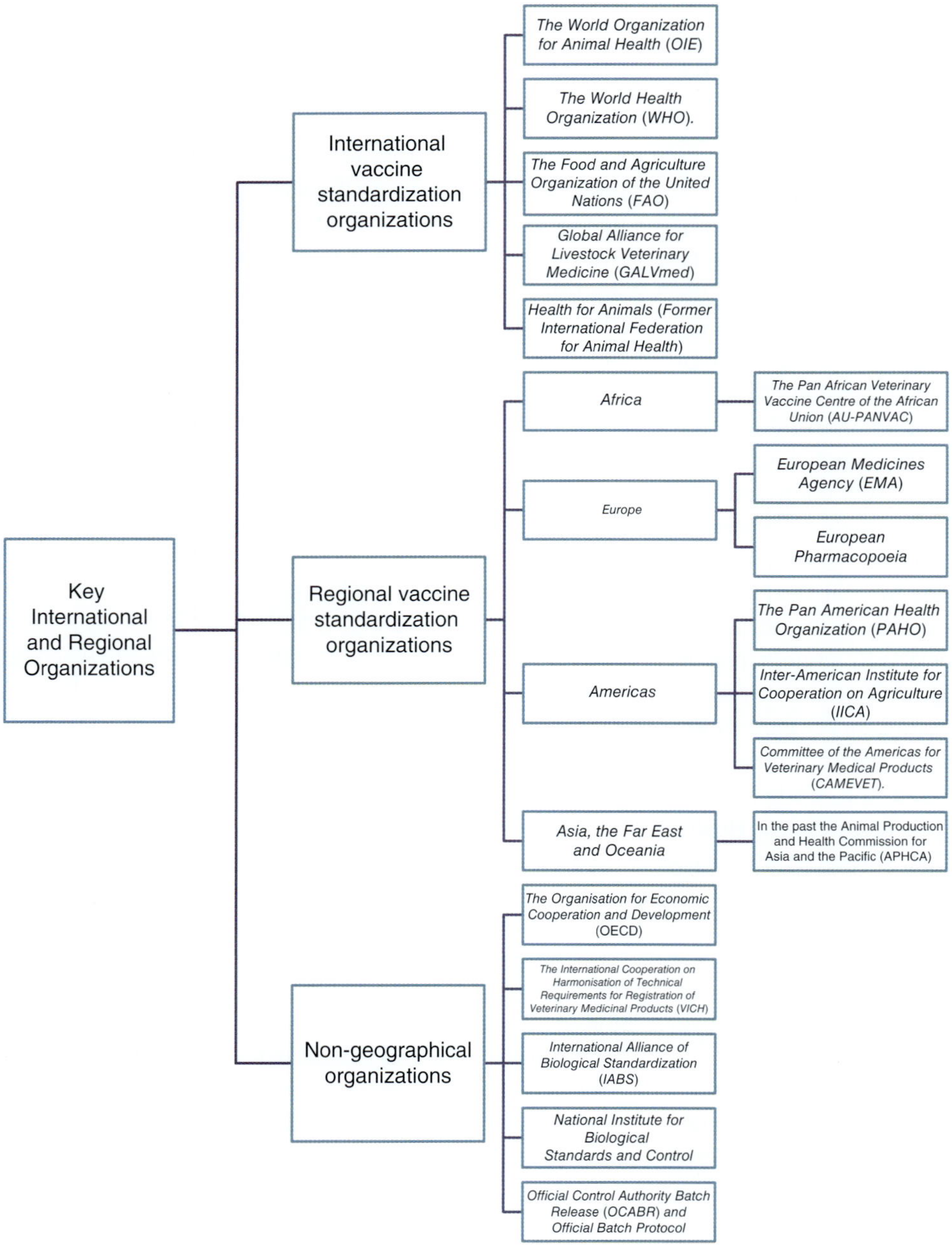

Figure 3.1 Key international and regional organizations.

historical acronym OIE. Currently (2020), the OIE has a total of 182 member countries and maintains permanent relations with 75 other international and regional organizations. It is responsible for setting standards for improving animal health and welfare worldwide and is recognized as a reference organization by the Agreement on Application of Sanitary and Phytosanitary Measures (SPS Agreement) of the World Trade Organization (WTO).

The OIE's financial resources are derived mainly from compulsory annual contributions, backed by voluntary contributions from member countries.

The OIE has four specialist commissions: Terrestrial Animal Health Standards Commission or Terrestrial Code Commission; Scientific Commission for Animal Diseases; Biological Standards Commission; and Aquatic Animal Health Standards Commission or Aquatic Code Commission. Their role is to use current scientific information to study problems of epidemiology and the prevention and control of animal diseases, to develop and revise OIE's international standards (including those for vaccines), and to address scientific and technical issues raised by members.

The OIE is committed to continuously improving the transparency of its standards development process in order to have the best scientific basis for its standards and to gain their widest possible support. All reports from OIE specialist commissions and accepted reports from relevant OIE working groups and *ad hoc* groups are published on the OIE public website and incorporated as appendices or chapters in publications.

3.3.1.2 Food and Agriculture Organization of the United Nations

The FAO was created in 1945 as an intergovernmental organization. Currently, the FAO has 194 member nations. The FAO is concerned with livestock development, including assisting its member countries in the control and eradication of animal diseases.

Based on its experience in the coordinated Global Rinderpest Eradication Programme (GREP) and through the European Commission for the Control of Foot and Mouth Disease, the FAO has been involved in the standardization of disease control tools, especially vaccines, and has defined major guidelines and standards for the use of vaccines which it insists must be high-quality internationally recognized vaccines, independently tested for efficacy and safety before use in coordinated mass vaccination campaigns.

Even though the FAO is not directly involved in testing vaccines for veterinary use, it established two auxiliary services to assist in matters related to veterinary vaccines. The Codex Alimentarius or "Food Code" was established jointly with the WHO in 1963 to promote standards to facilitate international trade in food commodities. The objective of the Codex Alimentarius is to develop harmonized international food standards, which protect consumer health and promote fair practices in food trade. The Joint Division of Nuclear Techniques in Food and Agriculture, operated jointly by the FAO and the International Atomic Energy Agency (IAEA), helps veterinary services and research institutes in developing countries to establish various immunoassays including radioimmunoassay (RIA), enzyme-linked immunosorbent assay (ELISA), and molecular techniques for monitoring vaccination campaigns, and for diagnosis and surveillance of animal diseases. This joint program is implemented by the Animal Production and Health Section and its laboratory respectively in Vienna and in Seibersdorf, Austria.

3.3.1.3 Global Alliance for Livestock Veterinary Medicine

The Global Alliance for Livestock Veterinary Medicines, formerly the Global Alliance for Livestock Vaccines, is a not-for-profit, livestock health product, development and access partnership. GALVmed's objectives are:

- to relieve financial hardship and promote good livestock health (including improving food security) among livestock keepers in developing countries through the promotion of affordable, accessible vaccines, pharmaceutical, and diagnostic products/services aimed at improving the health of their livestock
- to promote the effective use of resources to achieve the above charitable purposes through the identification, management, funding, and coordination of research into livestock products and services
- the development and delivery of these products and services at affordable prices, by working in partnership with others (whether charities, government, private bodies or institutions).

GALVmed achieves its objectives by facilitating the necessary dialogue and regulatory activities for vaccine registration harmonization arrangements in Africa, i.e. working to facilitate a process where vaccine registration in one country results in registration in other participating countries and also providing technical support in developing standardized tools and procedures to regulatory agencies. GALVmed works within the African Regional Economic Communities (RECs) framework to implement the mutual recognition framework in East Africa and engage other RECs in implementing appropriate activities.

3.3.1.4 Health for Animals (Formerly International Federation for Animal Health)

Health for Animals is a nonprofit, nongovernmental organization (NGO) based in Brussels representing the animal health sector, including manufacturers of veterinary pharmaceuticals, vaccines, and other animal health products throughout the world, as well as the associations that represent companies at national and regional levels. The mandates of Health for Animals are, among others, to:

- act as a unified global industry voice in dialogue with major international bodies (OIE, FAO, WHO, Codex, World Trade Organization, etc.), governments, animal health stakeholders, food industry partners, and consumers
- encourage and assist the development of predictable science-based regulatory processes and standards where authorization and approval to market medicines are firmly rooted in a thorough risk–benefit analysis
- promote international harmonization of testing requirements for animal health products to facilitate the availability and delivery of new and innovative products worldwide
- act as a source of information on the benefits of animal health products for animal health and welfare, food and safety, and public health
- actively promote the value of research-based medicines developed to the highest standards and authorized according to the regulatory criteria of quality, safety, and efficacy
- ensure the availability of all classes of veterinary medicines to the benefit of animal health and welfare, and promote their responsible use.

3.3.1.5 World Health Organization

The WHO is a specialized United Nations agency created in 1946 with its headquarters in Geneva (Switzerland). Its goal is to build better, healthier futures for people all over the world to ensure the highest attainable level of health.

The WHO budget is financed through a mix of assessed and voluntary contributions. It has more than 700 collaborating centers working on, among others, the standardization of terminology and nomenclature, of technology, of diagnostic, therapeutic and prophylactic substances, and of methods and procedures. The World Health Assembly is the decision-making body of WHO.

The WHO Expert Committee on Biological Standardization (ECBS) has issued general documents on standardization, which could apply to veterinary vaccines. Even though the major role of the WHO ECBS is not standardization of veterinary vaccines, it has issued reports on veterinary vaccines, most recently in 1992. The WHO catalogue entitled *Biological Substances: International Standards and Reference Reagents* (latest edition dated 1990) contains a list of some reference reagents for sera and vaccines against zoonoses (botulism, brucellosis, rabies) and against certain diseases confined to animals (e.g. canine distemper, classic swine fever, Newcastle disease).

3.3.2 Regional Vaccine Standardization Organizations

3.3.2.1 Africa: Pan African Veterinary Vaccine Centre of the African Union

The Pan African Veterinary Vaccine Centre of the African Union was founded in 1984 in support of the Pan African Rinderpest Campaign (PARC), as a result of the implementation of the recommendation of the FAO Expert Consultation on Rinderpest held in Rome (Italy) urging all vaccine-producing laboratories in Africa to participate in international and independent vaccine quality control schemes. The primary aim of this recommendation was to ensure the use of good-quality vaccines in the rinderpest vaccination campaigns. In 1986, the FAO established, through its Technical Cooperation Programme (TCP/RAF/6767 and 6766), two regional vaccine quality control and training centers, in Debre Zeit (Ethiopia) for eastern and southern Africa, and in Dakar (Senegal) for West and Central Africa, dedicated to improving the quality of the rinderpest vaccine produced in Africa. This initiative was followed, from 1988 to 1993, by a United Nations Development Programme (UNDP) funding (UNDP/RAF/88/050) of the two centers as a single project which became the Pan African Veterinary Vaccine Centre (PANVAC) under the responsibility of the then Organization of African Unity/Inter-African Bureau for Animal Resources (OAU/IBAR), with the FAO as the executing agency. In 1993, the two units merged and now perform the functions of PANVAC at one site in Debre Zeit. In 1994, the Fourth Conference of African Ministers responsible for Animal Resources held in Addis Ababa (Ethiopia) recommended the institutionalization of PANVAC as a technical center of the OAU, which later became the African Union. The Center was officially launched as an African Union Institution, with its headquarters located at Debre Zeit (Ethiopia) in 2004.

The major objective of the PANVAC is to promote the availability of safe, effective, and affordable veterinary vaccines. Its mandates are, among others, to provide international independent quality control of veterinary vaccines in Africa using the OIE standards, and facilitate the standardization of veterinary vaccines production and harmonization of their quality control techniques in Africa by establishing and maintaining a repository of well-characterized reference materials composed of cell, virus, and bacterial vaccine seed stocks, antisera, and antigens. The number of vaccines certified by PANVAC has continued to rise over the years as the disease priorities of the different regions in Africa change. Between 2010 and 2016, about 1318 batches of different veterinary vaccines, estimated at over 1.5 billion doses, were certified by PANVAC. Through its vaccine quality assurance systems, PANVAC was able to catalyze the adoption of improved methods for the production and quality control of priority vaccines in Africa. This is reflected by the fact that pass rates of vaccines from African laboratories are currently above 90% compared with about 30% in the 1980s.

Most vaccine production laboratories in Africa continue to benefit from supplies of reference repository materials in order to harmonize and standardize the quality of vaccines produced across the continent. This, in addition to the publishing of major vaccine standard operating procedures, contributes to the adoption of harmonized procedures for vaccine production and quality control in Africa. Through its training programs, PANVAC has trained hundreds of veterinarians and technicians from national vaccine production laboratories in Africa. These training sessions have been organized as annual workshops for vaccine-producing laboratories, fellowships or as in-house (*in situ*) arrangements. PANVAC also continues to provide technical expertise and to transfer new vaccine production technologies, when available, to vaccine-producing laboratories in order to improve their capacities and productivity.

PANVAC became an OIE collaborating center in vaccine quality control of veterinary vaccines in 2013 and an FAO reference center in 2015.

3.3.2.2 Europe

3.3.2.2.1 European Medicines Agency The European Medicines Agency (EMA) was set up in 1995, in London, to harmonize the work of existing national medicine regulatory bodies. Today, the EMA is a decentralized agency of the European Union (EU) responsible for the scientific evaluation, supervision, and safety monitoring of medicines developed by pharmaceutical companies for use in the EU.

EMA protects public and animal health in 28 EU member states, as well as the countries of the European Economic Area, by ensuring that all medicines available on the EU market are safe, effective, and of high quality.

The mission of the EMA is to foster scientific excellence in the evaluation and supervision of medicines, for the benefit of public and animal health in the EU. Its activities are to:

- facilitate development and access to medicines
- evaluate applications for marketing authorization
- monitor the safety of medicines across their lifecycle
- provide information on human and veterinary medicines to healthcare professionals and patients.

To fulfill its mission, the EMA works closely with national competent authorities in a unique partnership known as the European Medicines Regulatory Network. The network is composed of thousands of experts from across Europe grouped into seven EMA scientific committees and more than 30 working parties. Working together has encouraged the exchange of knowledge, ideas, and best practices, in order to ensure the highest standards in medicines regulation.

3.3.2.2.2 European Pharmacopoeia The European Pharmacopoeia was created in 1964 under the aegis of the Council of Europe by a treaty signed by eight nations: Belgium, France, Germany, Italy, Luxembourg, the Netherlands, Switzerland, and the UK. The objective of this institution is to harmonize national laws on the manufacture, circulation, and distribution of medicines in Europe. The role of the European Pharmacopoeia has been described by Artiges (1992).

The work of the European Pharmacopoeia is undertaken by two bodies: the European Pharmacopoeia Commission, which prepares and adopts the technical decisions relating to monographs, and the Public Health Committee of the Council of Europe, which exercises administrative authority over the Commission's activities and sets the date of application of the monographs but cannot interfere with their technical content.

3.3.2.2.3 Official Control Authority Batch Release and Official Batch Protocol Review: OCABR/OBPR for Immunological Veterinary Medicinal Products Article 82 of European Directive 2001/82/EC, as amended by Directive 2004/28/EC, of the European Parliament and the Council came into force throughout the EC in 2005. This article allows, for reasons of human or animal health, a member state to request samples of each batch of a given immunological veterinary product (IVMP) to be submitted to a Competent Authority (CA) for official testing by an Official Medicine Control Laboratory (OMCL) before it is placed on the market. It also establishes the conditions under which a restricted test list can be applied. This is referred to as Official Control Authority Batch Release (OCABR). OCABR performed by any given member state must be mutually recognized by all other member states requiring OCABR for that product.

Article 81 of European Directive 2001/82/EC allows a member state, where appropriate, to ask a Marketing Authorization Holder (MAH) to provide documentation to a control authority or an OMCL proving that control tests were carried out in accordance with the methods laid down in the marketing authorization (MA). This is referred to as an Official Batch Protocol Review (OBPR). A goodwill agreement has been adopted by the Veterinary Batch Release Network (VBRN) to mutually recognize OBPR certificates between member states, provided the procedure and rules codified by the network are followed.

The VBRN is an important forum for the confidential exchange of quality and technical information on IVMPs and related methods and is a key link in the regulatory chain. As mandated by the European Commission, the European Directorate for the Quality of Medicines (EDQMs) acts as its secretariat. The VBRN is a specific network within the general OMCL network, thus subject to its operating rules. It is supervised by an elected advisory group consisting of four representatives from different member states. A plenary meeting is held annually bringing together all the representatives to review the year's activities and discuss issues concerning the network. This meeting also serves as an opportunity to reconsider the need for testing different product types and to adopt officially the VBRN procedures and guidelines, which must be approved by all the network's members. A short list of IVMPs for which Article 82 may be applied using a restricted test list has been agreed upon. This short list is reviewed on a regular basis to ensure it continues to address product quality and safety needs appropriately. The current list can be found in annex I of the EU Administrative Procedure for Application of Article 82 for Official Control Authority Batch Release of Immunological Veterinary Medicinal Products (www.edqm.eu/en/ocabrobpr-immunological-veterinary-medicinal-products-ivmps).

3.3.2.3 Americas

Three major animal health organizations are involved in the standardization of veterinary vaccines at regional level for the Americas: Pan American Health Organization (PAHO), Inter-American Institute for Cooperation on Agriculture (IICA), and Latin-American Technical Committee for Harmonization of the Registration and Control of Veterinary Medicines.

3.3.2.3.1 Pan American Health Organization The PAHO, a specialized international health agency for the Americas, was created in 1920 to continue the work of the Pan American Sanitary Bureau established in 1902. It is composed of 48 member countries and territories, sets the regional health priorities and mobilizes action to address health problems that do not respect borders and that, in many cases, jeopardize the sustainability of health systems in the region. It is the specialized health agency of the Inter-American System and also serves as the WHO Regional Office for the Americas. The PAHO Headquarters is in Washington, DC (USA), and has three specialized centers, including the Pan American Foot and Mouth Disease Center (PANAFTOSA), involved in the standardization of foot and mouth disease (FMD) vaccines for the Americas.

The PANAFTOSA was opened in 1951 in Rio de Janeiro, Brazil, and provides training in vaccine production and control. It takes a direct and active part in defining quality control standards for FMD vaccine in every country of the region. It also advises on vaccine production and testing in local laboratories.

3.3.2.3.2 Inter-American Institute for Cooperation on Agriculture The IICA is a specialized agency in the region of the Americas. It was founded in 1942 and is now responsible for encouraging, facilitating, and supporting cooperation in agricultural development and rural prosperity among its 34 member states. Its Program V: Agricultural Health focuses on the development of equivalent compatible laws and regulations to facilitate trade within the region.

The activities of the PAHO, IICA, and the OIE with regard to the regulation and testing of vaccines in the Americas are coordinated by an Inter-American Cooperation Group on Animal Health. This body, made up of the international, regional, and subregional organizations and an associate member, the USDA-APHIS, provides technical cooperation in the field of animal health to the countries of the Americas. It meets once a year within the region to discuss action required by smaller regional structures, such as the International Regional Organization for Plant and Animal, the Junta del Acuerdo de Cartagena, the Caribbean Animal and Plant Health Information Network (CARAPHIN), and the Common Market of the South (MERCOSUR).

3.3.2.3.3 Committee of the Americas for Veterinary Medical Products The Committee of the Americas for Veterinary Medical Products (CAMEVET) is a working group for the harmonization of registration and control of veterinary medicines under the framework of the OIE, and has been working uninterruptedly since 1992, when the first seminar for the harmonization of rules governing the registration and control of veterinary medicines was held in the city of Buenos Aires, Argentina. The Committee has a unique nature, as it brings together government and private sector efforts in a framework of open and true discussion.

Its objectives, as indicated in the name of the opening seminars, have at all times been the harmonization of the rules governing the registration and control of veterinary medicines to ensure that products marketed in the region are manufactured, registered, and controlled using equivalent systems in order to facilitate their trade between the different countries. The deliverables from the group, in the form of rules applicable to the sphere of reference, constitute a set of documents that adapt the essential technical requirements for achieving effective, safe, and innocuous veterinary products to the actual circumstances of each member country, while keeping them equivalent to those recommended internationally.

3.3.2.4 Asia, the Far East, and Oceania

Currently no organization in the region is directly involved in activities aimed at the standardization of vaccines. In the past, the Animal Production and Health Commission for Asia and the Pacific, based since 1975 at the FAO Regional Office in Bangkok (Thailand), played an indirect role in testing vaccines for veterinary use.

The Commission, in collaboration with other units in the FAO and international partners OIE and WHO, continues to carry out a number of initiatives in the region: capacity building and training in technical measures and controls, assessments and planning, and regional information exchange.

3.3.3 Nongeographical Organizations

A number of organizations cover a group of countries with common problems. The major ones are the Organization for Economic Co-operation and Development (OECD); the VICH; the International Alliance of Biological Standardization (IABS); and the National Institute for Biological Standards and Control (NIBSC).

3.3.3.1 Organization for Economic Co-operation and Development

The organization was formed in 1960. It is concerned with the implications of biotechnology for agriculture, livestock, and the environment.

Although the OECD has no direct regulatory role in licensing or testing veterinary vaccines produced by biotechnological methods, it has produced many technical documents on good laboratory practice (GLP), which are widely used by vaccine manufacturers to ensure high quality production.

3.3.3.2 International Cooperation on Harmonization of Technical Requirements for Registration of Veterinary Medicinal Products

The VICH is an international program providing guidance on technical requirements for registration of veterinary medicinal products. The VICH was established in 1996 as a means of collaboration primarily between the regulatory authorities and the animal health industry of the EU, Japan, and the USA. It aims at harmonizing technical requirements for veterinary product registration. Its role is to establish and implement harmonized regulatory requirements for veterinary medicinal products in the VICH regions, as well as working toward providing a basis for wider international harmonization of registration requirements. This is done through the harmonization of technical requirements for data necessary for marketing authorization (also called "registration") of a veterinary medicinal product and by developing harmonized guidelines on the studies to be submitted in a marketing authorization application.

The VICH has an Outreach Forum (VICH 2014) composed of countries and regional organizations that have expressed an interest in the work of VICH and are motivated to participate in the activities of the VICH Outreach Forum. It aims at providing a basis for wider international harmonization of technical requirements, improving information exchange and raising awareness of VICH and VICH guidelines with non-VICH countries/regions.

The OIE provides support to VICH and considers that the international harmonization of technical requirements for pre- and postmarketing authorization of veterinary medicines is a necessity for animal health, public health, and facilitation of international trade and that the VICH is one of the necessary tools to achieve these aims.

3.3.3.3 International Alliance of Biological Standardization

The IABS was founded in 1955 to bring together controllers, manufacturers, and research workers interested in the control and standardization of biological products. The IABS is an independent, nonprofit scientific alliance, devoted to the scientific and medical advancement of biologicals, by facilitating communication among those who develop, produce, and regulate biological products for human and animal health. Its major objectives are:

- to create an ongoing interface among leaders in clinical and basic research, biological product development, public health, manufacturing and regulation, by organizing scientific conferences and publishing reports of such meetings and to facilitate the establishment of international reference materials
- the formulation of international guidance documents for biological substances used in human and veterinary medicine, through its conferences and publications
- to promote uniform methods for establishing the international quality of biological products
- to encourage research in connection with the characterization, standardization, quality, production, and clinical use of biological products.

3.3.3.4 National Institute for Biological Standards and Control

The NIBSC is a global leader in the characterization, standardization, and control of biological medicines for human health. The NIBSC began work in 1972 and plays a major role in assuring the quality of biological medicines worldwide through the provision of biological reference materials, by testing products, and carrying out research. As part of the Medicines and Healthcare products Regulatory Agency (MHRA), the NIBSC undertakes supporting research in regulatory science required for regulation of medicines. It is the UK's official medicines control laboratory.

3.4 Scope and Role/Functions of Reference and Regional Laboratories

3.4.1 OIE Reference Laboratories

OIE reference laboratories are designated to address all the scientific and technical problems relating to a specific disease and vaccines requirements. The role of a reference laboratory is to function as a center of expertise and standardization of diagnostic techniques for its designated disease. They may also provide scientific and technical training for personnel from members, and coordinate scientific and technical studies in collaboration with other laboratories or organizations (see OIE Criteria and Internal Rules for Reference Laboratories: www.oie.int/fileadmin/Home/eng/About_us/docs/pdf/basic_text/80%20SG19_basictexts_ANG%20part%205.pdf). In 2017, the OIE has a global network of 267 reference laboratories covering 118 diseases/topics in 38 countries.

The mandates of the reference laboratories are, among others:

- to recommend the prescribed and alternative diagnostic tests and vaccines as OIE standards
- to develop reference materials in accordance with OIE requirements, and implement and promote the application of OIE standards
- to store and distribute to national laboratories biological reference products and any other reagents used in the diagnosis and control of the designated pathogens or diseases
- to develop, standardize, and validate according to OIE standards new procedures for diagnosis and control of the designated pathogens or diseases.

The reference laboratory experts lead the production of OIE manuals of diagnostic tests and vaccines for terrestrial and aquatic animals.

3.4.2 OIE Collaborating Centers

OIE collaborating centers are centers of expertise in a specific designated sphere of competence relating to the management of general questions on animal health issues, including quality control of veterinary vaccines ("specialty"). In their designated specialty, they must provide their expertise internationally.

The mandates of the collaborating centers are, among others:

- to provide services to the OIE, in particular within the region, in the designated specialty, in support of the implementation of OIE policies and, where required, seek for collaboration with OIE reference laboratories
- to propose or develop methods and procedures that facilitate harmonization of international standards and guidelines applicable to the designated specialty.

In relation to livestock vaccines, there are OIE collaborating centers for:

- development and production of vaccines, pharmaceutical products, and veterinary diagnostic systems using biotechnology
- diagnosis of animal diseases and vaccine evaluation in the Americas
- quality control of veterinary vaccines
- validation, quality assessment, and quality control of diagnostic assays and vaccine for vesicular diseases in Europe
- veterinary medicinal products.

3.4.3 FAO Reference Centers

Currently, the FAO has more than 60 institutions, referred to as FAO reference centers and collaborating centers, which provide guidance on specific diseases and thematic areas. With the support of the reference centers, the FAO has published guidelines on vaccine standards, among which is the *Vaccine Manual: The Production and Quality Control of Veterinary Vaccines for Use in Developing Countries* that has been a major player in the OIE Standards Commission.

3.4.4 WHO Reference Laboratories

The WHO brings together international experts in specific fields through its biological standardization program to develop and revise specific recommendations for the production and quality control of vaccines of major international public health importance. These experts, who are drawn from various specialist areas including reference and collaborating centers, produce, on behalf of the WHO, a series of regularly updated position papers on vaccines and vaccine combinations against diseases that have an international public health impact. These papers, which are concerned primarily with the use of vaccines in large-scale immunization programs, summarize essential background information on the respective diseases and vaccines, and conclude with the current WHO position concerning their use in the global context. Authoritative, harmonized guidelines and recommendations, for use by manufacturers and regulatory authorities, are also published in the reports of the ECBS meetings in the WHO Technical Report Series. These include recommendations for individual vaccines, and also more general guidelines on technical or regulatory topics such as cell substrates, nonclinical evaluation, or clinical evaluation.

This program also establishes and distributes the WHO Biological Reference Materials required for the standardization of assays to laboratories around the world. These papers are reviewed by a number of experts within and outside the WHO and, since April 2006, have been reviewed and endorsed by WHO's Strategic Advisory Group of Experts (SAGE) on vaccines and immunization.

3.5 Development of Vaccine Standards and Establishment of Rules and Guidelines for Vaccine Standards

3.5.1 International Intergovernmental Standards: OIE Standards

The OIE procedures provide a basis for rapidity, responsiveness, scientific rigor, and transparency in the development of standards.

In the development and adoption of standards, each of the OIE member countries has an equal voice and each has a responsibility to engage with the OIE in this important work.

Requests for the development of a new standard or the revision of an existing one come to the OIE from various sources, including OIE delegates, OIE global conferences, international and regional organizations that have official agreements with the OIE, or other organizations, i.e. scientific, industry or NGOs. A specialist commission may propose new work to be undertaken by itself or by another specialist commission. Proposals for developing new or revised standards are identified in the work programs of the specialist commissions and permanent working groups, which are submitted to OIE delegates for information annually at the General Session. Specialist commissions play a central role in the OIE standard-setting procedures.

Recommendations on new standards and on significant revisions of existing standards are developed by small groups of independent experts (*ad hoc* groups), which report to a specialist commission. Reporting may be directly to the specialist commission or, depending on the topic, via a permanent OIE working group, which in turn reports to specialist commissions. Membership of working groups is proposed by the Director General and is endorsed by the Assembly. All draft texts are reviewed by the relevant specialist commission, then provided to OIE member countries for comments. All comments submitted by member countries are reviewed by the specialist commissions, who may deal with comments directly or may send them to an *ad hoc* or working group for consideration and advice, as appropriate. The reports of *ad hoc* groups submitted to specialist commissions, as well as the commission's review of member country comments are documented in the meeting report of the specialist commission, which is sent to member countries after each meeting and also placed on the OIE website. In March of each year, as part of the meeting report of the specialist commissions that have met by February, all texts proposed for adoption at the General Session (held in May) are sent to member countries for consideration prior to presentation to the Assembly for adoption.

Twice yearly, following distribution of specialist commission reports, OIE member countries have the opportunity (normally during a 60-day period) to submit written comments. Although there is no provision for written comments to be presented to the General Session, there is opportunity to make oral statements and to request clarification of texts before adoption.

In the case of emergency situations warranting a more rapid procedure, standards may be developed within a shorter period. Less significant modifications to existing texts may also be undertaken in a 1-year period, if member countries agree to the proposed modifications.

There is only one pathway for the adoption of OIE standards, i.e. approval by the Assembly, which meets annually at the OIE General Session. In almost all cases, standards are adopted by consensus. In a small minority of cases, where it is not possible to achieve consensus, standards have been adopted after a vote. A two-thirds majority is sufficient for the adoption of a standard. More than half the delegates representing member countries must be present in order to have a quorum for the adoption of standards.

Each OIE member country has an equal voice in the adoption of standards. Partner organizations may attend technical sessions of the General Session in an observer capacity but they do not have the right to participate in the adoption of standards. Discussion and decisions of the

Assembly on the adoption of standards are recorded in a report presented for adoption at the end of the General Session. This report is provided to delegates and is placed on the OIE website accessible to the public (Figure 3.2).

The OIE regularly updates its international standards as new scientific information comes to light, following its established transparent and democratic procedures.

3.5.2 Private Standards

In February 2010, the OIE convened a meeting with global private standard setting organizations, including Global Good Agricultural Practice and the Global Food Safety Initiative (GFSI). It was agreed that the basis for private standards on sanitary safety is the existing international standards of the OIE and Codex Alimentarius, as well as national and regional legislation.

3.6 Accessing Information and Guidance from Reference and Regional Laboratories

3.6.1 OIE

The OIE publishes two codes (Terrestrial and Aquatic) and two manuals (Terrestrial and Aquatic) as the main references for World Trade Organization members.

The *Terrestrial Manual* (OIE 2017a) and the *Aquatic Manual* (OIE 2017b) contain OIE international standards on quality management in testing laboratories, principles of validation and quality control of diagnostic assays, and diagnostic testing methods for specific diseases including official tests listed in the *Terrestrial* and *Aquatic Codes*.

The *Terrestrial Manual* also provides generic and specific guidance on vaccine quality. It provides general principles in vaccine production, requirements for vaccine seeds, the vaccine production, in-process and final products quality requirement tests. In addition to the *Manual*, the OIE publishes a list of approved standard sera (reagents) produced by OIE reference laboratories, validates and certifies commercially available diagnostic assays, and publishes a list of the tests certified "fit for purpose" in the OIE Register of Diagnostic Tests.

3.6.2 WHO

The WHO catalogue entitled *Biological Substances: International Standards and Reference Reagents* contains a list of some reference reagents for sera and vaccines against zoonoses (botulism, brucellosis, rabies) and against certain diseases confined to animals (e.g. canine distemper, classic swine fever, Newcastle disease).

Certain WHO texts apply to specific diseases common to human beings and animals, notably brucellosis and

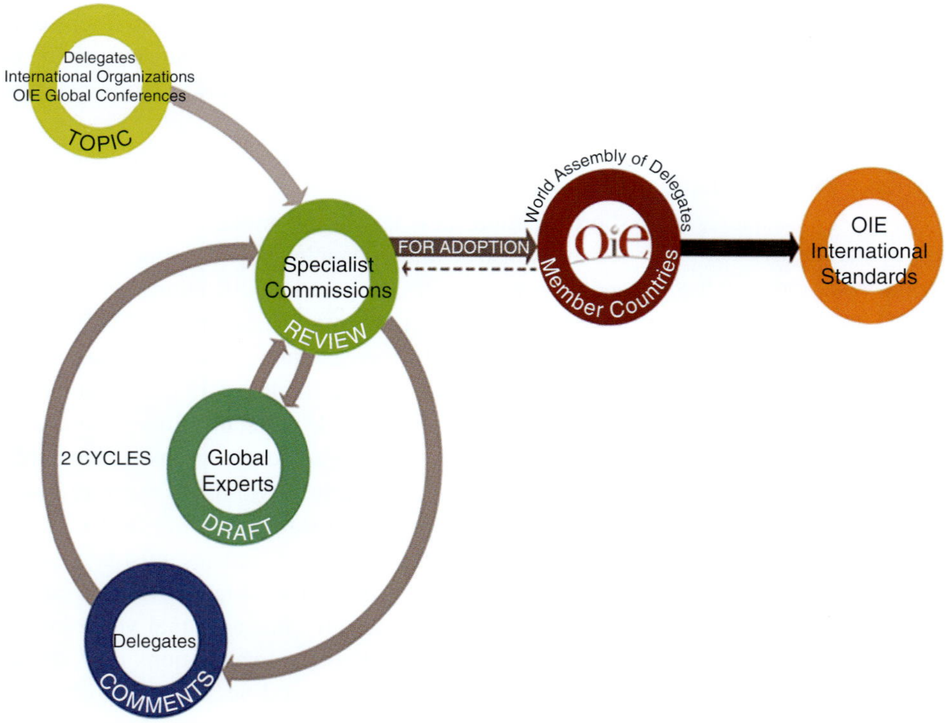

Figure 3.2 OIE standard setting process.

rabies. For example, chapters on veterinary vaccines against brucellosis are contained in the reports of the Joint FAO/WHO Expert Committee on Brucellosis, and chapters on veterinary vaccines against rabies are contained in the Eighth Report of the WHO Expert Committee on Rabies.

In every case, the WHO and OIE take care to ensure that the texts issued by both organizations are complementary (and not contradictory), and that reference reagents distributed by both organizations are of uniform quality.

3.6.3 FAO

The FAO produced a manual entitled Vaccine Manual: The Production and Quality Control of Veterinary Vaccines for Use in Developing Countries, published in 1997, as its response to the recommendation of an Expert Consultation on the Quality Control of Veterinary Vaccines in Developing Countries held in Rome in December 1991. This manual played an important role in improving the quality standards of vaccines during the rinderpest eradication campaign, through the establishment of the PANVAC in 1986.

The Codex Alimentarius standards (212), guidelines (73), codes of practice (51) and advisory texts are available from its list of standards. The Codex standards for food additives, veterinary drugs maximum residue levels, and pesticide maximum residue levels can also be accessed through its databases. The work of the Codex Alimentarius is governed by the Codex Alimentarius Commission (which meets every 2 years), the Secretariat of which is based at the FAO headquarters in Rome.

3.6.4 European Medicines Agency

The EU legislation and procedures for the regulation of veterinary medicines are compiled in the EMA document entitled *Rules Governing Medicinal Products in the EU* and more specifically in the following volumes.

- Volume 5 – EU pharmaceutical legislation for medicinal products for veterinary use.
- Volume 4 – Guidelines for good manufacturing practices for medicinal products for human and veterinary use.
- Volume 6 – Notice to applicants and regulatory guidelines for medicinal products for veterinary use.
- Volume 7 – Scientific guidelines for medicinal products for veterinary use.
- Volume 8 – Maximum residue limits.
- Volume 9 – Guidelines for pharmacovigilance for medicinal products for human and veterinary use.
- Volume 10 – Guidelines for clinical trials.

3.6.5 European Pharmacopoeia

The first edition of the EP was published in 1969 and comprised 120 texts. A new edition is published every 3 years. The 10th edition was published in 2019. It comprises 2376 monographs (legally binding to all member countries) describing individual quality standards (set of control tests applicable to one ingredient) and general quality standards applicable to families of ingredients or to dosage forms including vaccines, sera (human, veterinary), and general methods of analysis. The EP defines the minimum acceptable standards for products to be authorized within the EU because compliance with monographs is a mandatory requirement within Directive 2001/82/EC. It is a requirement that products must comply with the relevant specific monograph or with the general monographs where a specific one is not available.

3.6.6 Inter-American Institute for Cooperation on Agriculture

The IICA has published *Guidelines for the Use and Safety of Genetic Engineering Techniques or Recombinant DNA Technology* (IICA 1988), prepared in cooperation with the OIE, PAHO, and the Organization of American States. Another publication deals with the regulation of biotechnology, particularly the release into the environment of genetically modified organisms.

3.6.7 Organization for Economic Co-operation and Development

The OECD has published two documents on safety considerations in the field of biotechnology which could affect the testing of vaccines for veterinary use derived from this technology: Recombinant DNA Safety Considerations (www.oecd.org/sti/biotech/40986855.pdf) and OECD and Risk/Safety Assessment in Modern Biotechnology (www.oecd.org/chemicalsafety/biotrack/Risk-Safety-Assessment-in-Modern-Biotechnology.pdf).

3.7 Summary

The complex processes involved in the production of vaccines allow for variability which requires care to control batch-to-batch uniformity and to maintain the purity, safety, potency, and efficacy of the vaccine. In developed countries, quality control and biological standardization have always been a prerogative of the state, and quality standards have been developed at a national, regional, or international level. The globalization of trade and the introduction of technical barriers to trade dictate that harmonization and standardization of requirements for veterinary vaccines must be instituted at regional and international levels in order to safeguard the economic, environmental, and social welfare of the planet. Recent scientific and technical developments have led to a rapid expansion in the number and complexity of biologicals, with new products including vaccines and new biotechnologies posing new challenges for standardization. This review has examined the various international organizations responsible for addressing the issue of veterinary vaccine standardization, highlighting their various activities and the regulations and guidance produced to support the improvement of animal health.

The number of organizations involved in the formulation of standards and the number of regulations indicate the level of concern the global community attaches to standards relating to the production and use of biological products. However, due to the number of these standards and regulations, and the number of organizations involved, duplications and sometimes even disagreements and disparities in views do occur.

Even though these standards are numerous and sometimes cumbersome, they give national authorities ample opportunity to choose between the recommendations of the various international organizations, and to adopt the texts which are best suited to the local situation. They also give room for review and improvement of these standards in the light of current situations and gaps in the production and administration of biological products. Eventually, these regulations get restructured and incorporated into national laws and regulations. There is no doubt that as the international and national standards become increasingly harmonized, the rate of compliance with biological standards at national level will increase and at the same time the likelihood of substandard products being released into the market unnoticed will be greatly diminished. In the future, this convergence toward the harmonization of standards will be reflected not only between national authorities but also between the international organizations themselves, where mutual recognition and unity of purpose will lead to synergies in the development of better standards for biological production and use.

References

Artiges, A. (1992). The role of the European pharmacopoeia. *Dev. Biol. Stand.* 79: 87–93.

Blancou, J. and Truszczynski, M. (1995). The role of international and regional organisations in the regulation of veterinary biologicals. *Rev. Sci. Tech. Off. Int. Epiz.* 14 (4): 1193–1206. www.oie.int/doc/ged/D9021.PDF

IICA. (1988). *Guidelines for the Use and Safety of Genetic Engineering Techniques or Recombinant DNA Technology*, 1–134. Washington, DC: Inter-American Association for Cooperation on Agriculture. http://portal.oas.org/Portals/7/Ciencia_Tecnologia/documentos/Guidelines%20for%20the%20Use%20and%20Safety%20of%20Genetic%20Engineering.pdf

OIE. (2017a). Manual of Diagnostic Tests and Vaccines for Terrestrial Animals. www.oie.int/international-standard-setting/terrestrial-manual/access-online

OIE. (2017b). *Manual of Diagnostic Tests for Aquatic Animals.* www.oie.int/international-standard-setting/aquatic-manual/access-online

VICH. (2014). Terms of Reference for the VICH Outreach Forum. https://test.oie.int/fileadmin/Home/eng/Our_scientific_expertise/docs/pdf/VICH/Terms%20of%20Reference%20for%20Outreach%20Forum.pdf

4

Vaccination Strategies, Implementation, and Monitoring

Amanda Gibson[1], David Paton[2], and Dirk Werling[1]

[1] *Royal Veterinary College, Hatfield, Hertfordshire, UK*
[2] *The Pirbright Institute, Woking, Surrey, UK*

4.1 Introduction

Vaccination can be very effective, having been a cornerstone of the eradication of smallpox and rinderpest and providing protection against a wide range of other diseases as described in the different chapters of this book. Vaccines differ considerably in their production characteristics and physical properties, mode of application and action, the nature, breadth, and duration of the protection they provide, the target hosts they can be used in, the unwanted side effects and risks associated with their use, and their dependence upon complementary control measures. But in most cases, a common feature of vaccination is that it is a complex process that depends upon not only a good vaccine but also a correct strategy and implementation involving multiple steps, procedures, and players.

Problems can arise at many different stages in the production and application of vaccines, leading to suboptimal performance and failure to fully realize the potential of vaccination. Common problems with vaccination are: (i) loss of vaccine efficacy due to overheating or freezing of vaccines during storage, transport, or administration, (ii) failure to vaccinate and boost enough animals at the correct times, and (iii) failure to respond to vaccine by animals with maternally derived immunity. Therefore, it is vital not to underestimate what can go wrong, and to have the right staff, resources, training, awareness, procedures, and investigative tools to continuously monitor and periodically review the implementation and outcomes of all steps in the pathway from the selection of the vaccine and design of the vaccination strategy and regime, through the procurement, storage, transport, administration and recording of vaccination, to the measurement of what has been done, what has been achieved, and what has gone wrong (Table 4.1).

Many of these issues are covered in the disease-specific chapters (Section IV) while other chapters cover general aspects of the regulatory framework and quality control for the production and supply of veterinary vaccines. This chapter considers different vaccination strategies and important concepts for monitoring vaccine performance in the field, including vaccine coverage, herd immunity, and vaccine effectiveness studies.

4.2 Vaccine-Induced Protection

Vaccines act by reducing the susceptibility to infection, the extent of pathogen replication and shedding, the severity of clinical signs/disease, and the frequency of infection. The nature and strength of the immunity induced by vaccination may influence whether or not a sterile immunity is developed, in which animals become refractory to infection altogether (Pastoret and Jones 2004). For example, vaccines given by intramuscular or subcutaneous injection and that elicit a mainly systemic immunity may not prevent local replication at the mucosal entry points of many pathogens. However, by blocking or reducing internal replication and spread, or the actions of toxins, parenteral vaccines may prevent the agent reaching or affecting target organs for disease, transmission and persistence and reduce the levels of shedding and onward spread. A good example is inactivated foot and mouth disease (FMD) vaccines for which potency tests measure the ability of the parenterally administered vaccine to prevent an intradermolingual challenge leading to virus generalization and the development of vesicular lesions on the feet (OIE 2019).

For contagious diseases and livestock kept in groups, animals that have not been vaccinated will benefit from a

Veterinary Vaccines: Principles and Applications, First Edition. Edited by Samia Metwally, Gerrit Viljoen, and Ahmed El Idrissi.

Table 4.1 Some of the many steps and procedures to be established and reviewed in the vaccination process.

Vaccination strategy	Vaccine selection	Vaccination regime	Vaccination implementation	Vaccination monitoring and review
Objectives	Which vaccine and strain?	Who will vaccinate?	Procedures and training	Passive and active surveillance
Approaches	Potency and DIVA requirements	Eligibility criteria for vaccination	Storage and transport	Analysis of records
Targets	Quantities required	Vaccination schedules	Cold chain	Estimates of coverage
Cost–benefit	Procurement methods		Recording systems	Surveys of immunity
Feasibility	Quality control		Biosecurity	Surveys of infection
Sustainability				Vaccination effectiveness studies
Complementary requirements				Definition and follow-up of adverse effects and vaccine breakdowns
Awareness raising				Reviews of outcomes

DIVA, differentiating infected and vaccinated animals.

reduced likelihood of exposure to infection resulting from herd immunity generated by vaccination of their fellows (Fine et al. 2011). Meanwhile, failure to vaccinate enough animals in a group can increase the likelihood of vaccinated animals receiving an overwhelming infectious challenge exposure from their unprotected in-contacts. We expand on herd immunity later in this chapter.

Vaccine efficacy can be measured by potency tests or field studies. As well as the effectiveness of the vaccine itself, at the point of delivery, and the proportion of the herd that receive it, the success of vaccination depends upon many other influences, including the scheduling of primary and booster vaccinations, other factors which affect responsiveness to vaccination, the use of complementary control measures, the prevalence of challenge/infection, and the contact structures within the target population (Figure 4.1) (Heininger et al. 2012).

Vaccine epidemiology was explained in an editorial commentary by Weinberg and Szilagyi (2010). Here, the authors stated that “Each new vaccine considered for licensure must answer the most basic question regarding its effectiveness at disease prevention under field conditions.” Greenwood and Yule proposed more than 100 years ago the first mathematical concept to assess protective vaccine efficacy (Greenwood and Yule 1915). Vaccine efficacy is ideally assessed through double-blind, randomized, clinical controlled trials, which present a “best case scenario” to assess vaccine protectiveness under controlled conditions. In human medicine, such trials are required before a new vaccine is licensed by the regulatory

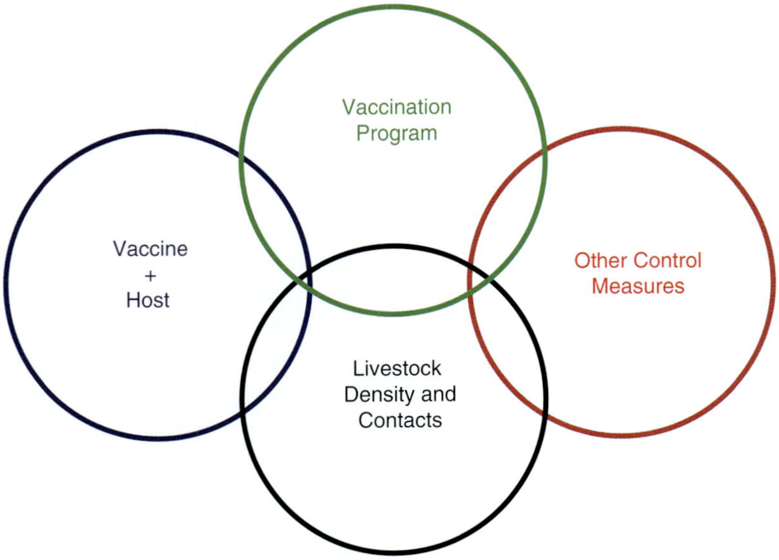

Figure 4.1 Determinants of vaccination program effectiveness for the control of contagious diseases.

authorities (Clemens et al. 1996). As Weinberg and Szilagyi define it, the outcome data (vaccine efficacy = VE) are expressed generally as a reduction in disease attack rate (AR) between the unvaccinated (ARU) and vaccinated (ARV) individuals, and this can be calculated from the relative risk (RR) of disease among the vaccinated group with use of the following formulas (Orenstein et al. 1985, 1988; Clemens et al. 1996):

$$VE = \frac{ARU - ARV}{ARU} \times 100$$

and

$$VE = \left(1 - RR\right) \times 100$$

The advantages of vaccine efficacy studies include rigorous controls for biases by sex/age, etc., as study individuals are randomly allocated into groups. Furthermore, they require recording of vaccination status and include a prospective, active monitoring phase for AR, including laboratory confirmation of the infectious status/outcome of interest and vaccine immunogenicity. However, VE trials have, in general, the disadvantage of being complex and expensive to run, especially if infection is uncommon, when large sample sizes are required to achieve clinically useful statistical power. In practice, for veterinary vaccines, potency tests are more commonly used than field studies of VE, which are more relevant to human medicine and can measure outcomes beyond AR, including hospitalizations, medical visits, and costs.

However, it should be remembered that the outcome of a VE study may differ compared with the vaccine's behavior in the whole population, as these trials often assess the performance of a vaccine under somewhat idealized conditions. This is mainly due to the set of inclusion/exclusion criteria applied to the study cohort (case definition), which may differ from those for the whole population and can give rise to a lower VE than the study cohort. Thus, the use of effectiveness trials should enable a more rational triaging of new vaccines for developing countries, thus accelerating the introduction of new vaccines and solving discussions regarding costs and benefits (Clemens et al. 1996).

4.3 Vaccination Strategies

4.3.1 Aims of Vaccination

Where infectious agents are endemic, with a high risk of exposure to infection, vaccination may be used to protect individual groups or animals from disease on a risk basis (RUMA 2007). Risk may be affected by diverse circumstances, such as season (e.g. abundance of arthropod vectors or transhumance activities), geography/proximity (e.g. anthrax in soil or spread from neighboring farms or countries), or related to the presence of a reservoir host (e.g. bat rabies, bovine tuberculosis in badgers, classic swine fever [CSF] in wild boar). The spread of agricultural areas into former wildlife habitats also increases the risk of reservoir hosts living in close proximity to farmed animals.

Where there is limited cooperative action to control the spread of infection, the decision to vaccinate may be at the discretion of animal owners, based on perceptions about the probability of infection, the consequences of disease, the availability of alternative treatments, and the cost and effectiveness of the vaccination. For example, some large intensive dairy cattle herds in Gulf States of the Middle East, where FMD is largely uncontrolled, are repeatedly vaccinated to prevent otherwise inevitable and catastrophic losses (Lyons et al. 2017). Other vaccines are targeted at specific individuals, such as heifers or pregnant animals, in order to prevent fetal infection (Williams et al. 2007) or to boost maternal transfer of antibodies in colostrum (Kurmann et al. 2011).

To maximize the indirect benefits of herd immunity, it is generally advisable to vaccinate as many as possible of the susceptible animals within each herd. This can lead to a "cocooning effect," protecting all newborns from day 1 onwards through a dramatically reduced risk of pathogen exposure, a concept already practiced in human medicine for pertussis (Swamy and Wheeler 2014). Take-up of discretionary or private vaccination may not be widespread or accompanied by complementary control measures and therefore tends not to prevent the spread and persistence of the pathogen in the population at large.

Alternatively, animals may be vaccinated as part of a concerted effort to raise wider population immunity and reduce the overall level of transmission of a pathogen. The classic approach is mass prophylactic vaccination as part of zonal, national, or regional disease eradication especially in the case of diseases with high economic impact (e.g. rinderpest [Roeder and Taylor 2007]), or if a disease possesses a high zoonotic importance (e.g. brucellosis [Singh et al. 2018]). This needs a high level of commitment and may be complicated by the risk of insufficient cross-protective coverage against different serotypes or strains, especially for RNA viruses such as avian influenza (AI), bluetongue, and FMD. As many herds as possible should be vaccinated and vaccination should be part of a package of control measures such as biosecurity, slaughter of affected or carrier animals, vector control, and especially control of animal movements.

Vaccination policies in different countries depend hugely on local animal health policies, and thus vary widely.

However, especially in the farming world, vaccination campaigns have to go hand in hand with educating the owners regarding the benefit of vaccination, which is often seen as an unnecessary cost, especially for diseases with rare outbreaks or for which, at least for now, antimicrobials are still available for treatment. Incentives offered by governments/levy boards include financial support for the purchase of vaccines, but these are often hampered by an inconsequent usage once this incentive is no longer paid. Where government funds are insufficient to sustain vaccination campaigns, priority may be given to ensuring the quality of vaccines available for purchase and pilot studies to demonstrate their cost-effectiveness to farmers.

Epidemiological and economic models are now widely used to study and compare the impact and resource requirements of different interventions, including vaccination, on changing the spread of different diseases (Huppert and Katriel 2013). This can help to develop and define vaccination strategies, to define vaccine needs and to decide when vaccination is or is not appropriate (Rawdon et al. 2018; Bitsouni et al. 2019; Casal et al. 2019), and explore the impact of vaccine-induced immunity that weakens over time.

4.3.2 Which Vaccines Are Needed and Where?

There is a clear differentiation between vaccines needed in the so-called developed countries, with high-intensity farming, and developing countries, which may contain a large number of animals kept in situations summarized under the term "backyard farming." In the former, the need for vaccines is driven by production-related diseases, such as mastitis, shipping fever, porcine circovirus, and *Eimeria* spp., for which currently existing antimicrobial treatment has become more limited due to changes in legislation and occurrence of more and more resistant strains. Vaccination in developing countries, however, is mainly used to impact highly contagious diseases that may have been eradicated in countries of the developed world, such as, for example, contagious bovine pleuropneumonia (CBPP), peste des petits ruminants (PPR), CSF, and FMD. These diseases are often accompanied by a high rate of morbidity/mortality, and are thus leading to substantial economic losses, due to replacement of culled animals, decreased production, treatment costs, and from transport and trade restrictions. A common problem in smallholder farming systems, in least in developed countries, is the availability of a reliable supply of vaccines of proven quality and demonstrated cost–benefit.

The genetic background of the animal population to be vaccinated should also be considered within the context of the biogeographical region. For example, a vaccine developed for animals with a fairly uniform and defined genetic background in the western world may not work as well in the more outbred populations that may be found in developing countries (Botros et al. 2006). Indeed, given the increasing evidence of differences in genetic resistance between *Bos indicus*- and *Bos taurus*-based breeds, as well as within subgenus of each breed, it becomes important to assess vaccine efficacy in the correct biogeographical setting (Glass 2004; Werling et al. 2009).

Managing vaccination in animal populations that live under nomadic conditions can be very challenging. In addition to a higher economic burden for nomadic groups, results may be affected by movement of pathogens between regions of high and low occurrence and problems in disease surveillance. Furthermore, there are potential implications for vaccine coverage, as animals/herds may be missed by national/regional vaccination programs or may originate in countries with different vaccination strategies. Disease surveillance in such nomadic herds may pose huge logistic problems, not only with respect to maintaining appropriate cold chains but also with tracking nomadic herds. Models can help to minimize the vaccination programs necessary to achieve the best success, as shown recently for PPR in Ethiopia (Fournie et al. 2018).

Despite these clear positive developments, there are no straightforward solutions to be offered. However, tiered pricing systems or bulk-buying of vaccines, local vaccine production (as for Newcastle disease vaccines in many North African nations), availability of heat-stable vaccines, reduction of vaccine dosage (one-shot regimes), combined with constant "in-field" further education may assist in more effective vaccination in nomadic and widespread communities. These can be delivered through coordinated international efforts assisted by development agencies, such as the AgResults Innovation in Research and Delivery Prizes that will support vaccine availability for brucellosis and FMD in developing countries (https://agresults.org/our-approach). In addition to these animal vaccine-specific approaches, vaccine campaigns for human and animal vaccination could be combined, sharing transport logistics and equipment, thus reducing total costs. Delivery of joint human and animal health services can be adapted to access hard-to-reach communities. By optimizing use of limited logistical and human resources, public health and veterinary services will become more effective, particularly at the local level.

4.3.3 Emergency Vaccination and Availability of Vaccines

Emergency vaccination, even in the form of a theraputic vaccination may be used in situations where an infectious agent is introduced into a naïve population, providing it with the means to spread rapidly, causing significant disease or economic losses and where a policy of nonvaccination is unacceptable and/or very costly (e.g. culling of affected livestock) or unlikely to succeed. It is a common contingency plan for diseases that may be reintroduced after eradication or in countries where the infection is sporadic (as for many contagious diseases, such as FMD or CSF). It may be used instead of or as a supplement to ongoing prophylactic vaccination. To be effective, it needs to be implemented quickly and to be well targeted, often requiring a stockpile of suitable vaccine (see Chapter 15) and good surveillance to define the correct vaccination area. If it is to prevent the spread of infection, as well as to limit losses from disease, then a high coverage is required and it must be accompanied by measures to control the movement of affected livestock beyond the vaccinated area. Great care must also be taken to avoid the spread of infection by vaccination teams.

As more countries have achieved eradication of different diseases and as public perception turns against culling and antibiotic treatments for controlling livestock diseases, emergency vaccination has become increasingly recognized as a preferred mechanism for dealing with disease incursions. Conditions that predispose to uncontrolled spread of infection tend to predispose to use of emergency vaccination, such as the presence of a relatively high-density population of vulnerable animals, or where the same agent has been introduced in different places (such as happened with the introduction of porcine epidemic diarrhea virus into the USA). Furthermore, emergency vaccination may be necessary in situations where the infection has not been detected fast enough, and therefore not controlled, leading to multifocal spread or uncontrollable spread of infection, especially in the case of airborne pathogens.

Finally, emergency vaccination may also be necessary in response to an act of bioterrorism targeted at livestock, especially for diseases with zoonotic potential. Within the European Commission, the Directorate D – Animal Health and Welfare (2010) has published an "Expert Opinion on Vaccine and/or Diagnostic Banks for Major Animal Diseases" as "Strategic Planning Option for Emergency Situations or Major Crisis," setting out the need for emergency vaccination to specified animal diseases, such as AI, CSF, etc. This document contains 13 key messages, clearly outlining when emergency vaccinations should be used (Directorate D – Animal Health and Welfare 2010).

1) Vaccination is a fundamental tool in a strategy to control and eradicate major emerging diseases.
2) Emergency vaccination has to be considered as one tool in a whole range of measures as a part of a complex strategy to control and eradicate major animal diseases.
3) Emergency vaccination for most relevant infectious diseases should in general be seen in a new light, directly linked to the availability of effective diagnostic tools substantiating that vaccinated animals, or meat and other products obtained from vaccinated animals, are free from pathogens and can be traded safely.
4) Emergency vaccination has to be understood as *vaccinate to live*, meaning that vaccinated animals are kept to the end of a normal production cycle, and that their meat and other products can be marketed.
5) Diagnostic banks supporting high-throughput testing for particular infectious diseases are necessary to supplement vaccine banks to enable a holistic strategy of disease control and eradication.
6) The establishment and maintenance of vaccine and diagnostic banks must be part of a strategic plan prepared during "peace time," ready for an emergency.
7) The issue of vaccine and diagnostic banks can only be treated in the context of a control and eradication strategy specific to each major animal disease (e.g. FMD, CSF, AI) and various outbreak scenarios.
8) For most of the relevant infectious diseases, existing legislation regarding emergency vaccination should be amended so that vaccination becomes a realistic option in the event of a crisis.
9) Trade issues regarding vaccinated animals or fresh meat and meat products obtained from vaccinated animals should be resolved.
10) Relevant legislation regarding veterinary medicinal products is not well suited to approve the use of vaccines in emergency situations.
11) The current review of legislation dealing with veterinary medicinal products is an ideal opportunity to introduce a mechanism to approve vaccines for emergency use at European level.
12) Proposals to be considered could include alternatives to vaccine banks, such as vaccine master seed stocks and "mock-up" authorizations for particular vaccines.
13) Vaccination and testing should replace unnecessary culling.

Emergency vaccination is also used to respond to outbreaks of highly contagious diseases that occur episodically in endemically affected countries, an example being responses to outbreaks of FMD in parts of Asia and Africa. In such cases, the emergency vaccination (also termed "reactive vaccination") may be used to reinforce immunity from earlier, prophylactic vaccination campaigns or as a stand-alone, risk-based measure to enable better targeting of vaccine, especially when it is in limited supply. Its effectiveness may be compromised by lack of surveillance, biosecurity, and movement controls.

4.4 Implementing Vaccination

4.4.1 Vaccine Selection

For many diseases, a choice of vaccines may be available and their different advantages and disadvantages, such as shelf-life, serotype or strain specificity, species suitability, cost, duration of immunity, safety in pregnant animals, etc., must be considered in the context of the aims and requirements of vaccination. Vaccine quality is of paramount importance and guidance on its control and on the necessary regulatory procedures for ensuring that it is in place is described in other chapters. Advice on tendering for FMD vaccine can be found in recent guidelines from the FAO and OIE (Ferrari et al. 2016). The steps described for rational procurement include: submitting outbreak viruses to a reference laboratory for characterization and vaccine matching; buying from reputable producers that adhere to prescribed standards; requesting a dossier of information from prospective suppliers; and seeking an independent evaluation of the manufacturer's claims or carrying out tests on their vaccine. Finally, checks should be made that the vaccine has worked before reordering it on a subsequent occasion. Opting for the cheapest vaccines may not be the most cost-efficient approach, given that the vaccine is only one element of the costs involved in vaccination campaigns and an ineffective vaccine is always the poorest value for money.

4.4.2 Vaccination Regimes and Procedures

Immunity induced by some live vaccines may be life-long, but for many vaccines, this is not the case and so immunity must be boosted to maintain protection. Advice on revaccination schedules may be obtained from vaccine manufacturers, but may depend upon a number of variables, such as the potency of the vaccines, the doses of vaccine already administered, and the severity of the subsequent challenge. The best time to vaccinate animals may be a balance between risk and convenience and procedures are needed to ensure the timely vaccination of new animals obtained by births and purchases. Interference with active immunization by maternal immunity means that in most cases, veterinary vaccines for use in food-producing animals are not administered until after newborns have lost their passive immunity and have developed the ability to mount their own adaptive immune response (van Oirschot et al. 1991; Ellis et al. 2001; McKeown et al. 2005; Opriessnig et al. 2008; Niewiesk 2014; Edwards 2015). Withdrawal periods for vaccines are regulated through national authorities, and are in most cases set at zero days.

Correct implementation of vaccination requires proper storage and transport conditions for the vaccine (maintaining the cold chain) and training of staff involved in the vaccination process, whether farmers, veterinarians, and/or animal health workers. Shelf-lives must be observed and administration must employ the correct route and dose targeted to the right species and ages of animals at the right time. Thermotolerance of some vaccines has been improved through specific strain selection, lyophilization techniques and use of a variety of stabilizing additives (Mariner et al. 2017; Dubrovina et al. 2018; Campbell et al. 2019) but not all vaccine formulations are compatible with freeze-drying and improving the thermotolerance of vaccines remains an important goal for further research (Porta et al. 2013).

Whereas vaccination documentation is fairly well established in industrial nations, it still remains difficult to implement in developing countries where even basic systems of animal identification may be lacking. According to the Responsible Use of Medicine in Agriculture Alliance (www.ruma.org.uk/farm/responsible-use-vaccines-vaccination-farm-animal-production), farmers must keep an animal medicine record book, and copies of relevant regulations and codes of good practice must be kept safely on every farm (in the UK, this relates to the Veterinary Medicines Directorate [VMD] Code of Practice on the Responsible Use of Animal Medicines on the Farm). Furthermore, accurate information must be kept with regard to the identity of the livestock vaccinated, which should include the date of administration of the vaccine, its batch number, the amount used and the expiry date of each batch used for each animal vaccinated, and, if applicable, if a withdrawal period must be observed. Such records should be kept for at least 5 years (even if the animals in question have been slaughtered or sold on). Information on all vaccines in use should be readily available to stock keepers, be kept on file, and should contain package inserts and safety data sheets.

A recent guideline on FMD vaccination provides examples of simple record-keeping sheets that can be used on farms and at vaccine distribution centers to help estimate the proportions of animals vaccinated and revaccinated and to calculate rates of consignment and utilization (Ferrari et al. 2016). Any suspected adverse reaction in livestock should be reported immediately to the VMD (in the UK) and the supplier, and should be accurately recorded in the on-farm medicine records (see Chapter 15). In the case of vaccines, a suspected failure to prevent disease also constitutes an adverse reaction. Investigations of the effectiveness of vaccines and vaccination and of vaccine breakdowns are greatly dependent upon vaccination records.

4.5 Monitoring and Evaluation of Vaccination

The process of vaccination involves multiple decisions and activities. Problems can arise due to poor strategy, inadequate implementation, or changes in the pathogen or the livestock industry. If not addressed, these problems can lead to ineffective vaccination, poor control, costly outbreaks of disease, and a loss of confidence in vaccination. The vaccination procedures and outcomes should therefore be monitored on an ongoing basis and reviewed periodically to check that the right measures are being performed and that the benefits are as expected. The fact that some diseases occur episodically can lead, temporarily, to a false sense of security if only outcomes are measured.

4.5.1 Monitoring the Implementation of Vaccination

Measuring vaccination coverage and postvaccination immunity are two key indicators establishing that vaccination has been applied correctly. Vaccine coverage can be estimated from vaccination records and is a measure of the proportion of animals that are vaccinated out of the total population, the latter being either all susceptible animals or only those species and individuals targeted for vaccination (Ferrari et al. 2016). Serology is the most widely used method to estimate immunity but varies in the accuracy with which it can predict protection (Plotkin 2010; Paton et al. 2019). Tests may be done on individual animals (e.g. to certify rabies immunity prior to travel for pets) or, more commonly for farm animals, on a representative sample from herds. It may be possible to distinguish between immunity due to vaccination and that due to infection if differentiating infected from vaccinated animals (DIVA) tests are available. Surveys need to take account of population heterogeneity, such as the fact that older animals are more likely to be immune. Coverage and immunity studies are synergistic and may be usefully combined; however, it has also to be stressed that serology for some diseases, such as vaccination against PCV2, may not be correlated to protection.

One of the epidemiological approaches that has been shown to be useful is the assessment of herd immunity, which was mentioned earlier in this chapter. Herd immunity is defined as a form of immunity that occurs when the vaccination of a significant portion of a herd/population provides a means of protection for individuals who have not (yet) developed immunity to a specific pathogen. Herd immunity arises when a high percentage of the population is protected through vaccination, making it difficult for a disease to spread as there are too few susceptible individuals left to contract the infection from. Application of herd immunity to a given population, within a geographic area, can effectively stop the spread of disease, making it an ideal tool to potentially protect nomadic herds without having to vaccinate them.

The number of individuals within a given population that must be vaccinated and develop immunity in order to achieve herd immunity varies for each disease, and even between pathogens causing the same disease. However, the underlying idea is simple: once enough individuals are protected, they help to protect vulnerable members of their communities by reducing the spread of the disease. This is termed the herd immunity threshold (HIT), and can be calculated by taking R_0 (average number of new infections caused by each case in an entirely susceptible population that is homogeneous and well mixed) (Garnett 2005; Perisic and Bauch 2009; Rodpothong and Auewarakul 2012), and multiplying it by S (proportion of the population who are susceptible to infection):

$$R_0 \times S = 1$$

S can be rewritten as (1−p, with p representing the proportion of the population that is immune and p+S = 1). Therefore, the equation can be rearranged to place "p" by itself as follows:

$$R_0 \times (1 - p) = 1,$$
$$\rightarrow 1 - p = 1 / R_0$$
$$\rightarrow p_c = 1 - 1 / R_0$$

With "p" being by itself on the left side of the equation, it can now be written as "p_c" to reflect the critical proportion of the population that needs to become immune to prevent disease transmission. This level is identified as HIT (Garnett 2005).

R_0 functions as a measure of contagiousness: low R_0 values are associated with lower HIT, whereas higher R_0 demand higher HIT to achieve population protection (Perisic and Bauch 2009; Rodpothong and Auewarakul 2012). For example, a disease with an R_0 of 2 theoretically needs only a 50% HIT to be eliminated, whereas a disease with an R_0 of 10 needs a 90% HIT (Rodpothong and Auewarakul 2012).

Whereas these calculations assume that the entire population is susceptible, the reality is in many cases very different, and we know that varying proportions of the population are immune to any given disease at any given time (Garnett 2005). Thus, the above formula needs adjusting for the average number of infections caused at a specific time. It would be outside the range of this chapter to discuss all necessary adjustments to estimate HIT, but one specific aspect needs further consideration within farmed animals. Assuming a vaccine is 100% effective, the equation used for calculating the HIT can be used to calculate the level of vaccination needed to eliminate a disease (V_c) (Fine 1993; Fine et al. 2011). As hardly any vaccines fulfill this requirement, the vaccine effectiveness "E" must be taken into account:

$$V_c = \frac{1 - 1/R_0}{E}$$

If E is less than $(1-1/R_0)$, it becomes impossible to eliminate a disease using a vaccine approach, even if the entire population is vaccinated (Fine 1993; Fine et al. 2011). Similarly, if vaccine-induced immunity is fading, more booster vaccine shots will be necessary to sustain herd immunity (Fine 1993; Fine et al. 2011; McGirr and Fisman 2015). Thus, once a disease has ceased to be endemic, natural infections no longer contribute to the reduction in the percentage of susceptible individuals; in this scenario, only vaccination will contribute to a further reduction (Garnett 2005). Using this approach, the relation between vaccine coverage, vaccine effectiveness, and disease incidence rate can be calculated (Garnett 2005).

4.5.2 Measuring Impact

If the aim of vaccination is to reduce disease and/or infection, then procedures must be in place to determine whether or not these outcomes are being achieved. A system of disease surveillance and reporting with proper case definitions, investigative procedures, and data recording and interrogation are all required along with the necessary vaccination records. In order to measure the impact of vaccination on the burden of infection and to demonstrate eventual freedom from infection, marker vaccines as well as the accompanying DIVA diagnostic tests are extremely useful (Uttenthal et al. 2010). Examples for this are the bovine herpesvirus (BHV) 1 marker vaccine (Scientific Committee on Animal Health and Animal Welfare 2000) and the use of serology to substantiate FMD freedom (Paton et al. 2014).

Disease in a vaccinated population does not necessarily mean the vaccine or vaccination policy is failing or underperforming – but it should be investigated in a systematic way to identify the cause of failure. A first step is to investigate whether or not the disease is actually caused by the pathogen in question. A systematic approach is required to examine different categories of problem, including vaccine failure (recipient or vaccine related) and failure to vaccinate properly (incorrect vaccine use and wider problems with the program) (Heininger et al. 2012).

Vaccine effectiveness (or "field efficacy") studies are conducted to find out how well vaccination is performing in a real-world population and should not be confused with vaccine efficacy, a distinctly different, although related, concept concerned with measuring how well the vaccine performs once properly administered (Orenstein et al. 1985, 1988; Comstock 1990; Moulton et al. 1995; Clemens et al. 1996; Halloran et al. 1997). Therefore, vaccine effectiveness can assess the net balance of benefits and adverse effects of a vaccination program (including cost–benefits), under more natural field conditions, rather than in a controlled clinical trial (Weinberg and Szilagyi 2010). Vaccine effectiveness should be proportional to vaccine potency (i.e. VE), but is also affected by herd immunity (according to the number/percentage of individuals immunized within a specific target group in the population).

In the literature, several study designs are described to measure vaccine effectiveness (Clemens and Shapiro 1984; Orenstein et al. 1985, 1988; Moulton et al. 1995; Clemens et al. 1996; Halloran et al. 1997) Perhaps the most familiar analysis is a retrospective case control analysis, in which the vaccination rate within a defined set of infected cases compared with the appropriate controls is calculated (Orenstein et al. 1985, 1988). The outcome data (vaccine effectiveness) are expressed as a rate difference, with use of the odds ratio (OR) for developing infection despite vaccination (Weinberg and Szilagyi 2010):

$$\text{Vaccine effectiveness} = (1 - \text{OR}) \times 100$$

Less frequently adopted designs to assess vaccine effectiveness are the indirect cohort or quasi-cohort study set-ups; here, different responses in the same vaccinated population are examined (Clemens and Shapiro 1984). This can involve, for example, assessment of serotype-specific disease assessment of vaccine effectiveness in a population cohort by comparing the rates of vaccine serotype infection and nonvaccine serotype infection, providing an indirect estimate of vaccine effectiveness (Broome et al. 1980). Another uncommon type of vaccine effectiveness study is the case-coverage or case-cohort method, in which vaccination rates among cases are compared with those in a similar cohort (which may include individuals who develop cases) over a defined period of time (Orenstein et al. 1988; Moulton et al. 1995; Szilagyi et al. 2008). The fourth type of vaccine effectiveness study is ecological or observational in nature, examining changes in disease burden over time (e.g. before and after introduction of routine vaccination) (Clemens et al. 1996). This type of study may use laboratory-based diagnostics methods using standardized assays as provided/described in VICH guidelines. Overall, this "real-world" view should be taken into account in planning animal health initiatives, specifically in the context of reducing/refining antimicrobial usage, as one cannot necessarily extrapolate vaccine effectiveness data obtained for a given population in one geographical setting to a different cohort/geographical setting.

The biggest advantage of such study designs, in connection with a simpler and less costly set-up, is their greater attractiveness and relevance. However, many biases (some of which are difficult to measure) can affect vaccine effectiveness studies. These include differential case definitions/selections for the vaccine and control groups, genetic differences in susceptibility or exposure of some individuals/groups within the defined population to infection, differences in general animal healthcare and welfare (unrelated to vaccination) between vaccinated and unvaccinated populations, undetected loss to follow-up from migration, and assumptions made during statistical analysis (Weinberg and Szilagyi 2010).

Thus, vaccine effectiveness studies have the benefit of using real-world outcomes but also possess challenges in distinguishing vaccine-related effects from other potential confounders that may affect outcomes (Weinberg and Szilagyi 2010). Indeed, it has become clear that the classic linear approach of vaccine design, research and development being performed in industrialized countries and only field evaluation performed in developing countries is no longer tenable, for both human and veterinary vaccine development (Pang 1999).

4.5.3 Confidence Gaps in Vaccination Campaigns

Farmers' decision making regarding the use of a vaccine is not only influenced by scientific evidence or economic considerations, but also by psychological, sociocultural, and political factors. Farmers' trust in vaccines is extremely variable, often depending on "hearsay" or perceptions, socioeconomic status, historical experiences, as well as religious or political influences. Although scientific evidence on the risk–benefit analysis of a vaccine is absolutely crucial, it may not be enough to close the gap between levels of farmer confidence in vaccines and the level of trust needed to ensure vaccine coverage. One clear example of how vaccination strategies can be negatively affected for years was the falsely made claim regarding the interaction of a measles-mumps-rubella (MMR) vaccine in humans with the occurrence of autism (Smeeth et al. 2004). This resulted in the development of a movement of so-called "anti-vaxxers" which has also started to affect veterinary medicine.

However, to enable farmers and veterinarians to decide which vaccine to use, strong evidence is required that a vaccine is efficacious, safe, and feasible. Interestingly, farmers seem to see veterinarians as an important source for the decision-making process (Richens et al. 2015, 2016). In view of the heterogeneity of the population involved, both on the animal as well as the farmer's side, it is essential to consider locally tailored approaches to vaccination, which need to be predicated on evidence-based approaches, taking public concerns into account and requiring good models of multidisciplinary research for vaccine introduction/usage. Gap analysis findings addressing the vaccine confidence gap in humans have been nicely summarized already (Larson et al. 2011), and these could be relatively easily implemented for veterinary vaccines as well. Finally, it is becoming imperative that all stakeholders work together to identify common denominators to identify what each party considers a vaccine campaign success.

4.6 Summary

It is becoming increasingly clear that a successful vaccination strategy should be designed carefully to address all aspects involved in vaccine effectiveness. These considerations not only include host–pathogen interaction in the specific geographical area but need to be far more tailored to the socioeconomic needs of the target audience. Indeed, vaccine design and delivery need to consider all participants involved in the system (pathogen, reservoir, immunizer, host, research community, funding bodies, etc.), the necessary actions (from identifying opportunities to vaccinate, characterization of pathogen, subsequent use of the generated vaccine, and the potential of the pathogen for co-evolution) as well as our growing understanding of vaccination, assets, and resources necessary to find a solution. Human vaccines are more and more developed according to "road maps," encompassing all the above criteria, and it is necessary that this is also done within the veterinary communities, especially for the topics discussed in this chapter. In addition, the increase in number of antimicrobials used in food-producing animals and heightened concerns about food safety and food security clearly emphasize the need for a faster harmonization of vaccination approaches, requiring further dialogue between developed and developing countries.

The underlying driving forces to answer these challenges will be the identification and acceptance of priorities, sustainability of programs, mutual benefit, and a sensitivity to national needs. This can be achieved through approaches involving multiple agencies working together at different levels with community involvement, the development of regional or country-specific vaccination strategies, and, most importantly, effective coordination (potentially with human vaccination programs) without duplication and competition.

References

Bitsouni, V., Lycett, S., Opriessnig, T., and Doeschl-Wilson, A. (2019). Predicting vaccine effectiveness in livestock populations: a theoretical framework applied to PRRS virus infections in pigs. *PLoS One* 14 (8): e0220738.

Botros, B., Omar, A., Elian, K. et al. (2006). Adverse response of non-indigenous cattle of European breeds to live attenuated Smithburn Rift Valley fever vaccine. *J. Med. Virol.* 78 (6): 787–791.

Broome, C.V., Facklam, R.R., and Fraser, D.W. (1980). Pneumococcal disease after pneumococcal vaccination: an alternative method to estimate the efficacy of pneumococcal vaccine. *N. Engl. J. Med.* 303 (10): 549–552.

Campbell, Z.A., Thumbi, S.M., Marsh, T.L. et al. (2019). Why isn't everyone using the thermotolerant vaccine? Preferences for Newcastle disease vaccines by chicken-owning households in Tanzania. *PLoS One* 14 (8): e0220963.

Casal, J., Saegerman, C., Bertagnoli, S. et al. (2019). A simple method to estimate the number of doses to include in a bank of vaccines. The case of lumpy skin disease in France. *PLoS One* 14 (1): e0210317.

Clemens, J.D. and Shapiro, E.D. (1984). Resolving the pneumococcal vaccine controversy: are there alternatives to randomized clinical trials? *Rev. Infect. Dis.* 6 (5): 589–600.

Clemens, J., Brenner, R., Rao, M. et al. (1996). Evaluating new vaccines for developing countries. Efficacy or effectiveness? *JAMA* 275 (5): 390–397.

Comstock, G.W. (1990). Vaccine evaluation by case-control or prospective studies. *Am. J. Epidemiol.* 131 (2): 205–207.

Directorate D – Animal Health and Welfare (2010). Expert opinion on vaccine and/or diagnostic banks for major animal diseases. European Commission Health & Consumers Directorate-General. SANCO/7070/2010.

Dubrovina, I.A., Kiseleva, I.V., Kireeva, E.V., and Rudenko, L.G. (2018). Composition of the stabilizer and conditions of Lyophilization for preserving infectious activity of influenza virus. *Bull. Exp. Biol. Med.* 165 (1): 52–56.

Edwards, K.M. (2015). Maternal antibodies and infant immune responses to vaccines. *Vaccine* 33 (47): 6469–6472.

Ellis, J., West, K., Cortese, V. et al. (2001). Effect of maternal antibodies on induction and persistence of vaccine-induced immune responses against bovine viral diarrhea virus type II in young calves. *J. Am. Vet. Med. Assoc.* 219 (3): 351–356.

Ferrari, G., Paton, D., Duffy, S. et al. (2016). *Foot and Mouth Disease Vaccination and Post-Vaccination Monitoring.* Rome: FAO/OIE.

Fine, P.E. (1993). Herd immunity: history, theory, practice. *Epidemiol. Rev.* 15 (2): 265–302.

Fine, P., Eames, K., and Heymann, D.L. (2011). "Herd immunity": a rough guide. *Clin. Infect. Dis.* 52 (7): 911–916.

Fournie, G., Waret-Szkuta, A., Camacho, A. et al. (2018). A dynamic model of transmission and elimination of peste des petits ruminants in Ethiopia. *Proc. Natl. Acad. Sci. U.S.A.* 115 (33): 8454–8459.

Garnett, G.P. (2005). Role of herd immunity in determining the effect of vaccines against sexually transmitted disease. *J. Infect. Dis.* 191 (Suppl 1): S97–S106.

Glass, E.J. (2004). Genetic variation and responses to vaccines. *Anim. Health Res. Rev.* 5 (2): 197–208.

Greenwood, M. and Yule, G.U. (1915). The statistics of anti-typhoid and anti-cholera inoculations, and the interpretation of such statistics in general. *Proc. R. Soc. Med.* 8 (Sect Epidemiol State Med): 113–194.

Halloran, M.E., Struchiner, C.J., and Longini, I.M. Jr. (1997). Study designs for evaluating different efficacy and effectiveness aspects of vaccines. *Am. J. Epidemiol.* 146 (10): 789–803.

Heininger, U., Bachtiar, N.S., Bahri, P. et al. (2012). The concept of vaccination failure. *Vaccine* 30 (7): 1265–1268.

Huppert, A. and Katriel, G. (2013). Mathematical modelling and prediction in infectious disease epidemiology. *Clin. Microbiol. Infect.* 19 (11): 999–1005.

Kurmann, J., Sydler, T., Brugnera, E. et al. (2011). Vaccination of dams increases antibody titer and improves growth parameters in finisher pigs subclinically infected with porcine circovirus type 2. *Clin. Vaccine Immunol.* 18 (10): 1644–1649.

Larson, H.J., Cooper, L.Z., Eskola, J. et al. (2011). Addressing the vaccine confidence gap. *Lancet* 378 (9790): 526–535.

Lyons, N.A., Ludi, A.B., Wilsden, G. et al. (2017). Evaluation of a polyvalent foot-and-mouth disease virus vaccine containing a Saudi-95 against field challenge on large-scale dairy farms in Saudi Arabia with the emerging a/ASIA/G-VII viral lineage. *Vaccine* 35 (49 Pt B): 6850–6857.

Mariner, J.C., Gachanja, J., Tindih, S.H., and Toye, P. (2017). A thermostable presentation of the live, attenuated peste des petits ruminants vaccine in use in Africa and Asia. *Vaccine* 35 (30): 3773–3779.

McGirr, A. and Fisman, D.N. (2015). Duration of pertussis immunity after DTaP immunization: a meta-analysis. *Pediatrics* 135 (2): 331–343.

McKeown, N.E., Opriessnig, T., Thomas, P. et al. (2005). Effects of porcine circovirus type 2 (PCV2) maternal antibodies on experimental infection of piglets with PCV2. *Clin. Diagn. Lab. Immunol.* 12 (11): 1347–1351.

Moulton, L.H., Wolff, M.C., Brenneman, G., and Santosham, M. (1995). Case-cohort analysis of case-coverage studies of vaccine effectiveness. *Am. J. Epidemiol.* 142 (9): 1000–1006.

Niewiesk, S. (2014). Maternal antibodies: clinical significance, mechanism of interference with immune responses, and possible vaccination strategies. *Front. Immunol.* 5: 446.

OIE. (2019). Manual of Diagnostic Tests and Vaccines for Terrestrial Animals. www.oie.int/standard-setting/terrestrial-manual/access-online

Opriessnig, T., Patterson, A.R., Elsener, J. et al. (2008). Influence of maternal antibodies on efficacy of porcine circovirus type 2 (PCV2) vaccination to protect pigs from experimental infection with PCV2. *Clin. Vaccine Immunol.* 15 (3): 397–401.

Orenstein, W.A., Bernier, R.H., Dondero, T.J. et al. (1985). Field evaluation of vaccine efficacy. *Bull. World Health Organ.* 63 (6): 1055–1068.

Orenstein, W.A., Bernier, R.H., and Hinman, A.R. (1988). Assessing vaccine efficacy in the field. Further observations. *Epidemiol. Rev.* 10: 212–241.

Pang, T. (1999). Vaccination in the third world. Contemporary issues. *C. R. Acad. Sci. III* 322 (11): 995–997.

Pastoret, P.P. and Jones, P. (2004). Veterinary vaccines for animal and public health. *Dev. Biol. (Basel)* 119: 15–29.

Paton, D.J., Fussel, A.E., Vosloo, W. et al. (2014). The use of serosurveys following emergency vaccination, to recover the status of "foot-and-mouth disease free where vaccination is not practised". *Vaccine* 32 (52): 7050–7056.

Paton, D.J., Reeve, R., Capozzo, A.V., and Ludi, A. (2019). Estimating the protection afforded by foot-and-mouth disease vaccines in the laboratory. *Vaccine* 37 (37): 5515–5524.

Perisic, A. and Bauch, C.T. (2009). Social contact networks and disease eradicability under voluntary vaccination. *PLoS Comput. Biol.* 5 (2): e1000280.

Plotkin, S.A. (2010). Correlates of protection induced by vaccination. *Clin. Vaccine Immunol.* 17 (7): 1055–1065.

Porta, C., Kotecha, A., Burman, A. et al. (2013). Rational engineering of recombinant picornavirus capsids to produce safe, protective vaccine antigen. *PLoS Pathog.* 9 (3): e1003255.

Rawdon, T.G., Garner, M.G., Sanson, R.L. et al. (2018). Evaluating vaccination strategies to control foot-and-mouth disease: a country comparison study. *Epidemiol. Infect.* 146 (9): 1138–1150.

Richens, I.F., Hobson-West, P., Brennan, M.L. et al. (2015). Farmers' perception of the role of veterinary surgeons in vaccination strategies on British dairy farms. *Vet. Rec.* 177 (18): 465.

Richens, I.F., Hobson-West, P., Brennan, M.L. et al. (2016). Factors influencing veterinary surgeons' decision-making about dairy cattle vaccination. *Vet. Rec.* 179 (16): 410.

Rodpothong, P. and Auewarakul, P. (2012). Viral evolution and transmission effectiveness. *World J. Virol.* 1 (5): 131–134.

Roeder, P.L. and Taylor, W.P. (2007). Mass vaccination and herd immunity: cattle and buffalo. *Rev. Sci. Tech.* 26 (1): 253–263.

RUMA. (2007). Responsible use of vaccines and vaccination in dairy and beef cattle production. A farm health planning initiative in partnership with DEFRA supported by the National Office of Animal Health (NOAH). www.ruma.org.uk/wp-content/uploads/2014/09/cattle-vaccine-long.pdf

Scientific Committee on Animal Health and Animal Welfare (SCAHAW). (2000). Report on bovine herpesvirus 1 (BHV1) marker vaccines and the accompanying diagnostic tests. Directorate C – Scientific Opinions, Health & Consumer Protection Directorate-General. SNCO/C3/R20/2000.

Singh, B.B., Kostoulas, P., Gill, J.P.S., and Dhand, N.K. (2018). Cost-benefit analysis of intervention policies for prevention and control of brucellosis in India. *PLoS Negl. Trop. Dis.* 12 (5): e0006488.

Smeeth, L., Cook, C., Fombonne, E. et al. (2004). MMR vaccination and pervasive developmental disorders: a case-control study. *Lancet* 364 (9438): 963–969.

Swamy, G.K. and Wheeler, S.M. (2014). Neonatal pertussis, cocooning and maternal immunization. *Expert Rev. Vaccines* 13 (9): 1107–1114.

Szilagyi, P.G., Fairbrother, G., Griffin, M.R. et al. (2008). Influenza vaccine effectiveness among children 6 to 59 months of age during 2 influenza seasons: a case-cohort study. *Arch. Pediatr. Adolesc. Med.* 162 (10): 943–951.

Uttenthal, A., Parida, S., Rasmussen, T.B. et al. (2010). Strategies for differentiating infection in vaccinated animals (DIVA) for foot-and-mouth disease, classical swine fever and avian influenza. *Expert. Rev. Vaccines* 9 (1): 73–87.

Van Oirschot, J.T. Bruin, G., de Boer-Luytze, E., and Smolders, G. (1991). Maternal antibodies against equine influenza virus in foals and their interference with vaccination. *Zentralbl. Veterinarmed. B* 38 (5): 391–396.

Weinberg, G.A. and Szilagyi, P.G. (2010). Vaccine epidemiology: efficacy, effectiveness, and the translational research roadmap. *J. Infect. Dis.* 201 (11): 1607–1610.

Werling, D., Jann, O.C., Offord, V. et al. (2009). Variation matters: TLR structure and species-specific pathogen recognition. *Trends Immunol.* 30 (3): 124–130.

Williams, D.J., Guy, C.S., Smith, R.F. et al. (2007). Immunization of cattle with live tachyzoites of Neospora caninum confers protection against fetal death. *Infect. Immun.* 75 (3) 1343–1348.

Section II

Current and Future Veterinary Vaccines

5

Viral Vaccines

Baptiste Dungu[1,2] *and Meritxell Donadeu*[2,3]

[1] *Onderstepoort Biological Products SOC Ltd, Onderstepoort, South Africa*
[2] *Initiative for Neglected Animal Diseases (INAND), Midrand, South Africa*
[3] *Faculty of Veterinary and Agricultural Sciences, University of Melbourne, Werribee, Australia*

5.1 Introduction

To date, vaccination is the most effective way of controlling animal and human viral diseases either through preventing mortality or reducing morbidity. While contributing immensely to improving animal health and productivity, veterinary viral vaccines also impact positively on the well-being and livelihood of animal owners. Vaccines for viral zoonotic diseases such as rabies have directly benefited both human and animal health.

Veterinary vaccines also can have a significant role in decreasing the use of veterinary pharmaceuticals and their residues in the food chain, by preventing disease, and thus the need for medication, or replacing prophylactic medication.

Viral vaccines have contributed to the eradication of infectious diseases globally or their elimination from specific areas. The case of smallpox and poliomyelitis can be mentioned for humans (WHO 1980; Fenner et al. 1988; The Global Polio Initiative 2014), while rinderpest in cattle has been eradicated from the planet through concerted vaccination efforts (OIE 2011). At a regional level, there have been a number of success stories with the elimination of diseases such as foot and mouth disease (FMD) in much of South America (Naranjo and Cosivi 2013).

Adding to the success achieved with traditional live attenuated and inactivated vaccines, novel approaches and biotechnology are being used extensively to generate safer and more efficacious viral vaccines. Several strategies are being used to generate vaccines that address specific challenges and fit the desired target product profile. These include:

- attenuation of pathogens by gene deletion or site-directed mutagenesis
- expression of pathogen proteins in eukaryotic (yeast, mammalian, insect) or bacterial cells
- expression of viral proteins that self-assemble into virus-like particles (VLPs)
- expression of pathogen antigens in viral vectors
- formation of viral chimeras (replicative machinery of one virus and protective antigens of another)
- organic synthesis of pathogen peptides
- production and administration of anti-idiotypic antibodies
- DNA vaccines.

5.2 Types of Viral Vaccines

Although generally, vaccines are classified into conventional (live attenuated and inactivated vaccines) and novel biotechnology-derived vaccines, in the present text, viral veterinary vaccines will be described in three categories: (i) replicating or live vaccines, (ii) nonreplicating or replication restricted vaccines, and (iii) DNA-based vaccines.

Replicating or live vaccines can be grouped into: (i) conventional attenuated live vaccines, (ii) live gene-deletion attenuation vaccines, and (iii) recombinant live vectored vaccines. Nonreplicating viral vaccines include (i) conventional inactivated vaccines and (ii) subunit vaccines.

It is also possible to differentiate vaccines based on specific properties, such as the ability to act as a marker vaccine, to prevent infection or disease, to be used therapeutically, etc.

Veterinary Vaccines: Principles and Applications, First Edition. Edited by Samia Metwally, Gerrit Viljoen, and Ahmed El Idrissi.

5.2.1 Replicating or Live Vaccines

5.2.1.1 Conventional Attenuated Live Vaccines

Vaccines based on the original principle of the Jenner smallpox vaccine, namely a weakened or attenuated strain of virus capable of multiplying sufficiently in the host to elicit a protective immune response without causing clinical disease, are highly effective. Examples of the successful use of such vaccines include the eradication of smallpox and control of many human diseases such as poliomyelitis, measles, and mumps, the eradication of rinderpest in cattle, and the effective control of Marek's disease and Newcastle disease in domestic poultry.

Conventional live viral vaccines should have little or no virulence in target animals. Most live virus vaccines are derived from attenuation of a pathogenic strain or from an already nonpathogenic strain of the pathogen. Some strains are also able to confer immunity on a nontarget host, for example the use of the measles virus against distemper in dogs.

The first bluetongue vaccine developed by Theiler in South Africa was based on a strain of the virus that he described as attenuated through passage in sheep, thus attenuated through passage in the host animal (Theiler 1908). It was used with reasonable success for several decades (Verwoerd and Erasmus 2004).

More commonly, viruses are passaged extensively through a nontarget cell culture line. This results in loss of specificity for a particular animal species or target tissue, thereby leading to loss of virulence.

Strategies for generating conventional live attenuated vaccines can therefore be grouped as follows.

5.2.1.1.1 Naturally Occurring Attenuated Strains Different approaches exist, including the use of a related organism from a different host (heterologous vaccines), the use of virulent organisms given by an unnatural route, and the use of wild-type pathogens with natural deletions or insertions, resulting in reduced or abolished virulence. One good example is the use of cowpox virus for human protection against smallpox. Other examples include the immunization of poultry with the herpesvirus of turkeys (HVT), which is a ubiquitous virus in turkeys, to protect chickens from Marek's disease (Okazaki et al. 1970) and an avirulent Rift Valley fever (RVF) virus isolated from a nonfatal human case of RVF in the Central African Republic which was identified as a good candidate vaccine. After adaptation of the RVF virus to cell culture through limited passage in mice and Vero cells, and then plaque purification to study the homogeneity of virus subpopulations, a clone designated 13 was found to be avirulent in mice, yet immunogenic. The attenuation appears to result from a large internal deletion in the NSs gene (Muller et al. 1995). It has since been proven safe and efficacious in sheep and cattle (Dungu et al. 2010; von Teichman et al. 2011), and has been licensed and widely used.

Attenuation in live vaccines can also be obtained with naturally occurring or artificially created mutant strains of an organism. Mutations can be introduced into wild virus strains through exposure to chemicals (phenol is widely used), or by the application of ultraviolet or x-ray radiation. The RVF MP-12 vaccine strain is a good example of a vaccine strain generated by 12 serial plaque passages in human diploid MRC-5 cells in the presence of the chemical mutagen 5-fluorouracil (Caplen et al. 1985).

5.2.1.1.2 Serial Passage in Heterologous Host Animals This could be achieved through passaging in rabbits or in hen's eggs. Using chick embryos as an example, the virus is grown in different embryos in a series. With each passage, the virus becomes better at replicating in chick cells, but loses its ability to replicate in mammalian cells. A virus targeted for use in a vaccine may be grown through – "passaged" through – upwards of 200 different embryos or cell cultures. Eventually, the attenuated virus will be unable to replicate well (or at all) in target animal cells, and can be used in a vaccine.

Examples of successful attenuation in heterologous host animals include rinderpest and hog cholera virus (classic swine fever [CSF]) vaccines that were attenuated through serial passages in rabbits.

5.2.1.1.3 Serial Passage in Cell Culture This is a common strategy for viral vaccines. It involves both primary or cell lines such as Vero cells and baby hamster kidney (BHK) cells. Examples include bluetongue and African horse sickness.

Live or attenuated vaccines have the advantage of being capable of generating early and long-lasting immunity in vaccinated animals. Compared with inactivated vaccines, live vaccines often elicit stronger mucosal immunity (Kagnoff 1996). They usually do not require frequent revaccination. Their costs are generally low because they can be produced in specific, scalable culture systems in large batches, with minimal downstream processing.

Disadvantages of live attenuated vaccines include the potential risk of reversion to virulence, the risk of reassortment with wild-type viruses (therefore, may not be recommended for use during disease outbreaks), residual virulence linked to the complex nature of the vaccine strain, or to higher susceptibility of a subpopulation of the host being vaccinated. This was seen with the live attenuated bluetongue vaccine used in Europe, although the same vaccine had been used successfully in southern Africa for decades (Dungu et al. 2004; Batten et al. 2008; Coetzee et al. 2012). There is also a potential risk of release into a new environment of new isolates (Ferrari et al. 2005; Batten et al. 2008).

For success to be achieved, careful selection of appropriate strains is required. Even then, the selection is laborious and unpredictable in order to achieve the correct balance between loss of virulence and the ability to multiply in the host sufficiently to elicit immune protection.

Safety concerns linked to cases and risks of reversion to virulence or reassortment of vaccine viruses with wild-type variants have led to a shift toward the use of inactivated viruses or viral antigens. Despite notable successes like the inactivated Newcastle disease and RVF vaccines, inactivated viruses are generally less immunogenic than their live attenuated vaccine counterparts.

Rift Valley fever is a good example where, for safety reasons linked to the widely used Smithburn vaccine strain, and its limited immunogenicity in cattle, an inactivated vaccine was developed. The need for two rounds of vaccination and subsequent high vaccination costs when using the inactivated vaccine have stimulated further efforts to develop different forms of replicating live RVF vaccines (Kortekaas et al. 2011).

5.2.1.2 Live Gene-Deleted Attenuated Vaccines

Several viral infections can only be prevented by the use of replicating attenuated virus vaccines. However, safety concerns have prevented the widespread use of attenuated virus vaccines, especially those with high potential for reassortment or reversion to virulence.

Advances in genetic engineering techniques and the advent of reverse genetics are making it more and more possible to not only identify the genes associated with the virulence of a pathogenic organism, but also to delete or inactivate these genes, thereby increasing the safety profile of potential vaccine candidates.

Vaccines made using this approach include the gene-deleted pseudorabies virus (Aujeszky's disease) marker vaccine, with a double gene deletion (gE and TK) now licensed for use in pigs (Ferrari et al. 2000; Meeusen et al. 2007), the RVF MP-12 with a deletion in the NSm gene (Morrill et al. 2013), and the gE deleted bovine herpesvirus-1 marker vaccine, now licensed for use in cattle (van Oirschot et al. 1996; Meeusen et al. 2007).

5.2.1.3 Recombinant Vectored Vaccines

Genetically modified bacteria or viruses can act as carriers, known as vectors, when genetic materials responsible for the stimulation of an immune response are cloned into them. The vectors therefore act as vaccine delivery vehicles. Administration of vector material triggers a natural immune response, including a response to the pathogen from which genetic material has been taken. They thus combine the benefits of a modified live vaccine with those of a subunit vaccine.

Initial work involved the use of vaccinia virus vectors to generate vaccines such as the rabies vaccines, where the G protein of the virus was expressed in a vaccinia vector. This vaccine was used extensively in Europe to stop the spread of rabies in wild animals (Pastoret and Brochier 1999).

A number of viruses have been transformed into vectors and successfully tested for the expression of foreign genes. The development at Onderstepoort Veterinary Institute of the Neethling strain of the lumpy skin virus as a vector for the expression of RVF glycoproteins and bovine ephemeral fever is an example of this approach (Wallace and Viljoen 2005).

Pox viruses have been studied extensively as virus vectors because their large genomes can accommodate relatively large inserts. The need for a species-restricted vector, as required by most regulators fearing the potential of expression in nontarget animals, has led to the use of vectors such as the canary pox, which does not further replicate in mammalian hosts after initial expression (Poulet et al. 2007). Examples of successfully commercialized pox vector vaccines include the canary pox vaccines for canine distemper and West Nile virus (Table 5.1).

5.2.2 Nonreplicating Vaccines

5.2.2.1 Conventional Inactivated Viral Vaccines

Inactivated viral vaccines are prepared by growing large amounts of the viruses in tissue culture cells, in embryonated hen's eggs, or sometimes in the target animal and then inactivating them either chemically or physically.

Inactivated vaccines are generally formulated with an adjuvant, whose effect is to modulate or improve the immune response that would have been generated by the vaccine antigen on its own. Understanding the type of protective immunity required for a specific disease is critical in designing inactivated vaccines and identifying the most appropriate type of adjuvant.

Methods of inactivation:

- Chemical inactivation of viruses has been the most common approach, relying on formaldehyde. Following serious concerns about the ability of formaldehyde to fully inactivate the poliomyelitis virus, and later on the FMD virus (Barteling and Vreeswijk 1991), alternative methods were evaluated such as use of phenol, β-propiolactone or an aziridine (commonly binary ethylenimine, BEI). Substances such as ethylene oxide or

Table 5.1 Examples of nonconventional new-generation veterinary vaccines.

Target pathogen	Target animal	Characteristics	Reference/examples
Replicating vaccines: live gene-deletion attenuated vaccines			
Pseudorabies virus	Pigs	gE and thymidine kinase-deleted marker vaccine	Ferrari et al. (2000)
BHV-1	Cattle	Live gE-deleted marker vaccine	Van Oirschot et al. (1996)
Rift Valley fever	Ruminants	RVF MP-12 strain with a deletion on the NSm segment	Morrill et al. (2013)
Replicating vaccines: recombinant live vectored vaccines			
MDV (HTV) and IBVD	Poultry	Live recombinant chimera virus expressing VP2 gene of IBD on HTV virus	Darteil et al. (1995)
West Nile virus	Horse	Live flavivirus chimera vaccine	Monath et al. (2001)
West Nile virus	Horse	Canarypox virus vectored vaccine	Minke et al. (2004)
Equine influenza virus	Horse	Canarypox virus vectored vaccine	Minke et al. (2004)
Canine distemper virus	Dogs	Canarypox virus vectored vaccine	RECOMBITEK® distemper (Boehringer Ingelheim)
Avian influenza virus	Poultry	Fowlpox virus vectored vaccine	Bublot et al. (2006)
Rabies	Wildlife, canines	Vaccinia virus recombinant	Pastoret and Brochier (1996)
Newcastle disease virus	Poultry	Fowlpox virus vectored vaccine	TROVAC-NDV® (a Boehringer Ingelheim product commercialized in the USA)
Nonreplicating vaccines: subunit vaccines			
Classic swine fever	Pigs	Baculovirus recombinant E2 protein	Van Aarle (2003) and Madera et al. (2016)
PCV2	Pigs	Subunit baculovirus expressed PCV2 ORF2 protein	Blanchard et al. (2003) PORCILIS PCV® (produced by MSD) CIRCUMVENT® PCV G2 (produced by Merck/MSD)
Nonreplicating vaccines: plant-made vaccines			
Newcastle disease virus	Poultry	HN recombinant produced in plant cell lines	Vermij and Waltz (2006)
Nonreplicating vaccines: synthetic peptide vaccines			
Parvovirus	Dogs	Peptides corresponding to the amino-terminal region of VP2 of the canine parvovirus	Langeveld et al. (1994)
DNA vaccines			
West Nile virus	Horses	DNA vaccine	Davis et al. (2001)
IHN	Salmon	DNA vaccine	Garver et al. (2005)

This list of vaccines does not represent any authentication of the quality or efficacy of the products.

β-propiolactone are popular, since they do not interfere with surface proteins and act directly on the viral nucleic acid.

- The most commonly studied physical method for virus inactivation has been UV irradiation. Due to the unreliability of the UV irradiation method to completely inactivate as well as the risk of loss of immunogenicity by overexposure, γ-irradiation has been considered (Yoichi 2012).

The main advantage of inactivated vaccines is safety as they are nonreplicating and should have no residual virulence risk or risk of release into the environment. Their major drawbacks include the short-term immunity generated, which requires booster doses and revaccination, thus increasing vaccination costs, especially for vaccination campaigns. Also, they are more expensive to produce than live vaccines, due to the need for a high antigen payload in the vaccine dose as well as additional downstream processing requirements, which include concentration, inactivation, and formulation with adjuvant (van Oirschot 1997). High vaccine and vaccination costs often compromise disease control programs in countries where resources are limited.

Typical examples of inactivated veterinary viral vaccines include FMD and some bluetongue vaccines.

5.2.2.2 Subunit Vaccines

The concept that the entire organism is not required to elicit protective immunity was demonstrated a century ago when it was shown that antiserum produced in animals against the toxins secreted by the agents causing diphtheria and tetanus would passively protect against these diseases.

This approach has been applied to viral and other vaccines when it has been possible to fractionate or purify protein or glycoprotein components of a pathogen, which have been identified as triggers of the protective immune response.

However, some antigens are too small to trigger an immune response unless coupled to carrier proteins, even if able to bind to the product of the immune response.

Over the past three decades, increasing pressure has been applied by the regulatory authorities, both human and veterinary, to specifically define the protective antigens and produce vaccines that would be free from pathogen-associated toxins, extraneous agents, and immunosuppressive components (Castle 2005). Subunit vaccines based on recombinant protein immunogens, DNA immunogens, and nonpathogenic vectors are currently the most cost-effective methods of producing antigens free from the exogenous material characteristic of conventional vaccines (Rogan and Babiuk 2005).

Specific proteins from pathogenic organisms responsible for triggering immune responses in host animals can be expressed in a host system. The gene that encodes the protective antigen is cloned into a secondary, preferably nonpathogenic organism that is capable of expressing the immunogen in its native form or with minimal alteration. This protein can then be expressed and harvested using traditional bacterial antigen production methods, or delivered by a live nonpathogenic vector (see section 5.2.1.3). If the protein is produced in prokaryotic systems, it can be tailored in such a way that the protein of interest is expressed on the surface of the bacteria, in the periplasm, as insoluble inclusion bodies, or secreted into the media (Rogan and Babiuk 2005; Wesley 2005).

To date, different prokaryotic and eukaryotic expression systems have been tried and used to produce commercial veterinary vaccines. Bacterial expression systems are excellent candidates for the production of nonglycosylated proteins. Bacteria such as *Escherichia coli*, *Bacillus brevis* (Ichikawa et al. 1993; Udaka and Yamagata 1993; Nagahama et al. 1996; Shiga et al. 2000; Yokomizo et al. 2002; Kashima and Udaka 2004) and *Salmonella typhimurium* (Husseiny and Hensel 2005; Yang et al. 2005; Salam et al. 2006; Hanna et al. 2008; Zekarias et al. 2008) have been used extensively for the expression of a wide variety of foreign genes and, as a result, many production, stabilization, and optimization strategies have been described. Although prokaryotic expression is efficient and affordable for the production of a broad range of antigens, including a few natively glycosylated proteins, production of many viral glycoproteins in prokaryotic systems does not result in immunologically protective proteins due to the lack of glycosylation, despite producing significant immune responses (Wesley 2005).

Eukaryotic expression systems include yeast, insect cells, plants, and mammalian cells. These expression systems are more suitable for the expression of glycoproteins and other modified proteins (Rogan and Babiuk 2005). The most commonly used yeast expression systems are *Saccharomyces cerevisiae* and *Pichia pastoris*. Notably, *S. cerevisiae* was used to produce the first ever subunit vaccine for hepatitis B (Valenzuela et al. 1982), which was later licensed and commercialized. Baculovirus and vaccinia virus have been commonly used to direct expression of veterinary vaccines in cell culture expression systems (Moss and Flexner 1987; Beljelarskaya 2011). Insect cell expression is based on infection of cultured caterpillar or lepidopteran cells with a recombinant baculovirus designed to express the gene product under the control of the strong polyhedron promoter, typically resulting in a high yield of immunologically active protein (O'Reilly et al. 1992; Beljelarskaya 2011). Proteins are expressed glycosylated. The major limitation of insect cell expression has been obtaining sufficient cell density and protein yields (Radford et al. 1997; Maranga et al. 2002; Ikonomou et al. 2003). An example of a successfully commercialized veterinary subunit vaccine for viral diseases is the baculovirus-expressed E2 vaccine against CSF.

5.2.2.3 Other Forms of Nonreplicating Particulate and Subunit Vaccines

These include a variety of vaccines, such as VLPs, plant-made vaccines, and synthetic peptide vaccines.

Virus-like particles are antigenic structures composed of one or several recombinantly expressed viral proteins which spontaneously assemble into supramolecular structures resembling infectious viruses or, in some cases, subviral particles. VLPs have many advantages since they are structurally similar to the virus and therefore highly immunogenic but they are safer, as they lack nucleic acid and are noninfectious.

Plant-made vaccines are based on expression of pathogen gene(s) encoding immunogenic protein(s) by transgenic plants or under the control of transient expression systems. The concept of cheap edible vaccines has been superseded by a realization that formulated, injectable products will often be needed (Rybicki 2010).

Synthetic peptide vaccines are based on the fact that it is possible to identify individual epitopes within protective proteins and develop peptide vaccines. These peptide epitopes represent the minimal immunogenic region of a protein antigen and allow for precise direction of immune responses. Although peptide vaccines have been seen for years as very promising, their implementation has been limited, mainly due to difficulties associated with instability, poor immunogenicity unless modified, and by inconsistent immunogenicity due to the major histocompatibility complex (MHC) polymorphism of the host species (Tam 1996). However, better understanding in inducing and maintaining efficient immune responses is making it possible to devise strategies to enhance both peptide immunogenicity and stability. A number of commercial companies are already in different stages of development for various human peptide vaccines (Purcell et al. 2007). On the animal health side, the first effective peptide vaccine has been developed against canine parvovirus (Langeveld et al. 1994).

5.2.3 DNA Vaccines

For decades during the twentieth century, it had been considered that it would be necessary to present the immunogenic protein (or carbohydrate–protein complex) to the host in order to elicit the appropriate immune response. In the late 1980s, however, work on several viruses showed that immune responses can be obtained by injecting the DNA coding for the protective antigens directly into the muscle tissue of mice (Ulmer et al. 1993).

Different approaches and innovative technologies have resulted in significant improvements in immune responses, such as specific targeting of the vaccine antigen to antigen-presenting cells (Kennedy et al. 2006), prime-boosting with CpG oligodeoxynucleotides (Liang et al. 2006), and *in vivo* electroporation of DNA (Scheerlinck et al. 2004).

The DNA vaccine technology has been particularly studied and used in the development of fish vaccines (Heppell and Davis 2000; Lorenzen and LaPatra 2005). The first DNA vaccine for a food-producing species (Apex-IHN), encoding a surface glycoprotein of the infectious hematopoietic necrosis virus, was registered in Canada to protect against this enzootic disease of wild salmon that can cause devastating outbreaks in farm-raised Atlantic salmon.

Meanwhile, a DNA vaccine, based on the DNA plasmid encoding for the West Nile virus outer coat proteins and administered with a proprietary adjuvant, has been licensed in the USA to protect horses against viremia with this virus (Powell 2004).

Refer to Chapter 10 for more details on DNA vaccines.

5.3 Immune Responses to Viral Vaccines

Key requirements for an effective vaccine generally include efficacy, safety, ease of administration, and cost-effectiveness. Put in different terms, modern vaccine design builds on the central concept of inducing quick, solid, and durable protective immunity against a disease by mimicking the naturally occurring immune response against the disease-causing pathogen, but without inducing the disease or serious side effects. Thus, vaccines aim at prophylactically inducing effector molecules and cells that are capable of eliminating a pathogen as quickly as possible. It is now well recognized that a range of primary immune responses is required by the host for this process of elimination to be successful (Schijns 2001; Mutwiri et al. 2007).

Effective protection against a variety of bacterial, viral, and parasitic infections can be provided by long-lived B lymphocytes that produce antigen-specific neutralizing antibodies (Bachmann et al. 1993). Cellular immunity, on the other hand, is critical for the control of certain intracellular pathogens (Schijns 2001). A major disadvantage of inactivated and subunit vaccines is that since they do not replicate in the host, they have a limited ability to elicit the same immune response that is induced by the pathogen they are expected to generate protection against. It is therefore critical that delivery techniques, including adjuvants, and vaccine formulation be designed in such a way that a suitable immune response is generated.

Although systemic immunization ensures that adequate amounts of antigen reach peripheral lymphoid tissues to elicit protection against infectious agents, it is largely ineffective for providing immunity at mucosal surfaces. Mucosal immunization through the nose, eye, and respiratory and gastrointestinal tracts may be needed to induce protective immunity, such as IgA, at mucosal tissues, which act as common portals of entry for most pathogenic organisms. An important point is that all mucosal sites are interconnected by a common mucosal immune system, and that administration of antigens at one primary site will stimulate antigen-specific lymphocytes that will provide immunity via their migration throughout the body (Mestecky 1987; McGhee et al. 1992). A number of veterinary live viral vaccines are delivered intranasally, in eye drops or as aerosols; the last two are commonly used in chickens to administer the Newcastle disease vaccine. Intranasal vaccines against viral respiratory diseases of cattle, such as infectious bovine rhinotracheitis (IBR), parainfluenza3 (PI3), and bovine respiratory syncytial virus (BRSV), are extensively used.

Due to the highly variable nature of some viruses, another consideration is the need to induce immunity against several serotypes or against current field strains. Immunity from vaccination is often serotype specific, with only partial protection or no protection at all against other serotypes. Good examples are the FMD and bluetongue vaccines. In the case of FMD, some serotypes are themselves highly variable, so it is necessary to ensure that the vaccine virus is antigenically matched to the predominant, circulating field strains. In the case of bluetongue, protective immunity is generally associated with the presence of type-specific neutralizing antibodies which may persist for years, but is not associated with the group-specific antibodies which usually disappear after a few months (Verwoerd and Erasmus 1994). So, immunization against one bluetongue serotype will not necessarily provide partial or complete protection against other serotypes. However, infection or immunization with more than one bluetongue virus type usually results in protection against a wider range of serotypes, even types against which no neutralizing antibodies are present (Dungu et al. 2004; Coetzee et al. 2012; Verwoerd 2012).

5.4 Characteristics and Immunity of Each Vaccine Type

The main characteristics and immunity for each type of vaccine are described below.

5.4.1 Replicating or Live Vaccines

Live attenuated virus vaccines, containing all viral antigens and replicating in the host, supply an extensive repertoire of appropriately presented epitopes that, in general, assure a broad range of protective immune responses within most members of an immunogenetically heterogeneous population. They generally elicit both antibodies and cell-mediated immunity (including cytotoxic T cells). Mucosal immunity is also very good in comparison to that induced by inactivated vaccines (Kagnoff 1996).

The peste des petits ruminants (PPR) vaccine provides a good example of solid immunity obtained with a live attenuated vaccine. The only currently available PPR vaccines are cell culture-attenuated strains of wild-type PPR virus (PPRV). The first vaccine, the Nigeria 75/1, has been used extensively in Africa and the Middle East, but other strains have also been developed. With the Nigeria 75/1 prescribed vaccine dose of $10^{2.5}$ $TCID_{50}$, a single injection induces cellular and humoral immune responses, and protection is long lasting (at least 3 years).

5.4.2 Nonreplicating Vaccines

In general, killed and subunit vaccines do not trigger an immune response similar to the one elicited during natural infection; their inability to infect cells and activate cytotoxic T cells makes them much less protective on their own. Being extracellular, they will generally trigger a humoral, antibody-mediated response. Extracellular antigens are presented by major histocompatibility class II (MHC class II) molecules to T helper 2 (Th2) cells, which secrete the cytokines IL-4, IL-5, IL-6, IL-10, and IL-13, stimulating B cells to produce antibody, including mucosal antibody (IgA or IgE). The response to inactivated and subunit vaccines is also short-lived. Consequently, they generally require strong adjuvants and several injections to induce the required level of immunity and are usually effective in controlling only clinical signs rather than infection (Minke et al. 2004). Adjuvants can stimulate the appropriate immune response through different mechanisms.

Inactivated adjuvanted vaccines also may pose a risk of causing autoimmune diseases, allergic disorders, and vaccine injection site sarcomas (Day 2006).

With FMD, cattle which have recovered from infection with one of the seven serotypes of FMD are not immune to the other serotypes but remain protected against the first serotype for a considerable period of time. However, further rounds of infection with other serotypes may result in less severe clinical responses or protection (Cottral and Gailiunas 1972) and the cross-neutralization titers in these cases tend to be consistent with the protection observed. In contrast, killed FMDV vaccines elicit a more short-lived and antigenically narrower protective immunity.

5.4.3 DNA Vaccines

Because they stimulate the synthesis of the antigen they encode within cells, DNA vaccines elicit a mostly cell-mediated immune response, which could be long-lived.

DNA immunization can elicit a range of helper T cell responses, including lymphoproliferation and the generation of a variety of cytokine profiles. A major advantage of DNA vaccines is the ease with which they can be manipulated to bias the type of T cell help toward a Th1 or Th2 response (Feltquate et al. 1997). Each type of response has distinctive patterns of lymphokine and chemokine expression, specific types of immunoglobulins expressed, patterns of lymphocyte trafficking, and types of innate immune responses generated.

5.5 Vaccine Type Selection

The choice of a certain type of vaccine over another will depend on various factors.

- *Options available for the disease of interest*: for some diseases, there might be only one type of vaccine developed. For example, for PPR there are only conventional attenuated live vaccines commercially available, while for Newcastle disease, there are several types of vaccines available on the market. Additionally, in some countries, only certain types of vaccines might be available due to logistic, commercial, or regulatory issues.
- *Circulating field strains*: vaccines against the specific serotype(s) or strain(s) circulating in the field might be only available as a specific type of vaccine. For example, certain combinations of bluetongue serotypes are only available as live vaccines, while other combinations are only available as inactivated vaccines.
- *Cost*: livestock keepers or local authorities and governments in different parts of the world will have different returns on their investment (in this case the investment in the vaccine), depending on the disease prevalence and disease impact. Bigger returns might justify the use of more expensive types of vaccines, as far as they still represent value for money. Awareness and perception of risk might also influence the choice of more expensive options.
- *Objectives of the vaccination*: different objectives such as disease control or disease elimination will influence the selection of vaccine type. This applies at herd level, but also at larger scale (regional, national, continental, etc.). A live (or inactivated) vaccine that does not prevent infection and only prevents clinical signs might not be the appropriate choice for disease elimination, but might be the best choice for disease control. A live attenuated vaccine that prevents transmission might be adequate for both purposes, for example the PPR vaccine.
- *Disease epidemiological situation*: linked to the previous point. In an endemic situation, the main objective might be to prevent mortality and limit losses, and live vaccines might produce more solid and long-lasting immunity. In an epidemic situation, live vaccines that have a tendency to recombine with the field virus (note this is not the case for all live vaccines) or might trigger abortion in pregnant animals (for example, the live attenuated Smithburn vaccine for RVF) might not be indicated. In an epidemic situation, the priority might be vaccines that have a rapid onset of immunity (for example, for hog cholera or CSF, a live vaccine might be preferred over a subunit vaccine), or vaccines that might favor the subsequent eradication of the disease, for example vaccines with differentiate between infected and vaccinated animals (DIVA) characteristics.
- *Logistics of delivery*: especially for livestock owners living in remote areas, or governments setting up vaccination campaigns in remote areas or with difficult access, aspects such as thermotolerance, in-use stability, number of vaccinations required to trigger protective immunity, frequency of boosters, and other characteristics that vary with the different type of vaccines are very relevant. The decision might not be easy, as for example, a subunit vaccine might have better thermotolerance than a live vaccine but might require frequent boosters.
- *Combinations*: in order to maximize the value of a vaccination, it might be desired to vaccinate the animal for several diseases at the same time. If a combined vaccine does not exist, then it might be possible to use several vaccines simultaneously (by injecting the vaccines in different sites). Some types of vaccines would be more acceptable for simultaneous use depending on the species and the disease targeted.
- *Local and/or regional legislation*: local regulations might not allow the use of a certain type of vaccine, for example, if there is a local control plan that requires a DIVA vaccine, or there is an elimination plan.

5.6 Summary

Viral vaccines have had great success in controlling diseases, and vaccines for livestock will continue to play a key role in disease control and elimination or eradication programs.

Currently there are different types of veterinary viral vaccines available: replicating vaccines (conventional attenuated live vaccines, live gene-deleted attenuated vaccines, and recombinant vectored vaccines), nonreplicating vaccines (conventional inactivated vaccines, subunit vaccines, and other forms of nonreplicating particulate and subunit vaccines such as VLP and synthetic peptide vaccines) and DNA-based vaccines. They all have different characteristics which are reflected in their advantages and disadvantages. Replicating vaccines usually trigger a broad range of protective immune responses similar to the ones elicited during natural infection, generally including both antibodies and cell-mediated immunity. Nonreplicating vaccines usually trigger a short-lived immunity, and generally require strong adjuvants and several presentations of the antigen to trigger the required level of immunity. DNA vaccines elicit a mostly cell-mediated immune response.

The choice of a certain type of vaccine over another depends on various factors including the options available, the circulating field strains, the cost of the vaccine, objectives of the vaccination, the disease epidemiological situation, and logistics of the delivery.

References

Bachmann, M.F., Rohrer, U.H., Kundig, T.M. et al. (1993). The influence of antigen organization on B cell responsiveness. *Science* 262 (5138): 1448–1451.

Barteling, S.J. and Vreeswijk, J. (1991). Developments in foot-and-mouth disease vaccines. *Vaccine* 9 (2): 75–88.

Batten, C.A., Maan, S., Shaw, A.E. et al. (2008). A European field strain of bluetongue virus derived from two parental vaccine strains by genome segment reassortment. *Virus Res.* 137: 56–63.

Beljelarskaya, S.N. (2011). Baculovirus expression systems for production of recombinant proteins in insect and mammalian cells. *Mol. Biol.* 45: 123–138.

Blanchard, P., Mahe, D., Cariolet, R. et al. (2003). Protection of swine against post-weaning multisystemic wasting syndrome (PMWS) by porcine circovirus type 2 (PCV2) proteins. *Vaccine* 21: 4565–4575.

Bublot, M., Pritchard, N., Swayne, D.E. et al. (2006). Development and use of fowlpox vectored vaccines for avian influenza. *Ann. N.Y. Acad. Sci.* 1081: 193–201.

Caplen, H., Peters, C.J., and Bishop, D.H. (1985). Mutagen-directed attenuation of Rift Valley fever virus as a method for vaccine development. *J. Gen. Virol.* 66: 2271–2277.

Castle, P. (2005). European pharmacopoeia (EP), USDA and MAFF standards – will they ever be harmonised under the VICH umbrella? *Dev. Biol.* 121: 227–234.

Coetzee, P., Stokstad, M., Venter, E.H. et al. (2012). Bluetongue: a historical and epidemiological perspective with the emphasis on South Africa. *J. Virol.* 9: 198.

Cottral, G.E. and Gailiunas, P. (1972). Experimental multiple infection of animals with foot-and-mouth disease viruses. *Proc. Annu. Mtg U.S. Anim. Hlth. Assoc.* 75: 441–465.

Darteil, R., Bublot, M., Laplace, E. et al. (1995). Herpesvirus of turkey recombinant viruses expressing infectious bursal disease virus (IBDV) VP2 immunogen induce protection against an IBDV virulent challenge in chickens. *Virology* 211: 481–490.

Davis, B.S., Chang, J.G., Cropp, B. et al. (2001). West Nile virus recombinant DNA vaccine protects mouse and horse from virus challenge and expresses in vitro a non-infectious recombinant antigen that can be used in enzyme-linked immunosorbent assays. *J. Virol.* 75: 4040–4047.

Day, M.J. (2006). Vaccine side effects: fact and fiction. *Vet. Microbiol.* 117 (1): 51–58.

Dungu, B., Potgieter, C., Von, T.B., and Smit, T. (2004). Vaccination in the control of bluetongue in endemic regions: the South African experience. *Dev. Biol.* 119: 463–472.

Dungu, B., Louw, I., Lubisi, A. et al. (2010). Evaluation of the efficacy and safety of the Rift Valley Fever Clone 13 vaccine in sheep. *Vaccine* 28 (29): 4581–4587.

Feltquate, D.M., Heaney, S., Webster, R.G., and Robinson, H.L. (1997). Different T helper cell types and antibody isotypes generated by saline and gene gun DNA immunization. *J. Immunol.* 158 (5): 2278–2284.

Fenner, F., Henderson, D.A., Arita, I. et al. (1988). *Smallpox and Its Eradication*. Geneva: World Health Organization. www.who.int/iris/handle/10665/39485

Ferrari, M., Brack, A., Romanelli, M.G. et al. (2000). A study of the ability of a TK-negative and gE/gI negative pseudorabies virus (PRV) mutant inoculated by different routes to protect pigs against PRV infection. *J. Vet. Med. B.* 47: 753–762.

Ferrari, G., de Liberato, C., Scavia, G. et al. (2005). Active circulation of bluetongue vaccine virus serotype-2 among unvaccinated cattle in central Italy. *Prev. Vet. Med.* 68: 103–113.

Garver, K.A., LaPatra, S.E., and Kurath, G. (2005). Efficacy of an infectious hematopoietic necrosis (IHN) virus DNA vaccine in Chinook *Oncorhynchus tshawytscha* and sockeye *O. nerka* salmon. *Dis. Aquat. Org.* 64 (1): 13–22.

Hanna, E.S., Roque-Barreira, M.C., Mendes, G.M. et al. (2008). Cloning, expression and purification of a glycosylated form of the DNA-binding protein Dps from *Salmonella enterica typhimurium*. *Protein Expression Purif.* 59: 197–202.

Heppell, J. and Davis, H.L. (2000). Application of DNA vaccine technology to aquaculture. *Adv. Drug Delivery Rev.* 43 (1): 29–43.

Husseiny, M.I. and Hensel, M. (2005). Rapid method for the construction of *Salmonella enterica* serovar Typhimurium vaccine carrier strains. *Infect. Immun.* 73: 1598–1605.

Ichikawa, Y., Yamagata, H., Tochikubo, K., and Udaka, S. (1993). Very efficient extracellular production of cholera toxin B subunit using *Bacillus brevis*. *FEMS Microbiol. Lett.* 111: 219–224.

Ikonomou, L., Schneider, Y.J., and Agathos, S.N. (2003). Insect cell culture for industrial production of recombinant proteins. *Appl. Microbiol. Biotechnol.* 62: 1–20.

Kagnoff, M.F. (1996). Mucosal immunology: new frontiers. *Immunol. Today* 17: 57–59.

Kashima, Y. and Udaka, S. (2004). High-level production of hyperthermophilic cellulase in the *Bacillus brevis* expression and secretion system. *Biosci. Biotechnol., Biochem.* 68: 235–237.

Kennedy, N.J., Spithill, T.W., Tennent, J. et al. (2006). DNA vaccines in sheep: CTLA-4 mediated targeting and CpG motifs enhance immunogenicity in a DNA prime/protein boost strategy. *Vaccine* 24 (7): 970–979.

Kortekaas, J., Zingeser, J., de Leeuw, P. et al. (2011). Rift Valley fever vaccine development, progress and constraints. *Emerg. Infect. Dis.* 17 (9): e1.

Langeveld, J.P., Casal, J.I., Osterhaus, A.D. et al. (1994). First peptide vaccine providing protection against viral infection in the target animal: studies of canine parvovirus in dogs. *J. Virol.* 68 (7): 4506–4513.

Liang, R., van den Hurk, J.V., Babiuk, L.A., and van Drunen Littel-van den Hurk S. (2006). Priming with DNA encoding E2 and boosting with E2 protein formulated with CpG oligodeoxynucleotides induces strong immune responses and protection from Bovine viral diarrhea virus in cattle. *J. Gen. Virol.* 87 (10): 2971–2982.

Lorenzen, N. and LaPatra, S.E. (2005). DNA vaccines for aquacultured fish. *Rev. Sci. Tech.* 24 (1): 201–213.

Madera, R., Gong, W., Wang, L. et al. (2016). Pigs immunized with a novel E2 subunit vaccine are protected from subgenotype heterologous classical swine fever virus challenge. *BMC Vet. Res.* 12 (1): 197.

Maranga, L., Cruz, P.E., Aunins, J.G., and Carrondo, M.J. (2002). Production of core and virus-like particles with baculovirus infected insect cells. *Adv. Biochem. Eng./ Biotechnol.* 74: 183–206.

McGhee, J.R., Mestecky, J., Dertzbaugh, M.T. et al. (1992). The mucosal immune system from fundamental concepts to vaccine development. *Vaccine* 2: 75–88.

Meeusen, E.N., Walker, J., Peters, A. et al. (2007). Current status of veterinary vaccines. *Clin. Microbiol. Rev.* 20: 489–510.

Mestecky, J. (1987). The common mucosal immune system and current strategies for induction of immune responses in external secretions. *J. Clin. Immunol.* 4: 265–276.

Minke, J.M., Audonnet, J.C., and Fischer, L. (2004). Equine viral vaccines: the past, present and future. *Vet. Res.* 35: 425–443.

Monath, T.P., Arroyo, J., Miller, C., and Guirakhoo, F. (2001). West Nile virus vaccine. *Curr. Drug Targets Infect. Disord.* 1: 37–50.

Morrill, J.C., Laughlin, R.C., Lokugamage, N. et al. (2013). Safety and immunogenicity of recombinant Rift Valley fever MP-12 vaccine candidates in sheep. *Vaccine* 31 (3): 559–565.

Moss, B. and Flexner, C. (1987). Vaccinia virus expression vectors. *Annu. Rev. Immunol.* 5: 305–324.

Muller, R., Saluzzo, J.F., Lopez, N. et al. (1995). Characterization of clone 13, a naturally attenuated avirulent isolate of Rift Valley fever virus, which is altered in the small segment. *Am. J. Trop. Med. Hyg.* 53: 405–411.

Mutwiri, G., Gerdts, V., Lopez, M., and Babiuk, L.A. (2007). Innate immunity and new adjuvants. *Rev. Sci. Tech.* 26: 147–156.

Nagahama, M., Michiue, K., and Sakurai, J. (1996). Production and purification of *Clostridium perfringens* alpha-toxin using a protein-hyperproducing strain, *Bacillus brevis* 47. *FEMS Microbiol. Lett.* 145: 239–243.

Naranjo, J. and Cosivi, O. (2013). Elimination of foot-and-mouth disease in South America: lessons and challenges. *Philos. Trans. R. Soc. London, Ser. B* 368 (1623): 20120381.

OIE. (2011). Global rinderpest eradication. www.oie.int/for-the-media/rinderpest/

Okazaki, W., Purchase, H.G., and Burmester, B.R. (1970). Protection against Marek's disease by vaccination with a herpesvirus of turkeys. *Avian Dis.* 14: 413–429.

O'Reilly, D.R., Miller, L.K., and Luckow, V.A. (1992). An overview of baculoviruses, choosing a transfer plasmid and parent virus, methods for vector construction and gene expression. In: *Baculo-expression Vectors: A Laboratory Manual* (eds. D.R. O'Reilly, L.K. Miller and V.A. Luckow), 1–36. New York: W.H. Freeman.

Pastoret, P.P. and Brochier, B. (1996). The development and use of a vaccinia-rabies recombinant oral vaccine for the control of wildlife rabies; a link between Jenner and Pasteur. *Epidemiol. Infect.* 16 (3): 235–240.

Pastoret, P.P. and Brochier, B. (1999). Epidemiology and control of fox rabies in Europe. *Vaccine* 17: 1750–1754.

Poulet, H., Minke, J., Pardo, M.C. et al. (2007). Development and registration of recombinant veterinary vaccines. The example of the canarypox vector platform. *Vaccine* 25 (30): 5606–5612.

Powell, K. (2004). DNA vaccines – back in the saddle again? *Nat. Biotechnol.* 22 (7): 799–801.

Purcell, A.W., McCluskey, J., and Rossjohn, J. (2007). More than one reason to rethink the use of peptides in vaccine design. *Nat. Rev. Drug Discovery* 6 (5): 404–414.

Radford, K.M., Reid, S., and Greenfield, P.F. (1997). Substrate limitation in the baculovirus expression vector system. *Biotechnol. Bioeng.* 56: 32–44.

Rogan, D. and Babiuk, L.A. (2005). Novel vaccines from biotechnology. *Rev. Sci. Tech.* 24: 159–174.

Rybicki, E.P. (2010). Plant-made vaccines for humans and animals. *Plant Biotechnol. J.* 8 (5): 620–637.

Salam, M.A., Katz, J., Zhang, P. et al. (2006). Immunogenicity of *Salmonella* vector vaccines expressing SBR of *Streptococcus mutans* under the control of a T7-*nirB* (dual) promoter system. *Vaccine* 24: 5003–5015.

Scheerlinck, J.P., Karlis, J., Tjelle, T.E. et al. (2004). In vivo electroporation improves immune responses to DNA vaccination in sheep. *Vaccine* 22 (13–14): 1820–1825.

Schijns, V.E.J.C. (2001). Activation and programming of adaptive immune responses by vaccine adjuvants. *Vet. Sci. Tomorrow* 3: 15.

Shiga, Y., Maki, M., Ohta, T. et al. (2000). Efficient production of N-terminally truncated biologically active human interleukin-6 by *Bacillus brevis*. *Biosci. Biotechnol. Biochem.* 64: 665–669.

Tam, J.P. (1996). Recent advances in multiple antigen peptides. *J. Immunol. Methods* 196 (1): 17–32.

The Global Polio Initiative. (2014). www.polioeradication.org/Polioandprevention/Thevaccines.aspx

Theiler, A. (1908). The innoculation of sheep against bluetongue and the results in practice. *Vet J* 64: 600–607.

Udaka, S. and Yamagata, H. (1993). Protein secretion in *Bacillus brevis*. *Antonie Van Leeuwenhoek* 64: 137–143.

Ulmer, J.B., Donnelly, J.J., Parker, S.E. et al. (1993). Heterologous protection against influenza by injection of DNA encoding a viral protein. *Science* 259 (5102): 1745–1749.

Valenzuela, P., Medina, A., Rutter, W.J. et al. (1982). Synthesis and assembly of hepatitis B virus surface antigen particles in yeast. *Nature* 298: 347–350.

Van Aarle, P. (2003). Suitability of an E2 subunit vaccine of classical swine fever in combination with the E(rns)-marker-test for eradication through vaccination. *Dev. Biol.* 114: 193–200.

Van Oirschot, J.T. (1997). Classical inactivated vaccines. In: *Veterinary Vaccinology* (eds. P.P. Pastoret, J. Blancou, P. Vannier and R. Verschueren), 89–97. Amsterdam: Elsevier Science.

Van Oirschot, J., Kaashoek, T.M.J., and Rijsewijk, F.A. (1996). Advances in the development and evaluation of bovine herpesvirus 1 vaccines. *Vet. Microbiol.* 53: 43–54.

Vermij, P. and Waltz, E. (2006). USDA approves the first plant-based vaccine. *Nat. Biotechnol.* 24 (3): 233–234.

Verwoerd, D.W. (2012). History of Orbivirus research in South Africa. *J. S. Afr. Vet. Assoc.* 83 (1): 532.

Verwoerd, D.W. and Erasmus, B.J. (1994). Bluetongue. In: *Infectious Diseases of Livestock with Special Reference to Southern Africa* (eds. J.A.W. Coetzer, G.R. Thomson and R.C. Tustin), 443–459. Cape Town: Oxford University Press.

Verwoerd, D.W. and Erasmus, B.J. (2004). Bluetongue. In: *Infectious Diseases of Livestock*, 2e (eds. J.A.W. Coetzer, G.R. Thomson and R.C. Tustin), 1201–1220. Cape Town: Oxford University Press.

Von Teichman, B., Engelbrecht, A., Zulu, G. et al. (2011). Safety and efficacy of Rift Valley fever Smithburn and Clone 13 vaccines in calves. *Vaccine* 29 (34): 5771–5777.

Wallace, D.B. and Viljoen, G.J. (2005). Immune responses to recombinants of the South African vaccine strain of lumpy skin disease virus generated by using thymidine kinase gene insertion. *Vaccine* 23: 3061–3067.

Wesley, T. (2005). Veterinary Vaccines. Animal Pharm Reports, T&F Informa. Latest update of this series (2015) at: https://store.agribusinessintelligence.informa.com/vet14.html.

WHO. (1980). The global eradication of smallpox. Final report of the Global Commission for the Certification of Smallpox Eradication. Geneva, December 1979.

Yang, X.L., Liu, W.C., Yang, W.W. et al. (2005). Oral immunization of mice with vaccine of attenuated *Salmonella typhimurium* expressing *Helicobacter pylori* urease B subunit. *Biomed. Environ. Sci.* 18: 411–418.

Yoichi, F. (2012). Return of inactivated whole-virus vaccine for superior efficacy. *Immunol. Cell Biol.* 90: 571–578.

Yokomizo, Y., Watanabe, F., Imada, Y. et al. (2002). Mucosal immunoadjuvant activity of the low toxic recombinant *Escherichia coli* heat-labile enterotoxin produced by *Bacillus brevis* for the bacterial subunit or component vaccine in pigs and cattle. *Vet. Immunol. Immunopathol.* 87: 291–300.

Zekarias, B., Mo, H., and Curtiss, R. (2008). Recombinant attenuated *Salmonella enterica* serovar Typhimurium expressing the carboxy-terminal domain of alpha toxin from *Clostridium perfringens* induces protective responses against necrotic enteritis in chickens. *Clin. Vaccine Immunol.* 15: 805–816.

6

Bacterial and *Mycoplasma* Vaccines

Abdelali Benkirane[1], Ahmed El Idrissi[2], and April Johnson[3]

[1] Department of Pathology and Veterinary Public Health, Institut Agronomique et Vétérinaire Hassan II, Rabat, Morocco
[2] Formerly, Animal Production and Health Division, Food and Agriculture Organization of the United Nations, Rome, Italy
[3] USDA APHIS, Veterinary Services, Field Operations, Alabama, USA

6.1 Introduction

The discovery of bacteria and the ability to culture them in the laboratory paved the way for the development of bacterial, live attenuated vaccines, using simple methods such as culture aging or chemical treatments. The Pasteurian era in the nineteenth century witnessed the advent of the first bacterial vaccines (fowl cholera, swine erysipelas, and anthrax) even before Louis Pasteur developed, in 1885, the first virus attenuated vaccine, was for rabies (Lombard et al. 2007). This led to the development of many types of vaccines aimed at preventing bacterial and viral infections.

However, the advent of antibacterial substances including sulfonamides and other antibiotics in the early twentieth century made it possible to treat bacterial diseases, with variable success. This reliance on antibiotics to treat and prevent bacterial infections has impacted the progression of research in the field of bacterial vaccinology, while viral vaccinology has attracted more attention given the absence of similarly effective antiviral therapies. Investment in research and development of viral vaccines exceeds by far the investment in bacterial vaccinology and, as a result, little is done in the development of a new generation of bacterial vaccines.

Although bacterial vaccines have shown good outcomes in the control of various types of animal diseases, many of those in use are of limited quality or nonexistent for certain bacterial pathogens. Vaccine development is not straightforward and there are significant challenges associated with research and development for bacterial vaccinology. The design of a vaccine is based on the identification of the antigens involved in protection, on their immunogenicity, and on the analysis of the respective efficacy of antibodies and cellular mechanisms of immunity. Unlike viruses, which have relatively limited numbers of surface antigens, bacteria have a much larger number of coding genes and a very complex antigenic structure made of external as well as internal antigens, including toxins. Predicting which antigens may produce an appropriate immune response is not straightforward in bacteria, so much effort is devoted to identifying vaccine candidates and vaccine formulations.

Despite the difficulties in developing novel vaccines, the use of bacterial vaccines has led to a significant reduction in the incidence of infectious diseases in the veterinary field. At the end of the twentieth century, the number of attenuated or inactivated classic bacterial vaccines remains much larger in the veterinary field than in the human field. The development of new vaccines could lead to further decreases in the incidence of infectious diseases, which could also lead to a reduction in use of antibiotics, which risks the development of antimicrobial resistance.

This chapter provides an overview of bacterial and *Mycoplasma* vaccines used in veterinary medicine and their role in reducing disease burdens in animals. The chapter deals with vaccines against enteric, respiratory, and reproductive diseases commonly used in the livestock industry, focusing on those not addressed in other chapters.

6.2 Types of Bacterial Vaccines

There are several types of bacterial vaccines being produced, based on the type of pathogen or bacterial component being targeted, how the bacteria cause infection and how the immune system responds. Bacterial vaccines can be classified into different groups: live attenuated vaccines, killed whole cell vaccines, toxoids, subunit vaccines, and

Veterinary Vaccines: Principles and Applications, First Edition. Edited by Samia Metwally, Gerrit Viljoen, and Ahmed El Idrissi.

recombinant vaccines. Each type of vaccine has its associated advantages and disadvantages (Table 6.1).

6.2.1 Live Attenuated Vaccines

Virulent microbes may lose some of their pathogenicity while retaining their protective effect as a result of random genetic mutations that occur spontaneously during replication. Most, but not all, attenuated whole cell vaccines are derived from strains with moderate virulence which is then selected for and stabilized through different methods. Live attenuated vaccines are often cheaper to produce than other vaccines produced with different methods.

There are several ways in which live organisms can become attenuated, or weakened.

- *Serial passage in culture media*: this approach involves multiple cycles of growth of the bacteria under cultivation conditions that ultimately lead to an accumulation of genetic mutations resulting in altered virulence. This process can be tedious, taking years, as was seen with the 13 years of serially passaging *Mycobacterium bovis* that resulted in attenuation and subsequent establishment of the *M. bovis* Calmette-Guérin strain (Oettinger et al. 1999). Serial passage has also been used to generate *Brucella* vaccine strains – for example, the *Brucella melitensis* Rev.1 (Elberg and Faunce 1957) vaccine which was derived from a streptomycin-dependent virulent strain cloned to select only reverse streptomycin-resistant mutants. Another example is the RB51 vaccine, a spontaneous rough mutant, derived using repeated passage of *Brucella abortus* strain 2308 *in vitro* (Schurig et al. 1991).
- *Serial passage in eggs or nontarget animal species*: an example of this approach in livestock is the contagious bovine pleuropneumonia (CBPP) vaccine produced from *Mycoplasma mycoides* subsp. *mycoides* small colony (Mmm SC) T1/44 (Sheriff and Piercy 1952). The attenuated strain was obtained after passaging a low-virulence strain of Mmm 44 times in embryonated eggs. *B. abortus* strain 19 (Buck 1930) was also produced with this method, undergoing 19 passages in guinea pigs.
- *Exposure to chemicals and/or low temperatures ("heat-sensitive mutants")*: an example of this method is the chemically induced temperature-sensitive mutant strain of *Chlamydia abortus* that grows at 35 °C but not at 39.5 °C, the body temperature of sheep (Rodolakis and Souriau 1986).
- *Directed mutation*: the genes involved in pathogenicity are modified or suppressed in such a way that the strain loses its pathogenicity. This type of attenuation usually involves deletion of essential virulence factors or mutation of genes encoding metabolic enzymes whose function is essential for survival outside the laboratory (Detmer and Glenting 2006)

Live attenuated vaccines produce immunity in most recipients with one dose, except those administered orally. They are very efficient in inducing long-lasting immunity via cell-mediated and humoral immune responses. These vaccines, however, do have disadvantages when given to animals that are immunocompromised, such as pregnant animals, since the organism can replicate in an uncontrolled manner if the immune system cannot respond. Local side effects are also possible, including pain, redness, swelling, and transient fever. Over time, there is a possibility for the organism to undergo mutations that could result in more pathogenic or virulent strains. However, reversion to the virulence of the original wild strain, as is the case with some viral vaccines, has never been reported with bacterial vaccines. The use of spontaneously mutant variants reduces the potential for reversion to virulence of bacterial live vaccines.

To produce an immune response, live attenuated vaccines must be able to replicate in the vaccinated individual and therefore must be viable when administered. Anything that either damages the live organism in the vial (e.g. excessive heat, exposure to ultraviolet light) or interferes with replication of the organism in the body (such as circulating antibody) can cause the vaccine to be ineffective. For this reason, appropriate storage (often refrigeration) and transportation is required to ensure vaccines remain effective.

6.2.2 Inactivated Vaccines

Inactivated vaccines consist of microorganisms that have undergone an inactivation process aimed at blocking their ability to replicate in the host while keeping intact the constituents that induce protection. The inactivation is generally carried out by a standardized protocol for heating the culture in the presence of oxidizing agents.

Chemicals or radiation can also be used for inactivation. The inactivation can be carried out on a crude mixed microbial culture (bacterin), but is done more often on purified organisms or even on antigens, such as to create toxoids from toxins.

Inactivated vaccines typically are not as immunogenic as live attenuated vaccines, so adjuvants are needed to enhance the immune response (antibodies and effector T cell functions). When adjuvants are used, a smaller amount of antigen can be used and in some cases fewer doses of vaccine are required to elicit the same response. Additionally, adjuvants can influence the type of immune response. Adjuvants can be a variety of materials including

Table 6.1 Characteristics of most common veterinary bacterial vaccines.

Type	Characteristics	Examples of vaccines
Live attenuated	**Advantages** Induce both humoral and cellular immunity Strong and long-lasting immunity One injection usually sufficient No adjuvant required **Disadvantages** May have side effects Need for refrigerated storage	*Salmonella gallinarum* 9R *Escherichia coli* F5 (K99) *Brucella abortus* S19 *Brucella melitensis* Rev. 1 *Bacillus anthracis* strain F34 *Mycoplasma mycoides* subsp. *mycoides* SC strain T1/44 *Mycoplasma gallinarum* strains F, ts-11, and 6/85 *Mycoplasma synoviae* strain MS-H *Chlamydophila abortus* TS1B, strain AB7
Bacterin vaccines	**Advantages** Do not replicate (safe vaccines) More stable during storage and transport **Disadvantages** Weakly immunogenic Require adjuvants Repeated doses required to maintain immunity over time Variable efficacy	Clostridial bacterins *Escherichia coli* F5/F41 *Pasteurella multocida* A, B and E *Mannheimia haemolytica* type A and T *Mycoplasma capricolum* subsp. *capripneumoniae*, strain F38 *Coxiella burnetii* phase I vaccine *Mycobacterium avium* subsp. *paratuberculosis*, strain 316F Autogenous vaccines (colibacillosis)
Toxoids	**Advantages** Well-defined composition **Disadvantages** Some may require high levels of biosafety during manufacture Usually require adjuvants *In vitro* production limitations	Clostridial toxoids *Clostridium tetani* toxoid
Subunit vaccines	**Advantages** Safe nonreplicating vaccines Good tolerance (purified immunogenic antigens) **Disadvantages** Require adjuvants Primarily induce a humoral immunity Require identification of immunogenic and protective antigen(s) Require repeated doses Poorly immunogenic (unless combined with toxoids)	*Salmonella typhi* *Escherichia coli* vaccines *Actinobacillus pleuropneumoniae*
Recombinant vaccines	**Advantages** Induce both cellular and humoral immune responses **Disadvantages** Require identification of immunogenic and protective antigen(s) May require repeat doses to maintain immunity over time	*Streptococcus equi* subsp. *equi* strain TW928 Fowlpox vectored *Mycoplasma gallisepticum*

aluminum salts, paraffin oil and surfactants, oil-in-water emulsions, and saponins.

Inactivated vaccines cannot replicate and are thus non-infectious which makes them safer to use than live attenuated vaccines as well as more stable for storage and transport. However, they also lack the ability to induce a long-lasting and comprehensive immune response, requiring repeated dosing to maintain immunity over time. Efficacy also varies greatly from vaccine to vaccine. They are thus often regarded as inferior in stimulating immunity than live attenuated vaccines.

Inactivated bacterial vaccines consist of bacterins (killed/inactivated whole bacteria), toxoids (inactivated toxins), or a combination thereof, depending on the capacity of the organism to produce harmful toxins.

6.2.2.1 Whole Cell Bacterin Vaccines

Whole cell bacterin vaccines contain killed cells of one or more bacteria. Because such vaccines do not undergo purification of antigen, immunity will be induced to almost all bacterial components so that antibodies will neutralize the pathogen and fight the infection. Killed vaccines have been widely used in veterinary medicine and are still used to protect animals against some bacteria, including *Clostridia*, *Pasteurella*, *Salmonella*, and coliforms. They offer an economical, and potentially safe, effective means of preventing disease.

Whole cell bacterin vaccines are also used in some circumstances for the preparation of autogenous vaccines for on-farm specific demands where no commercial vaccines are available or where commercial vaccines are ineffective or do not cover the current pathogen strains in the flock or herd. Autogenous vaccines are often used to address emergency situations or persisting problems at herd level such as endemic mastitis or septicemic colibacillosis, using an isolate obtained from the affected herd to create the vaccine. Autogenous bacterial vaccines can be live or inactivated, but in most cases they consist of whole cell bacterins of one or more bacterial species or serotypes. Commercial and licensed vaccines have advantages compared with autogenous vaccines, including obligatory good manufacturing practice (GMP) production (Hoelzer et al. 2018).

6.2.2.2 Toxoid Vaccines

For bacteria owing their pathogenicity principally to the presence of one or more toxins, toxoids are used to immunize the organism against that particular pathogen. Toxoids are normally produced from the crude toxin by treatment with formaldehyde. Toxoids retain the same structure as their parent compound, the harmful toxin, but can no longer damage the body, therefore becoming a useful vaccination tool. Such toxoids are normally adsorbed by an adjuvant, usually a mineral salt such as aluminum phosphate and aluminum or potassium sulfate. For cost reasons, the latter is usually the most popular for vaccines for veterinary use.

Toxoids, although efficient, present some production limitations. For example, the amount of toxin produced *in vitro* is unpredictable, and some toxins are potent biological agents that require high levels of biosafety (Arimitsu et al. 2004). The use of recombinant vaccines can overcome these limitations, since they can be produced efficiently in large amounts and usually present low toxicity (Jorge and Dellagostin 2017).

6.2.3 Subunit Vaccines

Unlike whole cell vaccines, subunit vaccines include only the antigens that best induce the immune response. Subunit vaccines are difficult to produce as it is sometimes difficult to identify which antigens best stimulate a protective immune response. But when the immunogenic antigens can be determined, the vaccine is easier to produce. The bacteria can be grown in the laboratory and then the subunits separated by chemically breaking down the organism and selecting for the specific components. Alternatively, recombinant technology can be used to insert the gene for the specific antigen into another organism to be grown, such as yeast. Polysaccharide-based vaccines are a type of subunit vaccine composed of pure cell wall polysaccharides from bacteria. The immune response to a pure polysaccharide vaccine is poor and multiple doses may be required. This problem has been overcome through polysaccharide–protein conjugate technology (conjugate vaccines).

6.2.4 Conjugate Vaccines

Conjugate vaccines are produced when the antigen is not sufficiently or strongly immunogenic. In this case, the antigen is chemically linked to a stronger antigen which in turn increases the strength of the immune response to the poorer antigen. As an example, conjugate polysaccharide vaccines contain polysaccharide that is chemically linked to a protein, typically an inactivated toxin. This linkage makes the polysaccharide a more potent vaccine and enables the change of the immune response from T independent (where B cells produce antibodies without T cell stimulation) to T dependent, with a stronger and faster response as well as the induction of immunological memory (Anon 2011).

6.2.5 Recombinant Vaccines

In comparison with viral diseases, bacterial diseases of animals have benefited little from the new vaccine production technologies and currently, the majority of licensed bacterial vaccines are conventional – either live attenuated or inactivated. However, efforts are being made to move toward the production of more efficient vaccines, which include recombinant toxoids. Attempts are ongoing to produce other recombinant vaccines by modification or deletion or addition of a gene or the introduction of a new gene which becomes a selectable marker to enable differentiation of infected from vaccinated animals (DIVA) but of the vaccine candidates under consideration, none has been licensed so far. The best targets for a bacterial genome are the genes associated with virulence determinants, biosynthesis, and regulatory genes which are critical for bacterial survival.

6.2.6 Combination Vaccines

Because of the complexity of many disease syndromes, the limited cross-protection between strains, and to avoid giving animals multiple injections, it is common to use mixtures of organisms in single vaccines. A combined vaccine is intended for immunization against more than one disease, pathogen, and/or antigen which is authorized by one marketing authorization. The requirements for manufacture and control of combined vaccines in terms of quality and safety are the same as those for a vaccine containing one active substance (European Medicines Agency 2013). The combined vaccine can be supplied in a single primary container or in several primary containers, the contents of which are mixed prior to administration (European Medicines Agency 2013).

Combined vaccines may include a mixture of different serotypes of a bacterial pathogen or different bacteria and viruses causing a disease complex in an animal species. For example, for bovine respiratory disease syndrome, combined vaccines are available for bovine respiratory syncytial virus, infectious bovine rhinotracheitis virus, bovine viral diarrhea virus, parainfluenza 3 virus, and *Mannheimia haemolytica*. Other examples of combining two or more bacterial strains or antigens include the anthrax-blackleg vaccine, *Pasteurella-Salmonella* vaccine, and clostridial vaccines which may include up to eight antigens. The impact of the historical combined vaccine (rinderpest and CBPP) includes the eradication of rinderpest and control over pleuropneumonia when vaccination was in practice.

While combination of vaccines may be considered as a useful vaccine delivery practice, it can be limited by interference in the immune response between different strains and the biological compatibility of immunogens (possible immunosuppression by some viruses) (European Medicines Agency 2013).

6.3 Bacterial Vaccines as Alternatives to Antibiotics

The growing prevalence of bacterial strains resistant against a broad spectrum of antibiotics poses a substantial problem in the treatment of bacterial diseases. There is a growing understanding that increased efforts are needed to prevent diseases through improved biosecurity and use of effective vaccines. Bacterial vaccines can help minimize the need for antibiotics by preventing and controlling infectious diseases in animal populations and their direct mitigating impact on antibiotic consumption has been demonstrated in a number of studies (Pang 2009; Lipsitch and Siber 2016).

Bacterial vaccines protect against susceptible and resistant strains alike and therefore can help limit the spread of antibiotic resistance. Due to the clonal spread of resistant strains, a vaccine approach targeting one or more antigens expressed by such clones might be a valid way to combat resistance (Henriques-Normark and Normark 2014). Effectiveness of bacterial vaccines in reducing disease and antibiotic resistance in human medicine has been reported. The pneumococcal conjugate vaccine, for instance, has led to reductions in resistant organisms and antibiotic prescribing (Clift and Salisbury 2017). New vaccines targeting resistant bacteria in animals are yet to be developed.

6.4 Immune Response to Bacterial Vaccines

Most bacterial vaccines were developed before tools enabling measurement of cellular immunity were discovered (Plotkin 2001). Hence, vaccine efficacy was solely correlated to neutralizing and/or opsonizing antibody titers. While this approach can be adequate for extracellular bacteria, it proves insufficient for facultative intracellular bacteria such as *Listeria*, *Brucella*, or *Salmonella*. Furthermore, vaccine trials seldom address mucosal immunity, even though the causal agents addressed often penetrate the organism through mucous membranes.

Intrinsic characteristics of bacteria, such as the lipopolysaccharides in gram-negative bacteria or lipoteichoic acid in gram-positive bacteria, which mediate different signaling pathways, resulting in the production of inflammatory cytokines and expression of other antimicrobial genes (Janeway and Medzhitov 2002). This innate immune response to bacterial pathogens and its influence on the adaptive immune system make attenuated live vaccines extremely efficient for stimulation of specific and long-term immune responses against the bacteria.

Repeated doses of inactivated vaccines can boost the antibody titer progressively. However, repeat doses of polysaccharide vaccines usually do not cause a booster response. Antibody induced with polysaccharide vaccines has less functional activity than that induced by protein antigens. This is because the predominant antibody produced in response to most polysaccharide vaccines is IgM, and little IgG is produced.

6.5 Vaccination Procedures

Vaccines can be administered by a variety of routes, including subcutaneously, intradermally, or intramuscularly. Some are also delivered through aerosols or administered conjunctivally, orally, or into the teats of dairy livestock. For neonatal diseases, pregnant females can be vaccinated so that passive immunity will be transferred to their offspring through colostrum and confer protection before their immune system becomes mature enough to develop active immunity after their own vaccination.

Vaccination procedures must be carefully analyzed and applied. It is necessary to assess the context under which vaccination is to be implemented and undertake a clinical examination of animals to be vaccinated. The choice of the most suitable vaccine when different options are available is also of paramount importance. For some notifiable diseases, there are regulatory aspects involved, which can forbid the use of a certain type of vaccine or define the legal framework within which a vaccine ought to be used (e.g. bovine paratuberculosis). Vaccination protocols must be clearly defined, taking into consideration the nature of the vaccines, the objectives of vaccination, and any indications and contraindications. It is important to ensure the quality and traceability of vaccinations (certificates and registries) in order to identify possible vaccine risks and failures and to plan for any necessary vaccination recalls.

6.6 Vaccines Against Enteric Diseases

Bacterial pathogens cause a wide range of enteric diseases in animals, some of which are zoonotic. In addition, some also contain antimicrobial resistance genes which pose a threat to animal and human health. Selection of vaccine type depends on the mechanism of pathogenicity. For bacteria where pathogenicity is mostly associated with the excretion of exotoxins, subunit vaccines made of formaldehyde extracted toxoids combined with adjuvants have proven their efficacy over decades and current efforts principally aim at better purifying these extracts. For other bacteria, essentially nonspore-forming gram-negative bacteria, exerting their virulence through somatic antigens, both inactivated whole cell bacterins and purified outer membrane polysaccharides are used. For intracellular bacteria such as *Salmonella*, live attenuated vaccines prove superior as they have the capacity to stimulate both humoral and cell-mediated immunity and to elicit mucosal immunity when administered orally.

6.6.1 Salmonellosis

Salmonellosis in animal species is commonly associated with serovars of *Salmonella* such as *S. enteritis*, *S. gallinarum*, *S. dublin*, *S. pullorum*, and *S. typhimurium*. Infection can result in either a carrier state or clinical disease which can be either a systemic septicemia or enteritis.

The immunity conferred by most commercial vaccines against salmonellosis prevents the colonization of the gut of the vaccinated animal, but rarely eliminates the presence of the bacteria in the herd/flock as a whole or prevents cross-contamination of meat products.

Various killed and live vaccines are commercially available for vaccination against disease and infection in animal species. Live vaccines are recognized to be more effective and induce optimal immune protection against disease; however, there is some evidence that inactivated bacterins can induce a sufficient level of protection. Live vaccine can be administered orally to induce mucosal immunity.

For poultry, there are at least 10 live *Salmonella* vaccines available for *S. enteritidis*, *S. typhimurium*, *S. dublin*, or *S. gallinarum* infection. Vaccines against fowl typhoid (*S. gallinarum*) and pullorum disease (*S. pullorum*) are currently commercialized by at least 12 manufacturers and licensed worldwide. Most of them are made of strain 9R of *S. gallinarum*. Some inactivated vaccines are also available on the market.

Partial cross-protection is induced by various *Salmonella* serovars. A live *S. gallinarum* vaccine is not only effective against fowl typhoid but also reduces the infection of laying hens challenged with *S. enteritidis*.

A combined inactivated *Salmonella-Pasteurella* vaccine which associates *Pasteurella multocida* A3 and D4, *M. haemolytica* and somatic (O) and flagellar (H) antigens of both *S. dublin* and *S. typhimurium* is used to protect cattle, sheep, and goats against enteric and respiratory infections.

6.6.2 Colibacillosis in Neonatal Ruminants

Escherichia coli is the most important bacterial cause of diarrhea in calves during the first week of life; at least two distinct types of diarrheal disease are produced by different strains of this organism.

One type of diarrheal disease in calves is associated with enterotoxigenic *E. coli* (ETEC), which has two virulence factors. One is the fimbrial antigens which enable the organism to attach to and colonize the villi of the small intestine of neonatal calves. The responsible strains in calves and lambs most commonly possess K99 (F5) or F41 fimbrial antigens, or both. More than 90% of the ETEC strains in farm animals belong to the F5 fimbrial antigen family (Hodgins et al. 2005). Other strains that affect calves possess F7 or F17 fimbrial antigens (Nguyen et al. 2011). The other virulence factor is a thermostable, non-antigenic enterotoxin (Sta) that influences intestinal ion and fluid secretion to produce a noninflammatory secretory diarrhea.

Another type of diarrheal disease in calves has been associated with enteropathogenic *E. coli* (EPEC) that adhere to the intestine to produce so-called attaching and effacing lesions, with dissolution of the brush border and loss of microvillous structure at the site of attachment, a decrease in enzyme activity, and changes in ion transport in the intestine. Some produce verotoxin, which may be associated with more severe hemorrhagic diarrhea.

Immunization of calves against colibacillosis by vaccination of pregnant dams can control enterotoxigenic colibacillosis. The pregnant dam is vaccinated 6 and 2 weeks before parturition to stimulate antibodies to strains of ETEC; these antibodies are then passed on to the newborn through the colostrum. A single booster is given to the dam in subsequent years.

Several maternal vaccines are on the market. They contain either inactivated bacteria with fimbriae or purified fimbriae (F5 adhesins). However, there are ETEC which produce colonization factors not included in the presently available vaccines, such as F17 fimbriae.

The most widely used vaccine is a subunit vaccine made of a purified preparation of the attachment pili. The antipilus antibodies protect animals by preventing bacterial attachment to the intestinal wall.

There are also antigens against the subunit of *E. coli* enterotoxin, generated by gene cloning. The cloned subunits are antigenic and function as effective toxoids. One or more valences of ETEC strains (K99 or F5, F41, F17, CS31A) are often combined with vaccines against other causes of newborn calf diarrhea, especially rotavirus and coronavirus. These vaccines confer excellent protection to the newborn calves of dams that have been vaccinated, provided they receive colostrum.

6.6.3 Clostridial Diseases

Clostridial diseases include a complex group of infections affecting many animal species. Enteritis and enterotoxemia due to *Clostridium perfringens* are by far the most important of the clostridial diseases in farm animals. Other *Clostridium* spp. such as *C. septicum*, *C. chauvoei*, *C. sordellii*, *C. novyi*, and *C. haemolyticum* are associated with a number of necrotic and gas gangrene infections in animal species. *Clostridium tetani* and *C. botulinum* respectively cause tetanus and botulism (El Idrissi and Ward 2010).

Ensuring correct husbandry methods combined with vaccination is the most effective way to prevent the occurrence of clostridial infections, and to reduce the losses they cause to livestock production. Clostridial vaccines are effective and protection is mostly by humoral immunity based on the circulating antibodies against clostridial toxins present in the body. Animals are immunized with vaccines containing a single antigen or more often a combination of 2–8 different immunogenic antigens. A large number of commercial vaccines are available; most are inactivated and consist of bacterins or toxoids or a combination of bacterins and toxoids adsorbed with aluminum hydroxide adjuvant and homogenized with formaldehyde as preservative. Toxoids generally confer better protection, except for *C. chauvoei* vaccine which requires a mixture of both somatic antigen and soluble toxins to produce effective protection (El Idrissi and Ward 2010).

Single vaccination with most clostridial vaccines does not provide adequate levels of protection and must be followed by a booster dose within 3–6 weeks. Vaccination of young animals does not yield adequate protective immunity until they are at least 1–2 months old. Therefore, most vaccination strategies target the pregnant dam during the last third of pregnancy so that maximal immunity is transferred to the neonate in colostrum. Tetanus toxoid is commonly used as a single vaccine in horses but is often used in combination in sheep, goats, and cattle (for example, with *C. perfringens* types C and D in sheep and goats) (Stämpfli 2016).

6.6.4 Paratuberculosis

Paratuberculosis, also called Johne's disease, is a chronic intestinal disease caused by *Mycobacterium avium* subsp.

paratuberculosis (MAP), a member of the genus *Mycobacteria*. Transmission is primarily by the fecal–oral route and the incubation period can be months to years.

Control of the disease is difficult and management focuses on decreasing transmission through separation of infected and susceptible animals, and improving farm hygiene. Vaccination is another possible strategy for control of the disease, but it is not a well-accepted control measure. These mycobacterial organisms multiply slowly and maintain a particular relation with the host immune system. Certain components such as liposaccharides modulate the immunity by stimulating or repressing it. These immune characteristics make the design of effective vaccines very difficult. It has been demonstrated that vaccination of young calves (around 1 month of age) reduces the incidence of clinical disease but does not prevent the excretion of the bacterium or the development of new cases within the herd. Furthermore, vaccinations may compromise eradication programs based on the detection and culling of infected animals as the vaccines are not DIVA, and therefore vaccinated animals may test positive when tested serologically for either paratuberculosis or bovine tuberculosis. Thus, the decision to resort to vaccination to combat paratuberculosis should be taken carefully and vaccination should be regarded as a means to complement sanitary measures when dealing with the disease. Furthermore, such vaccination is subject to regulatory aspects that must be adhered to in many countries across the world. The restrictions, however, do not apply to vaccination of sheep and goats.

One of the most widely used vaccines in sheep and goats consists of a suspension of inactivated MAP strain 316F. It is believed that vaccination reduces not only clinical signs of paratuberculosis, lesions, and mortality but also fecal excretion of the pathogen.

6.7 Bacterial Vaccines Against Abortifacient Diseases

There are several bacterial diseases that cause abortion in livestock for which there are vaccines available. Often these diseases are also zoonotic. Vaccination not only prevents reproductive failure, abortions, and stillbirths, thereby protecting and improving animal production, but also protects human health. It is important to vaccinate animals at the appropriate time, according to the product label, particularly with modified live vaccines, to ensure the safety of the fetus. Live vaccines should not be used in pregnant animals.

6.7.1 Coxiellosis (Q Fever)

Coxiella burnetii is the causative agent of Q fever, a zoonotic bacterial disease for which domestic ruminants are the main reservoir. The infection is usually asymptomatic in ruminants, but late-term abortions, stillbirths, and birth of weak offspring may occur in sheep and goats. In cattle, metritis, infertility, and abortions associated with the infection are sometimes reported.

Transmission of the disease to humans often results from the inhalation of aerosolized organisms, although ingestion of the organism such as from unpasteurized milk products can also lead to disease.

Coxiella burnetii is an obligate intracellular pathogen, and can form spore-like structures, which make the organism resilient and allow it to persist in the environment, be carried as a fomite and transmitted by wind. The organism also has two distinct antigenic phases (I and II), which are morphologically the same but differ biochemically including the lipopolysaccharide composition of the outer membrane.

Vaccination of cattle, goats, and sheep against Q fever uses an inactivated vaccine derived from the Nine Mile strain of *C. burnetii* in phase I, which reduces the clinical impact of the disease and the excretion of the pathogen to the environment. A study of the vaccine efficacy in dairy goats was performed during the outbreak of Q fever in the Netherlands which started in 2007 (Hogerwerf et al. 2011). The study found that following vaccination, fewer animals tested positive for the presence of bacteria by polymerase chain reaction (PCR) in uterine fluid, vaginal swabs, and milk. The bacterial load in animals that tested positive was lower than bacterial loads in unvaccinated animals. This study was consistent with other studies where vaccination does not always prevent disease but can reduce the bacterial load, which may reduce environmental contamination and human exposure.

6.7.2 Small Ruminant Chlamydiosis

Chlamydiae are obligate intracellular bacteria with a wide host range, several of which are zoonotic, causing a wide spectrum of diseases. The most important veterinary species are *Chlamydophila psittaci*, causing respiratory infections in poultry (psittacosis/ornithosis), and *C. abortus*, causing enzootic abortion, one of the most important causes of ovine and caprine abortion worldwide (Meeusen et al. 2007).

Currently, two types of vaccines (inactivated and attenuated live) against abortive chalmydiosis in sheep and goats are available commercially, to be administered intramuscularly or subcutaneously at least 4 weeks before breeding to aid in the prevention of abortion (Rank 1999). A multicomponent recombinant vaccine against *C. abortus* remains a future goal of chlamydial vaccine research (Longbottom and Livingstone 2006).

Inactivated vaccines can be prepared from infected yolk sacs or cell cultures (Jones et al. 1995) and incorporate whole organisms or fractions of them (Tan et al. 1990) using the appropriate biosecurity precautions to prevent human contamination. Inactivated vaccines are safe for administration during pregnancy and have been widely used in the control of enzootic abortion in sheep. However, although inactivated vaccines may reduce the abortion rate, they do not completely prevent bacterial shedding and reproductive failures may still occur (Rodolakis and Laroucau 2015).

The commercial live attenuated vaccine is a chemically induced temperature-sensitive mutant strain, TS1B, of the *C. abortus* reference strain AB7, obtained by nitrosoguanidine mutagenesis that grows at 35–38 °C but not at 39.5 °C, the body temperature of sheep. The vaccine induces good and long-lasting protection in sheep (Chalmers et al. 1997) and goats (Rodolakis and Souriau 1986). It is supplied lyophilized and must be reconstituted in diluent immediately before administration. Importantly, the live vaccine must not be given to animals being treated with antibiotics, particularly tetracyclines. Live chlamydial vaccines cannot be used in pregnant animals.

Both types of vaccine are used in controlling disease, but neither confers absolute protection against challenge or completely eliminates the shedding of infective organisms. No firm data are available, but revaccination is recommended every 1–3 years, according to the exposure risk. The live vaccine strain 1B has been detected in the placentas of vaccinated animals that have aborted as a result of ovine enzootic abortion, suggesting a possible role for the vaccine in causing disease (Sargison et al. 2015; Wheelhouse et al. 2010). Despite this disadvantage, the use of live vaccine remains the most effective method of protecting from the disease (Stuen and Longbottom 2011).

6.7.3 Brucellosis

Brucellosis is a zoonotic disease, endemic in some regions of the world such as Latin America, Middle East, Africa, and Asia. The disease in animals is responsible for abortion and infertility. Due to the public health importance of brucellosis and the economic losses that it causes to the livestock industry, much effort has been expended to control and eradicate the disease, particularly in domestic ruminants. Available vaccines are effective in controlling the disease but they have numerous drawbacks, such as interference with diagnostic tests, pathogenicity for humans and potential to cause abortion in pregnant animals (Dorneles et al. 2015). More details on *Brucella* vaccines and their use in brucellosis control in different animal species are provided in Chapter 22.

6.7.4 Bovine Leptospirosis

Leptospirosis is a bacterial infection caused by pathogenic species of the genus *Leptospira*, affecting humans and animals. It can be spread through direct contact with an infected animal or, more commonly, by exposure to water sources contaminated by the urine of an infected animal.

Leptospira interrogans serovars of major importance in cattle are Hardjo, Pomona, Grippotyphosa, Bratislava, Icterohaemorrhagiae, and Canicola. Cattle are maintenance hosts for serovar Hardjo, which has the ability to colonize and persist in the genital tract of infected cows and bulls.

Sheep and goats are considered resistant to leptospiral infection, with lower seroprevalence rates and only a small number of serogroups implicated in clinical disease.

Vaccines for veterinary use are widely available and most often are inactivated suspensions of multiple serovars of *L. interrogans* as vaccines are only protective against the serovar(s) included and perhaps closely related serovars. Most cattle vaccines include Hardjo, while the other serovars included may vary depending on the region and prevalent serovars. While a range of experimental vaccines based on cellular extracts has been tested, all commercial vaccines are whole cell products. Vaccines may contain various adjuvants.

A number of monovalent products used in cattle have been shown to produce clinical and microbiological protection for up to 1 year and a successful vaccination program requires epidemiological studies to assess the incidence of different *Leptospira* serovars in a given population (Adler and de la Peña Moctezuma 2010).

6.8 Bacterial Vaccines Against Respiratory Diseases

Respiratory tract infections are a major cause of morbidity and mortality among farm animals and poultry. Poor management practices, such as mixing of different age groups and multiple stresses, can intensify the impact of these conditions. Furthermore, certain diseases result from the interplay of several pathogens, and multiple agents must be represented in vaccines. Finally, whenever possible, vaccines against respiratory diseases should be administered so as to elicit a primarily mucosal immunity; unfortunately, for the time being, only a small number of such vaccines are available on the market.

6.8.1 Hemorrhagic Septicemia

Hemorrhagic septicemia (HS) is a peracute or acute, highly fatal disease of cattle and water buffalo caused by various serotypes of *Pasteurella multocida*, where serotypes are identified by a letter indicating the capsular antigen and a number indicating the somatic antigen. Types B:2 and E:2 are endemic in Asia and in Africa, respectively (corresponding to the newer 6:B and 6:E classification by the Namioka–Carter system). Type B is also present in some eastern and central African countries and it is therefore recommended to use a bivalent vaccine in these countries (Benkirane and de Alwis 2002). Other serotypes such as A:1 and A:3 have been associated with HS-like conditions in India (Kumar et al. 1996) and serotypes B1 and B:3,4 have also been associated with disease (Bastianello and Henton 2004).

There are three types of bacterins used against HS: alum-precipitated, oil-adjuvanted, and formalinized bacterins. Immunity subsequent to the use of bacterins is of short duration, lasting from 6 to 9 months on primary vaccination and 12 months after booster vaccination. Alum-precipitated vaccines are most commonly used, as they are easy to inject.

An intranasal, live vaccine of nonvirulent serotype B:3,4 was developed and used in Myanmar to control the disease in cattle and water buffaloes. While it seems to have been successful, it has not gained acceptance outside this country.

6.8.2 *Mannheimia haemolytica* Infection in Cattle

Mannheimia haemolytica is a normal constituent of the nasopharynx but can also be one of several pathogens associated with bovine respiratory disease. Bovine respiratory disease can be caused by one of several viruses or other stressful conditions, such as transport or changes in climate, which predispose animals to overgrowth of *M. haemolytica*, followed by inhalation and colonization of the lungs giving rise to a fibrinous and necrotizing lobar pneumonia and pleuropneumonia.

Over 20 serotypes of *M. haemolytica* have been identified to date, subdivided into two biotypes (A and T). Biotype A serotype 1 (A1) is most commonly associated with pneumonic lesions, but other serotypes can be involved, such as 2 and 6.

Shewen and Wilkie (1985) demonstrated that immunity against *M. haemolytica* requires antibodies against both the heat-labile leukotoxin (LKT) as well as antibodies against cell surface antigens. This discovery enabled the production of specific toxoids and paved the way for an intensive search for other protective antigens of *M. haemolytica* that is still continuing (Hodgins et al. 2005; Ayalew et al. 2011; Alvarez et al. 2015). Outer membrane proteins, neuraminidase, adhesins, lipopolysaccharides, and fusion proteins have all been investigated for vaccine use to increase the efficacy of vaccines composed of LKT.

Most of the *M. haemolytica* vaccines available commercially consist of culture supernatants or cell extracts (with or without LKT) and are used parenterally.

6.9 *Mycoplasma* Vaccines

Mycoplasma species cause a variety of diseases in various animal species, including pigs, poultry, and ruminants. In small ruminants, two clinical entities stand out due to their importance in terms of prevalence: contagious agalactia and contagious caprine pleuropneumonia (CCPP). In cattle, *Mycoplasma* infections include CBPP and *Mycoplasma bovis*. *M. bovis* is considered one of the more pathogenic species and is the most frequent *Mycoplasma* pathogen of pneumonia, mastitis, and arthritis in cattle.

Vaccines for important *Mycoplasma* diseases, including contagious bovine and caprine pleuropneumonia, have been used for centuries, consisting mainly of infected tissue or fluids which are inoculated into sites at which the risk of severe infection is slight, such as the tail and bridge of the nose. However, little progress has been made in developing safe and protective alternatives. Currently available vaccines commonly used consist of mildly attenuated strains serially passaged in eggs or in culture.

6.9.1 Contagious Bovine Pleuropneumonia

Contagious bovine pleuropneumonia (CBPP), caused by *Mycoplasma mycoides* subsp. *mycoides* (Mmm), remains one of the most important infectious diseases of cattle in sub-Saharan Africa. CBPP affects the lungs and can cause great economic loses if it is not controlled. Vaccination is an effective option for controlling the disease. However, it needs to be combined with other measures to keep the disease under complete control.

Several vaccines have been developed, and the effective ones are those based on live *Mycoplasma* organisms. However, they are of limited efficacy and duration of immunity and occasional postvaccinal reactions occur at the site of injection. An overview of vaccines currently used against CBPP is provided in Chapter 23.

6.9.2 Contagious Caprine Pleuropneumonia

Contagious caprine pleuropneumonia is a severe respiratory disease of goats caused by *Mycoplasma capricolum* subsp. *capripneumoniae* (Mccp). The acute form of the disease is characterized by unilateral serofibrinous pleuropneumonia with severe pleural effusion (Thiaucourt and Bölske 1996). Outbreaks of the disease can result in morbidity and mortality rates reaching 100%.

Transmission occurs as a result of inhalation of respiratory droplets when naïve animals are in close contact with infected animals. It has been hypothesized that a carrier state exists as outbreaks occur following introductions of healthy animals to a herd, but this remains unproven.

The disease occurs in many countries in Africa and Asia and the Middle East. Genetic studies have grouped Mccp isolates into major clusters that correlate to geographic regions. Its exact geographical distribution might be larger because it is often confused with other respiratory infections. Additionally, isolation of the organism is difficult as the organism is fastidious, so many laboratories are unable to isolate it or to differentiate it from other members of the "Mycoides cluster."

Commercially available vaccines are inactivated preparations containing saponin as an inactivating agent and adjuvant (Rurangirwa et al. 1987). This vaccine induces protection for a period exceeding 12 months. It is not recommended to vaccinate pregnant animals because of a possible reaction to saponin.

6.9.3 Contagious Agalactia

Contagious agalactia is a worldwide disease of sheep and goats characterized by mastitis, arthritis, and keratoconjunctivitis. It is mainly caused by *M. agalactiae* (Ma), but the taxonomy of *Mycoplasma* is changing and other mycoplasmas such as *M. capricolum* subsp. *capricolum* (Mcc), *M. mycoides* subsp. *capri* (Mmc), and, to a lesser extent, *M. putrefaciens* have been found to be associated with agalactia (Bergonier et al. 1997).

Vaccines for the prevention of contagious agalactia due to *M. agalactiae* are used widely in the Mediterranean countries of Europe and in western Asia. No single vaccine has been universally adopted, and no standard methods of preparation and evaluation have been applied.

In Europe, only formalin inactivated vaccines adsorbed with aluminum hydroxide in an oil emulsion are authorized. However, vaccines inactivated with phenol or with saponin have given superior protection against experimental infections (Tola et al. 1999).

Live attenuated vaccines against *M. agalactiae* have been used in Turkey for many years and have been reported to provide better protection in ewes and their lambs than inactivated vaccines (Nicholas et al. 2002). However, they can produce a transient infection with shedding of the pathogen. They should not be used in lactating animals. Saponized vaccines have been reported in India with a strong antibody response and some protection (Sunder et al. 2002).

A trivalent preparation containing *M. agalactiae*, Mcc, and Mmc is available but there are not enough data on its efficacy. Also, a multivalent formalin inactivated vaccine incorporating all four mycoplasmas, adsorbed with saponin and aluminum hydroxide, is available (Ramirez et al. 2001).

6.9.4 Avian Mycoplasmoses

Mycoplasma gallisepticum (MG) and *Mycoplasma synoviae* (MS) are considered to be the most important pathogenic mycoplasmas in poultry as they both occur worldwide. It should be noted, however, that *M. meleagridis* and *M. iowae* can also cause disease. The preferred method of control is to maintain MG- and MS-free flocks. Vaccination should be considered only in situations where field exposure is inevitable, such as on multi-age sites. Live vaccines available for the control of MG are produced from various low-virulent to nonvirulent MG strains including the following:

- The F strain of MG has been the most commonly used vaccine strain (Carpenter et al. 1981). It is a naturally occurring strain of mild to moderate virulence for chickens, but it is virulent for turkeys. It is safely administered in the nostrils of healthy birds, but when administered by aerosol or in the presence of other respiratory disease agents, such as Newcastle disease or infectious bronchitis virus, respiratory signs and air sacculitis may result. Nevertheless, aerosol or eye drop administration of the vaccine is preferred.
- Strains ts-11 and 6/85 are nonvirulent and spread to unvaccinated birds does not occur or occurs only to a limited extent, when birds are in very close contact (Ley et al. 1997). However, the level of protection they confer is less than with F strain vaccine. Strain ts-11 should be administered by eye drop and 6/85 is given as a fine spray. No postvaccination reaction should be observed with these two strains.
- A live vaccine for MS is available in several countries for use in broiler breeder and layer chickens. It is produced from a temperature-sensitive mutant, MS-H (Markham et al. 1998). Its characteristics and method of use are similar to those for the MG vaccine, ts-11.

Inactivated oil-emulsion MG bacterins are also available and prepared from a concentrated suspension of whole cells that is emulsified into an oil adjuvant.

6.10 Other Bacterial Vaccines

6.10.1 Caseous Lymphadenitis

Caseous lymphadenitis is a disease of sheep and goats caused by infection with the intracellular organism *Corynebacterium pseudotuberculosis*. Transmission occurs through contact with material or pus from subcutaneous abscesses or fomites contaminated with abscess material.

Commercial vaccines are available for caseous lymphadenitis, which can be used to reduce the within-herd incidence of disease. Vaccines commonly used are formalin inactivated, culture supernatants rich with phospholipase D gene, encoding an exotoxin characterized as a major virulence factor. Attenuated live vaccines and DNA vaccines are also used. Other genes are also being explored for their potential applications to vaccine development (Afonseca et al. 2008).

Efficacy is not 100% and vaccines should only be used in the species for which they are authorized (i.e. sheep vaccines should not be administered to goats) as adverse reactions may occur. Strict adherence to vaccine schedules as outlined by the manufacturer is also essential. Vaccination will not clear infected animals of the organism, so culling is recommended to decrease disease transmission.

6.10.2 Strangles in Horses

Strangles is a highly contagious rhinopharyngitis in horses caused by *Streptococcus equi* subsp. *equi*. Transmission occurs by direct contact with infected horses or subclinical shedders, or by indirect contact via contaminated equipment, feed, water, pastures, and other fomites. Younger horses are more commonly affected but horses of any age can be infected.

Safety and efficacy issues surrounding available vaccines are driving research efforts to develop improved vaccines for strangles. Modified live vaccines are available which are administered either intranasally or injected submucosally. These vaccines may have residual virulence leading to development of abscesses, nasal discharge, or purpura hemorrhagica. Foals less than 1 year of age should not be vaccinated as they have a higher risk of developing clinical disease. Horses that have had strangles in the previous year should not be vaccinated as they may be at increased risk of vasculitis (Boyle et al. 2018).

6.11 Summary

Veterinary bacterial vaccines continue to play an increasingly vital role in maintaining animal health and welfare. Conventional attenuated live and inactivated bacterial vaccines have been available for decades as prophylaxis against bacterial diseases. However, in many instances these vaccines have their limitations, necessitating the application of different technologies to fill the gaps.

Among the bacterial vaccines currently available, attenuated live vaccines have proven to be powerful tools in protecting animals against many bacterial diseases and, in many cases, represent superiority to subunit, killed, or recombinant vaccines. But the conventional attenuation method through repeated passaging *in vitro* may be time-consuming, somewhat unpredictable and challenging to find a balance between attenuation and immunogenicity.

Despite the difficulties in developing novel vaccines, the importance of using bacterial vaccines when possible should be encouraged. Bacterial vaccines are promising alternatives that can reduce the need to use antibiotics in food-producing animals and therefore vaccine research and development, especially for diseases with a potentially high impact on antibiotic use and antibiotic resistance, warrant more attention in the coming years.

Dedication

This chapter is dedicated to the memory of Professor Ali Benkirane who passed away during the writing of this chapter.

References

Adler, B. and de La Peña Moctezuma, A. (2010). *Leptospira* and leptospirosis. *Vet. Microbiol.* 140: 287–296.

Afonseca, V.D., Moraes, P.M., Dorella, F.A. et al. (2008). A description of genes of *Corynebacterium pseudotuberculosis* useful in diagnostics and vaccine applications. *Gen. Mol. Res.* 7 (1): 252–260.

Alvarez, A.H., Gutiérrez-Ortega, A., and Hernández-Gutiérrez, R. (2015). Identification of immunodominant proteins from *Mannheimia haemolytica* and *Histophilus somnii* by an immunoproteomic approach. *Can. J. Vet. Res.* 79 (4): 339–342.

Anon. (2011). Types of vaccines. Immunisation Advisory Centre, University of Auckland. www.immune.org.nz/types-vaccines.

Arimitsu, H., Lee, J.C., Sakaguchi, Y. et al. (2004). Vaccination with recombinant whole heavy chain fragments of *Clostridium botulinum* Type C and D neurotoxins. *Clin. Diagn. Lab. Immunol.* 11 (3): 496–502.

Ayalew, S., Shrestha, B., Montelongo, M. et al. (2011). Immunogenicity of *Mannheimia haemolytica* recombinant outer membrane proteins serotype 1-specific antigen, OmpA, OmpP2, and OmpD15. *Clin. Vaccine Immunol.* 18 (12): 2067–2074.

Bastianello, S.S. and Henton, M.M. (2004). Haemorrhagic septicaemia. In: *Infectious Diseases of Livestock*, vol. 3 (eds. J.A.W. Coetzer and R.C. Tustin), 1689–1694. Cape Town: Oxford University Press.

Benkirane, A. and de Alwis, M.C.L. (2002). Haemorrhagic septicaemia, its significance, prevention and control in Asia. *Vet. Med. Czech.* 47 (8): 234–244.

Bergonier, D., Bertholet, X., and Poumarat, F. (1997). Contagious agalactia of small ruminants: current knowledge concerning epidemiology, diagnosis and control. *Rev. Sci. Tech. Off. Int. Epiz.* 16: 848–873.

Boyle, A.G., Timoney, J.F., Newton, J.R. et al. (2018). *Streptococcus equi* infections in horses: guidelines for treatment, control and prevention of strangles – revised consensus statement. *J. Vet. Internal Med.* 32 (2): 633–647.

Buck, J.M. (1930). Studies on vaccination during calfhood to prevent bovine infectious abortion. *J. Agric. Res.* 41: 667–689.

Carpenter, T.E., Mallinson, E.T., Miller, K.F. et al. (1981). Vaccination with F-strain *Mycoplasma gallisepticum* to reduce production losses in layer chickens. *Avian Dis.* 25 (2): 404–409.

Chalmers, W.S., Simpson, J., Lee, S.J., and Baxendale, W. (1997). Use of a live chlamydial vaccine to prevent ovine enzootic abortion. *Vet. Rec.* 141: 63–67.

Clift, C. and Salisbury, D.M. (2017). Enhancing the role of vaccines in combatting antimicrobial resistance. *Vaccine* 35: 6591–6593.

Detmer, A. and Glenting, J. (2006). Live bacterial vaccines – a review and identification of potential hazards. *Microb. Cell Fact.* 5: 23. https://microbialcellfactories.biomedcentral.com/track/pdf/10.1186/1475-2859-5-23.

Dorneles, E.M., Sriranganathan, N., and Lage, A.P. (2015). Recent advances in *Brucella abortus* vaccines. *Vet. Res.* 46: 76.

El Idrissi, A.H. and Ward, D. (2010). Enterotoxemia and gas gangrene. In: *Infectious and Parasitic Diseases of Livestock* (eds. P.C. Lefevre, J. Blancou, R. Chermette and G. Uilenberg), 1207. Paris: Lavoisier.

Elberg, S.S. and Faunce, K. Jr. (1957). Immunization against *Brucella* infection. VI. Immunity conferred on goats by a nondependent mutant from a streptomycin-dependent mutant strain of *Brucella melitensis*. *J. Bacteriol.* 73 (2): 211–217.

European Medicines Agency (2013). Guideline on the requirements for combined vaccines and associations of immunological veterinary medicinal products (IVMPs). www.ema.europa.eu/en/documents/scientific-guideline/guideline-requirements-combined-vaccines-associations-immunological-veterinary-medicinal-products_en.pdf

Henriques-Normark, B. and Normark, S. (2014). Bacterial vaccines and antibiotic resistance. *Uppsala J. Med. Sci.* 119: 205–208.

Hodgins, D.G., Tuan, L., Parreno, V. et al. (2005). Mucosal veterinary vaccines: comparative vaccinology. In: *Mucosal Immunology*, 3e (eds. J. Mestecky, M.L. Lamm, W. Strober, et al.), 1085–1107. Cambridge: Academic Press.

Hoelzer, K., Bielke, L., Blake, D.P. et al. (2018). Vaccines as alternatives to antibiotics for food producing animals. Part 2: new approaches and potential solutions. *Vet. Res.* 49: 70.

Hogerwerf, L., van den Brom, R., Roest, H.I.J. et al. (2011). Reduction of *Coxiella burnetii* prevalence by vaccination of goats and sheep, the Netherlands. *Emerging Infect. Dis.* 17 (3): 379–386.

Janeway, C.A. Jr. and Medzhitov, R. (2002). Innate immune recognition. *Ann. Rev. Immunol.* 20: 197–216.

Jones, G.E., Jones, K.A., Machell, J. et al. (1995). Efficacy trials with tissue-culture grown, inactivated vaccines against chlamydial abortion in sheep. *Vaccine* 13 (8): 715–723.

Jorge, S. and Dellagostin, O.A. (2017). The development of veterinary vaccines: a review of traditional methods and modern biotechnology approaches. *Biotechnol. Res. Innovation* 1 (1): 6–13.

Kumar, A.A., Harbola, P.C., Rimler, R.B., and Kumar, P.N. (1996). Studies on *Pasteurella multocida* isolates of animal and avian origin from India. *Indian J. Comp. Microbiol. Immunol. Infec. Dis.* 17: 120–124.

Ley, D.H., McLaren, J.M., Miles, A.M. et al. (1997). Transmissibility of live *Mycoplasma gallisepticum* vaccine strains ts-11 and 6/85 from vaccinated layer pullets to sentinel poultry and identification by random amplified polymorphic DNA (RAPD) analysis. *Avian Dis.* 41: 187–194.

Lipsitch, M. and Siber, G.R. (2016). How can vaccines contribute to solving the antimicrobial resistance problem? *mBio* 7: 1–8. https://mbio.asm.org/content/mbio/7/3/e00428-16.full.pdf.

Lombard, M., Pastoret, P.P., and Moulin, A.M. (2007). A brief history of vaccines and vaccination. *Rev. Sci. Tech. Off. Int. Epiz.* 26 (1): 29–48.

Longbottom, D. and Livingstone, M. (2006). Vaccination against chlamydial infections of man and animals. *Vet. J.* 171 (2): 263–275.

Markham, J.F., Morrow, C.J., and Whithear, K.G. (1998). Efficacy of a temperature sensitive *Mycoplasma synoviae* live vaccine. *Avian Dis.* 42 (4): 671–676.

Meeusen, E.N.T., Walker, J., Peters, A. et al. (2007). Current status of veterinary vaccines. *Clin. Microbiol. Rev.* 20 (3): 489–510.

Nguyen, T.D., Vo, T.T., and Vu-Khac, H. (2011). Virulence factors in *Escherichia coli* isolated from calves with diarrhoea in Vietnam. *J. Vet. Sci.* 12: 159–164.

Nicholas, R.A., Ayling, R.D., and Stipkovits, L.P. (2002). An experimental vaccine for calf pneumonia caused by *Mycoplasma bovis*: clinical, cultural, serological and pathological findings. *Vaccine* 20 (29–30): 3569–3575.

Oettinger, T., Jørgensen, M., Ladefoged, A. et al. (1999). Development of *Mycobacterium bovis* BCG vaccine: review of the historical and biochemical evidence for a genealogical tree. *Tuber Lung Dis* 79 (4): 243–250.

Pang, T. (2009). Vaccination in developing countries: problems, challenges and opportunities. In: *Global Perspectives in Health, Vol II. Water and Health, Encyclopedia of Life Support Systems (EOLSS)* (ed. W.O.K. Grabow), 106–121. Oxford: EOLSS Publishers.

Plotkin, S.A. (2001). Immunologic correlates of protection induced by vaccination. *Pediatr. Infect. Dis. J.* 20: 63.

Ramirez, A.S., de la Fe, C., Assuncao, P. et al. (2001). Preparation and evaluation of an inactivated polyvalent vaccine against *Mycoplasma* spp on infected goats. In: *Mycoplasmas of Ruminants: Pathogenicity, Diagnostics, Epidemiology and Molecular Genetics*, vol. 5 (eds. J.B. Poveda, A. Fernandez, J. Frey and K.E. Johansson), 154–157. Brussels: European Commission.

Rank, R.G. (1999). Models of immunity. In: *Chlamydia: Intracellular Biology, Pathogenesis and Immunity* (ed. R.S. Stephens), 239–295. Washington, DC: American Society for Microbiology.

Rodolakis, A. and Laroucau, K. (2015). Review Chlamydiaceae and chlamydial infections in sheep or goats. *Vet. Microbiol.* 181 (1–2): 107–118.

Rodolakis, A. and Souriau, A. (1986). Response of goats to temperature-sensitive mutants of *Chlamydia psittaci* obtained by nitrosoguanidine mutagenesis. *Am. J. Vet. Res.* 47: 2627–2631.

Rurangirwa, F.R., McGuire, T.C., Kibor, A., and Chema, S. (1987). An inactivated vaccine for contagious caprine pleuropneumonia. *Vet. Rec.* 121: 397–402.

Sargison, N.D., Truyers, I.G., Howie, F.E. et al. (2015). Identification of the 1B vaccine strain of *Chlamydia abortus* in aborted placentas during the investigation of toxaemic and systemic disease in sheep. *N. Z. Vet. J.* 63 (5): 284–287.

Schurig, G.G., Roop, R.M., Bagchi, T. et al. (1991). Biological properties of RB51; a stable rough strain of *Brucella abortus*. *Vet. Microbiol.* 28: 171–188.

Sheriff, D. and Piercy, S.E. (1952). Experiments with an avianised strain of the organism of contagious bovine pleuropneumonia. *Vet. Rec.* 64: 615–621.

Shewen, P.E. and Wilkie, B.N. (1985). Evidence for the *Pasteurella haemolytica* cytotoxin as a product of actively growing bacteria. *Am. J. Vet. Res.* 46: 1212–1214.

Stämpfli, H.R. (2016). Clostridial vaccines. In: *Merk Veterinary Manual*, 11e (ed. S. Line). Kenilworth: Merck & Co. www.merckvetmanual.com/generalized-conditions/clostridial-diseases/clostridial-vaccines

Stuen, S. and Longbottom, D. (2011). Treatment and control of chlamydial and rickettsial infections in sheep and goats. *Vet. Clin. North Am. Food Anim. Pract.* 27 (1): 213–233.

Sunder, J., Srivastava, N.C., and Singh, V.P. (2002). Preliminary trials on development of vaccine against *Mycoplasma mycoides* subsp *mycoides* type LC infection in goats. *J. Appl. Anim. Res.* 21: 75–80.

Tan, T.W., Herring, A.J., Anderson, I.E., and Jones, G.E. (1990). Protection of sheep against *Chlamydia psittaci* infection with a subcellular vaccine containing the major outer membrane protein. *Infect. Immun.* 58 (9): 3101–3108.

Thiaucourt, F. and Bölske, G. (1996). Contagious caprine pleuropneumonia and other pulmonary mycoplasmoses of sheep and goats. *Rev. Sci. Tech.* 15 (4): 1397–1414.

Tola, S., Manunta, D., Rocca, S. et al. (1999). Experimental vaccination against *Mycoplasma agalactiae* using different inactivated vaccines. *Vaccine* 17 (22): 2764–2768.

Wheelhouse, N., Aithison, K., Laroucau, K. et al. (2010). Evidence of *Chlamydophila abortus* vaccine strain 1B as a possible cause of ovine enzootic abortion. *Vaccine* 28 (35): 5657–5663.

7

Protozoal and Rickettsial Vaccines*

Isabel Marcelino[1,2], Adela Chavez[1,2], Mohamed Gharbi[3], Marisa Farber[4], Philippe Holzmuller[2,5], Dominique Martinez[1], and Nathalie Vachiéry[1,2]

[1] *CIRAD, UMR ASTRE, Petit-Bourg, Guadeloupe, France*
[2] *CIRAD INRA, ASTRE, University of Montpellier, Montpellier, France*
[3] *Laboratoire de Parasitologie, Ecole Nationale de Médecine Vétérinaire de Sidi Thabet, University of Manouba, Sidi Thabet, Tunisia*
[4] *INTA, CONICET, Instituto de Biotecnología, Buenos Aires, Argentina*
[5] *CIRAD, UMR ASTRE, Montpellier, France*

7.1 Introduction

Vector-borne diseases (VBDs), important for both human and veterinary health, account for approximately 17% of the infectious disease burden globally, with Africa, Asia, and the Americas representing the largest zones at risk. Moreover, human activities (such as changes in land use and animal movements), emergence of acaricide/insecticide resistance, increases in international trade and travel, and other factors have a high impact on ecosystems, leading to the emergence and reemergence of VBDs (Faburay 2015). An important group of VBDs are those caused by protozoal and rickettsial pathogens, such as animal trypanosomiasis (AT), East Coast fever (ECF), tropical theileriosis (TT), bovine babesiosis (BB), bovine anaplasmosis (BA), and heartwater (HW).

These six diseases cause high levels of morbidity and mortality in livestock, mainly in developing countries, limiting productivity and reinforcing the vicious cycle of poverty. Ticks and tick-borne diseases (TBDs) affect 80% of the world's cattle population, with a widespread distribution, being particularly important in tropical and subtropical countries. The global economic losses caused by these diseases were estimated at about US$ 14–19 billion per year (as reviewed by Manjunathachar et al. 2014). BB is considered the most important TBD of cattle, from an economic point of view, as over half of the world's cattle (1.2 billion animals) are at risk of infection and disease (Bock et al. 2004). ECF is responsible for over 1 million cattle deaths per year in sub-Saharan Africa, at a cost of US$ 300 million (Tretina et al. 2015). For AT, the combined use of trypanocidal drugs and vector control is estimated to cost annually over US$ 4–5 billion in direct expenses and lost production (Angara et al. 2014). Moreover, AT and BB have been identified among the 12 diseases (zoonotic or in wildlife) most likely to increase in incidence and/or to expand their geographical range during the twenty-first century, due to predicted climate changes (Moore et al. 2012; Pérez de León et al. 2012). But VBDs not only represent an important economic burden to the countries where they are endemic, they also pose an important risk to adjacent and distant areas. In 2012, HW was categorized in the top 12 priority transboundary animal diseases and thus represents an important threat (Vachiery et al. 2013).

To limit losses incurred by these VBDs, several control measures have been used, including vector chemical control and traps, treatment of animals, chemoprophylaxis, and vaccination. For TBDs, chemical control is limited due to the development of acaricide resistance within tick populations (Manjunathachar et al. 2014). Moreover, pesticide residues in meat, milk, and the environment have raised public health and ecological concerns. Chemoprophylaxis can be effective, but only a short period of time and it is costly. In endemic areas, indigenous breeds have developed natural resistance, i.e. endemic stability, to the vectors and agents of VBDs. Nevertheless, this endemic stability is highly susceptible to variations in climate and host/pathogen phenotypes and therefore hard to maintain. More effective and sustainable integrated control methods, such as nonchemical-based vector control and vaccination, should be developed to manage these VBDs.

* All authors contributed equally to this chapter.

Veterinary Vaccines: Principles and Applications, First Edition. Edited by Samia Metwally, Gerrit Viljoen, and Ahmed El Idrissi.

Veterinary vaccines are considered as the most effective, economical and sustainable method to prevent and control several animal diseases. This chapter is intended to provide state-of-the-art information to the reader with an overview on the trends, advances, and perspectives in vaccines and vaccinology against fastidious microorganisms such as eukaryotic protozoans (*Trypanosoma* spp., *Theileria* spp., *Babesia* spp.) and obligate intracellular *Rickettsiales* (*Anaplasma marginale* and *Ehrlichia ruminantium*). We also provide a brief description of what is known about the immune responses triggered by different vaccine candidates for each pathogen. But first, we provide an overview of the complex life cycle of each pathogen, as this is the basis for vaccine research and development.

7.1.1 Life Cycle Features

7.1.1.1 Animal Trypanosomiasis

Animal trypanosomiasis is a protozoal disease that affects all species of domesticated livestock throughout several countries within the tropical and subtropical regions of the world, mainly in sub-Saharan Africa. *Trypanosoma evansi* and *T. vivax* are also found in North Africa, the Middle East, South Asia, Central and South America, and recently, cases have been reported in southern continental Europe. Two different types of trypanosomes exist, the stercorarian and the salivarian species, which present different life cycles (Carrea and Diambra 2016; Hochstetter and Pfohl 2016). *Trypanosoma theileri* (infective to cattle and transmitted by tabanid flies), *T. melophagium* (infective to sheep and transmitted by sheep keds), and *T. cruzi* (infective to humans and to wild and domestic animals and transmitted by reduviid bugs) are stercorarian trypanosomes. In the vector, these parasites develop in the posterior gut. During the blood meal, infective metacyclic trypanosomes are released in the feces and deposited on the skin of the host (illustrated for *T. cruzi* in Figure 7.1). Afterwards, they invade the surrounding host cells and differentiate into intracellular amastigotes. After multiplication by binary fission, the amastigotes redifferentiate into nonreplicative but infectious trypomastigotes, which are released into the circulatory system of the mammalian host, as bloodstream trypomastigotes. These can invade other host cell types and reinitiate a new replication cycle. A new vector becomes infected once it feeds on infected animals. Once in the insect midgut, the ingested trypomastigotes differentiate into epimastigotes and multiply (Carrea and Diambra 2016).

The salivarian trypanosomes *Trypanosoma brucei brucei*, *T. congolense*, *T. evansi*, and *T. vivax* are transmitted by tsetse flies (*Glossina* spp.). However, *T. evansi* and *T. vivax* can also be transmitted by hematophagous biting flies (tabanids and stomoxes) (Figure 7.2). These trypanosomes infect the insect during the blood meal and develop in its anterior gut.

During the life cycle of *T. brucei* (Figure 7.2), the infection of a host starts when an infected vector delivers growth-arrested metacyclic trypomastigotes to the mammalian bloodstream. Upon entry into the mammalian host, these nonreplicative forms differentiate into long slender forms that multiply, spreading throughout the body. In the bloodstream, some parasites transform into short stumpy, nonproliferative forms. When an infected host is bitten by a tsetse fly, the stumpy forms are taken up with the blood meal into the midgut, where they differentiate into replicative procyclic trypomastigotes to establish a midgut infection. From there, the parasites migrate toward the salivary glands and undergo a series of transformations, first into replicative epimastigotes and finally into nonproliferative

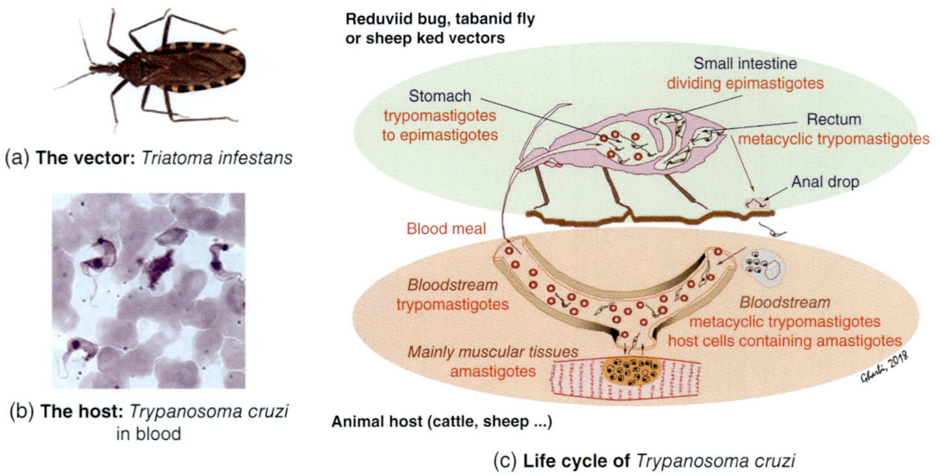

Figure 7.1 (a) Vector, (b) infected host cell morphology, and (c) life cycle of the stercorarian trypanosome *Trypanosoma cruzi*. Source: Photos by Dr Frédéric Lardeux, Institut de Recherche pour le Développement IRD, France.

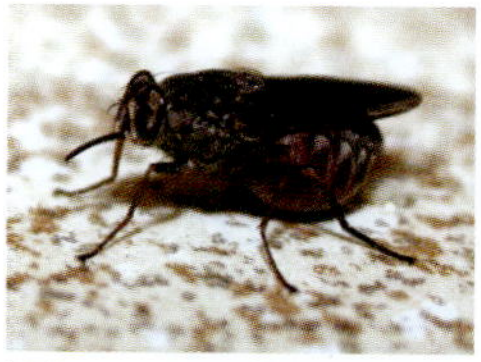

(a) **The vector:** *Glossina palpalis* (Tsetse fly)

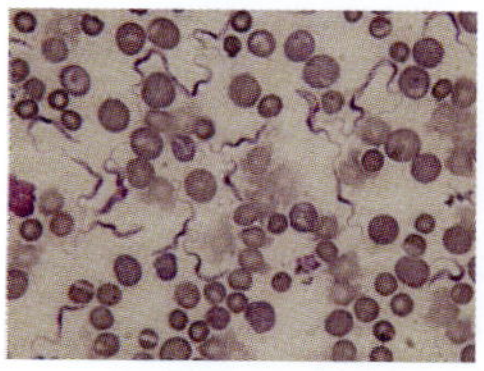

(b) **The host:** *Trypanosoma brucei brucei* in blood

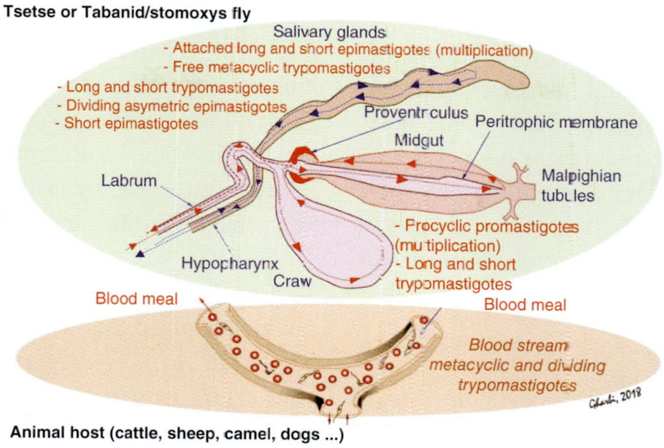

(c) **Life cycle of** *Trypanosoma brucei brucei*

Figure 7.2 (a) Vector, (b) infected host cell morphology, and (c) life cycle of the salivarian trypanosome *Trypanosoma brucei brucei*. Source: Photos by Dr P. Holzmuller and J. Javelle, Centre International de Recherche Agronomique pour le Développement (CIRAD), France.

metacyclic trypomastigotes. These will be injected into the mammalian host during blood feeding.

The life cycles of other salivarian trypanosomes are less complex: *T. congolense* does not infect salivary glands, and mechanical transmission of *T. evansi* and *T. vivax* occurs with a trypomastigote-epimastigote-trypomastigote differentiation in the esophagus of the vector (Hochstetter and Pfohl 2016).

7.1.1.2 East Coast Fever and Tropical Theileriosis

East Coast fever and TT are caused by the protozoans *Theileria parva* and *T. annulata*, respectively. *T. parva* is transmitted by *Rhipicephalus appendiculatus* ticks, while *T. annulata* is transmitted by several species of the *Hyalomma* genus (Figure 7.3). ECF occurs in eastern and southern Africa, while TT is reported in North Africa (from Mauritania to Egypt and Sudan), southern Europe (Portugal, Spain, and Turkey) and Asia (from the Mediterranean coast to China) (Lempereur et al. 2017).

In the animal host, *T. annulata* sporozoites attach to and enter into white blood cells (macrophages) (Figure 7.3). There, they develop into schizonts that turn the white blood cells into blastoid cells. Some of the schizonts develop into merozoite forms, which are then released into the bloodstream. In the blood, they invade erythrocytes and develop into piroplasms. When *Hyalomma* spp. larvae and nymph ticks feed on infected animals, they ingest erythrocytes containing the piroplasms. Once in the tick gut, the parasites

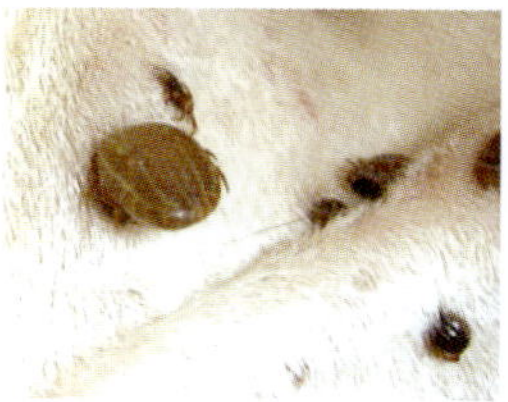

(a) **The vector:** different stages of *Hyalomma scupense* ticks attached to cattle skin

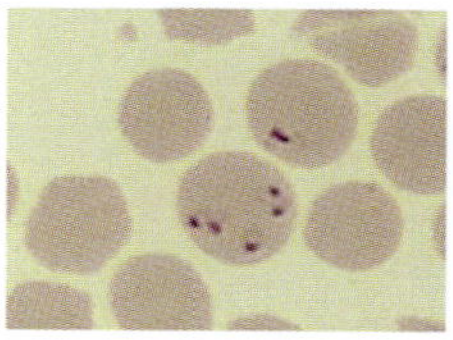

(b) **The host:** erythrocytes infected with schizonts

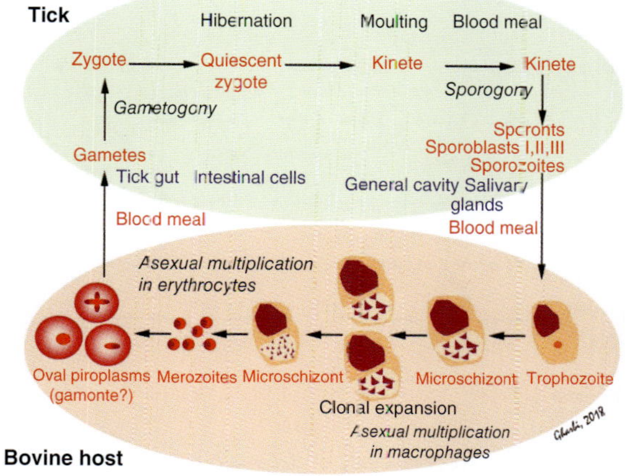

(c) **Life cycle of** *Theileria annulata*

Figure 7.3 (a) Vector, (b) infected host cell morphology, and (c) life cycle of the protozoan *Theileria annulata*. Source: Photos by Mohamed Gharbi, Ecole Nationale de Médecine Vétérinaire de Sidi Thabet, Tunisia.

differentiate into male and female gametocytes, which fuse to form zygotes. The zygotes differentiate into motile kinetes, which move to the salivary gland and enter into the acini cells. The sporozoites are injected into a cattle host through the salivary secretions, initiating a new cycle of parasite development. *T. parva* and *T. annulata* are only transmitted by adult ticks. Although *T. parva* has a similar life cycle, it preferentially infects lymphocytes (Nene et al. 2016; Nene and Morrison 2016).

7.1.1.3 Bovine Babesiosis

Bovine babesiosis is caused by intraerythrocytic protozoal parasites of the genus *Babesia*, which are transmitted by ticks of the Ixodidae family. The most common *Babesia* species infecting cattle are *Babesia bovis*, *B. bigemina*, and *B. divergens*. *B. divergens* can also infect humans, being considered an important zoonotic pathogen (Beugnet and Moreau 2015). *B. bovis* and *B. bigemina* are widespread but are primarily found in tropical and subtropical regions. *B. divergens* is localized in northern and southern Europe and in Tunisia (Lempereur et al. 2017).

Infected ticks inject sporozoites into the bovine host. The parasites enter into erythrocytes where they multiply by binary fission and undergo several changes until they become merozoites (Figure 7.4). After division, merozoites are released from the erythrocyte (mature merozoites). Mature merozoites can invade new erythrocytes to develop into trophozoites (mammalian cycling stage) or be picked up by adult ticks during the blood meal. Sexual stages (gametocytes) develop in the intestinal lumen of the tick to form a zygote with the capacity to penetrate the tick intestinal cells to give rise to motile kinetes. The kinetes destroy the intestinal cells, escape into the hemolymph and distribute into the different cell types. Infection of the tick ovaries allows transovarial transmission. During their first feeding, an infected larva attaches to a bovine host and the kinetes migrate to the salivary glands. In the salivary glands, they become sporozoites, which are injected into the mammalian host at the next blood meal. *B. bovis* is injected into cattle by larval ticks, whereas *B. bigemina* is injected by nymphal and adult ticks.

7.1.1.4 Bovine Anaplasmosis

Bovine anaplasmosis is caused by the obligate intracellular bacterium *A. marginale* and transmitted by hematophagous arthropods including ticks and hematophagous diptera (Figure 7.5). Procedures such as dehorning, castration, vaccination, and collection of blood samples may also spread the disease within a herd. Transplacental transmission from mother to calves can also occur. This disease occurs in all the Americas, Asia, Africa, and Oceania (Aubry and Geale 2011; Silaghi et al. 2017).

Ticks acquire the pathogen during the first 24 hours of blood feeding independently of the level of infection in the mammalian host. Once infected, erythrocytes are ingested by the tick vector (*Dermacentor* spp., *Rhipicephalus* spp.), *A. marginale* replicates in tick gut cells, muscle cells, and other tissues, and organisms can generally be visualized within 6 days of feeding. Two forms of *A. marginale*, reticulated and dense forms, are found in infected tick cells. Cattle become infected with *A. marginale* when the dense form is transmitted during tick feeding via the salivary glands (Figure 7.5). Once transmission occurs, the incubation period of the bacteria is between 24 and 26 days before the animals present signs of infection. Tick transmission can occur from stage to stage (transstadial) or within a stage (intrastadial), while transovarial transmission from one tick generation to the next does not appear

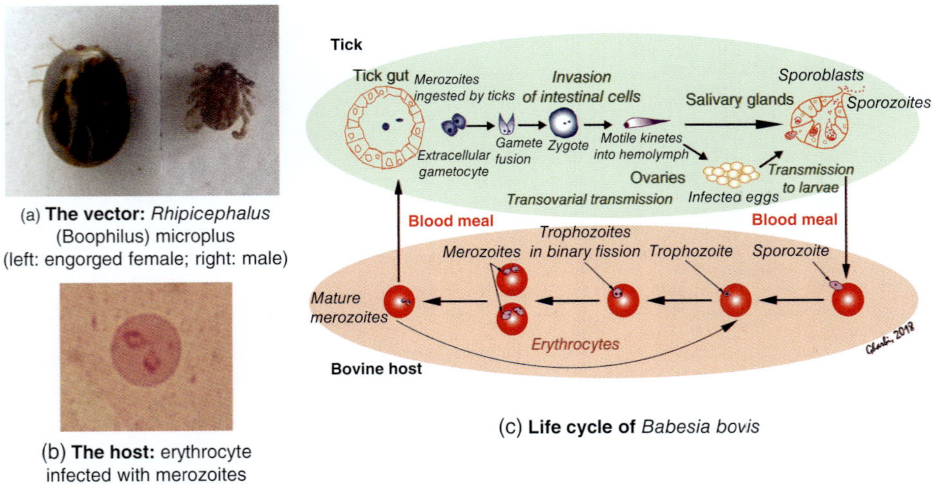

Figure 7.4 (a) Vector, (b) infected host cell morphology, and (c) life cycle of the protozoan *Babesia bovis*. Source: Photos by Marisa Farber, INTA, Argentina, and Manon Hamon, CIRAD, Guadeloupe.

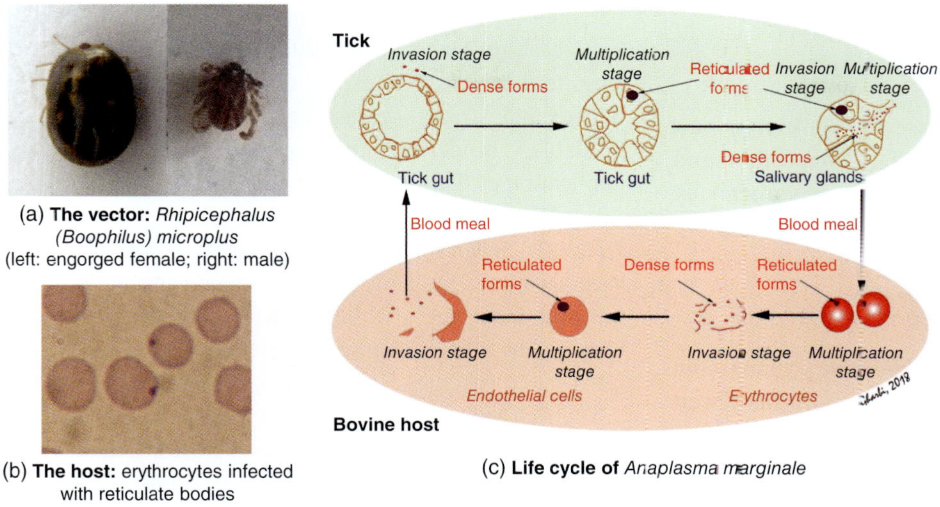

(a) **The vector:** *Rhipicephalus (Boophilus) microplus* (left: engorged female; right: male)

(b) **The host:** erythrocytes infected with reticulate bodies

(c) **Life cycle of** *Anaplasma marginale*

Figure 7.5 (a) Vector, (b) infected host cell morphology, and (c) life cycle of the rickettsial pathogen *Anaplasma marginale*. Source: Photos by Marisa Farber, INTA, Argentina, and Manon Hamon, CIRAD, Guadeloupe.

to occur. Both nymphs and adult ticks can transmit *A. marginale* (Aubry and Geale 2011; Atif 2015).

7.1.1.5 Heartwater

Heartwater, also called cowdriosis, is caused by the obligate intracellular bacterium *Ehrlichia ruminantium* and transmitted by ticks from the *Amblyomma* genus. HW is present in sub-Saharan Africa, the Indian Ocean (Madagascar, Comoro Islands, Mayotte, Réunion, Mauritius Island) and in two Caribbean islands (Guadeloupe and Antigua). The infection is particularly severe for nonindigenous livestock that are introduced into affected areas and it represents a threat for the American mainland (Marcelino et al. 2016).

In the tick, *E. ruminantium* initially develop in the gut epithelial cells and subsequently invade and develop in the salivary glands of the vector (Figure 7.6). The vertebrate host is infected via the saliva of the tick during a blood meal. Upon entry in the host, *E. ruminantium* proliferate in vascular endothelial cells, neutrophils, and macrophages, presenting a biphasic developmental cycle with two morphologically distinct forms: the extracellular infectious elementary bodies (EBs) and the intracellular metabolically active reticulate bodies (RBs). Organisms enter cells as EBs and divide within intracytoplasmic vacuoles, resulting in large colonies of RBs (morulae). *Amblyomma* ticks become infected during the larval and nymphal stages when they feed on infected hosts but only nymphal and adult ticks can transmit *E. ruminantium* to susceptible hosts, as transovarial transmission does not occur. The developmental cycle of the organism in the tick is poorly understood.

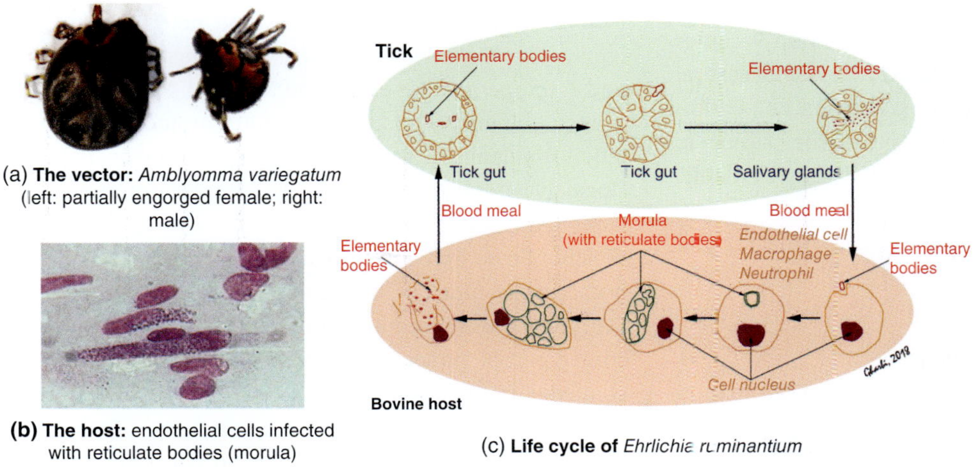

(a) **The vector:** *Amblyomma variegatum* (left: partially engorged female; right: male)

(b) The host: endothelial cells infected with reticulate bodies (morula)

(c) **Life cycle of** *Ehrlichia ruminantium*

Figure 7.6 (a) Vector, (b) infected host cell morphology, and (c) life cycle of the rickettsial pathogen *Ehrlichia ruminantium*. Source: Adapted from Marcelino et al. (2012). Photos by Nathalie Vachiéry and Willy Hilaire, CIRAD, Guadeloupe.

7.2 Types of Protozoal and Rickettsial Vaccines

This section describes the main classes of veterinary protozoal and rickettsial vaccine designs. The composition and performance of several vaccines (either commercially available or in experimental phase) are outlined.

7.2.1 Vaccines Against Trypanosomiasis

Trypanosoma cruzi is a stercorarian zoonotic trypanosome causing Chagas disease in humans. Many efforts have been made to develop vaccines against this particular pathogen (Rodriguez-Morales et al. 2015), targeting both preventive and curative vaccines (Arce-Fonseca et al. 2015; Biter et al. 2018). The strategies developed are as diverse as DNA or adenovirus-based vaccination (Arce-Fonseca et al. 2015; Pereira et al. 2015), gene-deleted live attenuated parasites (Sanchez-Valdez et al. 2015), or nanoparticle delivery system (Barry et al. 2016). Currently, clinical trials are under way with significant advances and promising results for a bivalent molecular vaccine, which consists of Tc24/TSA-1 recombinant antigens formulated on alum adjuvant together with the toll-like receptor (TLR) 4 agonist, E6020 (Sabin Vaccine Institute) (Dumonteil et al. 2012). The efficacy of the vaccine has been explained by the characteristics of the antigens used with limited antigenic variation (Knight et al. 2014) and induction of a Th1-mediated immune response. The memory immune response recall is associated with specific human leukocyte antigen (HLA) supertypes (Villanueva-Lizama et al. 2018). Moreover, other promising antigen candidates are under evaluation, such as the trans-sialidase adjuvanted by ISCOMATRIX™ (Bontempi et al. 2015; Prochetto et al. 2017) or the Tc52 in a prime-boost DNA-recombinant protein administration (Matos et al. 2016).

Many efforts have also been made to develop vaccines against salivarian trypanosomes (Table 7.1), testing several strategies that aimed at three different targets: the pathogen, the disease, and the transmission of the pathogen. Although no vaccine is currently commercially available, candidate vaccines continue to be evaluated for vaccination against pathogenic trypanosomes (Black and Mansfield 2016).

7.2.1.1 Vaccines Against the Pathogen

7.2.1.1.1 Live and Inactivated Vaccines The first vaccination trials against AT were performed using live pathogens. Trials of the infection and treatment method (ITM) in mice and cattle resulted in full to partial protection against homologous challenge (Table 7.1). The same results were obtained for inactivated vaccines (Table 7.1) (reviewed by La Greca and Magez (2011); Black and Mansfield (2016)). Despite these positive results, no data on protective effect of vaccinal strains against heterologous challenges are available, hindering the possibility of widespread application of these vaccines in the field.

7.2.1.1.2 Subunit and Recombinant Vaccines These vaccines aimed at using: (i) trypanosome-specific proteins purified from the pathogen, (ii) recombinant proteins obtained by a heterologous expression system, and/or (iii) DNA-based vaccines (Table 7.1).

The first subunit vaccine aimed at targeting the surface glycoprotein variable surface genes (VSG), which display a high antigenic variation. Intravenous administration of soluble or cell-bound VSG from *T. brucei* conferred full protection against homologous challenge in cattle but it induces only the production of short-lived IgM antibody isotypes, with limited cross-protection. Contrary to VSG, the flagellar pocket (FP), relevant in virulence, is composed of invariant proteins (Field and Carrington 2009). Immunization of cattle or mice with FP protein provided partial to no protection. Due to these results, studies with the FP vaccination were discontinued. Other proteins, native or recombinant (e.g. cysteine proteases [CPs] or tubulin), were tested as vaccine candidates on cattle and mice, conferring partial protection. A second strategy consisted of the development of DNA vaccines based on trans-sialidase, specific invariant surface glycoprotein (ISG) (Table 7.1). Only partial protection was observed in mice.

Structural molecules (i.e. actin and tubulin), proteins involved in cell division (microtubule-associated proteins [MAPs], and outer membrane-associated proteins [cation pumps]) were also tested as candidate vaccines. Immunization of mice with recombinant actin and β-tubulin from *T. brucei* or *T. evansi* conferred 60–80% protection, during both homologous and heterologous challenges with *T. brucei*, *T. rhodesiense*, *T. congolense*, *T. evansi*, and *T. equiperdum* (Li et al. 2009). In 2004, MAPp15 (native or recombinant) generated up to 100% protection against a lethal challenge with a heterologous strain of *T. brucei* (Rasooly and Balaban 2004). By contrast, immunization using the *T. brucei* cation pump Ca^{2+} ATPase (TBCA2), which is essential for trypanosome survival and cation homeostasis, failed to induce long-term protection (Ramey et al. 2009). More recently, calreticulin (CRT) was shown to confer partial protection against *T. congolense* infectious challenge in mice (Bossard et al. 2016). A second strategy was the development of DNA vaccines (Table 7.1). Immunization of mice with a plasmid encoding the catalytic and N-terminal domain of the *T. brucei* trans-sialidase, a major virulence factor of *T. cruzi*, or with *T. b. brucei*

Table 7.1 Vaccine candidates against salivarian trypanosome infections historically reported in the literature: antiparasite, antidisease, and antivector strategies

Antigen preparation	Antigen	Host	Vaccination route	Boosts	Time lapse last boost-challenge	Parasite load for infectious challenge	Immunological outcome
Inactivated parasite or ITM	Formalinized trypanosomes	Mouse	IV	1	21 and 42 d, respectively	Antilog 2.0	Partial to full protection
ITM	Live trypanosomes	Mouse	Infectious fly bites	1	21 d	Infectious fly bites	Stock-specific full protection
	Live trypanosomes	Cattle[a]	Infectious fly bites	1	3 wk	Infectious fly bites	Partial to full protection
Inactivated parasite	Alkylated trypanosomes	Mouse	IV	4	21 d	10^3	Full protection
	Irradiated trypanosomes	Cattle[a]	IV	1	14 d	10^3	Full protection
Parasite isolated	Soluble VSG	Cattle[a]	IV	1	43 d	10^4	Partial to full protection
	Soluble or cell-bound VSG	Mouse	IV	1	4–30 d	10^3	Full protection
	FP	Cattle[a]	IM	3	14 d or more	Natural exposure in the field	Partial protection
	FP	Mouse	IP	3	NI	500×	Partial/no protection
	Tubulin	Mouse	SC	3	NI	10^3	Partial protection
Recombinant protein	CP	Cattle[a]	SC[a]	4	1 mo	Experimental tsetse fly challenge	Partial protection
	Tubulin	Mouse	SC	3	6 d	10^3	Partial protection
	Actin	Mouse	SC	3	6 d	10^3	Partial protection
Recombinant protein	β-tubulin	Mouse	SC	2	35 d	10^3	Partial protection
Recombinant protein	CRT	Mouse	SC	3	15 d	10^3	Partial protection

(Continued)

Table 7.1 (Continued)

Antigen preparation	Antigen	Host	Vaccination route	Boosts	Time lapse last boost-challenge	Parasite load for infectious challenge	Immunological outcome
Plasmid DNA	Trans-sialidase	Mouse	IM	1	175 d	500	Partial protection
	ISG	Mouse	IP	1	175 d	500	Partial protection
Plasmid DNA	β-tubulin	Mouse	SC	2	21 d	10^2	Partial protection
Recombinant protein or plasmid DNA	Cation pump Ca^{2+} ATPase (TBCA2)	Mouse	IP	1	6 wk	10^6	Partial/no protection
Tsetse isolated	Tsetse fly midgut proteins	Rabbit for immunization/ tsetse fly	SC	1	NI	Infected blood	Partial protection to tsetse flies
Liposomes	GPI	Mouse	IP	2	3 wk	5×10^3	Partial protection

CP, cysteine protease; FP, flagellar pocket; GPI, glycosylphosphatidylinositol; IM, intramuscular; IP, intraperitoneal; ISG, invariant surface glycoprotein; ITM, infection and treatment method; IV, intravenous; NI, not indicated; SC, subcutaneous.

[a] Trials performed in natural host.

Source: Adapted from La Greca and Magez (2011), Kurup and Tewari (2012), Tabel et al. (2013), Black and Mansfield (2016), and Bossard et al. (2016).

bloodstream-stage trypanosome-specific, ISG or *T. evansi* tubulin, only conferred 40–60% survival rate after lethal challenge (Silva et al. 2009; Lanca et al. 2011; Kurup and Tewari 2012).

7.2.1.2 Vaccines Against the Disease: Subunit Vaccines

To eliminate or attenuate the pathophysiological effects of the infection, subunit vaccines were developed against enzymes from the CP family and the glycosylphosphatidylinositol (GPI) anchor that attaches the VSG molecules to the parasite's membrane (reviewed by La Greca and Magez 2011). The results showed that despite no effect on the early stages of the infection, animals immunized with CPs presented less severe anemia and even weight gain in posterior stages of the trypanosome infection. Inhibition of these enzymes by host-specific antibodies may alleviate the pathology associated with trypanosome infection. A second antidisease strategy consisted of a vaccine based on GPI molecules. This led to the reduction of the inflammatory response, prolonged time of animal survival, and alleviation of the clinical symptoms of the infection but the parasitaemia was not reduced. Despite the promising results, no additional results are currently available.

7.2.1.3 Vaccines Against the Transmission of the Pathogen

Transmission-blocking vaccines (TBVs) have given encouraging results after the immunization of rabbits against *Glossina* midgut extracts, which resulted not only in reduced trypanosome infection rates but also in reduced survival and fecundity of the flies themselves. However, protective antigens remain to be identified and characterized, to ensure natural boosting and success in field conditions.

More detailed information on the several vaccination strategies tested against AT can be read in reviews (La Greca and Magez 2011; Tabel et al. 2013; Black and Mansfield 2016).

7.2.2 Vaccines Against East Coast Fever and Tropical Theileriosis

For ECF and TT, live vaccines are currently commercially available and subunit vaccines are under development.

7.2.2.1 ECF: Infection and Treatment Method and Subunit Vaccines

The ITM against ECF is based on the inoculation of live *T. parva* sporozoites (extracted from ground-up, infected whole ticks) and simultaneous administration of oxytetracycline. This multivalent vaccine (called the Muguga Cocktail) contains three *T. parva* strains: Muguga, Kiambu 5, and Serengeti transformed. Originally developed by the East African Veterinary Research Organization (now the Kenya Agriculture Research Institute), it is now licensed and being produced by a commercial enterprise for distribution in Kenya, Tanzania, and Malawi (GALVmed; www.galvmed.org). Efforts are currently being made to scale up the production process of this vaccine in order to make it more widely available on a commercial basis. Efficacy of this ITM protocol is high and protection lasts at least 3 years, but sterile immunity is not achieved. As for many live vaccines, it requires a cold chain for transportation and risks introducing the parasites into ECF-free areas.

Alternatively, two antigens derived from the sporozoite surface antigen p67 have been tested as subunit vaccines: a partially complete (p67) and an 80 amino acid C-terminal section (p67C). Vaccination using p67 was tested against *T. parva* on cattle in Kenya. The reduction of ECF infection varied between 47% and 52%. Although p67 vaccination reduced the severity of infection after tick challenge, p67 is very unstable in both bacterial and eukaryotic expression systems. This made it necessary to look for alternative options. Bishop and co-workers showed that the p67C peptide confers protection against ECF comparable to p67, suggesting that a synthetic peptide vaccine might be achievable (Bishop et al. 2003).

A detailed review of all the vaccines and antigens tested against ECF is presented by Nene et al. (2016).

7.2.2.2 TT: Live Attenuated Vaccines

Because the ITM approach to *T. annulata* infection can lead to a carrier state infection, which is not suitable in farms with strong tick infestations, a live attenuated vaccine was developed. The vaccination strategy for this consists of the subcutaneous injection of attenuated *T. annulata* schizonts obtained by continuous *in vitro* culture in macrophages. This attenuation process, which is associated with loss of expression of parasite-induced matrix metalloproteinases, has been applied to many strains (Nene and Morrison 2016). Two commercially available live attenuated vaccines have been developed with this approach: Tayledoll® (DollVet company, Turkey) and Rakshavac-T® (Indian Immunologicals Ltd., India). Tayledoll is injected at a dose of 1×10^7 schizonts in 1.4% DMSO to cattle aged more than 3 months. The animals are protected after 45 days, and as such, the vaccine should be administered to susceptible animals at least 2 months before the tick season. Rakshavac-T is based on the strain Hisar and confers protection for up to 1 year in endemic regions. These vaccines show high efficacy

(>90%) and safety (100%), with little evidence of reversion to virulence. Immunity is cross-protective among strains. Vaccinal protection lasts at least 19 months in the field and although vaccine strains may cause cryptic infections, latent organisms are incapable of transmission to ticks. Table 7.2 summarizes the live attenuated vaccines currently available commercially or under experimental phase.

7.2.2.3 TT: Subunit Vaccines

Subunit vaccine development against *T. annulata* infection has focused on surface antigens such as SPAG-1 (present on sporozoites), Tams1 (present on merozoites), and TaSP (a highly antigenic *T. annulata* surface protein). These antigens have been tested individually, in combination regimes (as a cocktail or prime-boost strategy), or associated with a live attenuated vaccine (Gharbi et al. 2011; Jeyabal et al. 2012; Nene and Morrison 2016). Despite efforts in developing subunit and recombinant vaccines, none of these have so far replaced the conventional live-attenuated vaccines.

7.2.3 Babesiosis

Two main strategies have been used to develop vaccines against babesiosis: live attenuated and subunit vaccines. Commercially available live vaccines are presented in Table 7.3.

7.2.3.1 Live Attenuated Vaccines

Many BB vaccines are currently produced by governmental organizations around the world. These vaccines can be produced either by inoculation of calves with erythrocytes infected with selected strains, or by *in vitro* culture methods to produce parasites to be used as antigens (Table 7.3). Most vaccines are produced *in vivo* by injecting splenectomized calves with *B. bovis*, *B. bigemina*, or both species (Table 7.3). Vaccines derived from infected erythrocytes are produced in calves that are free from infectious agents with strains that are not tick transmissible, i.e. *B. bigemina* G, *B. bovis* R1A, and the South African strain *B. bovis* S24. Protective immunity develops 3–4 weeks after vaccination and normally lasts at least 4 years (OIE 2017b).

Vaccines can then be prepared in frozen or chilled forms depending on the demand, transport networks, and availability of liquid nitrogen or dry ice supplies (Table 7.3). Chilled vaccines (4 °C) have limited shelf-life (4–7 days) and safety and efficacy can only be tested retrospectively. Frozen vaccines allow long-term storage and each batch can go through postproduction testing. However, they are susceptible to damage after thawing, are more costly to produce, and more difficult to transport. These vaccines, however, carry a high risk of pathogen contamination (OIE 2017b).

In addition, many babesiosis vaccines may induce clinical disease. For example, a Cuban vaccine was reported to have a 2% rate of postvaccination disease incidence (McAllister 2014). This risk is higher in adult animals, so vaccinations are typically restricted to juveniles. If application is necessary in older animals, daily monitoring is suggested for up to 21 days and treatment is often needed (Shkap et al. 2005; de Waal and Combrink 2006).

A trivalent formula containing 10^7 erythrocytes infected with *Anaplasma centrale* is commercialized in areas with anaplasmosis (Table 7.3). This formula can be prepared in

Table 7.2 Specificity of available live attenuated vaccines against tropical theileriosis.

Country	Cell line	Number of passages	Dose (cells)	Vaccination route	Duration of immunity (year)
Turkey[a]	ND	–	1×10^7	SC	1
India[b]	Hisar	ND	ND	SC	3 (1 year in endemic areas)
China	–	95–98	10^6	IM	19 mo (1 year in endemic areas)
Iran	S15	–	$2.5–2.8\times10^6$	SC	More than 1 year
Uzbekistan	TAU-219	120	5.10^7	SC	ND
Tunisia	LC1	100	2.10^6	SC	2
Morocco (two vaccine strains)	Ghrab	3	10^2 to 10^8	SC	ND
	Doukala	256	10^4	SC	<6 mo

IM, intramuscular; ND: not determined; SC, subcutaneous.
Note: Trials were performed in cattle using a single injection.
[a] Tayledoll® commercialized by DollVet company (Turkey).
[b] Rakshavac-T® commercialized by Indian Immunologicals Ltd. (India).

either frozen or chilled form and is recommended to be applied to calves that are 4–10 months of age. Protective immunity develops 3–4 weeks after vaccination and normally lasts at least 4 years.

7.2.3.2 Subunit Vaccines

Due to the adverse reactions in highly susceptible animals and the difficulties in vaccine production and storage, subunit vaccines have been investigated. The discovery of candidate antigens to be used as a subunit vaccine has been extensively reviewed (Gohil et al. 2013; Florin-Christensen et al. 2014). Several antigens such as the rhoptry-associated protein 1 (RAP-1), the merozoite surface antigen-2c (MSA-2c), and the small heat shock protein 20 (HSP20) have been tested alone (i.e. RAP-1) or in combination with other proteins (i.e. MSA-2c). However, none of these antigens stimulated a protective immune response. In 2014, a recombinant modified vaccinia Ankara virus expressing a chimeric multi-antigen containing B and T cell epitopes from MSA-2c, RAP-1, and HSP20 antigens was evaluated in a mouse model. The results showed that the best vaccination strategy is a prime with a protein cocktail and a boost with the recombinant virus. These results open a window of opportunity for additional testing in cattle (Jaramillo Ortiz et al. 2014).

7.2.4 Bovine Anaplasmosis

Many vaccination trials have been tried to induce a protective immune response against *A. marginale* (Table 7.4). For this, two main strategies were followed: (i) develop vaccine against the pathogen and (ii) block the transmission of the pathogen. In the first case, live attenuated, subunit, DNA-based, and nano-vaccines have been developed. At the moment, only a live attenuated vaccine is commercially available, as will be discussed below.

Table 7.3 Vaccines available against bovine babesiosis.

Country	Vaccine name	Producer	Strains/production system	Storage conditions	Commercially available
Argentina	BioJaJa (trivalent)	Litoral Biológicos[a]	Bbo, Bbi/*in vitro* and Acent/*in vivo*	Ultrafreezing	Yes
	Babesan -Anacent	INTA Mercedes[b]	Bbo, Bbi, Acent/*in vivo*	+4 °C	
	Vacuna contra la Babesiosis y Anaplasmosis	INTA Rafaela[b]	Bbo, Bbi/*in vitro*, Acent/*in vivo*	+4 °C	
Australia	Combavac three in one live tick fever vaccine	Tick Fever Centre (TFC), Wacol[b]	Bbo, Bbi, Acent/*in vivo*	Ultrafreezing	
	Trivalent tick fever vaccine		Bbo, Bbi, Acent/*in vivo*	+4 °C	
South Africa	Frozen African Redwater	Onderstepoort Biological Products[c]	Bbi/*in vivo*	Ultrafreezing	
			Bbo/*in vivo*	Ultrafreezing	
Brazil	Embravac	EMBRAPA[b]	Bbo, Bbi, Acent/*in vivo*	Ultrafreezing	No
Columbia	Anabasan	Limor de Colombia SA[d]	Bbo, Bbi, Amarg/*in vivo*		
Israel	Israeli vaccine strains of *B. bovis*, *B. bigemina* and *A. centrale*	Kimron Veterinary Institute[b]	Bbo, Bbi, Acent/*in vivo*		
Mexico	Vacuna contra la Babesiosis Bovina	Cenid-Pavet- INIFAP[b]	Bbo, Bbi/*in vitro*		
Uruguay	Hemovacuna	Miguel C Rubino[b]	Bbo, Bbi, Acent/*in vivo*	+4 °C	

Bbo, Bbi, Acent, Amarg, bovine erythrocytes infected with *Babesia bovis*, *B. bigemina*, *Anaplasma centrale*, or *A. marginale* respectively; *in vitro*, *in vitro* produced Bbo and Bbi-infected erythrocytes; *in vivo*, infected erythrocytes obtained from splenectomized calves. NA, not available. Ultrafreezing is in liquid nitrogen.

[a] Private undertaking.

[b] Public institution.

[c] Public commercially driven enterprise.

[d] Public/private partnership.

7.2.4.1 Live Attenuated Vaccines

Live attenuated vaccines against BA can be obtained by *in vivo* passage on nontarget hosts, *in vitro* culture using tick cell lines, and by using a live-modified *A. marginale* (Aubry and Geale 2011; Silaghi et al. 2017). The level of protection induced by these different antigens varied from partial to full (Table 7.4).

At the moment, the only vaccine commercially available against BA contains *A. marginale* subsp. *centrale* and is called Anavac® (PHL Associates, USA). This is a naturally occurring strain that is less virulent when injected into susceptible animals, producing protective immunity against severe disease. Vaccination of animals is performed by injecting susceptible animals with blood from *A. marginale* subsp. *centrale*-infected cattle. This vaccine was used in several countries for over 100 years. However, due to the side effects inherent in live vaccines, its use has been restricted and it is now mainly commercialized in Zimbabwe, Argentina, Colombia, Israel, and Australia, where it is considered economically justified (OIE 2017a).

7.2.4.2 Subunit Vaccines

Several attempts have been made to develop effective subunit vaccines using antigens purified from the pathogen (outer membrane fractions) or recombinant proteins. Preparations of outer-membrane proteins (OMPs) were tested in cattle and complete protection against homologous challenge, with protection against anemia in heterologous challenges, was obtained (Tebele et al. 1991; Brown et al. 1998; Noh et al. 2013). As an alternative, *A. marginale* OM genes were cloned and expressed in a heterologous expression system. Initial attempts were directed against major surface proteins (MSPs). However, cross-protection was shown to be poor and limited as the proteins are highly variable (Agnes et al. 2011; Chavez et al. 2012). A second attempt was directed against Type IV secretion system (T4SS) proteins (VirB2, VirB7, VirB9-1, VirB9-2, VirB10, and VirB11) (Lopez et al. 2005; Sutten et al. 2010). Recombinant versions of these proteins were strongly recognized by both antibodies and T cells (Lopez et al. 2007). To boost immunogenicity of these proteins, VirB9-1 and VirB9-2 were combined with nanoparticles (silica vesicles SV-100) to increase the amount of repetitive antigens available and to improve the display by antigen-presenting cells (Zhao et al. 2016). However, as tests were done in mice, the real potential of these preparations as vaccines against *A. marginale* still needs to be evaluated in ruminants.

Table 7.4 Vaccination strategies tested for bovine anaplasmosis (Kocan et al. 2010; Aubry and Geale 2011; Quiroz-Castaneda et al. 2016; Silaghi et al. 2017).

Vaccine	Vaccination route	Boosts	Type of protection	Animal tested
Live *A. centrale* blood[a]	IV	No	Partial	Cattle
Attenuated *A. marginale*	IM	No	Partial	Cattle
	IV	No	Partial	Cattle
Deer attenuated *A. marginale*	IV	No	Partial to full	Cattle
Attenuated tick-cultured *A. marginale*	SC	4	Partial	Cattle
Purified *A. marginale*	SC	2	Partial to full	Cattle
Tick-cultured *A. marginale*	SC	2	Partial	Cattle
Tick-cultured *A. marginale*	SC	3	None	Cattle
Cross-linked *A. marginale* outer membranes	SC	3	Partial	Cattle
Live modified *A. marginale*	IV	No	Partial	Cattle
Purified outer membrane *A. marginale*	SC	3	Partial to full	Cattle
Subolesin-MSP1	IM	2	Partial	Cattle and sheep
Recombinant AM936	SC	4	None	Cattle
Recombinant AM854	SC	4	None	Cattle
DNA vaccine (pcDNA3.1/MSP1b)	IM	3	Partial	Cattle

IM, intramuscular; IV, intravenous; IM, intramuscular; SC, subcutaneous.
[a] Commercially available.

7.2.4.3 DNA Vaccines

DNA vaccines using *A. marginale* genes have also been tested. DNA vaccines using plasmids containing the complete coding sequence for Msp1β (de Andrade et al. 2004) and antigen CD205 fused with a domain that activates dendritic cells (Njongmeta et al. 2012) showed promise but the actual efficacy of the vaccines against homologous or heterologous challenges remains to be tested.

7.2.4.4 Vaccines Against the Transmission of the Pathogen (Subunit Vaccines)

Because of the difficulty in finding protective vaccine options within the bacterial protein repertoire, vaccination with tick proteins involved in pathogen–vector interactions is being explored (de la Fuente et al. 2016). Subolesin is a tick protein involved in *A. marginale* transmission. This vaccine candidate, as well as other tick antigens, led to reduction in the fertility of larvae molting to nymphs and engorged females. Chimeric vaccines composed of MSP1α-tick antigen produce higher immune response and a more cost-effective production of the antigen and resulted in reduced *A. marginale* strain diversity in endemic regions. Thus, the use of vaccines based on tick antigens for the control of *A. marginale* transmission is an important option that could be considered in the future for integrated management of both ticks and TBPs (de la Fuente et al. 2016).

The vaccines tested for BA have been extensively reviewed (Kocan et al. 2010; Aubry and Geale 2011; Quiroz-Castaneda et al. 2016; Silaghi et al. 2017).

7.2.5 Heartwater

Four immunization strategies against HW are currently available (Table 7.5): the ITM, *in vitro* attenuated or chemically inactivated *in vitro* grown bacteria, and recombinant DNA and/or protein (Marcelino et al. 2016).

Table 7.5 Vaccination strategies tested for heartwater.

Vaccine	Host	Vaccine isolate	Challenge isolate(s)[a]	Type of protection
ITM[b]	Cattle	Ball 3	Ball 3	Full
Live attenuated	Sheep/goat	Senegal	Senegal, Welg., Umpala, Lutale, Ball 3; Gardel Um Banein	None to full (for homologous challenge)
		Gardel	Gardel	Full
		Welgevonden	Welgevonden; Ball 3; Gardel; Mara 87/7, Blaauwkrans	Partial to full
Inactivated cell cultured organism (+ adjuvant)	Cattle/goat	Gardel	Gardel	Partial to full
	Sheep	Crystal Spring[c]	Crystal Spring; Crystal Spring (ticks) Beatrice (ticks)	Partial to full
		Mbizi	Mbizi, Beatrice Isiolo, Welgevonden; Beatrice (ticks)	
	Goats/sheep/cattle	Mbizi, Sunnyside, Lutale, Bathurst	Field tick challenge	Partial
Subunit/recombinant	Mice	*map-1* DNA vaccine (Crystal Spring)	Crystal Spring	Partial
	Sheep	Cocktail of genes (Welg.)	Welg.	Partial to full
	Mice/sheep	*cpg1* gene (Welg.)	Welg.	None to full
	Mice	*groEL, groES* genes (Welg.)	Welgevonden	None
	Mice	*E. coli* lysates expressing 5 different genes	Highway	Highly variable

[a] The challenge of vaccinated animals was intravenous (IV), unless stated otherwise (ticks; via ticks).
[b] The immunization by the "infection and treatment" method is less effective in goats and sheep than in cattle, and mortalities due to infection are observed despite treatment. This is the only commercially available vaccine.
[c] This strain is not highly pathogenic in cattle.
Source: Adapted from Marcelino et al. (2016); Faburay et al. (2017).

7.2.5.1 Infection and Treatment Method

In the ITM approach, animals are injected with blood infected with the highly virulent *E. ruminantium* Ball 3 strain and subsequently treated with long-acting oxytetracycline to prevent disease. Despite the low cross-protection levels of the Ball 3 blood vaccine strain against other *E. ruminantium* strains and the fact that it is a risky control method, it has been the only commercially available vaccine for more than 50 years, mainly in South Africa (Onderstepoort Biological Products SOC Ltd).

7.2.5.2 Live Attenuated Vaccines

Only three *E. ruminantium* strains have been attenuated by *in vitro* serial passages: the Senegal (from Senegal) and Gardel strains (from Guadeloupe) in bovine endothelial cells and the Welgevonden strain (from South Africa) in canine macrophages (Jongejan 1991; Zweygarth et al. 2005; Marcelino et al. 2015). These strains induced a total protection against homologous challenges and some heterologous challenges. These vaccines induced a strong, long-lasting immune protection without any additional treatment and limited postvaccinal clinical signs. The main drawbacks of the attenuated vaccine are their extreme liability that requires storage in liquid nitrogen and the risk of reversion to virulence. So far, the attenuation mechanisms of *E. ruminantium* remain unknown.

7.2.5.3 Inactivated Vaccine

The inactivated vaccine against HW is based on bovine endothelial cell culture-derived *E. ruminantium* organisms that are chemically inactivated and emulsified in oily adjuvants. Although this vaccine is not commercially available, a fully scalable bioprocess for the production has been developed. This bioprocess includes the purification and storage of the antigen, at reduced cost for widespread application (reviewed by Marcelino et al. 2016). As the level of cross-protection from inactivated vaccine is variable, depending on the strains circulating in the region, cocktails of *E. ruminantium* strains should be used according to the target region (Faburay et al. 2007; Adakal et al. 2010; Cangi et al. 2016).

7.2.5.4 Subunit and Recombinant Vaccines

Several genes and proteins have been tested for their ability to elicit a protective immune response in vaccinated animals. The *map1* gene was cloned and tested as a naked-DNA vaccine in a mouse model system. Other genes, such as *groE* operon (*groES* and *groEL)* and *cpg 1*, have also been cloned and tested as recombinant DNA vaccines to protect animals against death due to HW. Subunit vaccines using denatured *E. ruminantium* have also been tested, although no protection was acquired. Several recombinant vaccines based on DNA and the recombinant protein prime/boost approaches have been evaluated. The use of four ORFs (open reading frames) DNA/recombinant proteins prime-boost (Erum2540, Erum2550, Erum2580, and Erum2590 corresponding to four 1H12-derived proteins) resulted in a 100% survival rate after homologous needle challenge but lower survival rates (20% of protection) after field tick challenge. A prime-boost vaccination trial using the polymorphic *cpg1* gene and the recombinant protein also resulted in complete protection of vaccinated animals after homologous challenge. No trials with heterologous strains have yet been performed. Due to the polymorphic property of *cpg1*, a cocktail of *CpG1* proteins from different strains should be included in the vaccine before any field trial.

Although recombinant vaccines look promising under experimental conditions, field trial results have been less successful. Moreover, simple intramuscular immunization is not enough for a primary DNA injection to induce protection and so the use of a gene gun is necessary, which is expensive and not suitable for field use during a vaccination campaign.

Marcelino et al. (2016) recently reviewed the candidate vaccines tested against HW.

Recently, Faburay et al. (2017) evaluated the immune response of sheep after the injection of a glycosylated recombinant Map-1 protein emulsified in oil adjuvant. The results revealed that this recombinant vaccine can induce specific humoral and Th1 immune responses. Nevertheless, as no challenge was performed afterwards, it is difficult to evaluate its efficacy. Still, this opens a window of opportunity to the development of subunit vaccines based on glycosylated recombinant proteins.

7.3 Immune Responses to Protozoal and Rickettsial Vaccines

7.3.1 Animal Trypanosomiasis

From several vaccination experiments (Table 7.1), it has become clear that trypanosomes have developed refined mechanisms to escape from the immune system by either changing their own "antigen appearance" and/or actively eliminating the B cell memory compartment.

7.3.1.1 Trypanosomal Antigenic Variation

Antibodies raised against VSG proteins on whole trypanosomes are able to mediate an efficient opsonization and complement-mediated lysis of the parasites. Nevertheless, these antibodies targeting VSG are highly specific for only one variable antigen type (VAT) but not the subsequent variants produced. This allows these parasites to continuously evade the host antibody response for years, perpetuating the infection until the host succumbs to either secondary infections or infection-associated complications (Horn 2014; Hovel-Miner et al. 2015).

By contrast, antibodies induced by the injection of tubulin or actin were able to recognize several trypanosome species. Furthermore, passive transfer of antibodies through serum from immunized mice conferred partial protection. Intriguingly, antibody production during the immunization of rabbits against midgut proteins from tsetse flies not only affected the fitness and reproduction of the flies, but resulted in partial transmission blockage of trypanosomes (Tabel et al. 2013; Black and Mansfield 2016).

7.3.1.2 Immune Amnesia After a Trypanosome Infection

It has been suggested that trypanosomes have developed a defense mechanism that interferes with B cell homeostasis and impairs the host immune memory. Indeed, during trypanosome infection, the spleen is severely damaged with a drastic disappearance of B cells in the marginal zone. This cell subset is not only important for driving B cell memory, but is also the main mediator of T cell-independent immune responses. Depletion or hindered reactivation of efficient memory immunity could explain why monovalent vaccines failed to induce more than partial protection against trypanosomes and the observed failures in livestock vaccination campaigns (Bockstal et al. 2011; La Greca and Magez 2011).

7.3.1.3 Trypanotolerance

Some animals infected with trypanosomes can naturally survive the infection by becoming trypanotolerant. Twenty-three candidate genomic regions have been identified by comparing trypanotolerant cattle breeds to susceptible ones (Smetko et al. 2015). However, recent findings suggest that there are no clear genetic traits that can be identified (Alvarez et al. 2016) and that there is a relationship between the trypanosome species/genotype and the phenotype of disease in cattle (Auty et al. 2015).

7.3.2 Immune Response Against *Theileria parva* and *T. annulata* Vaccines

Theileria species parasites are the only eukaryotes known to modify eukaryotic host cells. It has been suggested that this complex and multi-step cellular transformation leads to the production of cancer-like cells that present modified signaling pathways, leading to immune deficiencies involving different molecular mechanisms (Tretina et al. 2015).

7.3.2.1 *Theileria parva*

From the ITM vaccination experiments, it was hypothesized that MHC class I $CD8^+$ cytotoxic T lymphocytes (CTLs) are directed against the schizont-infected lymphoblasts (Steinaa et al. 2012). These immune responses appear to be strain specific, as changes in the epitopes recognized by the CTLs between different strains resulted in lower recognition by the MHC class I and CTLs. This was particularly true for *T. parva* strains Muguga and Marikebuni. This antigenic variation is thought to play a role in immune evasion at the population level, inducing a very restricted CTL response.

Theileria parva-infected lymphocytes are also known to upregulate several immunoregulatory molecules, including IFN-γ, IL-2, and IL-10. IFN-γ and IL-10 improve the modification efficiency of host lymphocytes and IL-10 may have significant immunoregulatory roles during infection. It has been shown that *T. parva*-infected cells constitutively express MHC class II on their surface and have a higher molecular mass than those of uninfected cells. Because MHC class II molecules have conserved N-linked glycosylation sites, posttranslational modifications (PTMs) could play a crucial role in regulating immune responses against these pathogens (Tretina et al. 2015; Nene and Morrison 2016).

7.3.2.2 *Theileria annulata*

Theileria annulata infection results in the activation of humoral and cellular immunity. Vaccination with infected cells results in a broad, solid, and cell-mediated immunity that is lead by the activation of macrophages and natural killer cells. This macrophage activation results in the production of cytokines (TNF-α, IL-1, and IL-6) and nitrogen monoxide that leads to a Th1-type immune $CD4^+$ profile (Darghouth et al. 2010). The high levels of TNF-α in ill cattle explain most of the TT symptoms (fever, hyporexia, cachexia, etc.) (Darghouth et al. 2006). However, this immunity varies between breeds, especially in the activation of macrophages and the production of proinflammatory cytokines. Additionally, the immunity produced by vaccination has a short duration. For example, the CL1 vaccine candidate cell line confers a protection of 75.2% during 16 months (Darghouth 2008). Therefore, it is important that future research agendas explore the possibility of orientating the host immune response to its benefit, by genetic selection of resistant cattle populations or by developing new-generation vaccines (Glass et al. 2012; Nene and Morrison 2016).

7.3.3 Immune Response Against *Babesia bovis* and *B. bigemina* Vaccines

Host immune responses to anti-*Babesia* vaccines involve several factors. First, the spleen is essential for the protective cellular immune mechanisms against babesiosis, since it filters the infected erythrocytes; this phenomenon is highlighted by the resistance presented by calves under the age of 9 months and the severe diseases developed by splenectomized animals irrespective of their age. Both calves and adult animals respond with a Th1 immune response to primary infection. There is evidence that a delayed and systemic inflammatory response occurs in adult animals that is ineffectual and probably contributes to the pathogenesis. As such, humoral immunity is considered of importance for protection of adult animals while innate cellular immunity is sufficient for protection of calves.

It is of interest that an effective immunity is developed by animals that recover from infection. These animals are protected from disease but bear extremely low numbers of parasites in their blood. It is thought that protective, adaptive responses require IFN-γ producing $CD4^+$ T cells, and the production of opsonizing IgG2 and complement-fixing IgG1 antibody. Subsequent immunity lasts for a number of years but can be reduced by stress factors such as starvation or concurrent disease, in which case clinical signs may reappear. Repeated infections can result in permanent immunity. The roles of the innate system and the state of the art knowledge on the nature of protective immune responses have been extensively reviewed (Goff et al. 2010; Florin-Christensen et al. 2014).

7.3.4 Immune Response Against *Anaplasma marginale* Vaccines

7.3.4.1 Importance of Th1 in Protective Immunity

Because of the absence of lipopolysaccharides (LPS) and peptidoglycan in the membrane of *A. marginale,* TLR and other bacterial recognition patterns are not activated and the pathogen escapes some of the innate immune responses (Brayton et al. 2005). Thus, the adaptive immune response is the most important branch in the clearance of this pathogen. Protective immunity against *A. marginale* is believed to involve Th1 cells, inducing the secretion of IFN-γ and IL-2 (Noh et al. 2013). The secretion of these cytokines, in turn, has been associated with the production of IgG2, which is the antibody involved in opsonization, macrophage recognition, and nitric oxide production (Agnes et al. 2011).

7.3.4.2 Development of Persistent Infections

The development of persistent infection results from the rapid deletion of immune memory that occurs during *A. marginale* infection. It has been shown that the high loads of bacteria present during persistent infection result in the rapid depletion of $CD4^+$ T cells after immunization. This loss of T cell memory is probably due to apoptosis, mediated by the high abundance of antigen during bacteremia (Han et al. 2008) and persistent infection (Han et al. 2010). However, the exact mechanism by which *A. marginale* infection leads to T cell memory loss is not well understood. The fact that antigen abundance has a negative effect on the control of the disease is an important factor that should be taken into account when designing a protective vaccine.

7.3.5 Immune Response Against Heartwater Vaccines

High antibody titers are normally detected in infected animals at the height of the febrile reaction, and this led to the initial hypothesis that a humoral response might be involved in protection against HW. However, transfer of immune serum or γ-globulins from immunized to naïve animals failed to protect animals or even modify the course of the disease.

The apparent lack of an effective humoral response together with the report of a T cell-mediated response in experimentally infected mice then led to the hypothesis that immunity against HW is likely to be mediated by cellular responses, directed against infected cells. *E. ruminantium* has an important effect on endothelial cells. *In vitro*, it elicits the synthesis of several inflammatory cytokine transcripts such as IL-1β, IL-6, and IL-8 mRNA in infected host endothelial cells, and this effect appears to be potentiated by IFN-γ. IL-1 and IL-6 can act as co-stimulatory signals for T and B cell activation, while IL-8 might participate in the recruitment of neutrophils toward brain endothelial cells, with potentially deleterious effects. Additionally, infection of endothelial cells with *E. ruminantium* strongly affects the expression of IFN-γ induced MHC class I and MHC class II molecules at the surface of the host cells. Therefore, endothelial cells may have a pivotal role in the development of a protective immune response against HW.

To understand which cell subsets and antigens could be involved in the immune response against HW, *in vitro* lymphocyte proliferation studies were performed. The results revealed that the proliferative responses were characterized by a mixture of $CD4^+$, $CD8^+$, and γδ T cells, and strong expression of IFN-γ, (TNF-α/β), and IL-2 was observed, all of which are strong indicators of a Th1-driven immune response. However, in another study, it was not possible to associate INF-γ production in antigen-stimulated blood from vaccinated animals with protection (Vachiery et al. 2006).

Another issue that should be considered in evaluating the efficacy of a vaccine against HW is the impact of *Amblyomma* tick saliva on the host immune response during tick feeding. Indeed, it has been recently shown that tick saliva has a high impact on the host immune response by decreasing lymphoproliferation *in vitro* and has antiinflammatory and immune suppressive properties (Rodrigues et al. 2018). Thus, vaccine efficacy should also be evaluated after tick challenge, either under controlled conditions or in the field, whenever possible.

The nature of protective immune responses against HW was thoroughly reviewed in Marcelino et al. (2016).

7.4 Toward Improved Vaccines

Despite the numerous failures from all the vaccination trials described in this chapter (Tables 7.1–7.5), the knowledge obtained has lead to the development of an important concept: a subunit vaccine that would efficiently interfere with the infections caused by any of these pathogens should be multivalent, target all life cycle stages, and potentially block transmission. In the case of trypanosomes, it should also include antigens that help to avoid the development of the disease. This “super-vaccine” should also elicit a strong and long-lasting immune response.

To identify suitable antigens, it is necessary to improve our knowledge of the biology of the pathogen and the host–pathogen–vector interactions. Indeed, all these pathogens present different forms (intracellular, extracellular, infectious, noninfectious), have a wide genetic and/or antigenic diversity, and can have different levels of virulence. Different hosts have been shown to respond differently to infections by the same pathogens. Thus, it is important to elucidate the molecular mechanisms underlying these phenomena.

In order to better understand the biology of these pathogens and the infection that they produce, high-throughput technologies have been employed. For instance, the genome sequences of *T. brucei* (Berriman et al. 2005), *T. cruzi* (El-Sayed et al. 2005), *T. parva* (Gardner et al. 2005), *T. annulata* (Pain et al. 2005), *B. bovis* (Brayton et al. 2007), *B. bigemina* (Jackson et al. 2014), *A. marginale* (Brayton et al. 2006; Dark et al. 2011; Pierle et al. 2014), and *E. ruminantium* (Collins et al. 2005; Frutos et al. 2006; Nakao et al. 2016) are available. The sequence of the bovine genome is also currently available (Liu et al. 2009; Zimin et al. 2009) as is that of the tsetse fly (International Glossina Genome Initiative 2014). However, despite the rapid advances in molecular acarology, genomic information is only available for two tick species: *Ixodes scapularis* (Gulia-Nuss et al. 2016) and *Rhipicephalus* (*Boophilus*) *microplus* (Ullmann et al. 2005; Nene 2009). Although in most cases, comparison between different strains and organisms is necessary for the identification of potential vaccines, the information obtained from a single genome can lead to the identification of potential virulence factors, immune pathways not known before, and molecules that may play roles in disease transmission. These insights, along with post-genomic tools such as transcriptomics, proteomics, metabolomics, and systems biology, can lead to a better understanding of the biology of the parasites and the interaction between vectors and mammalian hosts (Marcelino et al. 2012; Chetouhi et al. 2015).

Furthermore, it is necessary to explore new technologies that are already available for the development of human vaccines, such as the use of delivery systems to enhance specific parts of the immune response. Some vaccine delivery systems that have shown promising results, including poly(lactic-co-glycolic acid) (PLGA) particles that increase the immunogenicity of subunit vaccines (Silva et al. 2016) or the use of biodegradable polymeric nanoparticle-based subunit vaccines that have been shown to activate the germinal center and result in enhanced antibody production (Vela Ramirez et al. 2016). These molecules are used not only as delivery systems but also as potential adjuvants (Boraschi and Italiani 2015), as has been shown with the use of liposomes in the development of veterinary vaccines and the study of their effects in several animal models (Schwendener 2014).

Furthermore, the addition of natural ligands or antibodies to nanoparticles can lead to a better association of the antigens with antigen-presenting cells, which could improve the development of immunity and immune memory. This has already been tested in the bovine system with the addition of monoclonal antibodies for the CD205 receptor, which led to an increased uptake of nanoparticles by dendritic cells in cattle (Walters et al. 2015). This approach has already been shown to work in cancer treatment in humans and could be further explored in the development of vaccines in different animals and against different pathogens. It was recently tested in the development of a subunit vaccine against *A. marginale* (Zhao et al. 2016), representing an encouraging advance that may lead to its adoption in the other systems discussed herein.

Alternative approaches for VBDs control involve the development of antivector vaccines. Control of ticks by host vaccination has the advantages of being cost-effective, and healing the direct pathogenic effect of ticks, controlling several TBDs, reducing human, animal health and environmental impact of acaricides, and preventing the selection of acaricide-resistant ticks that result from repeated application. The feasibility of controlling vector infestations through immunization of hosts with selected vector antigens was previously demonstrated for ticks using recombinant antigens such as Bm86, Bm95, Fer2, subolesin, EF1a, UBQ, and chimeric antigens (Almazan et al. 2012), but also for tsetse flies using gut extracts as antigens. In some cases, these vaccines also reduced the transmission of vector-borne pathogens. At the moment, three vaccines based on the Bm86 antigen are commercially available: TickGARD® and TickGARD plus® (in Australia) and GAVAC® (in Cuba and parts of South America), but they are not fully effective. As for vaccines against TBPs, the identification of tick antigens inducing host protective response remains the limiting step in the development of effective vaccines limiting tick infestation in hosts. The development of anti-tick vaccines has been recently reviewed (de la Fuente et al. 2016; Morrison and Tomley 2016; Rodriguez-Mallon 2016).

7.5 Summary

Although several experimental vaccines have been tested against AT, ECF, TT, BB, BA, and HW (Tables 7.1–7.5), few vaccines are commercially available. Moreover, most of these are still blood-derived or attenuated organisms that present many drawbacks, such as the requirements of a cold chain, a short shelf-life, potential for transmission of other pathogens, and reversion to virulence. Of those available, few are affordable for farmers in developing countries. Progress in the development of reasonably priced and effective vaccines is hindered by poor understanding of the different factors that play a role in the infection process of many of these pathogens and in the development of an effective immunity that can stop the progress of infection.

It is thus important to integrate different approaches to improve the bulk of information available to vaccine developers. This can be achieved by using "omics" approaches (such as genomics, transcriptomics, proteomics, metabolomics) and systems biology tools as well as technologies used to explore the development of human vaccines and cancer therapy, such as the use of nanoparticles.

However, lack of funding is often the limiting factor to pursue vaccine development. Indeed, many vaccine candidates do not go further, beyond validation experiments, due to the lack of financial support but also the lack of interest by industry, as in some cases the vaccine candidates are not cost-effective enough for them. This becomes particularly critical when dealing with diseases impacting cattle in developing countries, which might not be the main priority of government and funding agencies.

There is a need for funding agencies and governments to understand that the lack of vaccines against VBDs affecting developing countries is not just a matter of local demand but of global security for food and agriculture. Thus, it is important that the public and private sectors make a joint effort to tackle these important problems, which is an achievable task. One successful example that should be followed is the effort run by the Ministry of Agriculture, Livestock and Fisheries in Argentina, which launched a program for the prevention of BB and BA (MAGyP Resolución 227/20130) with the goal of improving livestock productivity in their northern region. The program is based on the free distribution of 420 000 doses of the trivalent frozen vaccine (*B. bovis*, *B. bigemina*, and *A. centrale*) produced by a private undertaking (Litoral Biológicos, www.litoralbiologicos.com.ar) free of charge to farmers.

Acknowledgments

Isabel Marcelino and Adela Chavez acknowledge financial support from EPIGENESIS RegPot European project (no 315 988).

References

Adakal, H., Stachurski, F., Konkobo, M. et al. (2010). Efficiency of inactivated vaccines against heartwater in Burkina Faso: impact of *Ehrlichia ruminantium* genetic diversity. *Vaccine* 28 (29): 4573–4580.

Agnes, J.T., Brayton, K.A., LaFollett, M. et al. (2011). Identification of *Anaplasma marginale* outer membrane protein antigens conserved between *A. marginale* sensu stricto strains and the live *A. marginale* subsp. *centrale* vaccine. *Infect. Immun.* 79: 1311–1318.

Almazan, C., Moreno-Cantu, O., Moreno-Cid, J.A. et al. (2012). Control of tick infestations in cattle vaccinated with bacterial membranes containing surface-exposed tick protective antigens. *Vaccine* 30 (2): 265–272.

Alvarez, I., Perez-Pardal, L., Traore, A. et al. (2016). Lack of haplotype structuring for two candidate genes for trypanotolerance in cattle. *J. Anim. Breed. Genet.* 133 (2): 105–114.

Angara, T.E.E., Ismail, A.A., and Ibrahim, A.M. (2014). An overview on the economic impacts of animal trypanosomiasis. *Global J. Res. Anal.* 3 (7): 275–276.

Arce-Fonseca, M., Rios-Castro, M., Carrillo-Sanchez Sdel, C. et al. (2015). Prophylactic and therapeutic DNA vaccines against Chagas disease. *Parasites Vectors* 8: 121.

Atif, F.A. (2015). *Anaplasma marginale* and *Anaplasma phagocytophilum*: *Rickettsiales* pathogens of veterinary and public health significance. *Parasitol. Res.* 114: 3941–3957.

Aubry, P. and Geale, D.W. (2011). A review of bovine anaplasmosis. *Transbound. Emerg. Dis.* 58 (1): 1–30.

Auty, H., Torr, S.J., Michoel, T. et al. (2015). Cattle trypanosomosis: the diversity of trypanosomes and implications for disease epidemiology and control. *Rev. Sci. Tech.* 34 (2): 587–598.

Barry, M.A., Wang, Q., Jones, K.M. et al. (2016). A therapeutic nanoparticle vaccine against *Trypanosoma cruzi* in a BALB/c mouse model of Chagas disease. *Hum. Vaccin. Immunother.* 12 (4): 976–987.

Berriman, M., Ghedin, E., Hertz-Fowler, C. et al. (2005). The genome of the African trypanosome *Trypanosoma brucei*. *Science* 309: 416–422.

Beugnet, F. and Moreau, Y. (2015). Babesiosis. *Rev. Sci. Tech.* 34 (2): 627–639.

Bishop, R., Nene, V., Staeyert, J. et al. (2003). Immunity to East Coast fever in cattle induced by a polypeptide fragment of the major surface coat protein of *Theileria parva* sporozoites. *Vaccine* 21: 1205–1212.

Biter, A.B., Weltje, S., Hudspeth, E.M. et al. (2018). Characterization and stability of *Trypanosoma cruzi* 24-C4 (Tc24-C4), a candidate antigen for a therapeutic vaccine against Chagas disease. *J. Pharm. Sci.* 107 (5): 1468–1473.

Black, S.J. and Mansfield, J.M. (2016). Prospects for vaccination against pathogenic African trypanosomes. *Parasite Immunol.* 38 (12): 735–743.

Bock, R., Jackson, L., de Vos, A., and Jorgensen, W. (2004). Babesiosis of cattle. *Parasitology* 129 (Suppl): S247–S269.

Bockstal, V., Guirnalda, P., Caljon, G. et al. (2011). *T. brucei* infection reduces B lymphopoiesis in bone marrow and truncates compensatory splenic lymphopoiesis through transitional B-cell apoptosis. *PLoS Pathog.* 7: e1002089.

Bontempi, I.A., Vicco, M.H., Cabrera, G. et al. (2015). Efficacy of a trans-sialidase-ISCOMATRIX subunit vaccine candidate to protect against experimental Chagas disease. *Vaccine* 33 (10): 1274–1283.

Boraschi, D. and Italiani, P. (2015). From antigen delivery system to adjuvanticy: the board application of nanoparticles in vaccinology. *Vaccines* 3: 930–939.

Bossard, G., Grebaut, P., Thevenon, S. et al. (2016). Cloning, expression, molecular characterization and preliminary studies on immunomodulating properties of recombinant *Trypanosoma congolense* calreticulin. *Infect. Genet. Evol.* 45: 320–331.

Brayton, K.A., Kappmeyer, L.S., Herndon, D.R. et al. (2005). Complete genome sequencing of *Anaplasma marginale* reveals that the surface is skewed to two superfamilies of outer membrane proteins. *Proc. Natl. Acad. Sci. U.S.A.* 102: 844–849.

Brayton, K.A., Palmer, G.H., and Brown, W.C. (2006). Genomic and proteomic approaches to vaccine candidate identification for *Anaplasma marginale*. *Expert Rev. Vaccines* 5 (1): 95–101.

Brayton, K.A., Lau, A.O., Herndon, D.R. et al. (2007). Genome sequence of *Babesia bovis* and comparative analysis of apicomplexan hemoprotozoa. *PLoS Pathog.* 3 (10): 1401–1413.

Brown, W.C., Shkap, V., Zhu, D. et al. (1998). CD4(+) T-lymphocyte and immunoglobulin G2 responses in calves immunized with *Anaplasma marginale* outer membranes and protected against homologous challenge. *Infect. Immun.* 66 (11): 5406–5413.

Cangi, N., Gordon, J.L., Bournez, L. et al. (2016). Recombination is a major driving force of genetic diversity in the Anaplasmataceae *Ehrlichia ruminantium*. *Front. Cell. Infect. Microbiol.* 6: 111.

Carrea, A. and Diambra, L. (2016). Systems biology approach to model the life cycle of *Trypanosoma cruzi*. *PLoS One* 11: e0146947.

Chavez, A.S., Felsheim, R.F., Kurtti, T.J. et al. (2012). Expression patterns of *Anaplasma marginale* Msp2 variants change in response to growth in cattle, and tick cells versus mammalian cells. *PLoS One* 7: e36012.

Chenouhi, C., Panek, J., Bonhomme, L. et al. (2015). Cross-talk in host-parasite associations: what do past and recent proteomics approaches tell us? *Infect. Genet. Evol.* 33: 84–94.

Collins, N.E., Liebenberg, J., de Villiers, E.P. et al. (2005). The genome of the heartwater agent *Ehrlichia ruminantium* contains multiple tandem repeats of actively variable copy number. *Proc. Natl. Acad. Sci. U.S.A.* 102 (3): 838–843.

Darghouth, M.A. (2008). Review on the experience with live attenuated vaccines against tropical theileriosis in Tunisia: considerations for the present and implications for the future. *Vaccine* 26 (Suppl 6): G4–G10.

Darghouth, M.A., Boulter, N.R., Gharbi, M. et al. (2006). Vaccination of calves with an attenuated cell line of *Theileria annulata* and the sporozoite antigen SPAG-1 produces a synergistic effect. *Vet. Parasitol.* 142: 54–62.

Darghouth, M.A., Preston, P.M., Bouattour, A., and Kilani, M. (2010). Theileriosis. Tropical theileriosis (*Theileria annulata* infection of cattle). In: *Infectious and Parasitic Diseases of Livestock* (eds. P. Lefèvre, J. Blancou, R. Chermette and G. Uilenberg). Wallingford: CABI.

Dark, M.J., Al-Khedery, B., and Barbet, A.F. (2011). Multistrain genome analysis identifies candidate vaccine antigens of *Anaplasma marginale*. *Vaccine* 29: 4923–4932.

de Andrade, G.M., Machado, R.Z., Vidotto, M.C., and Vidotto, O. (2004). Immunization of bovines using a DNA vaccine (pcDNA3.1/MSP1b) prepared from the Jaboticabal strain of *Anaplasma marginale*. *Ann. N.Y. Acad. Sci.* 1026: 257–266.

de la Fuente, J., Kopacek, P., Lew-Tabor, A., and Maritz-Olivier, C. (2016). Strategies for new and improved vaccines against ticks and tick-borne diseases. *Parasite Immunol.* 38 (12): 754–769.

de Waal, D.T. and Combrink, M.P. (2006). Live vaccines against bovine babesiosis. *Vet. Parasitol.* 138: 88–96.

Dumonteil, E., Bottazzi, M.E., Zhan, B. et al. (2012). Accelerating the development of a therapeutic vaccine for human Chagas disease: rationale and prospects. *Expert Rev. Vaccines* 11 (9): 1043–1055.

El-Sayed, N.M., Myler, P.J., Bartholomeu, D.C. et al. (2005). The genome sequence of *Trypanosoma cruzi*, etiologic agent of Chagas disease. *Science* 309: 409–415.

Faburay, B. (2015). The case for a 'one health' approach to combating vector-borne diseases. *Infect. Ecol. Epidemiol.* 5: 28132.

Faburay, B., Geysen, D., Ceesay, A. et al. (2007). Immunisation of sheep against heartwater in the Gambia using inactivated and attenuated *Ehrlichia ruminantium* vaccines. *Vaccine* 25 (46): 7939–7947.

Faburay, B., McGill, J., and Jongejan, F. (2017). A glycosylated recombinant subunit candidate vaccine consisting of *Ehrlichia ruminantium* major antigenic protein1 induces specific humoral and Th1 type cell responses in sheep. *PLoS One* 12: e0185495.

Field, M.C. and Carrington, M. (2009). The trypanosome flagellar pocket. *Nat. Rev. Microbiol.* 7: 775–786.

Florin-Christensen, M., Suarez, C.E., Rodriguez, A.E. et al. (2014). Vaccines against bovine babesiosis: where we are now and possible roads ahead. *Parasitology*: 1–30.

Frutos, R., Viari, A., Ferraz, C. et al. (2006). Comparative genomic analysis of three strains of *Ehrlichia ruminantium* reveals an active process of genome size plasticity. *J. Bacteriol.* 188 (7): 2533–2542.

Gardner, M.J., Bishop, R., Shah, T. et al. (2005). Genome sequence of *Theileria parva*, a bovine pathogen that transforms lymphocytes. *Science* 309 (5731): 134–137.

Gharbi, M., Darghouth, M.A., Weir, W. et al. (2011). Prime-boost immunisation against tropical theileriosis with two parasite surface antigens: evidence for protection and antigen synergy. *Vaccine* 29: 6620–6628.

Glass, E.J., Crutchley, S., and Jensen, K. (2012). Living with the enemy or uninvited guests: functional genomics approaches to investigating host resistance or tolerance traits to a protozoan parasite, *Theileria annulata*, in cattle. *Vet. Immunol. Immunopathol.* 148: 178–189.

Goff, W.L., Bastos, R.G., Brown, W.C. et al. (2010). The bovine spleen: interactions among splenic cell populations in the innate immunologic control of hemoparasitic infections. *Vet. Immunol. Immunopathol.* 138: 1–14.

Gohil, S., Herrmann, S., Gunther, S., and Cooke, B.M. (2013). Bovine babesiosis in the 21st century: advances in biology and functional genomics. *Int. J. Parasitol.* 43 (2): 125–132.

Gulia-Nuss, M., Nuss, A.B., Meyer, J.M. et al. (2016). Genomic insights into the *Ixodes scapularis* tick vector of Lyme disease. *Nat. Commun.* 7: 10507.

Han, S., Norimine, J., Palmer, G.H. et al. (2008). Rapid deletion of antigen-specific CD4+ T cells following infection represents a strategy of immune evasion and persistence for *Anaplasma marginale*. *J. Immunol.* 181: 7759–7769.

Han, S., Norimine, J., Brayton, K.A. et al. (2010). *Anaplasma marginale* infection with persistent high-load bacteremia induces a dysfunctional memory CD4+ T lymphocyte response but sustained high IgG titers. *Clin. Vaccine Immunol.* 17: 1881–1890.

Hochstetter, A. and Pfohl, T. (2016). Motility, force generation, and energy consumption of unicellular parasites. *Trends Parasitol.* 32 (7): 531–541.

Horn, D. (2014). Antigenic variation in African trypanosomes. *Mol. Biochem. Parasitol.* 195 (2): 123–129.

Hovel-Miner, G., Mugnier, M., Papavasiliou, F.N. et al. (2015). A host-pathogen interaction reduced to first principles: antigenic variation in *T. brucei*. *Results Probl. Cell Differ.* 57: 23–46.

International Glossina Genome Initiative (2014). Genome sequence of the tsetse fly (*Glossina morsitans*): vector of African trypanosomiasis. *Science* 344: 380–386.

Jackson, A.P., Otto, T.D., Darby, A. et al. (2014). The evolutionary dynamics of variant antigen genes in Babesia reveal a history of genomic innovation underlying host-parasite interaction. *Nucleic Acids Res.* 42: 7113–7131.

Jaramillo Ortiz, J.M., del Medico Zajac, M.P., Zanetti, F.A. et al. (2014). Vaccine strategies against *Babesia bovis* based on prime-boost immunizations in mice with modified vaccinia Ankara vector and recombinant proteins. *Vaccine* 32 (36): 4625–4632.

Jeyabal, L., Kumar, B., Ray, D. et al. (2012). Vaccine potential of recombinant antigens of *Theileria annulata* and *Hyalomma anatolicum anatolicum* against vector and parasite. *Vet. Parasitol.* 188: 231–238.

Jongejan, F. (1991). Protective immunity to heartwater (Cowdria ruminantium infection) is acquired after vaccination with in vitro-attenuated rickettsiae. *Infect. Immun.* 59 (2): 729–731.

Knight, J.M., Zingales, B., Bottazzi, M.E. et al. (2014). Limited antigenic variation in the *Trypanosoma cruzi* candidate vaccine antigen TSA-1. *Parasite Immunol.* 36 (12): 708–712.

Kocan, K.M., de la Fuente, J., Blouin, E.F. et al. (2010). The natural history of *Anaplasma marginale*. *Vet. Parasitol.* 167: 95–107.

Kurup, S.P. and Tewari, A.K. (2012). Induction of protective immune response in mice by a DNA vaccine encoding

Trypanosoma evansi beta tubulin gene. *Vet. Parasitol.* 187: 9–16.

La Greca, F. and Magez, S. (2011). Vaccination against trypanosomiasis: can it be done or is the trypanosome truly the ultimate immune destroyer and escape artist? *Hum. Vaccines* 7: 1225–1233.

Lanca, A.S., de Sousa, K.P., Atouguia, J. et al. (2011). *Trypanosoma brucei*: immunisation with plasmid DNA encoding invariant surface glycoprotein gene is able to induce partial protection in experimental African trypanosomiasis. *Exp. Parasitol.* 127: 18–24.

Lempereur, L., Beck, R., Fonseca, I. et al. (2017). Guidelines for the detection of *Babesia* and *Theileria* parasites. *Vector Borne Zoonotic Dis.* 17 (1): 51–65.

Li, S.Q., Yang, W.B., Ma, L.J. et al. (2009). Immunization with recombinant actin from *Trypanosoma evansi* induces protective immunity against *T. evansi*, *T. equiperdum* and *T. b. brucei* infection. *Parasitol. Res.* 104 (2): 429–435.

Liu, Y., Qin, X., Song, X.Z. et al. (2009). *Bos taurus* genome assembly. *BMC Genomics* 10: 180.

Lopez, J.E., Siems, W.F., Palmer, G.H. et al. (2005). Identification of novel antigenic proteins in a complex *Anaplasma marginale* outer membrane immunogen by mass spectrometry and genomic mapping. *Infect. Immun.* 73: 8109–8118.

Lopez, J.E., Palmer, G.H., Brayton, K.A. et al. (2007). Immunogenicity of *Anaplasma marginale* type IV secretion system proteins in a protective outer membrane vaccine. *Infect. Immun.* 75: 2333–2342.

Manjunathachar, H.V., Saravanan, B.C., Kesavan, M. et al. (2014). Economic importance of ticks and their effective control strategies. *Asian Pac. J. Trop. Dis.* 4 (Suppl 2): S770–S779.

Marcelino, I., de Almeida, A.M., Ventosa, M. et al. (2012). Tick-borne diseases in cattle: applications of proteomics to develop new generation vaccines. *J. Proteomics* 75: 4232–4250.

Marcelino, I., Ventosa, M., Pires, E. et al. (2015). Comparative proteomic profiling of *Ehrlichia ruminantium* pathogenic strain and its high-passaged attenuated strain reveals virulence and attenuation-associated proteins. *PLoS One* 10: e0145328.

Marcelino, I., Holzmuller, P., Stachurski, F. et al. (2016). *Ehrlichia ruminantium*: the causal agent of heartwater. In: *Rickettsiales: Biology, Molecular Biology, Epidemiology, and Vaccine Development* (ed. S. Thomas), 241–280. New York: Springer International Publishing.

Matos, M.N., Sanchez Alberti, A., Morales, C. et al. (2016). A prime-boost immunization with Tc52 N-terminal domain DNA and the recombinant protein expressed in *Pichia pastoris* protects against *Trypanosoma cruzi* infection. *Vaccine* 34 (28): 3243–3251.

McAllister, M.M. (2014). Successful vaccines for naturally occurring protozoal diseases of animals should guide human vaccine research. A review of protozoal vaccines and their designs. *Parasitology* 141: 624–640.

Moore, S., Shrestha, S., Tomlinson, K.W., and Vuong, H. (2012). Predicting the effect of climate change on African trypanosomiasis: integrating epidemiology with parasite and vector biology. *J. R. Soc. Interface* 9: 817–830.

Morrison, W.I. and Tomley, F. (2016). Development of vaccines for parasitic diseases of animals: challenges and opportunities. *Parasite Immunol.* 38 (12): 707–708.

Nakao, R., Jongejan, F., and Sugimoto, C. (2016). Draft genome sequences of three strains of *Ehrlichia ruminantium*, a tick-borne pathogen of ruminants, isolated from Zimbabwe, the Gambia, and Ghana. *Genome Announc.* 4 (3): 00453-16.

Nene, V. (2009). Tick genomics – coming of age. *Front. Biosci.* 14: 2566–2673.

Nene, V. and Morrison, W.I. (2016). Approaches to vaccination against *Theileria parva* and *Theileria annulata*. *Parasite Immunol.* 38 (12): 724–734.

Nene, V., Kiara, H., Lacasta, A. et al. (2016). The biology of *Theileria parva* and control of East Coast fever – current status and future trends. *Ticks Tick Borne Dis.* 7 (4): 549–564.

Njongmeta, L.M., Bray, J., Davies, C.J. et al. (2012). CD205 antigen targeting combined with dendritic cell recruitment factors and antigen-linked CD40L activation primes and expands significant antigen-specific antibody and CD4(+) T cell responses following DNA vaccination of outbred animals. *Vaccine* 30: 1624–1635.

Noh, S.M., Turse, J.E., Brown, W.C. et al. (2013). Linkage between *Anaplasma marginale* outer membrane proteins enhances immunogenicity but is not required for protection from challenge. *Clin. Vaccine Immunol.* 20: 651–656.

OIE (2017a). Chapter 2.4.1 – Bovine Anaplasmosis. In: *Manual of Diagnostic Tests and Vaccines for Terestrial Animals*, 599–610. Paris: OIE.

OIE (2017b). Chapter 2.4.2 – Bovine Babesiosis. In: *Manual of Diagnostic Tests and Vaccines for Terestrial Animals*, 611–623. Paris: OIE.

Pain, A., Renauld, H., Berriman, M. et al. (2005). Genome of the host-cell transforming parasite *Theileria annulata* compared with *T. parva*. *Science* 309 (5731): 131–133.

Pereira, I.R., Vilar-Pereira, G., Marques, V. et al. (2015). A human type 5 adenovirus-based *Trypanosoma cruzi* therapeutic vaccine re-programs immune response and reverses chronic cardiomyopathy. *PLoS Pathog.* 11: e1004594.

Pérez de León, A.A., Teel, P.D., Auclair, A.N. et al. (2012). Integrated strategy for sustainable cattle fever tick eradication in USA is required to mitigate the impact of global change. *Front. Physiol.* 3: 195.

Pierle, S.A., Rosshandler, I.I., Kerudin, A.A. et al. (2014). Genetic diversity of tick-borne rickettsial pathogens; insights gained from distant strains. *Pathogens* 3 (1): 57–72.

Prochetto, E., Roldan, C., Bontempi, I.A. et al. (2017). Trans-sialidase-based vaccine candidate protects against *Trypanosoma cruzi* infection, not only inducing an effector immune response but also affecting cells with regulatory/suppressor phenotype. *Oncotarget* 8: 58003–58020.

Quiroz-Castaneda, R.E., Amaro-Estrada, I., and Rodriguez-Camarillo, S.D. (2016). *Anaplasma marginale*: diversity, virulence, and vaccine landscape through a genomics approach. *Biomed. Res. Int.* 2016: 9032085.

Ramey, K., Eko, F.O., Thompson, W.E. et al. (2009). Immunolocalization and challenge studies using a recombinant *Vibrio cholerae* ghost expressing *Trypanosoma brucei* Ca(2+) ATPase (TBCA2) antigen. *Am. J. Trop. Med. Hyg.* 81: 407–415.

Rasooly, R. and Balaban, N. (2004). Trypanosome microtubule-associated protein p15 as a vaccine for the prevention of African sleeping sickness. *Vaccine* 22: 1007–1015.

Rodrigues, V., Fernandez, B., Vercoutere, A. et al. (2018). Immunomodulatory effects of *Amblyomma variegatum* saliva on bovine cells: characterization of cellular responses and identification of molecular determinants. *Front. Cell. Infect. Microbiol.* 7: 521.

Rodriguez-Mallon, A. (2016). Developing anti-tick vaccines. *Methods Mol. Biol.* 1404: 243–259.

Rodriguez-Morales, O., Monteon-Padilla, V., Carrillo-Sanchez, S.C. et al. (2015). Experimental vaccines against Chagas disease: a journey through history. *J. Immunol. Res.* 2015: 489758.

Sanchez-Valdez, F.J., Perez Brandan, C., Ferreira, A., and Basombrio, M.A. (2015). Gene-deleted live-attenuated *Trypanosoma cruzi* parasites as vaccines to protect against Chagas disease. *Expert Rev. Vaccines* 14 (5): 681–697.

Schwendener, R.A. (2014). Liposomes as vaccine delivery systems: a review of the recent advances. *Ther. Adv. Vaccines* 2: 159–182.

Shkap, V., Leibovitz, B., Krigel, Y. et al. (2005). Vaccination of older *Bos taurus* bulls against bovine babesiosis. *Vet. Parasitol.* 129: 235–242.

Silaghi, C., Santos, A.S., Gomes, J. et al. (2017). Guidelines for the direct detection of *Anaplasma* spp. in diagnosis and epidemiological studies. *Vector Borne Zoonotic Dis.* 17 (1): 12–22.

Silva, M.S., Prazeres, D.M., Lanca, A. et al. (2009). Trans-sialidase from *Trypanosoma brucei* as a potential target for DNA vaccine development against African trypanosomiasis. *Parasitol. Res.* 105 (5): 1223–1229.

Silva, A.L., Soema, P.C., Slutter, B. et al. (2016). PLGA particulate delivery systems for subunit vaccines: linking particle properties to immunogenicity. *Hum. Vaccin. Immunother.* 12 (4): 1056–1069.

Smetko, A., Soudre, A., Silbermayr, K. et al. (2015). Trypanosomosis: potential driver of selection in African cattle. *Front. Genet.* 6: 137.

Steinaa, L., Saya, R., Awino, E., and Toye, P. (2012). Cytotoxic T lymphocytes from cattle immunized against *Theileria parva* exhibit pronounced cross-reactivity among different strain-specific epitopes of the Tp1 antigen. *Vet. Immunol. Immunopathol.* 145: 571–581.

Sutten, E.L., Norimine, J., Beare, P.A. et al. (2010). *Anaplasma marginale* type IV secretion system proteins VirB2, VirB7, VirB11, and VirD4 are immunogenic components of a protective bacterial membrane vaccine. *Infect. Immun.* 78: 1314–1325.

Tabel, H., Wei, G., and Bull, H.J. (2013). Immunosuppression: cause for failures of vaccines against African trypanosomiases. *PLoS Negl.Trop. Dis.* 7: e2090.

Tebele, N., McGuire, T.C., and Palmer, G.H. (1991). Induction of protective immunity by using *Anaplasma marginale* initial body membranes. *Infect. Immun.* 59 (9): 3199–3204.

Tretina, K., Gotia, H.T., Mann, D.J., and Silva, J.C. (2015). Theileria-transformed bovine leukocytes have cancer hallmarks. *Trends Parasitol.* 31 (7): 306–314.

Ullmann, A.J., Lima, C.M., Guerrero, F.D. et al. (2005). Genome size and organization in the blacklegged tick, *Ixodes scapularis* and the Southern cattle tick, *Boophilus microplus*. *Insect Mol. Biol.* 14 (2): 217–222.

Vachiery, N., Lefrancois, T., Esteves, I. et al. (2006). Optimisation of the inactivated vaccine dose against heartwater and in vitro quantification of *Ehrlichia ruminantium* challenge material. *Vaccine* 24 (22): 4747–4756.

Vachiery, N., Marcelino, I., Martinez, D., and Lefrancois, T. (2013). Opportunities in diagnostic and vaccine approaches to mitigate potential heartwater spreading and impact on the American mainland. *Dev. Biol.* 135: 191–200.

Vela Ramirez, J.E., Tygrett, L.T., Hao, J. et al. (2016). Polyanhydride nanovaccines induce germinal center B cell formation and sustained serum antibody responses. *J. Biomed. Nanotechnol.* 12 (6): 1303–1311.

Villanueva-Lizama, L.E., Cruz-Chan, J.V., Aguilar-Cetina, A.D.C. et al. (2018). *Trypanosoma cruzi* vaccine candidate antigens Tc24 and TSA-1 recall memory immune response associated with HLA-A and -B supertypes in Chagasic chronic patients from Mexico. *PLoS Negl. Trop. Dis.* 12: e0006240.

Walters, A.A., Somavarapu, S., Riitho, V. et al. (2015). Assessment of the enhancement of PLGA nanoparticle uptake by dendritic cells through the addition of natural receptor ligands and monoclonal antibody. *Vaccine* 33 (48): 6588–6595.

Zhao, L., Mahony, D., Cavallaro, A.S. et al. (2016). Immunogenicity of outer membrane proteins VirB9-1 and VirB9-2, a novel nanovaccine against *Anaplasma marginale*. *PLoS One* 11: e0154295.

Zimin, A.V., Delcher, A.L., Florea, L. et al. (2009). A whole-genome assembly of the domestic cow, *Bos taurus*. *Genome Biol.* 10 (4): R42.

Zweygarth, E., Josemans, A.I., van Strijp, M.F. et al. (2005). An attenuated *Ehrlichia ruminantium* (Welgevonden stock) vaccine protects small ruminants against virulent heartwater challenge. *Vaccine* 23 (14): 1695–1702.

8

Parasite Vaccines

Anton Pernthaner[1], Heather Simpson[2], and Saleh Umair[1]

[1] AgResearchLtd, Hopkirk Research Institute, Grasslands Research Centre, Palmerston North, New Zealand
[2] School of Veterinary Science, Massey University, Palmerston North, New Zealand

8.1 Introduction

Multicellular ecto- and endoparasitism affect the health of companion and farmed animals, reduce the productivity of livestock, with losses estimated to be in the multibillion dollar range worldwide per annum, and cause important zoonoses (Robinson and Dalton 2009). Parasites damage internal tissues and organs either directly or indirectly through inflammation. Gut helminths cause diarrhea, dehydration, and loss of appetite, lungworms cause bronchitis and bronchopneumonia, flukes damage the bile ducts and liver, and anemia may result from blood sucking by hookworms, ticks, and *Haemonchus* spp. Some are also vectors of other diseases, for example ticks transmit the protozoa *Anaplasma*, *Babesia*, and *Theileria* (Nuttall et al. 2006). As natural immunity is slow to develop, ill health as a result of parasitism predominantly occurs between weaning and adulthood. Chemical anthelmintic drenches have been successfully used to control internal parasites, as have insecticide/acaricides for ticks and fleas, but increasing drug resistance and concerns about chemical residues in food have further stimulated the development of vaccines. These ideally would provide maximum protection during the period of susceptibility, without the requirement for revaccination.

While there are many vaccines that protect from viral and bacterial diseases, developing effective subunit vaccines against multicellular organisms has been more difficult and few have been commercialized. The focus for developing veterinary vaccines has understandably been directed at helminths, particularly nematodes, and the blood-sucking ticks, which are the principal parasites responsible for economic losses in livestock. This has resulted in five commercial vaccines, only three of which are still available in a restricted number of countries. A major contributor to this slow progress has been lack of knowledge of the complexity of protective immunity and of the role of adjuvants in enhancing and determining the balance between antibody- and cell-mediated responses. Assessment of antigens in experimental vaccines has thus been hampered by suboptimal adjuvants and immunization protocols, as well as a poor choice of antigens, so negative results from trials should not necessarily result in discounting the future inclusion of those antigens. Further progress in vaccine development is, therefore, likely to be an iterative process, whereby improved adjuvants and delivery systems allow better assessment of the suitability of the antigens and vice versa. This chapter explores the issues to be addressed in parasite vaccine development, which are summarized in Figure 8.1.

8.2 Types of Vaccines

8.2.1 Live Attenuated Parasites

These vaccines are based on the concept that infective larvae can be attenuated sufficiently with γ-rays, x-rays, or UV light to promote the induction of protective immune responses after oral delivery, but parasite development and thus the associated host pathology are limited. These products have a relatively short shelf-life and have specific temperature requirements for storage. There are also safety concerns of possible contamination of eggs isolated from feces. Animal welfare is also an issue, because of the inability to culture parasites *in vitro* through the whole life cycle, necessitating susceptible donor animals to provide eggs for larval culture.

This method was the basis of the earliest attempts to produce vaccines to prevent internal parasitism by helminths and resulted in the 1950s in the first commercial vaccine,

Veterinary Vaccines: Principles and Applications, First Edition. Edited by Samia Metwally, Gerrit Viljoen, and Ahmed El Idrissi.

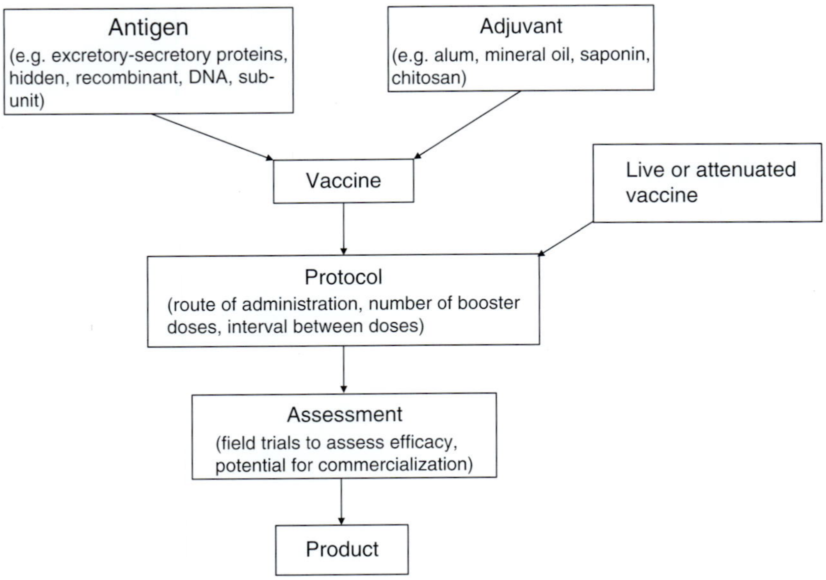

Figure 8.1. Design of vaccines – from antigens to a product.

Huskvac™, which contained irradiated L3 of the cattle lungworm *Dictyocaulus viviparus* (Jarrett and Sharp 1963). This vaccine is still available in Europe. For protection, two doses of irradiated larvae are required, the second dose at least 2 weeks before exposure to infective larvae, and natural challenge on pasture is required to maintain protective immunity. The vaccine prevents clinical disease but sterile immunity usually is not achieved. A second vaccine containing live attenuated parasites of the canine hookworm *Ascaris caninum* was available commercially only from 1973 to 1975 in the USA (Miller 1978).

Vaccine trials have shown partial protection in ruminants using irradiated schistosomula of *Schistosoma japonicum* and *S. bovis* (Bickle 2009) or larval *Onchocerca ochengi* (Tchakouté et al. 2006) and in horses with L3 *Strongylus vulgaris* (Monahan et al. 1994). More variable results were obtained with L3 *Haemonchus contortus* (Benitez-Usher et al. 1977), *Nematodirus battus* (Winter et al. 2000), and *Trichostrongylus colubriformis* (Windon et al. 1980). No further products have appeared, because of the disadvantages of high cost, short shelf-life, and incomplete protection.

8.2.2 Native Antigens

Although native antigens have many of the same limitations as irradiated parasites, a vaccine against *H. contortus*, Barbervax™, was developed and commercialized by the Moredun Institute in 2014 for use in lambs. It requires three priming doses to achieve protection, which lasts for 6 weeks, so that revaccination is required throughout the danger period (Kearney et al. 2016). The vaccine was also partially protective in calves (Bassetto et al. 2014b), but not in ewes (Bassetto et al. 2014a). The vaccine antigens are predominantly the "hidden" antigens H11 and H-gal-GP of the gut microvilli of adult worms, which were successful in the native forms but could not be successfully produced as recombinant antigens (Knox et al. 2003).

Significant protection was obtained with some helminth antigens, such as a native activation-associated secreted protein of *Cooperia oncophora* (van Meulder et al. 2015) and a cysteine proteinase-enriched fraction from the gut of *H. contortus* (Redmond and Knox 2006). There are generally more equivocal results with soluble antigens, such as whole homogenates (Adams et al. 1982) or a somatic fraction (p26/23) from *H. contortus* (Dominguez-Toraño et al. 2000), larval or adult somatic extract from *S. vulgaris* (Monahan et al. 1994), or surface antigens of *H. contortus* (Piedrafita et al. 2012). The carbohydrate larval antigen CarLA of sheep strongylid parasites (Harrison et al. 2008) failed to induce an antibody response (Harrison, pers. com.), but there may be more success with peptide mimotopes (Umair et al. 2016). Vaccines based on larval surface molecules may be limited by the variation in the surface epitopes within parasite species (Maass et al. 2009) and by the changing expression at each life cycle stage, a strategy which helminths use to evade host immunity (Blaxter et al. 1992). In addition, antibodies and immune cells bound to trematodes and nematodes can be actively shed (Caulfield et al. 1980; McKeand and Kennedy 1995).

8.2.3 Recombinant Vaccines

The use of defined antigens is desirable for cost of production, greater safety, and delivering a more uniform product.

Commercial parasite vaccines of the future will probably be based on recombinant proteins or DNA technology, but alternatively could target parasite glycans. Multivalent vaccines may be more effective, targeting more than one biological process or two points in a metabolic pathway simultaneously (Zhu et al. 2011). Mimotopes of the antigenic epitopes of native enzymes that cannot yet be synthesized may be able to be substituted as antigens in tick vaccines (Prudencio et al. 2010) or for the carbohydrate antigen CarLA of trichostrongylid parasites of sheep (Umair et al. 2016).

Two commercial bovine tick vaccines, both based on the recombinant gut glycoprotein antigen Bm86 of *Rhipicephalus microplus*, were launched in the 1990s: TickGUARD™ in Australia (Willadsen et al. 1995) and Gavac™ in Mexico and Latin America (de la Fuente et al. 1998). TickGUARD is no longer available, but Gavac is still in use. These vaccines had an efficiency of about 50%, depending on the tick species. The focus of the next generation of vaccines against hard and soft ticks is the incorporation of subunit antigens (Díaz-Martín et al. 2015). A similar protein, Bm95, is proving effective for tick strains refractory to vaccination with Bm86 (García-García et al. 2000). Partial success has been achieved with several other recombinant antigens (Nuttall et al. 2006), including Bm86 in combination with other proteins such as ferritin, aquaporin, metalloproteases, and the intracellular signaling molecule subolesin (Díaz-Martín et al. 2015).

The recombinant cestode vaccines aim to interrupt the life cycle in the intermediate host. The first effective vaccine was a *Taenia ovis* vaccine (To45), registered by the New Zealand Animal Remedies Board in 1994, although it has not resulted in a commercial product. The 45 kDa oncosphere antigen, which was expressed in *Escherichia coli* as a fusion protein with *S. japonicum* glutathione-S-transferase (GST), gave very strong protection in the sheep intermediate host (Johnson et al. 1989); two further protective antigens, To16 and To18, have been subsequently identified (Harrison et al. 1996). All three antigens are produced by the oncospheral penetration glands, are present in secretory blebs after oncosphere activation and later on the surface of the oncosphere and after *in vitro* culture (Jabbar et al. 2011).

Homologous antigens from related cestodes have also been used in highly effective recombinant vaccines (Gauci and Lightowlers 2013). Echinococcosis is a serious zoonosis worldwide, caused by the intermediate stage of *Echinococcus granulosus* for which vaccination programs are planned. The *E. granulosus* antigen EG95 also originates from penetration glands of oncospheres (Jabbar et al. 2011) and is protective in sheep (Larrieu et al. 2015) and cattle (Heath et al. 2012). A recent development has been fusion of EG95 to the orf virus to produce a bivalent vaccine (Tan et al. 2012). Immunization with *Taenia saginata* TSA-9 and TSA-18 oncosphere antigens resulted in >99% protection in cattle (Lightowlers et al. 1996).

Taenia solium cysticercosis is a zoonosis that can be prevented by interrupting the parasite life cycle by vaccination of pigs with the oncosphere antigens TSOL16 and TSOL18 (Jayashi et al. 2012). The vaccine was completely effective when combined with anthelmintic administration to remove existing parasites at the time of vaccination (Assana et al. 2010). A novel approach to reducing the cost of mass vaccination programs is attempting to develop an oral vaccine using TSOL18 expressed in carrot cells (Monreal-Escalante et al. 2016).

Development of recombinant vaccines for other animal parasites is making slow progress, for example for the bovine parasite *Ostertagia ostertagi* where there has been no success with recombinant proteins and variable results using native antigens, the best of which were cysteine proteases and thiol subfractions of excretory-secretory (ES) products (Rinaldi and Geldhof 2012). This is not surprising, given that the much greater research effort to produce vaccines against human flukes, filarial parasites, and hookworms has not been successful and only Bilhvax and Sm142 have entered clinical trials (McManus and Loukas 2008). Human vaccines may also lead to the development of similar products against the liver flukes *Fasciola hepatica* and *F. gigantica*, which cause both economic losses in ruminants and human diseases (Mas-Coma et al. 2005). Further advances are expected to result from using multivalent antigen vaccines and better adjuvants and routes of delivery for these antitrematode products (Molina-Hernández et al. 2015). As about 75% of cases of Asian schistosomiasis, which is caused by *S. japonicum*, are transmitted by water buffaloes, a vaccine to control infection in buffaloes is considered an important part of public health campaigns to control this parasite (Wu et al. 2005). Vaccines are also being developed to control the related fluke *S. bovis*, which infects sheep and goats as well as bovine species and causes significant production losses (Zhu et al. 2011).

8.2.4 DNA Vaccines

These vaccines incorporate gene sequences of selected antigens and offer the possibility of cheap vaccines which are stable at room temperature. So far, there have been mixed results against multicellular parasites. Partial protection resulted from DNA vaccination with a range of parasite enzymes: *H. contortus* glutathione peroxidase (Sun et al. 2011), *H. contortus* (Han et al. 2012), and *Onchocerca volvulus* glyceraldehye-3-phosphate dehydrogenase (GAPDH)

(Steisslinger et al. 2015), *S. japonicum* triose-phosphate isomerase, *F. hepatica* phosphoglycerate kinase (Wesolowska et al. 2016), and the *Ancylostoma ceylanicum* metalloprotease 7Ace-mep-7 (Wiśniewski et al. 2016). As with protein antigens, adjuvants are required to increase their antigenicity, and novel adjuvants or the combination of DNA with cytokines (Zhu et al. 2004) or prime boosting with recombinant proteins (Thirugnanam et al. 2007) may lead to success.

8.3 Antigens for Subunit Vaccines

There are numerous possible vaccine targets in parasites, including molecules involved in feeding, reproduction and development, enzymes of metabolism, and structural components, both on the surface or located internally. These are not mutually exclusive, as additional "moonlighting" activities have been ascribed to many metabolic enzymes (Copley 2012) and structural components, such as paramyosin (Sun et al. 2015). ES products which contribute to pathophysiology or interact with the host immune system could also be protective antigens. Prediction of likely vaccine candidates is most profitably based on understanding parasite biology and critical processes and is supported by recent progress in parasite genomics. As some promising candidate proteins are proving hard to express, it may be possible to use truncated molecules carrying sequences for active sites on the molecules, rather than the complete protein.

As it is not clear if cellular or structural components of parasites can be accessed by the host immune system unless they are on the external surface or on gut membranes, externally released molecules have been viewed more favorably as vaccine antigens. It is encouraging, however, that internal targets may be able to be neutralized, since host immunoglobulins can be taken up by both blood- and nonblood-feeding nematodes (Murray and Smith 1994) and ticks (Wang and Nuttall 1994). The ES products released by most parasites *in vitro* contain 100–200 proteins, glycolipids, glycoproteins, and polysaccharides (Yatsuda et al. 2003). These are enzymes, structural components, and molecules which mimic many pathophysiological effects of parasitism (Su et al. 2011), as well as immunomodulators of different arms of the immune system (Hewitson et al. 2009). Immunization with ES products or subfractions can be protective (Bakker et al. 2004) and several proteins commonly found in ES products have provided partial protection. Recombinant antigens showing promise for several parasite species include proteinases, protein inhibitors, glycolytic enzymes, GSTs, paramyosin, calreticulin, and fatty acid-binding proteins, while other antigens have been examined in isolated species, such as the recombinant 17 kDa antigen, which was protective against *T. colubriformis* (McClure 2009). Examples of partially protective antigens are given in Table 8.1.

Table 8.1 Recombinant vaccine antigens which confer partial protection against multicellular parasites.

Antigen	Parasite	Host	Reference
Glutathione S-transferase	*Fasciola gigantica*	Buffalo	Kumar et al. (2012)
	Schistosoma bovis	Sheep	Boulanger et al. (1999)
	Schistosoma bovis	Cattle	Bushara et al. (1993)
Fatty acid binding protein	*Fasciola gigantica*	Buffalo	Kumar et al. (2012)
Leucine aminopeptidase	*Fasciola hepatica*	Sheep	Maggioli et al. (2011)
Cysteine proteinase			Li et al. (2013)
Cysteine proteinase	*Trichinella spiralis*	Mouse	Muleke et al. (2007)
	Haemonchus contortus	Goat	Martín et al. (2015)
Cysteine proteinase	*Haemonchus contortus*	Sheep	
Calreticulin	*Necator americanus*	Mouse	Winter et al. (2005)
Paramyosin	*Schistosoma japonicum*	Buffalo	McManus et al. (2002)
	Dictyocaulus viviparus	Cattle	Joekel et al. (2015)
Enolase	*Fasciola gigantica*	Sheep	Mahana et al. (2016)
	Ascaris suum	Pig	Chen et al. (2012)
	Haemonchus contortus	Sheep	Kalyanasundaram et al. (2015)
Fructose-1,6 biphosphate aldolase	*Onchocerca ochengi*	Cattle	Makepeace et al. (2009)

8.4 Immune Responses to Parasitic Vaccines

Parasites are well adapted to survive in the hostile environment within the host and have developed many ways of evading and escaping host defenses. Consequently, protective immune responses to parasites are very complex and involve numerous means of controlling the infestation, many of which are not well understood. Some individuals are genetically more resistant to parasitism (McManus and Loukas 2008) and immunity can be compromised by poor nutrition (Coop and Kyriazakis 1999) and pregnancy (O'Sullivan and Donald 1970). After repeated natural infections and when they reach adulthood, animals normally develop a degree of immunity which increases the ability of the host to reject incoming larvae and to eliminate existing infections (Watson et al. 1994).

Vaccines against endoparasites primarily aim to reduce parasite numbers and secondly to limit parasite transmission by impairing their fecundity. In the case of schistosomes, decreased egg production would also reduce the pathology, which is largely caused by the host reaction to eggs (McManus and Loukas 2008). Selecting appropriate adjuvants and routes of delivery for antiparasite vaccines should be aided by understanding the distinguishing features of natural resistance to parasites, which may not be the same for all parasites or even within groups of related parasites.

8.4.1 Natural Immunity

8.4.1.1 Protective Immune Responses

The protective immune response to helminths is generally of the Th2 type, which includes both innate and adaptive Th2 cell components. Th1-type responses often cause disease, although this dichotomy is less pronounced in sheep and cattle than in some experimental laboratory animals (Almeria et al. 1998; Pernthaner et al. 2005a). The Th2 response is characterized by secretion of cytokines, particularly IL-4 from $CD4^{+}$ T cells, antigen-specific IgE and IgG, and antiinflammatory cytokines. Cells involved in the response to helminths include eosinophils, mast cells, basophils, and macrophages, as well as neutrophils where granulomas are formed around worms or eggs. Effectors at mucosal surfaces also include products of macrophages and epithelial cells, such as intelectins, resistin-like molecules, chitinases and arginases, changes in mucous biology, and smooth muscle contraction, which contributes to mechanical expulsion of parasites.

8.4.1.2 Immunomodulation

Common to many parasites is the ability to modulate numerous host responses which ultimately enhance parasite survival within the host. Luminal dwelling helminth parasites secrete yet to be identified molecules that increase the permeability of the tight junctions of the epithelium (Su et al. 2011; Rehman et al. 2016), which enables ES products to enter the host and directly modulate host responses, including antigen-presenting cell (APC) function. ES products alter the release from APC of cytokines that influence the polarization of T cells (Rehman et al. 2015). Parasites have also developed effective ways to prevent activation of complement, which is involved in protection (Alba-Hurtado and Muñoz-Guzmán 2013). Several proteins in ES products, such as GAPDH and calreticulin, interact with the host complement cascade (Suchitra and Joshi 2005), suggesting that inactivation of complement would be beneficial for nematode survival.

8.4.1.3 Antibodies in Antiparasite Immune Responses

An important feature of host responses to parasites is the generation of antibodies to molecules expressed in the different developmental stages of the parasite. Antibodies are also reported to be involved in the rejection of incoming larvae. Antibodies of the IgA, IgG, and IgE subclasses are implicated in resistance to parasitic nematodes, but the mechanisms by which antibodies protect against infestations are not well understood. This is complicated by the fact that antibody responses include binding to nonfunctional epitopes or antigens, which are only expressed for a short period of time during the various stages of the life cycle. Many parasite molecules are present in multiple isoforms that differ in size or isoelectric point when separated by gel chromatography. This may allow the parasite to escape immune surveillance, as all forms are not necessarily recognized by the immune host; for example, only six of 20 spots identified as the H15 antigen of *H. contortus* were recognized by immune serum (Yatsuda et al. 2003).

Elevated IgA and IgG levels are characteristic of nematode parasitism, including infection with *H. contortus* (Gill et al. 1993) and *T. colubriformis* (Pernthaner et al. 2006). Whereas correlation of serum antibody levels and the immune status of the host remains inconclusive, mucosal antibody levels are a much better correlate of protection (Shaw et al. 2012), presumably because local immune effectors are required to control infections, especially with luminal dwellers. The antibody repertoire of an immune host includes antibodies that may inactivate or neutralize vital metabolic enzymes, directly affecting worm survival (Moreau and Chauvin 2010). A negative correlation between the magnitude of an IgA response to sheep parasites and worm length suggests that IgA interferes with worms feeding (McCririe et al. 1997).

A characteristic feature of helminth infections is an increase in IgE, as seen in infections of sheep (Pernthaner et al. 2005b) or calves (Baker and Gershwin 1993). IgE responses are predominantly directed against adult parasite antigens and no significant changes in IgE levels occurred during larval infection (Huntley et al. 1998). IgE activation of mast cells via Fc-receptor binding, followed by cross-linking by parasite antigens, generates effectors against gastrointestinal parasites (Kawakami and Galli 2002). Parasites appear to be able to counter mast cell activation through the generation of large amounts of nonspecific IgE which may outcompete receptor binding by antigen-specific IgE.

Antibodies generated by the presence of parasites are not necessarily protective for the host and may fail to prevent parasite establishment or to cause expulsion. In these cases, the generation of large amounts of antibodies, such as by *F. hepatica* or the intermediate stages of cestodes, may be useful only as diagnostic tools. The mucosal polyclonal anti-CarLA IgA response to the glycan antigen CarLA on the epicuticle of L3 of many parasitic nematode species is a marker which reflects the immune status of the animal, as measured by fecal egg counts (Shaw et al. 2012). While exposure of L3 to mucosal polyclonal anti-CarLA IgA *in vitro* reduces their motility, causes clumping and prevents their subsequent establishment in recipient sheep (Harrison et al. 2008), vaccination with CarLA failed to induce an antibody response (Harrison, pers. comm.).

8.4.2 Vaccination-Induced Immune Response

The aim of many vaccines is to induce strong antigen-specific antibody responses that ultimately result in the elimination of the infection. The desired response may not simply mimic natural immunity, which in many cases is permissive of long-term infections, and it may vary with different parasites and hosts. Knowing the characteristics of naturally resistant individuals may be important in designing vaccines. Whereas outbred sheep genetically resistant to *H. contortus* had elevated serum IgG1 and IgA responses (Gill et al. 1993), resistant Merino lambs had an enhanced parasite-specific cell-mediated immune response (Gill 1994). The natural resistance of some humans in Brazil to infection with schistosomes involves both a Th1 and Th2 response (Viana et al. 1995) and it is believed that a vaccine to induce protection against *Schistosoma mansoni* infection or reinfection should have an appropriate adjuvant to induce both humoral and cellular responses (Corrêa-Oliveira et al. 2000). Many antiparasite vaccines induce strong serum antibody responses, which for a variety of reasons are not protective. It is likely that novel vaccines that consist of a cocktail of relevant antigens formulated with optimal adjuvants and administered via the most appropriate route will need to be developed for each host and parasite species to overcome these issues.

Vaccines against blood-feeding parasites, such as *Haemonchus* spp., hookworms and ticks, act through antibodies and other serum proteins ingested with each blood meal. This makes even more remarkable the ability of blood and lymphatic helminths to evade the host immune response and survive for decades in these environments. The tick vaccine causes antibody-mediated interference with the digestion of blood, as well as complement-mediated lysis of the gut epithelium (Willadsen et al. 1989). Similarly, the *H. contortus* antigen H11 induces the generation of IgG1, which appears to neutralize that enzyme and also act via the complement system. Similarly, antibodies have also been shown to be the major vehicle for protection of sheep against the intermediate stages of the cestodes *T. ovis* and *E. granulosus*. The recombinant vaccine antigens provoke both antibody- and complement-mediated lysis of oncospheres (Johnson et al. 1989).

Effective immunity to luminal parasites can be induced artificially by multiple infections with large numbers of gastrointestinal nematodes. Repeated experimental infection of sheep with L3 larvae, followed by drug treatment at a later stage of parasite development, induced high antibody levels and protective immunity to *T. colubriformis* and *Teladorsagia circumcincta* (Stankiewicz et al. 1996). While vaccinations typically induce the generation of high titers of serum IgG, IgA is not normally produced and secreted on to the mucosal surfaces, which may be a disadvantage, assuming effective mucosal immune responses may be essential.

8.4.3 Adjuvants

The role of adjuvants in vaccines against multicellular parasites is largely unknown, unlike those developed for viral and bacterial pathogens. Adjuvants enhance the immune response and affect the balance between antibody- and cell-mediated responses; this can be beneficial but may in some cases be detrimental to the induction of protective immune responses. A small number of the traditional adjuvants have been used in most trials, particularly alum, QuilA, and Montanide 888. The currently registered vaccines use aluminum hydroxide (Huskvac), 10% Montanide 888 in a mineral oil emulsion (TickGUARD and GAVAC), QuilA (EG95), and saponin (Barbervax). Aluminum adjuvants (which are registered for use in humans), which promote a predominant Th2-type response, would be expected to be desirable in vaccines against parasites; however, alum was used with limited effect in experimental studies (Piedrafita et al. 2013). A novel adjuvant, DEAE-dextran, induced significant protection under controlled conditions (Piedrafita et al. 2013), which needs replicating in field trials. Chitosans have been used successfully in vaccines against influenza and bacteria, as well as cestode parasites (Umair et al. 2017). They are thermosensitive biopolymers which form gels at body temperature and provide sustained-release depots of antigens (Kojarunchitt et al. 2015). Selection of a suitable adjuvant, possibly in connection with a co-adjuvant, will be a crucial component in the development of effective antiparasite vaccines.

8.5 Summary

Veterinary vaccines against multicellular parasites have largely been directed at ticks and helminths, particularly nematodes, which are the principal parasites responsible for economic losses in livestock. Vaccines to control cestodes in intermediate hosts and *S. japonicum* in buffaloes, which are reservoirs for zoonotic diseases, are considered an important part of public health campaigns. Three commercial vaccines are currently available in selected countries: Gavac (cattle ticks), Barbervax (*H. contortus*), and Huskvac (*D. viviparus*), whereas TickGUARD (cattle ticks) and an *A. caninum* dog hookworm vaccine are now withdrawn. Live attenuated parasites are used in Huskvac and in experimental vaccines against a number of species, but have the disadvantages of the need for donor animals, a relatively short shelf-life, specific temperature requirements for storage, and the risk of contamination. Vaccines based on native antigens, such as Barbervax, suffer from many of these limitations.

Development of commercially viable subunit vaccines has proved to be difficult, particularly the generation of recombinant antigens which are appropriately expressed, folded, and posttranslationally modified. The successful vaccines are the bovine tick vaccines, based on the recombinant gut glycoprotein antigen Bm86 of *R. microplus*, and the cestode vaccines using recombinant antigens from the oncospheral penetration glands. Future vaccines are likely to depend on selection of recombinant antigens, DNA technology, more appropriate adjuvants or novel methods of delivery.

Acknowledgments

We thank Drs Bryce Buddle and Neil Wedlock for reviewing the chapter and providing helpful suggestions.

References

Adams, D.B., Beh, K.J., and Davies, H.I. (1982). The response of sheep to parenteral vaccination and immunizing infections against the abomasal nematode, *Haemonchus contortus*. *Int. J. Parasitol.* 12: 445–449.

Alba-Hurtado, F. and Muñoz-Guzmán, M.A. (2013). Immune responses associated with resistance to haemonchosis in sheep. *BioMed Res. Int.* 2013: 162158.

Almeria, S., Canals, A., Gomez-Munoz, M.T. et al. (1998). Characterization of protective immune responses in local lymphoid tissues after drug-attenuated infections with *Ostertagia ostertagi* in calves. *Vet. Parasitol.* 80: 53–64.

Assana, E., Kyngdon, C.T., Gauci, C.G. et al. (2010). Elimination of *Taenia solium* transmission to pigs in a field trial of the TSOL18 vaccine in Cameroon. *Int. J. Parasitol.* 40: 515–519.

Baker, D.G. and Gershwin, L.J. (1993). Inverse relationship between IgE and worm burdens in cattle infected with *Ostertagia ostertagi*. *Vet. Parasitol.* 47: 87–97.

Bakker, N., Vervelde, L., Kanobana, K. et al. (2004). Vaccination against the nematode *Haemonchus contortus* with a thiol-binding fraction from the excretory/secretory products (ES). *Vaccine* 22: 618–628.

Bassetto, C.C., Picharillo, M.É., Newlands, G.F.J. et al. (2014a). Attempts to vaccinate ewes and their lambs against natural infection with *Haemonchus contortus* in a tropical environment. *Int. J. Parasitol.* 44: 1049–1054.

Bassetto, C.C., Silva, M.R.L., Newlands, G.F.J. et al. (2014b). Vaccination of grazing calves with antigens from the intestinal membranes of *Haemonchus contortus*: effects against natural challenge with *Haemonchus placei* and *Haemonchus similis*. *Int. J. Parasitol.* 44: 697–702.

Benitez-Usher, C., Armour, J., Duncan, J.L. et al. (1977). A study of some factors influencing the immunization of sheep against *Haemonchus contortus* using attenuated larvae. *Vet. Parasitol.* 3: 327–342.

Bickle, Q.D. (2009). Radiation-attenuated schistosome vaccination – a brief historical perspective. *Parasitology* 136: 1621–1632.

Blaxter, M.L., Page, A.P., Rudin, W., and Maizels, R.M. (1992). Nematode surface coats: actively evading immunity. *Parasitol. Today* 8: 243–247.

Boulanger, D., Schneider, D., Chippaux, J.-P. et al. (1999). *Schistosoma bovis*: vaccine effects of a recombinant homologous glutathione S-transferase in sheep. *Int. J. Parasitol.* 29: 415–418.

Bushara, H.O., Bashir, M.E.N., Malik, K.H.E. et al. (1993). Suppression of *Schistosoma bovis* egg production in cattle by vaccination with either glutathione *S*-transferase or keyhole limpet haemocyanin. *Parasite Immunol.* 15: 383–390.

Caulfield, J.P., Korman, G., Butterworth, A.E. et al. (1980). Partial and complete detachment of neutrophils and eosinophils from schistosomula: evidence for the establishment of continuity between a fused and normal parasite membrane. *J. Cell Biol.* 86: 64–76.

Chen, N., Yuan, Z.-G., Xu, M.-J. et al. (2012). *Ascaris suum* enolase is a potential vaccine candidate against ascariasis. *Vaccine* 30: 3478–3482.

Coop, R.L. and Kyriazakis, I. (1999). Nutrition-parasite interaction. *Vet. Parasitol.* 84: 187–204.

Copley, S.D. (2012). Moonlighting is mainstream: paradigm adjustment required. *Bioessays* 34: 578–588.

Corrêa-Oliveira, R., Caldas, I.R., and Gazzinelli, G. (2000). Natural versus drug-induced resistance in *Schistosoma mansoni* infection. *Parasitol. Today* 16: 397–399.

Díaz-Martín, V., Manzano-Román, R., Obolo-Mvoulouga, P. et al. (2015). Development of vaccines against *Ornithodoros* soft ticks: an update. *Ticks Tick-borne Dis.* 6: 211–220.

Domínguez-Toraño, I.A., Cuquerella, M., Gómez-Muñoz, M.T. et al. (2000). Vaccination of Manchego lambs against *Haemonchus contortus* with a somatic fraction (p26/23) of adult parasites. *Parasite Immunol.* 22: 131–138.

de la Fuente, J., Rodríguez, M., Redondo, M. et al. (1998). Field studies and cost-effectiveness analysis of vaccination with Gavac™ against the cattle tick *Boophilus microplus*. *Vaccine* 16: 366–373.

García-García, J.C., Montero, C., Redondo, M. et al. (2000). Control of ticks resistant to immunization with Bm86 in cattle vaccinated with the recombinant antigen Bm95 isolated from the cattle tick, *Boophilus microplus*. *Vaccine* 18: 2275–2287.

Gauci, C. and Lightowlers, M.W. (2013). Genes encoding homologous antigens in taeniid cestode parasites. Implications for development of recombinant vaccines produced in *Escherichia coli*. *Bioengineered* 4: 168–171.

Gill, H.S. (1994). Cell-mediated immunity in Merino lambs with genetic resistance to *Haemonchus contortus*. *Int. J. Parasitol.* 24: 749–756.

Gill, H.S., Gray, G.D., Watson, D.L., and Husband, A.J. (1993). Isotype-specific antibody responses to *Haemonchus contortus* in genetically resistant sheep. *Parasite Immunol.* 15: 61–67.

Han, K., Xu, L., Yan, R. et al. (2012). Vaccination of goats with glyceraldehyde-3-phosphate dehydrogenase DNA vaccine induced partial protection against *Haemonchus contortus*. *Vet. Immunol. Immunopathol.* 149: 177–185.

Harrison, G.B.L., Heath, D.D., Dempster, R.P. et al. (1996). Identification and cDNA cloning of two novel low molecular weight host-protective antigens from *Taenia ovis* oncospheres. *Int. J. Parasitol.* 26: 195–204.

Harrison, G.B.L., Pulford, H.D., Doolin, E.E. et al. (2008). Antibodies to surface epitopes of the carbohydrate larval antigen CarLA are associated with passive protection in Strongylid nematode challenge infections. *Parasite Immunol.* 30: 577–584.

Heath, D.D., Robinson, C., Shakes, T. et al. (2012). Vaccination of bovines against *Echinococcus granulosus* (cystic echinococcosis). *Vaccine* 30: 3076–3081.

Hewitson, J.P., Grainger, J.R., and Maizels, R.M. (2009). Helminth immunoregulation: the role of parasite secreted proteins in modulating host immunity. *Mol. Biochem. Parasitol.* 167: 1–11.

Huntley, J.F., Schallig, H.D., Kooyman, F.N. et al. (1998). IgE antibody during infection with the ovine abomasal nematode, *Teladorsagia circumcincta*: primary and secondary responses in serum and gastric lymph of sheep. *Parasite Immunol.* 20: 565–571.

Jabbar, A., Jenkins, D.J., Crawford, S. et al. (2011). Oncospheral penetration glands are the sources of the EG95 vaccine antigen against cystic hydatid disease. *Parasitology* 138: 89–99.

Jarrett, W.F.H. and Sharp, N.C.C. (1963). Vaccination against parasitic disease: reactions in vaccinated and immune hosts in *Dictyocaulus viviparus* infection. *J. Parasitol.* 49: 177–189.

Jayashi, C.M., Kyngdon, C.T., Gauci, C.G. et al. (2012). Successful immunization of naturally reared pigs against porcine cysticercosis with a recombinant oncosphere antigen vaccine. *Vet. Parasitol.* 188: 261–267.

Joekel, D., Hinse, P., Raulf, M.K. et al. (2015). Vaccination of calves with yeast- and bacterial-expressed paramyosin from the bovine lungworm *Dictyocaulus viviparus*. *Parasite Immunol.* 37: 614–623.

Johnson, K.S., Harrison, G.B.L., Lightowlers, M.W. et al. (1989). Vaccination against ovine cysticercosis using a defined recombinant antigen. *Nature* 338: 585–587.

Kalyanasundaram, A., Jawahar, S., Ilangopathy, M. et al. (2015). Comparative immunoprophylactic efficacy of *Haemonchus contortus* recombinant enolase (rHcENO) and ConA purified native glycoproteins in sheep. *Exp. Parasitol.* 154: 98–107.

Kawakami, T. and Galli, S.J. (2002). Regulation of mast-cell and basophil function and survival by IgE. *Nat. Rev. Immunol.* 2: 773–786.

Kearney, P.E., Murray, P.J., Hoy, J.M. et al. (2016). The 'toolbox' of strategies for managing *Haemonchus contortus* in goats: what's in and what's out. *Vet. Parasitol.* 220: 93–107.

Knox, D.P., Redmond, D.L., Newlands, G.F. et al. (2003). The nature and prospects for gut membrane proteins as vaccine candidates for *Haemonchus contortus* and other ruminant trichostrongyloids. *Int. J. Parasitol.* 33: 1129–1137.

Kojarunchitt, T., Baldursdottir, S., Dong, Y.-D. et al. (2015). Modified thermoresponsive Poloxamer 407 and chitosan sol-gels as potential sustained-release vaccine delivery systems. *Eur. J. Pharm. Biopharm.* 89: 74–81.

Kumar, N., Anju, V., Gaurav, N. et al. (2012). Vaccination of buffaloes with *Fasciola gigantica* recombinant glutathione S-transferase and fatty acid binding protein. *Parasitol. Res.* 110: 419–426.

Larrieu, E., Mujica, G., Gauci, C.G. et al. (2015). Pilot field trial of the EG95 vaccine against ovine cystic echinococcosis in Rio Negro, Argentina: second study of impact. *PLoS Negl.Trop. Dis.* 9: e0004134.

Li, X., Yao, J.-p., Pan, A.-h. et al. (2013). An antigenic recombinant serine protease from *Trichinella spiralis* induces protective immunity in BALB/c mice. *Parasitol. Res.* 112: 3229–3238.

Lightowlers, M.W., Rolfe, R., and Gauci, C.G. (1996). *Taenia saginata*: vaccination against cysticercosis in cattle with recombinant oncosphere antigens. *Exp. Parasitol.* 84: 330–338.

Maass, D.R., Harrison, G.B., Grant, W.N. et al. (2009). Intraspecific epitopic variation in a carbohydrate antigen exposed on the surface of *Trichostrongylus colubriformis* infective L3 larvae. *PLoS Pathog.* 5: e1000597.

Maggioli, G., Acosta, D., Silveira, F. et al. (2011). The recombinant gut-associated M17 leucine aminopeptidase in combination with different adjuvants confers a high level of protection against *Fasciola hepatica* infection in sheep. *Vaccine* 29: 9057–9063.

Mahana, M., Abd-Allah, H.A.-S., Salah, M., and El Ridi, R. (2016). *Fasciola gigantica* enolase is a major component of worm tegumental fraction protective against sheep fasciolosis. *Acta Trop.* 158: 189–196.

Makepeace, B.L., Jensen, S.A., Laney, S.J. et al. (2009). Immunisation with a multivalent, subunit vaccine reduces patent infection in a natural bovine model of onchocerciasis during intense field exposure. *PLoS Negl. Trop. Dis.* 3: e544.

Martín, S., Molina, J.M., Hernández, Y.I. et al. (2015). Influence of immunoprotection on genetic variability of cysteine proteinases from *Haemonchus contortus* adult worms. *Int. J. Parasitol.* 45: 831–840.

Mas-Coma, S., Bargues, M.D., and Valero, M.A. (2005). Fascioliasis and other plant-borne trematode zoonoses. *Int. J. Parasitol.* 35: 1255–1278.

McClure, S.J. (2009). Mucosal delivery of native and recombinant protein vaccines against *Trichostrongylus colubriformis*. *Int. J. Parasitol.* 39: 599–606.

McCririe, L., Bairden, K., Britton, C. et al. (1997). Heterogeneity in the recognition of *Ostertagia circumcincta* antigens by serum antibody from mature, infected sheep. *Parasite Immunol.* 19: 235–242.

McKeand, J.B. and Kennedy, M.W. (1995). Shedding of surface-bound antibody by adult *Dictyocaulus viviparus*. *Int. J. Parasitol.* 25: 1255–1258.

McManus, D.P. and Loukas, A. (2008). Current status of vaccines for schistosomiasis. *Clin. Microbiol. Rev.* 21: 225–242.

McManus, D.P., Wong, J.Y.M., Zhou, J. et al. (2002). Recombinant paramyosin (rec-Sj-97) tested for immunogenicity and vaccine efficacy against *Schistosoma japonicum* in mice and water buffaloes. *Vaccine* 20: 870–878.

Miller, T.A. (1978). Industrial development and field use of the canine hookworm vaccine. *Adv. Parasitol.* 16: 333–342.

Molina-Hernández, V., Mulcahy, G., Pérez, J. et al. (2015). *Fasciola hepatica* vaccine: we may not be there yet but we're on the right road. *Vet. Parasitol.* 208: 101–111.

Monahan, C.M., Taylor, H.W., Chapman, M.R., and Klei, T.R. (1994). Experimental immunization of ponies with *Strongylus vulgaris* radiation-attenuated larvae or crude soluble somatic extracts from larval or adult stages. *J. Parasitol.* 80: 911–923.

Monreal-Escalante, E., Govea-Alonso, D.O., Hernández, M. et al. (2016). Towards the development of an oral vaccine against porcine cysticercosis: expression of the protective HP6/TSOL18 antigen in transgenic carrots cells. *Planta* 243: 675–685.

Moreau, E. and Chauvin, A. (2010). Immunity against helminths: interactions with the host and the intercurrent infections. *J. Biomed. Biotech.* 10: 428593.

Muleke, C.I., Yan, R., Sun, Y. et al. (2007). Vaccination of goats against *Haemonchus contortus* with a recombinant cysteine protease. *Small Rum. Res.* 73: 95–102.

Murray, J. and Smith, W.D. (1994). Ingestion of host immunoglobulin by three non-blood-feeding nematode parasites of ruminants. *Res. Vet. Sci.* 57: 387–389.

Nuttall, P.A., Trimnell, A.R., Kazimirova, M., and Labuda, M. (2006). Exposed and concealed antigens as vaccine targets for controlling ticks and tick-borne diseases. *Parasite Immunol.* 28: 155–163.

O'Sullivan, B.M. and Donald, A.D. (1970). A field study of nematode parasite populations in the lactating ewe. *Parasitology* 61: 301–315.

Pernthaner, A., Cole, S.A., Morrison, L., and Hein, W.R. (2005a). Increased expression of interleukin-5 (IL-5), IL-13, and tumor necrosis factor alpha genes in intestinal lymph cells of sheep selected for enhanced resistance to nematodes during infection with *Trichostrongylus colubriformis*. *Infect. Immun.* 73: 2175–2183.

Pernthaner, A., Shaw, R.J., McNeill, M.M. et al. (2005b). Total and nematode-specific IgE responses in intestinal lymph of genetically resistant and susceptible sheep during infection with *Trichostrongylus colubriformis*. *Vet. Immunol. Immunopathol.* 104: 69–80.

Pernthaner, A., Cole, S.A., Morrison, L. et al. (2006). Cytokine and antibody subclass responses in the intestinal lymph of sheep during repeated experimental infections with the nematode parasite *Trichostrongylus colubriformis*. *Vet. Immunol. Immunopathol.* 114: 135–148.

Piedrafita, D., de Veer, M., Sherrard, J. et al. (2012). Field vaccination of sheep with a larval-specific antigen of the gastrointestinal nematode, *Haemonchus contortus* confers significant protection against an experimental challenge infection. *Vaccine* 30: 7199–7204.

Piedrafita, D., Preston, S., Kemp, J. et al. (2013). The effect of different adjuvants on immune parameters and protection following vaccination of sheep with a larval-specific antigen of the gastrointestinal nematode, *Haemonchus contortus*. *PLoS One* 8: e78357.

Prudencio, C.R., Marra, A.O.M., Cardoso, R., and Goulart, L.R. (2010). Recombinant peptides as new immunogens for the control of the bovine tick *Rhipicephalus (Boophilus) microplus*. *Vet. Parasitol.* 172: 122–131.

Redmond, D.L. and Knox, D.P. (2006). Further protection studies using recombinant forms of *Haemonchus contortus* cysteine proteinases. *Parasite Immunol.* 28: 213–219.

Rehman, Z.U., Knight, J.S., Koolaard, J. et al. (2015). Immunomodulatory effects of adult *Haemonchus contortus* excretory/secretory products on human monocyte-derived dendritic cells. *Parasite Immunol.* 37: 657–669.

Rehman, Z.U., Deng, Q., Umair, S. et al. (2016). Excretory/secretory products of adult *Haemonchus contortus* and *Teladorsagia circumcincta* which increase the permeability of Caco-2 cell monolayers are neutralised by antibodies from immune hosts. *Vet. Parasitol.* 221: 104–110.

Rinaldi, M. and Geldhof, P. (2012). Immunologically based control strategies for ostertagiosis in cattle: where do we stand? *Parasite Immunol.* 34: 254–264.

Robinson, M.W. and Dalton, J.P. (2009). Zoonotic helminth infections with particular emphasis on fasciolosis and other trematodiases. *Philos. Trans. R. Soc. London, Ser. B* 364: 2763–2776.

Shaw, R.J., Morris, C.A., Wheeler, M. et al. (2012). Salivary IgA: a suitable measure of immunity to gastrointestinal nematodes in sheep. *Vet. Parasitol.* 186: 109–117.

Stankiewicz, M., Cabaj, W., Pernthaner, A., and Hadas, E. (1996). Immunisation of sheep by drug-abbreviated infections of *Ostertagia circumcincta* and *Trichostrongylus colubriformis* against field challenge of gastro-intestinal nematodes. *Vet. Parasitol.* 67: 121–132.

Steisslinger, V., Korten, S., Brattig, N.W., and Ertmann, K.D. (2015). DNA vaccine encoding the moonlighting protein *Onchocerca volvulus* glyceraldehyde-3-phosphate dehydrogenase (Ov-GAPDH) leads to partial protection in a mouse model of human filariasis. *Vaccine* 33: 5861–5867.

Su, C., Cao, Y., Kaplan, J. et al. (2011). Duodenal helminth infection alters barrier function of the colonic epithelium via adaptive immune activation. *Infect. Immun.* 79: 2285–2294.

Suchitra, S. and Joshi, P. (2005). Characterization of *Haemonchus contortus* calreticulin suggests its role in feeding and immune evasion by the parasite. *Biochim. Biophys. Acta* 1722: 293–303.

Sun, W., Song, X., Yan, R. et al. (2011). Vaccination of goats with a glutathione peroxidase DNA vaccine induced partial protection against *Haemonchus contortus* infection. *Vet. Parasitol.* 182: 239–247.

Sun, R., Zhao, X., Wang, Z. et al. (2015). *Trichinella spiralis* paramyosin binds human complement C1q and inhibits classical complement activation. *PLoS Negl.Trop. Dis.* 9: e0004310.

Tan, J.L., Ueda, N., Heath, D. et al. (2012). Development of orf virus as a bifunctional recombinant vaccine: surface display of *Echinococcus granulosus* antigen EG95 by fusion to membrane structural proteins. *Vaccine* 30: 398–406.

Tchakouté, V.L., Graham, S.P., Jensen, S.A. et al. (2006). In a bovine model of onchocerciasis, protective immunity exists naturally, is absent in drug-cured hosts, and is induced by vaccination. *Proc. Natl. Acad. Sci. U.S.A.* 103: 5971–5976.

Thirugnanam, S., Pandiaraja, P., Ramaswamy, K. et al. (2007). *Brugia malayi*: comparison of protective immune responses induced by Bm-alt-2 DNA, recombinant Bm-ALT-2 protein and prime-boost vaccine regimens in a jird model. *Exp. Parasitol.* 116: 483–491.

Umair, S., Deng, Q., Roberts, J.M. et al. (2016). Identification of peptide mimics of a glycan epitope on the surface of parasitic nematode larvae. *PLoS One* 11: e0162016.

Umair, S., Pernthaner, A., Deng, Q. et al. (2017). Preliminary evaluation of a thermosensitive chitosan hydrogel for *Echinococcus granulosus* vaccine delivery. *Vet. Parasitol.* 236: 117–120.

Van Meulder, F., Ratman, D., van Coppernolle, S. et al. (2015). Analysis of the protective immune response following intramuscular vaccination of calves against the intestinal parasite *Cooperia oncophora*. *Int. J. Parasitol.* 45: 637–646.

Viana, I.R.C., Corrêa-Oliveira, R., Dos Santos Carvalho, O. et al. (1995). Comparison of antibody isotype responses to *Schistosoma mansoni* antigens by infected and putative resistant individuals living in an endemic area. *Parasite Immunol.* 17: 297–304.

Wang, H. and Nuttall, P.A. (1994). Comparison of the proteins in salivary glands, saliva and haemolymph of *Rhipicephalus appendiculatus* female ticks during feeding. *Parasitology* 109: 517–523.

Watson, D.L., Colditz, I.G., Andrew, M. et al. (1994). Age-dependent immune response in Merino sheep. *Res. Vet. Sci.* 57: 152–158.

Wesolowska, A., Zawistowska-Deniziak, A., Norbury, L.J. et al. (2016). Immune responses in rats and sheep induced by a DNA vaccine containing the phosphoglycerate kinase gene of *Fasciola hepatica* and liver fluke infection. *Acta Parasitol.* 61: 212–220.

Willadsen, P., Reding, G.H., McKenna, R.V., and Kemp, D.H. (1989). Immunological control of a parasitic arthropods. Identification of a protective antigen from *Boophilus microplus*. *J. Immunol.* 143: 1346–1351.

Willadsen, P., Bird, P., Cobon, G.S., and Hungerford, J. (1995). Commercialisation of a recombinant vaccine against *Boophilus microplus*. *Parasitology* 110: S43–S50.

Windon, R.G., Dineen, J.K., and Kelly, J.D. (1980). The segregation of lambs into 'responders' and 'non-responders': response to vaccination with irradiated *Trichostrongylus colubriformis* larvae before weaning. *Int. J. Parasitol.* 10: 65–73.

Winter, M.D., Wright, C., and Lee, D.L. (2000). Vaccination of young lambs with *Nematodirus battus* using gamma irradiated larvae. *Int. J. Parasitol.* 30: 1173–1176.

Winter, J.A., Davies, O.R., Brown, A.P. et al. (2005). The assessment of hookworm calreticulin as a potential vaccine for necatoriasis. *Parasite Immunol.* 27: 139–146.

Wiśniewski, M., Jaros, S., Bąska, P. et al. (2016). Hamsters vaccinated with ace-mep-7 DNA vaccine produced protective immunity against *Ancylostoma ceylanicum* infection. *Exp. Parasitol.* 163: 1–7.

Wu, Z.-D., Lü, Z.-Y., and Yu, X.-B. (2005). Development of a vaccine against *Schistosoma japonicum* in China: a review. *Acta Trop.* 96: 106–116.

Yatsuda, A.P., Krijgsveld, J., Cornelissen, A.W.C.A. et al. (2003). Comprehensive analysis of the secreted proteins of the parasite *Haemonchus contortus* reveals extensive sequence variation and differential immune recognition. *J. Biolumin. Chemilumin.* 278: 16941–16951.

Zhu, Y., Ren, J., Da'dara, A. et al. (2004). The protective effect of a *Schistosoma japonicum* Chinese strain 23 kDa plasmid DNA vaccine in pigs is enhanced with IL-12. *Vaccine* 23: 78–83.

Zhu, L., Liu, H.-F., Lu, M.-B. et al. (2011). Construction, purification, and evaluation of multivalent DNA vaccine against *Schistosoma japonicum*. *Parasitol. Res.* 108: 115–121.

9

Fish Vaccines

Alexandra Adams[1] *and Rohana Subasinghe*[2]

[1] *Institute of Aquaculture, University of Stirling, Stirling, Scotland*
[2] *FUTUREFISH, Rajagiriya, Sri Lanka*

9.1 Introduction

In 2014, the contribution of aquaculture to supply food for human consumption overtook that for wild-caught fish for the first time (FAO 2016). China has played a major role in this growth, as it represents more than 73% of world aquaculture production today (FAO 2018). Aquaculture currently contributes approximately 80 million tonnes of aquatic animals (including marine and freshwater finfish, crustaceans, and shellfish) with a value of US$ 232 billion. With an annual percent rate of growth of 5.8% since 2001, aquaculture still represents the fastest growing animal production sector in the world (FAO 2018). Twenty-seven finfish species make up 90% of global aquatic animal production, with Atlantic salmon (*Salmo salar*) being the number one fish species in terms of economic value and in the top 10 species in terms of volume (FAO 2018).

Fish diseases are considered to be a major constraint to aquaculture globally, with all finfish aquaculture sectors affected to some extent by infectious disease (Rodger 2016). It has been estimated that 10% of all cultured aquatic animals are lost because of infectious diseases alone, amounting to >10 billion US$ in losses annually on a global scale (Evensen 2016).

Although many bacterial diseases are now effectively controlled by the use of vaccines, viral diseases still present significant infectious disease challenges for salmonid and marine finfish, and there are only a limited number of effective vaccines commercially available for these (Rodger 2016). Bacterial pathogens still present some major challenges for rainbow trout, carp, tilapia, and catfish. In addition, these pose problems for "cleanerfish," i.e. ballan wrasse (*Labrus bergylta*) and lumpsucker (*Cyclopterus lumpus*), which are currently being used in the biological control of sea lice (*Lepeophtheirus salmonis*) in Atlantic salmon aquaculture. Ectoparasites (including sea lice and *Paramoeba perurans* which causes amoebic gill disease, AGD) currently pose the most significant disease threat for the Atlantic salmon industry and there are no commercial vaccines available at present for these, nor for fungi or fungi-like organisms. The more common "water molds" in fish, such as *Saprolegnia* and *Aphanomyces*, are not in fact true fungi but oomycetes and are now considered to be opportunistic facultative parasites, e.g. *Saprolegnia parasitica* and *Aphanamyces invadans*. The former, fungal-like oomycete causes significant economic losses to salmonid aquaculture (both eggs and fish) while the latter causes epizootic ulcerative syndrome (EUS) in many freshwater and brackish species in the Asia-Pacific region and Australia.

Vaccines are recognized as important tools for the prevention and control of diseases in fish. The number of fish vaccines commercially available has grown in recent years but there are still numerous diseases where no vaccines are available or cases where existing vaccines do not perform well. Atlantic salmon and rainbow trout aquaculture in the UK, Norway, and USA expanded in the 1980s with a concurrent increase in disease. This led to the use of large amounts of antibiotics and consequently concerns grew with regard to antibiotic resistance. This stimulated the development of vaccines against bacterial pathogens and led to the first commercially available fish vaccines against vibriosis and enteric redmouth (ERM), followed by furunculosis vaccines. Commercial vaccines for fish have expanded from two in the 1980s to 24 currently, with one vaccine also available for lobsters (Assefa and Abunna 2018), with many of these now being multivalent. For example, heptavalent vaccines exist for use in Atlantic salmon and the use of antibiotics has been reduced by over 99%. In comparison, although carp and tilapia are

Veterinary Vaccines: Principles and Applications, First Edition. Edited by Samia Metwally, Gerrit Viljoen, and Ahmed El Idrissi.

well-established cultured species, there are few vaccines available for them.

9.2 Current Fish Vaccines

Commercial fish vaccines are available for a wide range of fish species (reviewed by Evensen 2016; Assefa and Abunna 2018), including Atlantic salmon, rainbow trout, sea bass (*Dicentrarchus labrax*) and sea bream (*Sparus aurata*), tilapia (*Oreochromis niloticus/mossambicus*), amberjack (*Seriola dumerili*), and yellowtail (*Seriola quinqueradiata*) in Japan, catfish (*Ictalurus punctatus*), and Vietnamese catfish (*Pangasionodon hypophthalmus*). The majority of commercial fish vaccines are formalin killed whole cell vaccines although live attenuated vaccines are licensed in the USA for use in catfish (Klesius and Pridgeon 2014). The latter are not currently allowed to be used in Europe. In addition, a DNA vaccine against infectious hematopoietic necrosis (IHN) is licensed in Canada for use in Atlantic salmon (Alonso and Leong 2013). There is also currently one commercial subunit vaccine (peptide; VP2) used in Norway (against infectious pancreatic necrosis virus, IPNV) and one recombinant vaccine against infectious salmon anemia virus (ISAV) in Chile.

In the European Union (EU), the cost of fish vaccine production is high as there are stringent requirements for vaccine manufacturers, although vaccines for use in small markets may take advantage of the Minor Use Minor Species Limited Market (MUMS) where the regulatory requirements are reduced (Cowan et al. 2016).

There are a number of important considerations for the use of vaccines in fish, including fish species, status of the immune system, production cycle and life history, when a disease occurs, farming technology (handling, mechanization, etc.), environment (e.g. temperature, salinity), stress factors, nutrition, and cost benefits. Guidelines on the use of fish vaccines are provided by the Responsible Use of Medicines in Agriculture Alliance (RUMA 2006).

9.3 Methods of Administration

Fish vaccines are administered by injection, immersion, or orally. Each of these methods has advantages and drawbacks (Table 9.1).

9.3.1 Injection Vaccination

The majority of commercial vaccines are administered to fish by injection (normally intraperitoneal injection, IP). This requires catching and anesthetizing the fish prior to vaccination. This is either performed by hand, normally by an injection team on site (Figure 9.1), or automated machines are now available and used widely in some countries. Vaccination by injection can potentially cause stress but no mortality is usually associated with the vaccination process *per se*, although some weak fish may die due to the handling process. Vaccine (usually 0.1–0.2 mL) is injected in the abdominal area of each anesthetized fish (>50 g), although microdoses of vaccines (0.025 or 0.05 mL) are also now being used. Fish are held ventral side up for vaccination and the needle is inserted into the peritoneal cavity using an automated injection gun (Figure 9.2). A team of four people can vaccinate approximately 5000 salmon per hour. Fish are often graded at the same time.

Table 9.1 Advantages and disadvantages of different methods of fish vaccine delivery.

Delivery method	Advantages	Disadvantages
Injection	Exact dose known, good immune response, adjuvants available	Fish need to be caught and anesthetized, cannot use with small fry
Dip immersion	Exact dose known. Used with small fry, little handling needed – net the fish and dip in vaccine for 30 s	Do not always get a good immune response (depends on vaccine), cannot be used with larger fish. No adjuvants available, therefore protection short-lived
Bath immersion	Exact dose known. Used with larger fish. Can also be useful with small fry if dip vaccination is too stressful, e.g. with ballan wrasse	Do not always get a good immune response, fish need to be closely watched and water aerated. No adjuvants available, therefore protection short-lived
Oral	Vaccine given with feed so no fish handling	Do not always get a good immune response; normally used as booster vaccination and vaccine needs to be protected. Vaccine dose per fish not known

Vaccination by injection provides a long duration of protection (>12 months) and multiple antigens can be combined in a single administration. In addition, each fish receives the vaccine at the correct dose; 10 000 fish (>25 g) can be vaccinated per liter of vaccine by IP injection. Injections are in general superior to any other vaccine application method, but they normally can only be applied to fish of 10 g or more (usually larger), although vaccination machines are being developed for smaller fish. One major

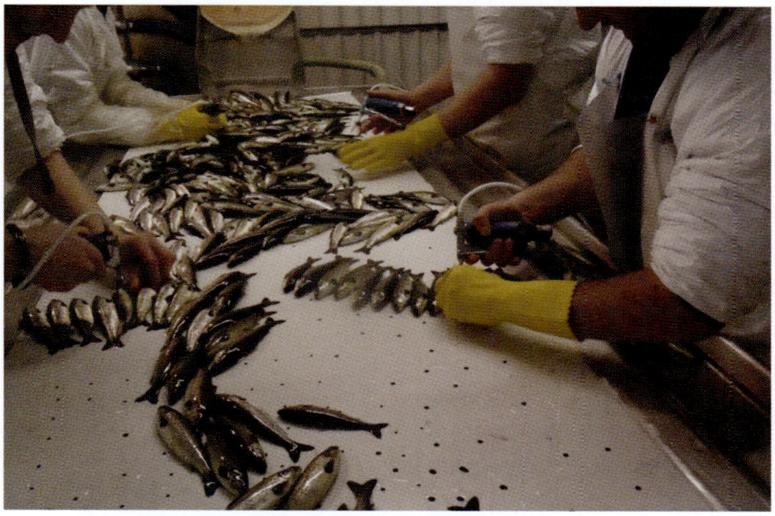

Figure 9.1 Vaccination of sedated fish is performed by hand, normally by an injection team on site. Source: Photograph courtesy of Pharmaq.

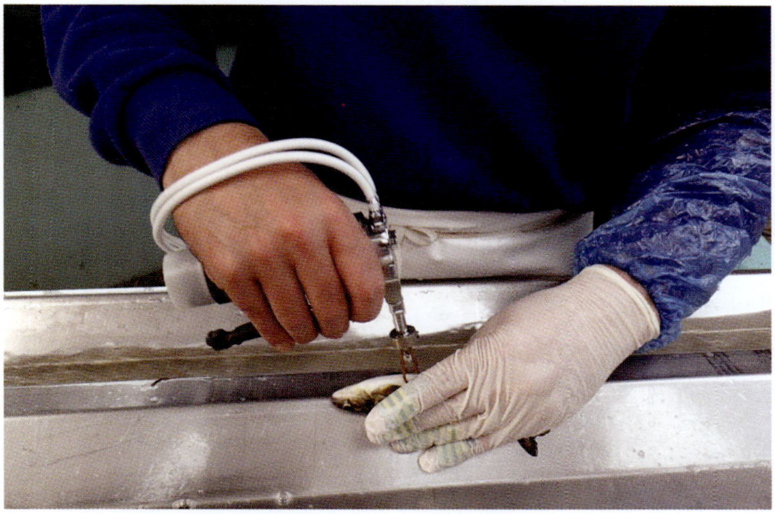

Figure 9.2 Fish are held ventral side up for vaccination and the needle is inserted into the peritoneal cavity using an automated injection gun. Source: Photograph courtesy of Pharmaq.

advantage of injection vaccination is that adjuvants can be included and there are a good range of adjuvants commercially available. Retention of antigens at the injection site is believed to be a prerequisite for long-term protection in fish, also known as the depot effect (Evensen et al. 2005).

9.3.2 Immersion Vaccination

There are two application methods for immersion vaccination: dip and bath. ERM and *Vibrio* vaccines are routinely administered to rainbow trout by immersion.

Dip vaccination is more widely used and involves immersing small fish for a short time (30 seconds) in a highly concentrated vaccine solution (one part vaccine to nine parts water). Large numbers of fish can be vaccinated using this method (up to 100 kg of fish per liter of vaccine) and it is widely used for vaccination of fry from 1 to 5 g. This method of vaccination is effective and provides relatively good protection. It is, however, limited in that there is a short duration of immunity (approximately 3 months) and a booster vaccination is required when the threat of disease persists. This method is impractical for larger fish due to cost-effectiveness and the stress of vaccination. In addition, in fish smaller than 1 g, the immune system may still be immature and therefore the vaccine efficacy may be reduced.

Bath vaccination is used for larger fish and they are exposed for a longer period, usually one to several hours, in a lower concentration of vaccine (normally 1/100). Large groups of fish are cut off from the rest in a cage and a low dose of diluted anesthetic is added. Air or oxygen needs to be continuously pumped in to avoid anoxia.

Following immersion vaccination, suspended antigens are adsorbed by the skin and gills. Specialized cells, such as antibody-secreting cells, in the skin and gill epithelium are activated and protect the fish when they are exposed to the live pathogen at a later stage. Other cells in the epithelium of skin and gills, such as antigen-presenting cells (macrophages), also absorb vaccine antigens and transport them to specialized tissues where the systemic immune response builds up.

9.3.3 Oral Vaccination

This is the most suitable method for mass vaccination but the amount eaten by individual fish is uncertain and poor potency can be a problem due to antigen destruction in the stomach. Thus, the vaccine needs to be protected in some way. Vaccine can be mixed with the feed, coated on top of the feed (top dressed), or bio-encapsulated. Stability in the feed as well as stability due to destruction in the stomach can both be an issue. Most vaccines are either incorporated in an "antigen-protecting vehicle" (*Yersinia ruckeri*, *Vibrio anguillarum*, and IPNV vaccines, MSD-Animal Health) or in a patented MicroMatrix™ delivery system (*Piscirickettsia salmonis*, ISAV, and IPNV, Centrovet) (Embregts and Forlenza 2016). When antigens are to be incorporated in feed, the heat sensitivity of the antigen has to be taken into consideration. Potency can be affected due to the low pH of the stomach. When vaccines are used as top dressing in feed, a coating agent is usually applied, to prevent either leaching of the antigen from the pellets or breakdown of the antigen in the acidic environment of the stomach. There are few oral vaccines on the market, and currently these are used as booster vaccines. Administration methods for oral vaccines still require optimization.

9.4 Nonfish Vaccines

Crustaceans (shrimp) are a very important species group in aquaculture with regard to value and volume. Although no commercial vaccines are available for aquatic animals other than fish (with the exception of the lobster gaffkemia vaccine), there has been some research effort on the development of shrimp vaccines. The mode of action of these is not fully known and it is thought that they could simply be stimulating the shrimp rather than vaccinating them as such (Musthaq and Kwang 2014). Further research to determine which alternative protection mechanisms can be found in crustaceans (especially shrimp) should be pursued. Development of specific pathogen-free (SPF) and specific pathogen-resistant (SPR) stocks are currently providing some hope for control of viral pathogens, but complete protection in open systems is currently not possible.

9.5 Immune Response to Vaccines

Fish differ from mammals in that they lack bone marrow and lymph nodes (Press and Evensen 1999). The major lymphoid tissues in teleost fish are the (head) kidney, thymus, spleen, and mucosa-associated lymphoid tissues (Press and Evensen 1999), including the gills (Haugarvoll et al. 2008), skin (Xu et al. 2013), and nostrils (Tacchi et al. 2014).

The fish immune system comprises both innate and adaptive immune responses, as in all vertebrates, with the latter playing the key role in providing protection following vaccination. A detailed review of the adaptive immune system in teleost fish and how this responds to vaccination has been recently published by Secombes and Belmonte (2016). The adaptive immune response is mediated by T and B lymphocytes, with T cells produced in the thymus and migrating to other tissue sites to induce responses. The B cells are produced at different sites in different vertebrate groups; in teleost fish this is mainly the kidney (akin to the bone marrow in mammals). Other differences between mammals and fish include immunoglobulin (Ig) classes – fish have no IgG, but instead have mainly IgM, IgD, and IgT. Significant advances have been made in understanding the fish immune system, with detailed knowledge of many of the cytokines involved in its regulation and assays developed to measure immune responses to vaccination and infection. This has assisted in the development of new vaccines.

9.6 Future Prospects and Challenges for Fish Vaccines

Fish vaccines have been very successful in reducing the use of antibiotics in the salmonid industry but additional vaccines are required for other fish species. Although the number of fish vaccines commercially available has grown in recent years, there are still numerous diseases where no vaccines are available or cases where existing vaccines do not perform well. Fish vaccine development is a very active research area (Evensen 2016). It is possible to measure with precision the responses elicited by vaccination (Secombes and Belmonte 2016), thus assisting the development of new vaccines for the future. The most crucial step in developing an effective vaccine is identification of "potentially" protective antigens and confirming their protective response in the host species by efficacy testing. The most effective approach taken depends on the type of pathogen and the final end-use envisaged for the vaccine (e.g. cost, fish species, immersion versus injection).

Fish vaccines have in general become much more sophisticated in recent years. Technologies such as recombinant and DNA vaccines are powerful tools for vaccine development as these enable the separation of potential protective antigens from suppressive ones. These are being developed because the simpler approach of using inactivated whole cell vaccines did not succeed for many important diseases, and attempts at developing attenuated vaccines in general have not been encouraged from a safety point of view. Recently, the use of DNA vaccines has been authorized in Europe, representing a major step forward. In addition, there is much current research focused on the development of mucosal vaccines (immersion and oral) and novel vaccine strategies following the discovery of IgT as a mucosal antibody in fish (Zhang et al. 2010, 2011). Discovery and optimization of the use of novel adjuvants is another area where improvements can be made. A variety of adjuvants exist for use by injection but none have so far been effective by immersion. In addition, the injectable adjuvants still cause concern with regard to fish welfare due to adhesions forming between organs in the fish, a long period after vaccination.

9.7 Summary

In conclusion, although many fish vaccines are commercially available and are effective, improvements are still required for some of the traditional inactivated vaccines with regard to vaccine efficacy (identification and optimization of antigen components), improved adjuvants, and oral administration. Development of successful vaccines against intracellular bacterial pathogens and viruses may require the use of live attenuated vaccines and application as oral vaccines, although there are safety concerns with the use of live vaccines in the aquatic environment. Vaccines against parasites and fungi-like organisms are also in development and these may need to rely on recombinant or DNA vaccine technology. There is also still a requirement for basic information on pathogenesis, immune response, and identification of potentially protective antigens for parasites and fungi. Autogenous vaccines are currently used in aquaculture, for example to prevent rainbow trout fry syndrome, and these are now also being developed against parasite diseases in Atlantic salmon (e.g. AGD).

References

Alonso, M. and Leong, J.A. (2013). Licensed DNA vaccines against infectious hematopoietic necrosis virus (IHNV). *Recent Pat. DNA Gene Seq.* 7 (1): 62–65.

Assefa, A. and Abunna, F. (2018, 2018). Review article: maintenance of fish health in aquaculture: review of epidemiological approaches for prevention and control of infectious disease of fish. *Vet. Med. Int.*: 5432497.

Cowan, G., Smith, P., and Christofilogiannis, P. (2016). Fish vaccines: the regulatory process and requirements from the laboratory bench to a final commercial product, including field trials. In: *Fish Vaccines* (ed. A. Adams), 105–118. Basel: Springer.

Embregts, C. and Forlenza, M. (2016). Oral vaccination of fish: lessons from humans and veterinary species. *Dev. Comp. Immunol.* 64: 118–137.

Evensen, O. (2016). Development of fish vaccines: focusing on methods. In: *Fish Vaccines* (ed. A. Adams), 53–74. Basel: Springer.

Evensen, O., Bruceseth, B., and Mutoloki, S. (2005). The vaccine formulation and its role in inflammatory processes in fish – effects and adverse effects. *Dev. Biol. (Basel)* 121: 117–125.

FAO (2016). *The State of World Fisheries and Aquaculture. Contributing to Food Security and Nutrition for All*. Rome: FAO. www.fao org/3/a-i5555e.pdf

FAO (2018). *The State of World Fisheries and Aquaculture 2016. Meeting the Sustainable Development Goals*. Rome: FAO. www.fao.org/3/i9540en/I9540EN.pdf

Haugarvoll, E., Bjerkas, I., Nowak, B.F. et al. (2008). Identification and characterization of a novel intraepithelial lymphoid tissue in the gills of Atlantic salmon. *J. Anat.* 213: 202–209.

Klesius, P.H. and Pridgeon, J.W. (2014). Vaccination against enteric septicemia of catfish. In: *Fish Vaccination*, 1e (eds. R. Gudding, A. Lillehaug and O. Evensen), 25. Chichester: Wiley Blackwell.

Musthaq, S.K. and Kwang, J. (2014). Evolution of specific immunity in shrimp – a vaccination perspective against white spot syndrome virus. *Dev. Comp. Immunol.* 46: 279–290.

Press, C.M. and Evensen, O. (1999). The morphology of the immune system in teleost fishes. *Fish Shellfish Immunol.* 9 (4): 309–318.

Rodger, H.D. (2016). Fish disease causing economic impact in global aquaculture. In: *Fish Vaccines* (ed. A. Adams), 1–34. Basel: Springer.

RUMA (2006). *Responsible Use of Vaccines and Vaccination in Fish Production*, 1–23. Leominster: RUMA. www.ruma.org.uk/fish/responsible-use-vaccines-vaccination-fish-production.

Secombes, C.J. and Belmonte, R. (2016). Overview of the fish adaptive immune system in fish. In: *Fish Vaccines* (ed. A. Adams), 35–52. Basel: Springer.

Tacchi, L., Musharrafieh, R., Larragoite, E.T. et al. (2014). Nasal immunity is an ancient arm of the mucosal immune system of vertebrates. *Nat. Commun.* 5: 5205.

Xu, Z., Parra, D., Gomez, D. et al. (2013). Teleost skin, an ancient mucosal surface that elicits gut-like immune responses. *Proc. Natl. Acad. Sci. U.S.A.* 110: 13097–13102.

Zhang, Y.A., Salinas, I., Li, J. et al. (2010). IgT, a primitive immunoglobulin class specialized in mucosal immunity. *Nat. Immunol.* 11 (9): 827–835.

Zhang, Y.A., Salinas, I., and Oriol Sunyer, J. (2011). Recent findings on the structure and function of teleost IgT. *Fish Shellfish Immunol.* 31 (5): 627–634.

10

Novel Developments and Next-Generation Vaccines

Gerrit Viljoen, Hermann Unger, Viskam Wijewardana, and Ivancho Naletoski

Joint FAO/IAEA Division of Nuclear Techniques in Food and Agriculture, Department of Nuclear Sciences and Applications, International Atomic Energy Agency, Vienna, Austria

10.1 Introduction

Vaccine development in its original form, as pioneered by Jenner and Pasteur, was based on a relatively simple principle of introducing an attenuated or inactivated antigen (pathogen or protein) into a host organism, in order to simulate infection and induce immunity, without causing disease. This approach was exceptionally successful in the control of many infectious diseases and has led to reductions (over 95%) of the harmful consequences of infectious disease outbreaks (Roush et al. 2007). This so-called classic vaccine approach still has the lion's share of the vaccine market. However, it often entails the use of harmful chemicals to inactivate pathogens, before administration to animal hosts, to stimulate a protective immune response. Moreover, the empirical approach of vaccine design has not been successful with certain pathogens for which, for instance, the mode of immune protection remains obscure. Therefore, rational design of vaccines is desired to curb immune evasion by pathogens and also to enhance host responses. This is built on three pillars: (i) antigen discovery, (ii) novel vaccine platforms, and (iii) adjuvant technologies.

Since the late 1980s, technological developments have fostered new and alternative vaccine approaches, which quickly grabbed the imagination as potential avenues to safer and more balanced protective immune responses. The era of recombinant derived vaccines started. This concept was introduced to the scientific community as a new way to induce an immune response, after expression of the protective gene products of a given pathogen. Despite this strong start, very little has been achieved since then, in terms of products reaching the market. However, technological developments during the last decades have led to a much better understanding of host–pathogen interactions and the mechanisms involved in immune responses to infections. Advances in molecular biology have, additionally, contributed to greater understanding of the genetic basis for antigenic phenotypes, underpinning specific and targeted gene transfer and expression, or deletion of specific gene fragments.

The trends in animal production, especially industrialized animal farming, the rapid increase in transport of people, animals, and animal products, as well as the spread of diseases facilitated by climate changes (FAO 2012), are demanding technologically advanced solutions throughout the whole chain of disease prevention and control. Consequently, the development of new-generation vaccines and methods for concomitant quality assurance are in great demand.

Use of recombinant technologies brings with it the need for the application of a risk–benefit assessment framework with respect to safety. The first veterinary recombinant vaccines were introduced in the 1990s to control Aujeszky's disease (Bruchhof and Straub 1992) and rabies in wildlife (Brochier et al. 1990) and are the forerunners of similar products that will be available in the future. The concept of recombinant vaccines is especially valuable in the implementation of vaccination strategies which require the differentiation of infected from vaccinated animals (DIVA strategy), based on advanced recombinant technologies to delete, modify (mutation), or combine the surface proteins of pathogens. The DIVA strategy enables pathogen circulation to be monitored among vaccinated animals and reservoir hosts and infected populations to be identified. This can greatly enhance the utility of emergency vaccination to rapidly stop the spread of highly contagious diseases, such as foot and mouth disease (FMD).

This chapter discusses some recent approaches in the development of new-generation vaccines with special

Veterinary Vaccines: Principles and Applications, First Edition. Edited by Samia Metwally, Gerrit Viljoen, and Ahmed El Idrissi.

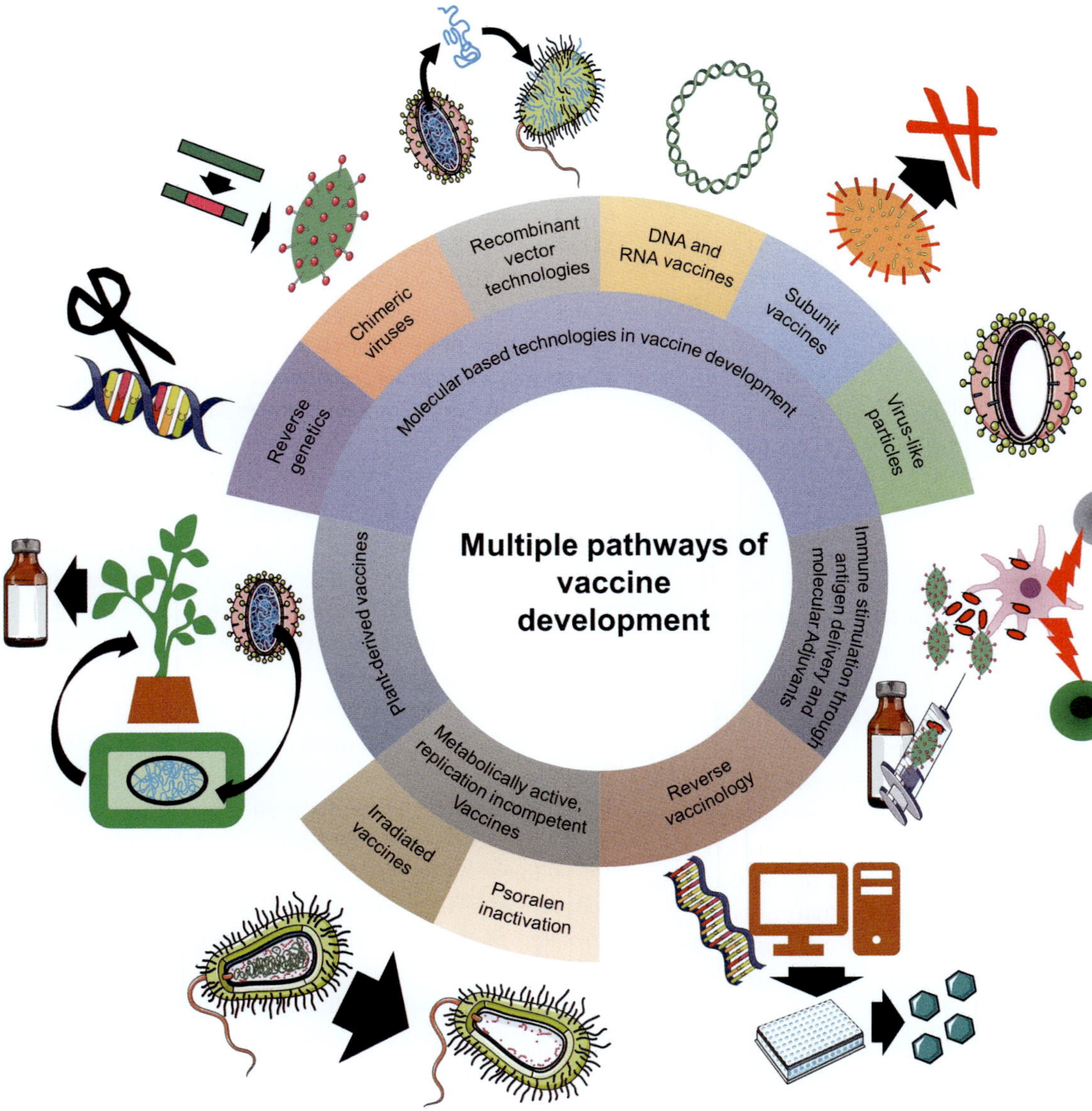

Figure 10.1 Multiple pathways of vaccine development. Rational design of vaccine development has utilized multiple approaches that range from molecular-based technologies to plant-derived vaccines. These technologies have developed rapidly during the past few decades and keep evolving to create new-generation vaccines. Source: Based on a modified version of images from Servier Medical Art, licensed under a Creative Commons Attribution 3.0 Generic License.

emphasis on viral vaccines as summarized in Figure 10.1, and their possible impact on the design and modulation of new vaccines or new approaches for their administration.

10.2 Molecular-Based Technologies in Vaccine Development

10.2.1 Reverse Genetics

Rapid developments in genetic sequencing and bioinformatics have created large amounts of genetic data associated with the phenotypic properties of specific pathogens. Reverse genetics (RG) can be used to match phenotypic properties to their genetic background. In this approach, using various techniques, genetic perturbations are introduced into a gene of interest, and the impacts are investigated through phenotypic and functional analyses. The technologies employed in RG have rapidly evolved in recent years from conventional methods to use of clustered regularly interspaced short palindromic repeat (CRISPR)/associated protein 9 (Cas9) technology, which is revolutionizing genome editing approaches. In terms of pathogen characterization, RG has contributed to an understanding of viral replication, transcription and translation, assembly and budding, virus–host cell protein interactions, identification and characterization of viral determinants of fitness, and investigation of the mechanisms by which viruses counteract host antiviral defenses. Moreover, it has helped us to understand gene functions in many other pathogens ranging from bacteria to more complex organisms such as nematodes.

In the area of vaccine development, recombinant DNA tools and RG have provided an in-depth understanding of virus replication and pathogenesis and enabled targeted genetic modifications in virus genomes aimed at attenuating or neutralizing the pathogenicity of microorganisms, as well as providing DIVA vaccines to support disease surveillance and epidemiological investigation. The proof of principle for the RG technology was initially demonstrated using bacteriophage Q-Beta and poliovirus (Taniguchi 1978). Later on, the RG system for negative-strand RNA (influenza) viruses was developed (Pleschka et al. 1996). Since then, RG has been used to develop an infectious clone of the transmissible gastroenteritis virus, which was able to induce lactogenic immunity in immunized pigs (Sola et al. 2003), infectious bovine rhinotracheitis/infectious pustular vulvovaginitis vaccine (IBR/IPV) (Kerkhofs et al. 2003), and a modified, deleted vaccine against porcine respiratory and reproductive syndrome virus (de Lima et al. 2008). Of these studies, the last two resulted in the development of DIVA markers. Vaccines against FMD (Li et al. 2012), classic swine fever (CSF) (Liu et al. 2009), Newcastle disease (Hu et al. 2009), and bluetongue virus (Boyce et al. 2008) have also been developed using RG.

Reverse genetics has proved helpful in vaccine research of highly pathogenic avian influenza (HPAI) virus, allowing changes to be targeted at the cleavage site of the virus (Stech and Klenk 2006), and by development of high-yield viral strains (Liu et al. 2006) and vaccine suited to emergency response strategies (Meng et al. 2013).

One of the applications of RG is the development of viral vectors with deleted genes (McGettigan 2010). The deleted target genes code for proteins associated with virulence, causing irreversible attenuation, or code for proteins, which induce antibodies that are not associated with protection. Gene-deleted vaccines have been developed against bovine herpes virus-1 (Bosch et al. 1997), pseudorabies virus (Swenson et al. 1993), *Salmonella choleraesuis* (Chu et al. 2007), and rabies (McGettigan et al. 2014).

Another application of RG is in the development of viruses which lack an essential gene and are therefore unable to undergo multicycle replication in vaccinated hosts, called disabled infectious single cycle (DISC) viruses (Zecchini and Smith 1999). Such viruses, upon entry into a host cell, can replicate for only one cycle, thereby stimulating the immune response of the host, with no possibility of conventional infection. This approach has been used in efforts to develop vaccines against herpes simplex virus (Zecchini and Smith 1999), bluetongue virus (Celma et al. 2013), and equine arteritis virus (Zevenhoven-Dobbe et al. 2004).

10.2.2 Chimeric Viruses

The term "chimeric virus" is used for recombinant viruses that consist of a combination of the genomes of two viruses (i.e. recombinantly mixed viruses) and which may display biological properties of both parent viruses. They are actually hybrid microorganisms created by joining nucleic acid fragments from two or more different microorganisms containing essential genes necessary for replication. Therefore, a chimeric virus can contain parts of the genome from different members belonging to the same virus family or different subtypes of the same virus genus. The main advantage of this approach is a backbone that provides predictable growth characteristics, while ensuring low pathogenicity and presenting vaccine antigens to the appropriate arm of the immune system. A single dose of chimeric virus can deliver a wide palette of closely related antigens, which can induce protective immune responses against multiple serotypes of the same pathogen.

Chimeric viruses have been constructed using the classic swine fever virus (CSFV) and the bovine viral diarrhea virus (BVDV) genome backbones, by replacing the BVDV E2 coding sequence with the CSFV E2 coding sequence of the Alfort 187 strain (Reimann et al. 2004) and, conversely, by replacing the CSFV E2 coding sequence of the vaccine C strain with the E2 coding sequence of the BVDV (van Gennip et al. 2000). These viruses induce protection against CSFV challenge and allow discrimination between vaccinated and infected pigs, thereby facilitating DIVA vaccination strategies. A similar approach has been used to induce significantly higher levels of cross-neutralizing antibodies in pigs against a heterologous porcine respiratory reproductive syndrome virus (PRRSV) strain FL-12 (Zhou et al. 2012). In chickens, chimeric, virus-like particles containing the spike glycoprotein of infectious bronchitis virus (Lv et al. 2013) have induced high levels of neutralizing antibody. In mouse models, a chimeric hepatitis B virus carrier expressing a specific influenza cytotoxic T lymphocyte (CTL) epitope (Cheong et al. 2009) was used to induce T and B cell immune responses against influenza A, while Moloney murine leukemia chimeric virus which contains glycoproteins G(N), G(C), nucleoprotein N, and the gag protein of Rift Valley fever virus (RVFV) (Mandell et al. 2010) was used to induce protective immunity against lethal challenge with RVFV.

Chimeric platforms have also been used for the development of human vaccines against zoonotic diseases. Some examples are Japanese encephalitis virus (Gromowski et al. 2014) and West Nile fever virus (WNV), reviewed by Dayan et al. (2013).

10.2.3 Recombinant Vector Technologies

Recombinant vector vaccines are based on the use of a vector carrier, a nonpathogenic vehicle (virus or bacteria) which transports and expresses a specific/targeted DNA sequence of the pathogen into the host cells. The selected DNA sequence should code for an immune-protective antigen of a targeted pathogen and should be able to induce a protective immune response. The carrier microorganism is actually a "helper which mimics an infection with a harmful microbe," inducing an immune response in the host.

The availability of bacterial and viral genome sequences has facilitated the rapid construction of defined deletions in the genomes of a wide variety of pathogens, which may not only result in attenuation, but can also create space for the insertion of foreign genes coding for antigens from heterologous pathogens.

Recombinant vector technologies can fill many gaps of the conventional vaccine approaches, because they offer well-characterized virulence-attenuating mutations, regulation of the quantity and *in vivo* localization of antigen expression. They can be combined with multiple vaccine delivery routes and potent innate and adaptive immune system stimulators. Additional advantages include combining "heterologous prime-boost" (different vaccine types used in the first and subsequent doses) strategies with other types of vaccines such as recombinant antigens or DNA vaccines.

Until recently, bacterial vector vaccines have not been extensively used in animal health. However, during the last decade, vector systems have been developed for many diseases of veterinary importance, such as the porcine circovirus type 2 (PCV2), using *Streptococcus equi* ssp. *zooepidemicus* as a vector (Wei et al. 2012), *Mycoplasma hyopneumoniae* using *Actinobacillus pleuropneumoniae* as a vector (Zou et al. 2011), and the causative agent of ovine footrot, *Dichelobacter nodosus*, using *Corynebacterium pseudotuberculosis* as a vector (Moore et al. 2001). More as a proof of principle, a number of other bacterial vectors have been developed, based on commensal microorganisms such as *Lactobacillus* (Stoeker et al. 2011) and *Streptococcus* (Mayer et al. 2009), or attenuated pathogenic bacteria such as *Vibrio* (Keller et al. 2010) and *Bordetella* (Stevenson and Roberts 2002), both of which have been evaluated for their ability to induce protective immunity.

Most viral vectors are developed using viruses that are associated with mild or no clinical disease potential or viruses attenuated by deletion of virulence genes. A number of viral vectors have been developed from adenoviruses (Greenall et al. 2010), herpesviruses (Donofrio et al. 2007), Newcastle disease virus (NDV) (Ferreira et al. 2014), and pox viruses (Kyriakis et al. 2009).

Licensed poxvirus vector vaccines based on a canary pox virus were developed for equine influenza (EPAR, EMEA/V/C/073 2008), and for the herpes virus of Turkey's vector backbone with an infectious bursal disease insert (EPAR, EMEA/V/C/065 2007).

A major drawback of this approach is the relatively low amount of antigen carried or presented by these vectors. Despite a good immune induction after the first application, a booster immunization will primarily stimulate a response toward the vector and only marginally against the "payload."

10.2.4 DNA and RNA Vaccines

The concept of DNA vaccines is a promising approach which brings immunization into a new technological dimension. DNA vaccines are designed to deliver the targeted genes to the host cell through a plasmid. The plasmid DNA instructs the host cell to produce antigen, which effectively converts the cells into "a vaccine production facility." As the presentation of the antigen to specific host cells is critical for induction of the immune response, significant efforts have been made not only to deliver DNA of disease-specific antigens, but also to enrich the vaccines with specific adjuncts that target the DNA toward a specific organ or cells and act as adjuvants in stimulating or directing the immune response. Limited research has been done to target specific organs using nanoparticles as vehicles for delivery of the DNA vaccines. Spherical nanoparticles with anionic charges, coated with γ-polyglutamic acid, have been used to deliver a plasmid DNA vaccine to the marginal zone of the spleen, where high gene expression has been measured (Kurosaki et al. 2013). In another study, the authors have observed enhanced T and B cell immune responses after percutaneous vaccination of mice with polycation nanocomplexes coated with DNA vaccine against the hepatitis B virus (Yin et al. 2013). Gold nanoparticles have also been used as nontoxic carriers of DNA vaccines, coated with adjuvant substances (poly-diallydimethylammonium chloride and polyethyleneimine) for the treatment of HIV-1 infections (Xu et al. 2012).

The first DNA vaccines for use in animal production and health were licensed between 2005 (WNV in USA and infectious hematopoietic virus for salmon in Canada) and 2006 (melanoma for dogs in the USA) (Kutzler and Weiner 2008).

Recently, the first online database for recording and querying DNA vaccines and vaccine candidates, with organized cross-referencing to third data sources, was established

(Racz et al. 2014). It currently contains 3130 entries (as of March 2020: www.violinet.org/dnavaxdb/) and is searchable by all attributes entered in the database.

An accepted DNA vaccine "prime-boost" strategy is to prime the animal with a DNA vaccine intradermally followed by a boost regime using purified or recombinantly expressed proteins (see also section 10.2.5) from the same pathogen, in order to elicit an enhanced humoral and cellular immune response.

Despite the great advantages of DNA vaccination, such as the relative ease of selecting the DNA and producing it in large quantities, the majority of experiments have only been done in mice and did not come up with tangible results in the target species due to differences in immune mechanisms of the species. In recent years, attention has been paid to RNA-based vaccines which have several advantages over DNA vaccines: (i) RNAs are directly recognized by receptors of the innate immune system, (ii) unlike DNA, potential detrimental integrations into chromosomal DNA do not take place, (iii) recombination between single-stranded RNA molecules is rare, and (iv) they do not suffer from antivector immune interference. On the other hand, RNA is notoriously unstable and this negatively affects its use in vaccine strategies without cold chains. However, this problem has been addressed and methods to stabilize RNA are emerging. Self-replicating RNA vaccines (RNA replicons) have emerged as a promising strategy for nucleic acid vaccine development. In 2014, a porcine epidemic diarrhea vaccine became the first RNA particulate vaccine to receive a conditional US Department of Agriculture license (Kim et al. 2016).

10.2.5 Subunit Vaccines

Subunit vaccines consist of antigens (basically proteins) responsible for triggering a protective immune response against a specific pathogen. They may contain antigenic complexes or purified epitopes recognized by host antibodies or T cells. Because they do not contain the whole pathogen, the risks of adverse reactions are much lower, and there are practically no biosecurity concerns in their application.

Subunit vaccines can be produced in two ways: (i) by physical or chemical separation and purification of the antigens (antigenic complexes) from pathogens grown *in vitro*, and (ii) using recombinant DNA technology (described above) in which a vector expresses the required antigens, followed by separation and purification. In order to distinguish between the two methods of production, it is commonly accepted to refer to the second approach as "recombinant subunit vaccines." To express the subunit proteins, bacteria, viruses, and plants can be used.

Subunit vaccines may contain 1–20 or more antigens; however, it is desirable to select the most appropriate antigen or antigen complexes which will induce the most appropriate immune response (National Institute of Allergy and Infectious Diseases 2012). Substantial research has been done to develop subunit vaccines against many animal and zoonotic diseases, including Aujeszky's disease (Motha et al. 1994), CSF (Lin et al. 2012), respiratory syncytial virus (Garg et al. 2014), tuberculosis (Windish et al. 2011), and others. Subunit vaccines have also been developed or are under development, for emerging and reemerging zoonotic diseases, such as ebola virus (Phoolcharoen et al. 2011) and Hendra virus (Pallister et al. 2011). Despite all these efforts, subunit antigen approaches for immunization have often been ineffective by themselves, as they present only a limited number of epitopes or possess a critical size and conformation, unrecognized by the host immune system. Therefore, most of the researchers mentioned above use different types of adjuvants to boost the immune response.

Advances in bioinformatics have also made it possible to develop synthetic peptide vaccines. The peptide epitopes represent a minimal immunogenic region of a protein antigen and allow for precise direction of immune responses. This type of vaccine offers significant advantages such as ease of characterization (important during the process of licensing), storage, transport and distribution, as well as ease of reformulation, important in highly variable viruses, such as influenza A. However, problems with stability and immunogenicity have still not been fully solved. Peptide vaccines have successfully been developed for low-pathogenic H5 avian influenza in poultry (Jackwood et al. 2009), group A streptococcal infection in a mouse model (Olive et al. 2002), and parvovirus infection in dogs (Langeveld et al. 1994). However, limited success has been observed in protection against FMD (Zhang et al. 2011).

Polysaccharides are also used as vaccine antigens but they have limited immunogenicity. Therefore, they are conjugated to a carrier protein to make fusion vaccines that yield long-term protective immunity; *Haemophilus influenzae* type b (Hib) was the first of such vaccines (Austrian 1989).

10.2.6 Virus-Like Particles

The term "virus-like particles" (VLP) refers to empty structures of viral origin with no coding nucleic acids, infectious viruses with chemically or genetically introduced structure modifications and noninfectious, self-assembled gene products resulting from the cloning and expression of viral structural genes in heterologous host systems. In the context of this chapter, VLPs are considered as multiprotein structures that mimic the organization and conformation of authentic native viruses but lack the viral genome (i.e. looking like the virus but without its genetic material, rendering it replication deficient) and potentially yielding safer and cheaper vaccine candidates (Roldão et al. 2010). Viral ghost vaccines are a part of this group.

They are robust, chemically programmable protein assemblies which may be used not only as vaccines or vaccine vehicles, but also as core nanoparticles, offering significant advantages over conventional synthetic particles: (i) they are stable self-assembled structures at nanometer level with sizes ranging from 10 to 200 nm, (ii) three-dimensional structures can be characterized at nearly atomic resolution, (iii) the composition and surface properties of the viruses can be controlled using molecular tools, (iv) they can be purified inexpensively on a large scale, and (v) for each type of virus and virus-like protein assembly, all the particles are identical (Andrew Lee et al. 2009).

Virus-like particles offer several advantages as vaccine candidates, including a high safety profile, their similarity to viral structures, compatibility for large-scale production, the possibility of combining with other adjuvants, and that they can induce rapid and strong antibody responses. A simple trick to induce or increase immune stimulation is to allow for the production of a truncated core protein which can bind small noncoding RNAs. After "virus" entry and disintegration, these induce the PKR–IFN system, attracting a T cell response. VLPs expressing the nucleocapsid gene have provided an efficient vaccine against RVFV (Pichlmair et al. 2010).

Research on the use of VLPs as vaccines in veterinary medicine has and is being done for numerous diseases. A VLP vaccine derived from the matrix, and hemagglutin or fusion protein of peste des petits ruminants virus (PPRV), produced through baculovirus transfected cells, induced protection comparable to conventional vaccines, without using an adjuvant. The PPRV VLPs were generated to selectively express the matrix (M) protein, and the hemagglutinin (H) or fusion (F) protein, making them DIVA compatible (Li et al. 2014). A plant-derived, enveloped VLP vaccine of influenza H1N1 based on the ectodomain of the HA protein and heterologous sequences has induced an enhanced immune response compared with the soluble antigen (Shoji et al. 2015). A high-yielding cloned cell line continuously producing VLPs of the envelope glycoprotein and the membrane protein of the Japanese encephalitis virus could induce 100% protective immunity against lethal challenge in mice (Hua et al. 2014). A chimeric VLP incorporating HA and M1 proteins of the H3N2 influenza virus and the GP5 PRRSV has stimulated humoral and cellular responses, comparable to those induced by an inactivated vaccine in a mouse model (Xue et al. 2014). VLPs composed of the VP2 protein of the canine parvovirus, expressed through a baculovirus expression system, could induce a systemic immune response and long-lasting immunity (Feng et al. 2014). Rabies virus glycoprotein VLPs, expressed through lentivirus transduced HEK293 cells, have induced antibody response in mice (Fontana et al. 2014). Additionally, Guo et al. (2013) used VLPs composed of capsid proteins (VP0, VP1, and VP3) produced in *Escherichia coli* to elicit antibodies and T cell responses that were 100% protective against FMD in guinea pigs, swine, and cattle.

Virus-like particle vaccines have also been developed for rabbit hemorrhagic disease (Chen et al. 2014), infectious bronchitis of chickens (Lv et al. 2013), ebola virus (Ayithan et al. 2014), bluetongue virus (Thuenemann et al. 2013), porcine reproductive and respiratory system (PRRS) virus (Wang et al. 2012), NDV (Schmidt et al. 2012), and others. With their ability to self-assemble in a structure most similar to the intact pathogens, with minimal or no biosafety concerns, and their ability to induce a rapid onset of both B and T cell immunity, VLPs have the potential to be ideal vaccines. They will probably attract even more attention in future and be more commonly present as commercially marketed products.

A very similar "empty particle" approach was developed for gram-negative bacteria (bacterial ghosts). These are empty bacterial envelopes produced by lysing bacterial pores through an expression of the bacteriophage gene E protein. Thus, the cytoplasm and parts of the bacterial DNA are ejected, rendering the ghost replication incompetent (Szostaka et al. 1996). Despite their capacity to carry immunogenic DNA, most efforts are directed toward empty particles of a specific pathogen like *Salmonella gallinarum*, which protects against fowl typhoid (Jawale et al. 2014).

Ghost vaccines have also been shown to protect piglets against *Haemophilus parasuis* (Hu et al. 2013). In the fish industry, ghost vaccines, in comparison with conventional counterparts, have induced equal or better protection against *Edwardsiella tarda* in tilapia fish (Kwon et al. 2006) and the olive flounder (Se Ryun Kwona et al. 2007), and also against infection with *Aeromonas hydrophila* in carp (Tu et al. 2009).

In human medicine, ghost vaccines have been used as recombinant vector vaccines against African trypanosomiasis, using *Vibrio cholerae*-expressing *Trypanosoma brucei* antigens Ca(2+) ATPase (TBCA2) (Ramey et al. 2009).

10.3 Immune Stimulation Through Antigen Delivery and Molecular Adjuvants

Adjuvants are substances that sensitize the host immunological environment to enhance the responses (humoral/cellular) when co-administered with antigens. They are a critical component of inactivated or nonreplicating recombinant and subunit vaccines, which are often poorly immunogenic.

Adjuvants can be classified into two groups: (i) enhancing delivery systems, and (ii) immune-stimulatory compounds. Adjuvant modulatory delivery systems include many types such as oil adjuvants, oil/water adjuvants, emulsion/protein adjuvants, and particulate adjuvants that will be discussed separately below. Despite the importance of adjuvants in vaccines and their clear immune-stimulating effect, their mechanisms of action remain poorly understood. Recent advances in the understanding of innate and acquired immunity have provided molecular pathways that help to elucidate their action. Thus, immune cells express a variety of receptors, collectively termed pattern recognition receptors (PRRs), that broadly detect conserved microbial components referred to as pathogen-associated molecular patterns (PAMPs). Several PRRs have been described, including toll-like receptors (TLRs). TLR2 recognizes diverse bacterial products (Lien et al. 1999). Natural agonists of TLR7/8, single-stranded viral RNA (oligoribonucleotides, ORN), strongly activate innate immune responses in mice and humans and are particularly potent in cattle (Buza et al. 2008). TLR4 agonists, such as lipopolysaccharide (LPS), are known for their powerful immunostimulatory and adjuvant properties but unfortunately this molecule is highly toxic (Needham et al. 2013). In addition, nucleotide oligomerization domain (NOD)-like receptor, retinoic acid-inducible gene-like receptors, and C-type lectin receptors (CLRs) are involved in pathogen recognition (Kawai and Akira 2014). Engagement of these receptors by their agonists leads to a cascade of molecular and cellular events that result in activation of innate immunity, which directs antigen-specific adaptive immunity.

Of these receptors, TLR agonists are the most widely explored and have shown great promise as adjuvants. Interestingly, the live attenuated yellow fever vaccine 17D, one of the most successful vaccines available, activates TLR2, 7, 8, and 9 (Querec et al. 2006), suggesting that the success of at least some of the live vaccines may be the result of their ability to activate TLRs. In addition, the "one adjuvant–one vaccine" approach by vaccine manufacturers is driven partly by costs associated with including more than one adjuvant in a vaccine. Evidence is slowly accumulating that multiple adjuvants may offer more than can be achieved with a single adjuvant. For example, although CpG ODNs are a good adjuvant, they can have even greater adjuvant activity if formulated or co-administered with other compounds, such as particulates, mineral salts, saponins, liposomes, cationic peptides, polysaccharides and bacterial toxins, and the synthetic polyphosphazene polymers.

The adjuvant effect of microparticles has been known for some time and has been previously reviewed (Mutwiri et al. 2005). Particulate delivery systems are thought to promote trapping and retention of antigens in local lymph nodes. In addition, microparticles facilitate antigen presentation by antigen-presenting cells (APCs) via both major histocompatibility complex (MHC) class I and MHC class II restricted processing and presentation pathways. One of the main advantages of microparticles for targeted antigen delivery is that they can be a flexible delivery platform that can be used to deliver both antigens and immunostimulatory molecules. Nano-scale liposomes and liposome-derived nanovesicles offer an attractive mechanism to direct antigens toward APCs and stimulate different immune pathways, as mentioned above. They are particularly used to deliver subunit antigens and nucleic acids and for mucosal as well as parenteral delivery of vaccines in livestock. Nano-scale particles have been used for efficient delivery of antigens in livestock species (Mahony et al. 2015).

Other potential antigen delivery systems include polyphosphazenes, a class of synthetic polymers consisting of a backbone with alternating phosphorus and nitrogen atoms and organic side groups attached to each phosphorus molecule (Mutwiri et al. 2007). Immune-stimulating complexes (ISCOMs), which are small 40 nm nanoparticles composed of saponin (adjuvant), lipids, and antigen, have been described as an antigen delivery system having not only adjuvant activity, but also the ability to target APC (Morein et al. 2004). A commercial ISCOM-based vaccine against equine influenza has been licensed for many years (Heldens et al. 2009).

10.4 Plant-Derived Vaccines

Vaccine production includes multiple technological steps for production, concentration, purification, packing, and delivery of the vaccines. Moreover, implementation of vaccination requires significant organizational and financial resources, such as capacity for storage (cold chain), transport, and trained human resources for performing the vaccination campaigns. Additionally, in most cases, vaccination requires direct contact with and manipulation of individual animals.

Recombinant technologies have enabled the expression of subunit antigens on vector carriers, thus offering a wide range of vaccine production possibilities. The use of plants as vaccine production and delivery systems has attracted much scientific attention, as they offer possibilities for antigen expression on different parts of the plant (root, seed, grain, fruit/vegetable, or leaf), and they allow for simplified and large-scale production, thus decreasing the price per unit produced (Streatfield 2005). Additionally, the thermostability of the antigens (especially in grains) gives rise to significantly extended shelf-life (Hammond and

Nemchinov 2009), the oral application enables a better stimulation of mucosal immunity, specifically important in ruminants (Rigano et al. 2003), and safety concerns are minimized, as there is no manipulation with highly contagious animal pathogens.

As plants must be genetically modified to produce these immunogens, planting these will need close supervision to avoid spillover into the natural vegetation. An alternative to overcome this limitation is the use of transfected chloroplasts which do not transfer the altered genes to next generations via pollination (Verma and Daniell 2007). An additional limitation of plant-derived vaccines is the low level of antigen expression, which should be improved by chloroplast transformation, plant breeding, or food processing technology.

Since the first report of successful immunization using plant-derived antigens (*Streptococcus mutans* surface protein A on tobacco leaf) in the early 1990s (Curtiss and Cardineau 1990), there have been many reports on the adaptation and improvement of the system to other animal and human diseases, such as avian influenza (Landry et al. 2010), peste des petits ruminants (PPR) (Khandelwal et al. 2011), transmissible gastroenteritis virus (Lamphear et al. 2004), bovine pasteurellosis (Lee et al. 2008), *Fasciola hepatica* (Legocki et al. 2005), and many others. Moreover, during 2006, the first vaccine expressed on a plant cell culture was approved for commercial use in the USA by the USDA (Das et al. 2008). It is a vaccine against Newcastle disease in poultry.

The advanced expression systems have significantly improved the potential for the production of plant-derived vaccines in terms of: (i) increased amount of expressed antigen for more consistent and better antigen delivery (Ling et al. 2010), (ii) improved immunogenicity through the capacity to express complex viral proteins (empty viral capsids) (Santos and Wigdorovitz 2005), and the possibility to co-express immunomodulatory molecules in the plant (Farran et al. 2010). However, there are still significant problems to be solved in order to facilitate the use of already developed plant-derived vaccines in prophylactic programs for animal diseases, such as antigen selection, efficiency of antigen production by plants, choice of plants, delivery, dosage, safety, the public's perception, quality control and licensing, and compatibility with government policies on genetically modified food.

10.5 Metabolically Active, Replication Incompetent Vaccines

10.5.1 Irradiated Vaccines

Irradiation has been extensively used for the attenuation or inactivation of viruses, bacteria, parasites, and toxins used for immunization of animals since the 1960s. Irradiation technology at that time was rather limited and tools for measuring attenuation were nonexistent. It was not until the 1990s, when molecular tools and testing systems became available, that cellular immune responses could be properly measured. Today with high-dose x-ray machines and electron beam irradiation, microbial cultures can be treated to selectively affect their genes and not their surface structures. This, for instance, can still allow virus entry into cells and initiation of their "metabolic activity" leading to normal intracellular response reactions and the attraction of immune cells. Protocols for subcutaneous and intramuscular vaccination against Venezuelan equine encephalitis using the γ-irradiated virus subtype IA/B-Trinidad Donkey strain (V3526) led to 100% protection (Martin et al. 2010). Results obtained with γ-irradiated influenza vaccine have identified the importance of the recognition of cytosolic receptors, which correspond with the ability of γ-irradiated influenza virus to induce cross-reactive and cross-protective cytotoxic T cell responses (Furuya et al. 2011). Additionally, γ-irradiated influenza A vaccine (γ-flu) has been used as an adjuvant for stimulation of the immune response for the Semliki Forest virus (γ-SFV) in mice. Co-vaccination resulted in enhanced SFV-specific antibody responses, in terms of neutralization titers increased by sixfold and greater, when compared with vaccination with γ-SFV alone (Babb et al. 2014).

γ-Irradiation has been used to attenuate bacterial pathogens for use as orally administered vaccines, for example to protect against *E. coli* H10407 (078:H11) in rats (Dima et al. 1992). γ-Irradiated *Brucella melitensis* with inhibited replication capability and retained "live-brucella" protective features (possession of metabolic and transcriptional activity), persisted in macrophages, induced antigen-specific cytotoxic T cells and protected mice against virulent bacterial challenge (Magnani et al. 2009). Similar results, with cross-protective immunity against *Brucella abortus*, *B. melitensis* and *B. suis* challenge, have been observed when vaccinating mice with irradiation-inactivated *Brucella neotomae* (Moustafa et al. 2011). Subunit immunogens that can generate enhanced CD8 T cell and Th1 responses against *Mycobacterium tuberculosis* combined with irradiated *M. tuberculosis* have been used to elicit elevated IFN-γ responses, with the hybrid showing significant increases over the native proteins in mice (Walton et al. 2008). Irradiation-inactivated *Listeria monocytogenes*, unlike heat-killed vaccine, efficiently activated dendritic cells via TLR and induced protective T cell responses in mice (Datta et al. 2006).

In the field of parasitology, extensive research has been done on the use of irradiated vaccines for malaria and schistosomiasis, although there are also published reports on successful immunization against other parasitic diseases. *Plasmodium falciparum* sporozoite surface protein 2 has been found to stimulate CTL in two HLA-B8+ volunteers immunized with irradiated *P. falciparum* sporozoites. The data indicated that there are two CTL epitopes among *P. falciparum* isolates, one conserved and the other variant (Wizel et al. 1995). The vaccine produced from radiation-attenuated *Plasmodium berghei* and *P. yoelii* sporozoites induces specific cytotoxic T lymphocytes ($CD8^+$) that recognize malaria antigens on the surface of malaria-infected hepatocytes (Hoffman et al. 1990). Immunization with 54, 55, 224, 663, and 715 infective bites of irradiated mosquitoes (200 Gy) did not protect volunteers from parasitemia, although the patency was delayed in the volunteer with the highest antibody response (Herrington et al. 1990). Blood irradiated with a dose of 28 kilorads (280 Gy) has successfully protected nonimmune cattle from infection with *Babesia divergens*, when pasturing in high-risk areas in cohabitation with negative controls (Purnell et al. 1981).

Vaccine prepared from irradiated trophozoites of *Toxoplasma gondii* from the peritoneal cavities of mice (10, 15, and 20 kiloroentgens, equivalent to 87, 130, and 174 Gy respectively) protected all mice from virulent challenge 3 weeks post vaccination (Seah and Hucal 1975). Radiation attenuation of the cercariae of *Schistosoma mansoni*, a platyhelminth parasite, has been successfully used to produce protective vaccines in mouse (El Amir 2008), guinea pig (Xu et al. 1991), pig (Bickle et al. 2001), and nonhuman primate (Yole et al. 1996) models.

Irradiated vaccines have also been tested for other parasitic worms, such as lungworm-*Dictyocaulus* spp. (Johnson et al. 2003) and *Ancylostoma ceylanicum* (Menon and Bhopale 1985), fungal diseases such as coccidioidomycosis (Pulliam et al. 1967) and against bacterial endotoxins, such as the *Salmonella* enterotoxin, the common, serotype nonspecific, virulence factor among the *Salmonella* spp. (Begum et al. 2011).

The process of attenuation or inactivation of pathogens for vaccine formulation using ionizing radiation is targeted to damage the pathogen genome. However, depending on the dose delivered, the ionizing radiation may damage surface proteins, including epitopes, which is an adverse consequence in the process of vaccine development. The manganese peptide complex (Mn-DP-Pi complex) from the radiation-resistant bacterium *Deinococcus radiodurans* has been shown to protect protein epitopes from radiation-induced damage and uncouple it from genome damage and organism killing. The principle of protection is based on the ability of the Mn-DP-Pi complexes to act as superoxide dismutase and catalyze the decomposition of H_2O_2 produced during the process of irradiation (Gaidamakova et al. 2012).

This property of Mn-DP-Pi complexes has been tested and proven on bacterial (methicillin-resistant *Staphylococcus aureus* – MRSA, up to 25 kGy) and viral (Venezuelan equine encephalitis virus, up to 50 kGy) pathogens for the possibility to use immensely increased doses. However, enzymes were protected only up to 70 kGy after γ-irradiation in non-frozen aqueous conditions (Gaidamakova et al. 2012).

This achievement may significantly improve the development of irradiated vaccines, especially when considering pathogens of different phylogenetic categories (viruses, bacteria, protozoa, parasitic worms, etc.). Additionally, the work may contribute to better "fine-tuning" of the dose aimed for production of metabolically active but nonreplicating pathogens.

In order to protect proteins from radiation damage, stabilizing and protecting solutions have been tested with many biological compounds, such as antibodies, viruses, vaccines and others, and have proven beneficial. Additionally, these approaches can be complemented with other preservation techniques, such as spray drying and spray freeze drying processes, in order to maintain the molecular integrity and function to physical influences (high pressure and elevated temperatures), extreme energy input during irradiation and extended storage. These achievements are opening different perspectives in the development of irradiated vaccines and the biotechnological applications of irradiation in general, as they separate the irradiation damage to DNA and protein, thereby allowing the use of much higher irradiation doses for sterilization of biological materials and for the production of thermostable biological compounds, such as vaccines, sera, etc.

10.5.2 Psoralen Inactivation

An alternative to disrupting genes by irradiation is the use of intercalating substances. Psoralens are photoreactive compounds that freely permeate phospholipid membranes and intercalate between nucleic acids. Following exposure to UV-A radiation, the intercalated psoralen covalently cross-links pyrimidine residues, leading to the inhibition of genome transcription and replication. The interaction of psoralen with viral nucleic acids leaves their immunogenic surface epitopes intact (Groene and Shaw 1992).

The production of such vaccines is rather trivial. The virus culture is supplemented with a psoralen solution and after a short incubation, the solution is cured with UV light, polymerizing the psoralen and thus inactivating the free-floating residues and fixing the DNA or RNA strands, abrogating replication. Vaccinia virus was one of the first to be inactivated with psoralens, after which early gene expression was still possible, but no cytopathic effect occurred (Tsung et al. 1996).

Listeria trials showed that there was still metabolic activity after psoralen treatment, but replication was abrogated. Immunized mice were completely protected against challenge (Brockstedt et al. 2005). Since then a number of experimental vaccines against anthrax (Skoble et al. 2009), dengue fever in monkeys (Maves et al. 2011), and HIV (Glenn 2013) have been published. How this technology can be adapted for large-scale vaccine production has still to be determined.

10.5.3 Hydrogen Peroxide (H_2O_2)-Inactivated Vaccines

Inactivation of pathogens by H_2O_2 is not new and has been practiced for a long time, for instance to clean wounds. Only recently, however, has an approach to inactivate pathogens for vaccine use been published and patented. The addition of H_2O_2, to a final concentration of 3%, inactivated pathogens so that, for instance, mice immunized with H_2O_2-inactivated lymphocytic choriomeningitis virus (LCMV) generated cytolytic, multifunctional virus-specific $CD8^+$ T cells that conferred protection against chronic LCMV infection (Walker et al. 2012). Other studies have proven that H_2O_2-inactivated vaccinia and West Nile fever viruses can induce protective immunity in mice (Amanna et al. 2012). More recently, a recombinant, replication-deficient ebola vaccine inactivated with H_2O_2 was protective against a lethal challenge with the ebola virus in macaques (Marzi et al. 2015).

10.6 Reverse Vaccinology

Development of molecular biological techniques has revealed full genome information and the genome of the first free-living organism was published in 1995 by Craig Venter (Fleischmann et al. 1995). The availability of this new wealth of information allowed scientists to rationally design vaccines using computers, starting with information present in the genome, without the need to grow the specific microorganisms. This new approach was called reverse vaccinology (RV) and Rino Rappuoli developed the first vaccine using RV against serogroup B *Meningococcus* (Rappuoli 2000). Later, this technique was applied to develop vaccines against group B and group A *Streptococcus* (Maione et al. 2005) and a vaccine which uses this approach against *Chlamydia* has also been described (Thorpe et al. 2007).

In essence, reverse vaccinology techniques include predicting protective antigens/epitopes using algorithms that interrogate the whole genome of pathogens, synthesizing peptides and proteins, and then *in vitro* analysis of such antigens prior to *in vivo* studies. Hence, epitope mapping software sits in a key position in this strategy and several software tools to map T cell and B cell epitopes are available. "Vaxign" is a freely available web-based software to map both MHC class I and class II restricted antigens (www.violinet.org/vaxign/) (He et al. 2010).

The RV approach has shortened the development process of vaccines to 1–3 years, compared with classic vaccine development approaches which take 5–15 years. Several candidate vaccines have been developed using the RV approach in the livestock industry. With the failure of anti-tick vaccines due to diverse *Rhipicephalus (Boophilus) microplus* found in different geographical locations, interest has grown in developing vaccines using RV (Maritz-Olivier et al. 2012). Research conducted at the International Livestock Research Institute (ILRI) showed promising results, after vaccination with *Mycoplasma mycoides* protein genes protected against contagious bovine pleuropneumonia (CBPP). The team used RV technology to design 66 candidate vaccine proteins (Nkando et al. 2016). A small-scale experimental trial showed a positive trend of protection against swine dysentery (Song et al. 2009) with a vaccine developed using this technology. In an early stage study, vaccine candidates were developed using RV for *Histophilus somni* (Madampage et al. 2015) which is associated with the bovine respiratory disease (BRD) complex and for which the available vaccines are suboptimal. Polysaccharide antigens cannot be identified by RV, but operons coding for the biosynthesis of polysaccharides can be identified (Sette and Rappuoli 2010). This can lead to discovery of novel carbohydrate antigens.

10.7 Summary

Many diseases that have plagued humans and animals have been controlled by vaccination over the last two centuries and some have even been eradicated, a remarkable accomplishment of humankind. However, the empirical approach that was employed to develop these early vaccines could not overcome some of the devastating diseases that still scourge humans and animals alike. Hence, the rational design of vaccines is needed to address immune evasion by certain pathogens and also to address other factors that prevent vaccine effectiveness.

The innovations taking place in different disciplines of science have already made an impact. Rapid development of molecular biological techniques during the latter part of the last century and the data obtained using such techniques changed the paradigm of vaccine research. RG and recombinant DNA technology approaches delivered the much-needed technology to attenuate pathogens in a targeted manner rather than culturing *in vitro* or passaging through various animal models to induce unpredicted attenuation. These approaches were extended to deliver vaccine antigens through vectored viruses and the development of chimeric viruses and VLPs. Another product of the molecular biology revolution was DNA and RNA vaccines which use the vaccine as a vehicle to produce the necessary antigens within the host cells. In parallel to the development of genomics, the rapid advancement in proteomics saw an influx of subunit vaccines with improved safety characteristics.

Another key area that vaccinologists struggled with during past decades and continue to address is how to improve recognition and induce a long-lasting protective immunity. A large number of novel vaccine adjuvants and cutting-edge delivery systems have been designed to increase vaccine efficacy in this context. Discovery of pattern recognition receptors in immune cells is playing a major role in the design of these novel adjuvants, while delivering vaccines through nano-scale particles has yielded enhanced immunity. Delivering vaccines through edible plants is a new approach for delivering vaccines on a large scale. The unique combination of molecular biology and computational technologies has led to the development of vaccines through RV which can shorten the discovery of vaccine antigens from decades to months.

While unprecedented novel discoveries are turning the wheels of vaccine development, scientists still continue to revisit, renew, and refine the older technologies for their continued use in vaccine research and development. One such technology that surfaced in the field of vaccinology is use of irradiation to produce metabolically active yet non-replicating pathogens to utilize as vaccine candidates.

References

Amanna, I.J., Raué, H.P., and Slifka, M.K. (2012). Development of a new hydrogen peroxide-based vaccine platform. *Nat. Med.* 18 (6): 974–979.

Andrew Lee, L., Niu, Z., and Wang, Q. (2009). Viruses and virus-like protein assemblies – chemically programmable Nanoscale building blocks. *Nano Res.* 2 (5): 349–364

Austrian, R. (1989). Pneumococcal polysaccharide vaccines. *Rev. Infect. Dis.* 11 (3): 598–602.

Ayithan, N., Bradfute, S.B., Anthony, S.M. et al. (2014) Ebola virus-like particles stimulate type I interferons and proinflammatory cytokine expression through the toll-like receptor and interferon signaling pathways. *J. Interferon Cytokine Res.* 34 (2): 79–89.

Babb, R., Chan, J., Khairat, J.E. et al. (2014). Gamma-irradiated influenza a virus provides adjuvant activity to a co-administered poorly immunogenic SFV vaccine in mice. *Front. Immunol.* 5: 267.

Begum, R.H., Rahman, H., and Ahmed, G. (2011). Development and evaluation of gamma irradiated toxoid vaccine of salmonella enterica var typhimurium. *Vet. Microbiol.* 153 (1–2): 191–197.

Bickle, Q.D., Bøgh, H.O., Johansen, M.V., and Zhang, Y. (2001). Comparison of the vaccine efficacy of gamma-irradiated *Schistosoma japonicum* cercariae with the defined antigen Sj62(IrV-5) in pigs. *Vet. Parasitol.* 100 (1–2): 51–62.

Bosch, J.C., Frankena, K., and van Oirschot, J.T. (1997). Effect on milk production of vaccination with a bovine herpesvirus 1 gene-deleted vaccine. *Vet. Rec.* 140 (8): 196–199.

Boyce, M., Celma, C.C., and Roy, P. (2008). Development of reverse genetics systems for bluetongue virus: recovery of infectious virus from synthetic RNA transcripts. *J. Virol.* 82 (17): 8339–8348.

Brochier, B.M., Languet, B., Artois, M. et al. (1990). Efficacy of a baiting system for vaccinating foxes against rabies with vaccinia-rabies recombinant virus. *Vet. Rec.* 127 (7): 165–167.

Brockstedt, D.G., Bahjat, K.S., Giedlin, M.A. et al. (2005). Killed but metabolically active microbes: a new vaccine paradigm for eliciting effector T-cell responses and protective immunity. *Nat. Med.* 11 (8): 853–860.

Bruchhof, B.R. and Straub, O.C. (1992). Vaccination of sheep against Aujeszky's disease with a gI-deleted mutant. *Dtsch. Tierarztl. Wochenschr.* 99 (8): 322–325.

Buza, J., Benjamin, P., Zhu, J. et al. (2008). CD14+ cells are required for IL-12 response in bovine blood mononuclear cells activated with toll-like receptor (TLR) 7 and TLR8 ligands. *Vet. Immunol. Immunopathol.* 126 (3–4): 273–282.

Celma, C.P., Boyce, M., van Rijn, P.A. et al. (2013). Rapid generation of replication-deficient monovalent and multivalent vaccines for bluetongue virus: protection against virulent virus challenge in cattle and sheep. *J. Virol.* 87 (17): 9856–9864.

Chen, M., Song, Y., Fan, Z. et al. (2014). Immunogenicity of different recombinant rabbit hemorrhagic disease virus-like particles carrying $CD8^+$ T cell epitope from chicken ovalbumin (OVA). *Virus Res.* 183: 15–22.

Cheong, W.S., Reiseger, J., Turner, S.J. et al. (2009). Chimeric virus-like particles for the delivery of an inserted conserved influenza A-specific CTL epitope. *Antiviral Res.* 81 (2): 113–122.

Chu, C.Y., Wang, S.Y., Chen, Z.W. et al. (2007). Heterologous protection in pigs induced by a plasmid-cured and crp gene-deleted *Salmonella choleraesuis* live vaccine. *Vaccine* 25 (41): 7031–7040.

Curtiss, R.I. and Cardineau, C.A. (1990). Oral immunisation by transgenic plants. International Application Published Under the Patent Cooperation Treaty (PCT) WO 90/02484.

Das, V., Peter, W.B., Phillips, P.W.B. et al. (2008). Commercialization of plant-derived vaccines in Canada: a distant dream? *Health Law Rev.* 16 (4): 25–29.

Datta, S.K., Okamoto, S., Hayashi, T. et al. (2006). Vaccination with irradiated listeria induces protective T cell immunity. *Immunity* 25: 143–152.

Dayan, G.H., Pugachev, K., Bevilacqua, J. et al. (2013). Preclinical and clinical development of a YFV 17 D-based chimeric vaccine against West Nile virus. *Viruses* 5 (12): 3048–3070.

de Lima, M., Kwon, B., Ansari, I.H. et al. (2008). Development of a porcine reproductive and respiratory syndrome virus differentiable (DIVA) strain through deletion of specific immunodominant epitopes. *Vaccine* 26: 3594–3600.

Dima, V.F., Ionescu, M.D., Dima, V.S. et al. (1992). Development of an irradiated vaccine that protects against enterotoxigenic *Escherichia coli* diarrhoea. *Roum. Arch. Microbiol. Immunol.* 51 (1–2): 5–16.

Donofrio, G., Sartori, C., Ravanetti, L. et al. (2007). Establishment of a bovine herpesvirus 4 based vector expressing a secreted form of the bovine viral diarrhoea virus structural glycoprotein E2 for immunization purposes. *BMC Biotech.* 7: 68.

El Amir, A. (2008). Effect of mouse strain on humoral responses to *Schistosoma mansoni* irradiated cercariae vaccine. *Egypt. J. Immunol.* 15 (1): 51–63.

European Public Assessment Report (EPAR) EMEA/V/C/065. (2007). VAXXITEK HVT+IBD. www.ema.europa.eu/docs/en_GB/document_library/EPAR_-_Summary_for_the_public/veterinary/000065/WC500069346.pdf

European Public Assessment Report (EPAR) EMEA/V/C/073. (2008). PROTEQFLU. www.ema.europa.eu/docs/en_GB/document_library/EPAR_-_Summary_for_the_public/veterinary/000073/WC500065182.pdf

FAO. (2012). Building Resilience for Adaptation to Climate Change in the Agriculture Sector. Proceedings of a Joint FAO/OECD Workshop, 23–24 April 2012. www.fao.org/docrep/017/i3084e/i3084e.pdf

Farran, I., McCarthy-Suárez, I., Río-Manterola, F. et al. (2010). The vaccine adjuvant extra domain a from fibronectin retains its proinflammatory properties when expressed in tobacco chloroplasts. *Planta* 231 (4): 977–990.

Feng, H., Hu, G.Q., Wang, H.L. et al. (2014). Canine parvovirus VP2 protein expressed in silkworm pupae self-assembles into virus-like particles with high immunogenicity. *PLoS One* 9 (1): e79575.

Ferreira, H.L., Rauw, F., Pirlot, J.F. et al. (2014). Comparison of single 1-day-old chick vaccination using a Newcastle disease virus vector with a prime/boost vaccination scheme against a highly pathogenic avian influenza H5N1 challenge. *Avian Pathol.* 43 (1): 68–77.

Fleischmann, R.D., Adams, M.D., White, O. et al. (1995). Whole-genome random sequencing and assembly of *Haemophilus influenzae* Rd. *Science* 269 (5223): 496–512.

Fontana, D., Kratje, R., Etcheverrigaray, M., and Prieto, C. (2014). Rabies virus-like particles expressed in HEK293 cells. *Vaccine* 32 (24): 2799–2804.

Furuya, Y., Chan, J., Wan, E.C. et al. (2011). Gamma-irradiated influenza virus uniquely induces IFN-I mediated lymphocyte activation independent of the TLR7/MyD88 pathway. *PLoS One* 6 (10): e25765.

Gaidamakova, E.K., Myles, I.A., McDaniel, D.P. et al. (2012). Preserving immunogenicity of lethally irradiated viral and bacterial vaccine epitopes using a radio-protective Mn^{2+}-peptide complex from Deinococcus. *Cell Host Microbe* 12 (1): 117–124.

Garg, R., Latimer, L., Simko, E. et al. (2014). Induction of mucosal immunity and protection by intranasal immunization with a respiratory syncytial virus subunit vaccine formulation. *J. Gen. Virol.* 95 (2): 301–306.

Glenn, L.L. (2013). Limited effectiveness of psoralen- and ultraviolet-inactivated Vaccinia virus on SHIV infection. *Front. Immunol.* 4: 327.

Greenall, S.A., Tyack, S.G., Johnson, M.A., and Sapats, S.I. (2010). Antibody fragments, expressed by a fowl adenovirus vector, are able to neutralize infectious bursal disease virus. *Avian Pathol.* 39 (5): 339–348.

Groene, W.S. and Shaw, R.D. (1992). Psoralen preparation of antigenically intact noninfectious rotavirus particles. *J. Virol. Methods* 38: 93–102.

Gromowski, G.D., Firestone, C.Y., Hanson, C.T., and Whitehead, S.S. (2014). Japanese encephalitis virus vaccine candidates generated by chimerization with dengue virus type 4. *Vaccine* 32 (25): 3010–3018.

Guo, H.C., Sun, S.Q., Jin, Y. et al. (2013). Foot-and-mouth disease virus-like particles produced by a SUMO fusion protein system in *Escherichia coli* induce potent protective immune responses in Guinea pigs, swine and cattle. *Vet. Res.* 44: 48.

Hammond, R.W. and Nemchinov, L.G. (2009). Plant production of veterinary vaccines and therapeutics. *Curr. Top. Microbiol. Immunol.* 332: 79–102.

He, Y., Xiang, Z., and Mobley, H.L. (2010). Vaxign: the first web-based vaccine design program for reverse vaccinology and applications for vaccine development. *J. Biomed. Biotechnol.* 2010: 297505.

Heldens, J.G., Pouwels, H.G., Derks, C.G. et al. (2009). The first safe inactivated equine influenza vaccine formulation adjuvanted with ISCOM-matrix that closes the immunity gap. *Vaccine* 27 (40): 5530–5537.

Herrington, D.A., Clyde, D.F., Davis, J.R. et al. (1990). Human studies with synthetic peptide sporozoite vaccine (NANP)3-TT and immunization with irradiated sporozoites. *Bull. World Health Organ.* 68 (Suppl): 33–37.

Hoffman, S.L., Weiss, W., Mellouk, S., and Sedegah, M. (1990). Irradiated sporozoite vaccine induces cytotoxic T lymphocytes that recognize malaria antigens on the surface of infected hepatocytes. *Immunol. Lett.* 25 (1–3): 33–38.

Hu, S., Ma, H., Wu, Y. et al. (2009). A vaccine candidate of attenuated genotype VII Newcastle disease virus generated by reverse genetics. *Vaccine* 27 (6): 904–910.

Hu, M., Zhang, Y., Xie, F. et al. (2013). Protection of piglets by a Haemophilus parasuis ghost vaccine against homologous challenge. *Clin. Vaccine Immunol.* 20 (6): 795–802.

Hua, R.H., Li, Y.N., Chen, Z.S. et al. (2014). Generation and characterization of a new mammalian cell line continuously expressing virus-like particles of Japanese encephalitis virus for a subunit vaccine candidate. *BMC Biotech.* 14: 62.

Jackwood, M.W., Bogoch, S., Bogoch, E.S. et al. (2009). Efficacy of a replikin peptide vaccine against low-pathogenicity avian influenza H5 virus. *Avian Dis.* 53 (4): 613–617.

Jawale, C.V., Chaudhari, A.A., and Lee, J.H. (2014). Generation of a safety enhanced *Salmonella gallinarum* ghost using antibiotic resistance free plasmid and its potential as an effective inactivated vaccine candidate against fowl typhoid. *Vaccine* 32 (9): 1093–1099.

Johnson, M., Labes, R.E., Taylor, M.J., and Mackintosh, C.G. (2003). Efficacy trial of an irradiated cattle lungworm vaccine in red deer (*Cervus elaphus*). *Vet. Parasitol.* 117 (1–2): 131–137.

Kawai, T. and Akira, S. (2014). The roles of TLRs, RLRs and NLRs in pathogen recognition. *Int. Immunol.* 21 (4): 317–337.

Keller, R., Hilton, T.D., Rios, H. et al. (2010). Development of a live oral attaching and effacing *Escherichia coli* vaccine candidate using *Vibrio cholerae* CVD 103-HgR as antigen vector. *Microb. Pathog.* 48 (1): 1–8.

Kerkhofs, P., Renjifo, X., Toussaint, J.F. et al. (2003). Enhancement of the immune response and virological protection of calves against bovine herpesvirus type 1 with an inactivated gE-deleted vaccine. *Vet. Rec.* 152 (22): 681–686.

Khandelwal, A., Renukaradhya, G.J., Rajasekhar, M. et al. (2011). Immune responses to hemagglutinin-neuraminidase protein of peste des petits ruminants virus expressed in transgenic peanut plants in sheep. *Vet Immunol. Immunopathol.* 140 (3–4): 291–296.

Kim, H., Lee, Y.K., Kang, S.C. et al. (2016). Recent vaccine technology in industrial animals. *Clin. Exp. Vaccine Res.* 5 (1): 12–18.

Kurosaki, T., Kodama, Y., Muro, T. et al. (2013). Secure splenic delivery of plasmid DNA and its application to DNA vaccine. *Biol. Pharm. Bull.* 36 (11): 1800–1806.

Kutzler, M.A. and Weiner, D.B. (2008). DNA vaccines: ready for prime time? *Nat. Rev. Genet.* 10: 776–788.

Kwon, S.R., Nam, Y.K., Kim, S.K., and Kim, K.H. (2006). Protection of tilapia (*Oreochromis mossambicus*) from edwardsiellosis by vaccination with *Edwardsiella tarda* ghosts. *Fish Shellfish Immunol.* 20 (4): 621–626.

Kyriakis, C.S., de Vleeschauwer, A., Barbé, F. et al. (2009). Safety, immunogenicity and efficacy of poxvirus-based vector vaccines expressing the haemagglutinin gene of a highly pathogenic H5N1 avian influenza virus in pigs. *Vaccine* 27 (16): 2258–2264.

Lamphear, B.J., Jilka, J.M., Kesl, L. et al. (2004). A corn-based delivery system for animal vaccines: an oral transmissible gastroenteritis virus vaccine boosts lactogenic immunity in swine. *Vaccine* 22 (19): 2420–2424.

Landry, N., Ward, B.J., Trépanier, S. et al. (2010). Preclinical and clinical development of plant-made virus-like particle vaccine against avian H5N1 influenza. *PLoS One* 5 (12): e15559.

Langeveld, J.P., Casal, J.I., Osterhaus, A.D. et al. (1994). First peptide vaccine providing protection against viral infection in the target animal: studies of canine parvovirus in dogs. *J. Virol.* 68 (7): 4506–4513.

Lee, R.W., Cornelisse, M., Ziauddin, A. et al. (2008). Expression of a modified Mannheimia haemolytica GS60 outer membrane lipoprotein in transgenic alfalfa for the development of an edible vaccine against bovine pneumonic pasteurellosis. *J. Biotechnol.* 135 (2): 224–231.

Legocki, A.B., Miedzinska, K., Czaplińska, M. et al. (2005). Immunoprotective properties of transgenic plants expressing E2 glycoprotein from CSFV and cysteine protease from *Fasciola hepatica*. *Vaccine* 23 (15): 1844–1846.

Li, P., Bai, X., Sun, P. et al. (2012). Evaluation of a genetically modified foot-and-mouth disease virus vaccine candidate generated by reverse genetics. *BMC Vet. Res.* 8: 57.

Li, W., Jin, H., Sui, X. et al. (2014). Self-assembly and release of peste des petits ruminants virus-like particles in an insect cell-baculovirus system and their immunogenicity in mice and goats. *PLoS One* 9 (8): e104791.

Lien, E., Sellati, T.J., Yoshimura, A. et al. (1999). Toll-like receptor 2 functions as a pattern recognition receptor for diverse bacterial products. *J. Biolumin. Chemilumin.* 274 (47): 33419–33425.

Lin, G.J., Deng, M.C., Chen, Z.W. et al. (2012). Yeast expressed classical swine fever E2 subunit vaccine candidate provides complete protection against lethal challenge infection and prevents horizontal virus transmission. *Vaccine* 30 (13): 2336–3341.

Ling, H.Y., Pelosi, A., and Walmsley, A.M. (2010). Current status of plant-made vaccines for veterinary purposes. *Expert Rev. Vaccines* 9 (8): 971–982.

Liu, M., Zhang, Y., Liu, C.G. et al. (2006). Generation high yield vaccine strain wholly derived from avian influenza viruses by reverse genetics. *Sheng Wu Gong Cheng Xue Bao* 22 (5): 720–726.

Liu, D., Sun, Y., and Qiu, H. (2009). Applications of reverse genetics in studying classical swine fever virus. *Sheng Wu Gong Cheng Xue Bao* 25 (10): 1441–1448.

Lv, L., Li, X., Liu, G. et al. (2013). Production and immunogenicity of chimeric virus-like particles containing the spike glycoprotein of infectious bronchitis virus. *J. Vet. Sci.* 15 (2): 209–216.

Madampage, C.A., Rawlyk, N., Crockford, G. et al. (2015). Reverse vaccinology as an approach for developing *Histophilus somni* vaccine candidates. *Biologicals* 43 (6): 444–451.

Magnani, D.M., Harms, J.S., Durward, M.A., and Splitter, G.A. (2009). Nondividing but metabolically active gamma-irradiated *Brucella melitensis* is protective against virulent *B. melitensis* challenge in mice. *Infect. Immun.* 77 (11): 5181–5189.

Mahony, D., Mody, K.T., Cavallaro, A.S. et al. (2015). Immunisation of sheep with bovine viral diarrhoea virus, E2 protein using a freeze-dried hollow silica mesoporous nanoparticle formulation. *PLoS One* 10 (11): e0141870.

Maione, D., Margarit, I., Rinaudo, C.D. et al. (2005). Identification of a universal group B streptococcus vaccine by multiple genome screen. *Science* 309 (5731): 148–150.

Mandell, R.B., Koukuntla, R., Mogler, L.J. et al. (2010). A replication-incompetent Rift Valley fever vaccine: chimeric virus-like particles protect mice and rats against lethal challenge. *Virology* 397 (1): 187–198.

Maritz-Olivier, C., van Zyl, W., and Stutzer, C.A. (2012). Systematic, functional genomics, and reverse vaccinology approach to the identification of vaccine candidates in the cattle tick, *Rhipicephalus microplus*. *Ticks Tick-borne Dis.* 3 (3): 179–187.

Martin, S.S., Bakken, R.R., Lind, C.M. et al. (2010). Comparison of the immunological responses and efficacy of gamma-irradiated V3526 vaccine formulations against subcutaneous and aerosol challenge with Venezuelan equine encephalitis virus subtype IAB. *Vaccine* 28 (4): 1031–1040.

Marzi, A., Halfmann, P., Hill-Batorski, L. et al. (2015). An Ebola whole-virus vaccine is protective in nonhuman primates. *Science* 348 (6233): 439–442.

Maves, R.C., Oré, R.M., Porter, K.R., and Kochel, T.J. (2011). Immunogenicity and protective efficacy of a psoralen-inactivated dengue-1 virus vaccine candidate in *Aotus nancymaae* monkeys. *Vaccine* 29 (15): 2691–2696.

Mayer, M.L., Phillips, C.M., Townsend, R.A. et al. (2009). Differential activation of dendritic cells by toll-like receptor agonists isolated from the gram-positive vaccine vector *Streptococcus gordonii*. *Scand. J. Immunol.* 69 (4): 351–356.

McGettigan, J.P. (2010). Experimental rabies vaccines for humans. *Expert Rev. Vaccines* 9 (10): 1177–1186.

McGettigan, J.P., David, F., Figueiredo, M.D. et al. (2014). Safety and serological response to a matrix gene-deleted rabies virus-based vaccine vector in dogs. *Vaccine* 32 (15): 1716–1719.

Meng, W., Pan, W., Zhang, A.J. et al. (2013). Rapid generation of human-like neutralizing monoclonal antibodies in urgent preparedness for influenza pandemics and virulent infectious diseases. *PLoS One* 8 (6): e66276.

Menon, S. and Bhopale, M.K. (1985). Efficacy of UV-irradiated larval vaccine of *Ancylostoma ceylanicum* (Looss, 1911) in golden hamsters (*Mesocricetus auratus*). *J. Helminthol.* 59 (4): 287–293.

Moore, R.J., Stewart, D.J., Lund, K., and Hodgson, A.L. (2001). Vaccination against ovine footrot using a live bacterial vector to deliver basic protease antigen. *FEMS Microbiol. Lett.* 194 (2): 193–196.

Morein, B., Hu, K.F., and Abusugra, I. (2004). Current status and potential application of ISCOMs in veterinary medicine. *Adv. Drug Delivery Rev.* 56: 1367–1382.

Motha, M.X., Atkinson, G., and Hoyle, F.P. (1994). Progress towards the eradication of Aujeszky's disease in New Zealand by vaccination with a subunit vaccine. *Vet. Rec.* 135 (9): 204–206.

Moustafa, D., Garg, V.K., Jain, N. et al. (2011). Immunization of mice with gamma-irradiated *Brucella neotomae* and its recombinant strains induces protection against virulent B. abortus, B. melitensis, and B. suis challenge. *Vaccine* 29 (4): 784–794.

Mutwiri, G., Bowersock, T.L., and Babiuk, L.A. (2005). Microparticles for oral delivery of vaccines. *Expert Opin. Drug Deliv.* 2 (5): 791–806.

Mutwiri, G., Benjamin, P., Soita, H. et al. (2007). Poly [di(sodium carboxylateethylphenoxy) phosphazene] (PCEP) is a potent enhancer of mixed Th1/Th2 immune responses in mice immunized with influenza virus antigens. *Vaccine* 25 (7): 1204–1213.

National Institute of Allergy and Infectious Diseases. (2012). Vaccines types. www.niaid.nih.gov/research/vaccine-types

Needham, B.D., Carroll, S.M., Giles, D.K. et al. (2013). Modulating the innate immune response by combinatorial engineering of endotoxin. *Proc. Natl. Acad. Sci. U.S.A.* 110 (4): 1464–1469.

Nkando, I., Perez-Casal, J., Mwirigi, M. et al. (2016). Recombinant *Mycoplasma mycoides* proteins elicit protective immune responses against contagious bovine pleuropneumonia. *Vet. Immunol. Immunopathol.* 171: 103–114.

Olive, C., Clair, T., Yarwood, P., and Good, M.F. (2002). Protection of mice from group A streptococcal infection by intranasal immunisation with a peptide vaccine that contains a conserved M protein B cell epitope and lacks a T cell autoepitope. *Vaccine* 20 (21–22): 2816–2825.

Pallister, J., Middleton, D., Wang, L.F. et al. (2011). A recombinant Hendra virus G glycoprotein-based subunit vaccine protects ferrets from lethal Hendra virus challenge. *Vaccine* 29 (34): 5623–5630.

Phoolcharoen, W., Dye, J.M., Kilbourne, J. et al. (2011). A nonreplicating subunit vaccine protects mice against lethal Ebola virus challenge. *Proc. Natl. Acad. Sci. U.S.A.* 108 (51): 20695–20700.

Pichlmair, A., Habjan, M., Unger, H., and Weber, F. (2010). Virus-like particles expressing the nucleocapsid gene as an efficient vaccine against Rift Valley fever virus. *Vector Borne Zoonotic Dis.* 10 (7): 701–703.

Pleschka, S., Jaskunas, R., Engelhardt, O.G. et al. (1996). A plasmid-based reverse genetics system for influenza A virus. *J. Virol.* 70 (6): 4188–4192.

Pulliam, J.D., Converse, J.L., Snyder, E.M. et al. (1967). Experimental irradiated arthrospore vaccine against coccidioidomycosis in mice. *J. Bacteriol.* 94 (5): 1394–1399.

Purnell, R.E., Lewis, D., Brabazon, A. et al. (1981). Field use of an irradiated blood vaccine to protect cattle against Redwater (*Babesia divergens* infection) on a farm in Dorset. *Vet. Rec.* 108 (2): 28–31.

Querec, T., Bennouna, S., Alkan, S. et al. (2006). Yellow fever vaccine YF-17D activates multiple dendritic cell subsets via TLR2, 7, 8, and 9 to stimulate polyvalent immunity. *J. Exp. Med.* 203 (2): 413–424.

Racz, R., Li, X., Patel, M. et al. (2014). DNAVaxDB: the first web-based DNA vaccine database and its data analysis. *BMC Bioinf.* 15 (Suppl. 4): S2.

Ramey, K., Eko, F.O., Thompson, W.E. et al. (2009). Immunolocalization and challenge studies using a recombinant *Vibrio cholerae* ghost expressing *Trypanosoma brucei* Ca(2+) ATPase (TBCA2) antigen. *Am. J. Trop. Med. Hyg.* 81 (3): 407–415.

Rappuoli, R. (2000). Reverse vaccinology. *Curr. Opin. Microbiol.* 5: 445–450.

Reimann, I., Depner, K., Trapp, S., and Beer, M. (2004). An avirulent chimeric *Pestivirus* with altered cell tropism protects pigs against lethal infection with classical swine fever virus. *Virology* 322 (1): 143–157.

Rigano, M.M., Sala, F., Arntzen, C.J., and Walmsley, A.M. (2003). Targeting of plant-derived vaccine antigens to immunoresponsive mucosal sites. *Vaccine* 21 (7–8): 809–811.

Roldão, A., Mellado, M.C., Castilho, L.R. et al. (2010). Virus-like particles in vaccine development. *Expert Rev. Vaccines* 9 (10): 1149–1176.

Roush, S.W., Murphy, T.V., and Vaccine-Preventable Disease Table Working Group (2007). Historical comparisons of morbidity and mortality for vaccine-preventable diseases in the United States. *JAMA* 298 (18): 2155–2163.

Santos, M.J.D. and Wigdorovitz, A. (2005). Transgenic plants for the production of veterinary vaccines. *Immunol. Cell Biol.* 83 (3): 229–238.

Schmidt, M.R., McGinnes, L.W., Kenward, S.A. et al. (2012). Long-term and memory immune responses in mice against Newcastle disease virus-like particles containing respiratory syncytial virus glycoprotein ectodomains. *J. Virol.* 86 (21): 11654–11662.

Se Eyun Kwona, S.R., Eun Hye Leea, E.H., Yoon Kwon Namb, Y.K. et al. (2007). Efficacy of oral immunization with *Edwardsiella tarda* ghosts against edwardsiellosis in olive flounder (*Paralichthys olivaceus*). *Aquaculture* 269 (1–4): 84–88.

Seah, S.K. and Hucal, G. (1975). The use of irradiated vaccine in immunization against experimental murine toxoplasmosis. *Can. J. Microbiol.* 21: 1379–1385.

Sette, A. and Rappuoli, R. (2010). Reverse vaccinology: developing vaccines in the era of genomics. *Immunity* 33 (4): 530–541.

Shoji, Y., Prokhnevsky, A., Leffet, B. et al. (2015). Immunogenicity of H1N1 influenza virus-like particles produced in *Nicotiana benthamiana*. *Hum. Vaccin. Immunother.* 11 (1): 118–123.

Skoble, J., Beaber, J.W., Gao, Y. et al. (2009). Killed but metabolically active bacillus anthracis vaccines induce broad and protective immunity against anthrax. *Infect. Immun.* 77 (4): 1649–1663.

Sola, I., Alonso, S , Zúñiga, S. et al. (2003). Engineering the transmissible gastroenteritis virus genome as an expression vector inducing lactogenic immunity. *J. Virol.* 77: 4357–4369.

Song, Y., La, T., Phillips, N.D. et al. (2009). A reverse vaccinology approach to swine dysentery vaccine development. *Vet. Microbiol.* 137 (1–2): 111–119.

Stech, J. and Klenk, H.D. (2006). A new approach to an influenza life vaccine: haemagglutinin cleavage site mutants generated by reverse genetics. *Berl. Munch. Tierarztl. Wochenschr.* 119 (3–4): 186–191.

Stevenson, A. and Roberts, M. (2002). Use of a rationally attenuated *Bordetella bronchiseptica* as a live mucosal vaccine and vector for heterologous antigens. *Vaccine* 20 (17–18): 2325–2335.

Stoeker, L., Nordone, S., Gunderson, S. et al. (2011). Assessment of *Lactobacillus gasseri* as a candidate oral vaccine vector. *Clin. Vaccine Immunol.* 18 (11): 1834–1844.

Streatfield, S.J. (2005). Oral hepatitis B vaccine candidates produced and delivered in plant material. *Immunol. Cell Biol.* 83 (3): 257–262.

Swenson, S.L., McMillen, J., and Hill, H.T. (1993). Diagnostic compatibility of a thymidine kinase, inverted repeat, gI, and gpX modified live gene-deleted PRV vaccine with three differential ELISAs. *J. Vet. Diagn. Invest.* 5 (3): 347–350.

Szostaka, M.P., Hensela, A., Ekoa, F.O. et al. (1996). Bacterial ghosts: non-living candidate vaccines. *J. Biotechnol.* 44 (1–3): 161–170.

Taniguchi, T. (1978). Site-directed mutagenesis on bacteriophage Qbeta RNA (author's transl). *Tanpakushitsu Kakusan Koso.* 23: 159–169.

Thorpe, C., Edwards, L., Snelgrove, R. et al. (2007). Discovery of a vaccine antigen that protects mice from *Chlamydia pneumoniae* infection. *Vaccine* 25 (12): 2252–2260.

Thuenemann, E.C., Meyers, A.E., Verwey, J. et al. (2013). A method for rapid production of heteromultimeric protein complexes in plants: assembly of protective bluetongue virus-like particles. *Plant Biotechnol. J.* 11 (7): 839–846.

Tsung, K., Yim, J.H., Marti, W. et al. (1996). Gene expression and cytopathic effect of vaccinia virus inactivated by psoralen and long-wave UV light. *J. Virol.* 70 (1): 165–171.

Tu, F.P., Chu, W.H., Zhuang, X.Y., and Lu, C.P. (2009). Effect of oral immunization with *Aeromonas hydrophila* ghosts on protection against experimental fish infection. *Lett. Appl. Microbiol.* 50 (1): 13–17.

van Gennip, H.G., van Rijn, P.A., Widjojoatmodjo, M.N. et al. (2000). Chimeric classical swine fever viruses containing envelope protein E(RNS) or E2 of bovine viral diarrhoea virus protect pigs against challenge with CSFV and induce a distinguishable antibody response. *Vaccine* 19: 447–459.

Verma, D. and Daniell, H. (2007). Chloroplast vector systems for biotechnology applications. *Plant Physiol.* 145 (4): 1129–1143.

Walker, J.M., Raué, H.P., and Slifka, M.K. (2012). Characterization of $CD8^+$ T cell function and immunodominance generated with an H_2O_2-inactivated whole-virus vaccine. *J. Virol.* 86 (24): 13735–13744.

Walton, C.B., Inos, A.B., Andres, O.A. et al. (2008). Immunization with hybrid recombinant *Mycobacterium tuberculosis* H37Rv proteins increases the TH1 cytokine response in mice following a pulmonary instillation of irradiated mycobacteria. *Vaccine* 26 (34): 4396–4402.

Wang, W., Chen, X., Xue, C. et al. (2012). Production and immunogenicity of chimeric virus-like particles containing porcine reproductive and respiratory syndrome virus GP5 protein. *Vaccine* 30 (49): 7072–7077.

Wei, Z., Fu, Q., Liu, X., and Chen, Y. (2012). Attenuated *Streptococcus equi* ssp. *zooepidemicus* as a bacterial vector for expression of porcine circovirus type 2 capsid protein. *FEMS Microbiol. Lett.* 332 (1): 20–26.

Windish, H.P., Duthie, M.S., Misquith, A. et al. (2011). Protection of mice from *Mycobacterium tuberculosis* by ID87/GLA-SE, a novel tuberculosis subunit vaccine candidate. *Vaccine* 29 (44): 7842–7848.

Wizel, B., Houghten, R.A., Parker, K.C. et al. (1995). Irradiated sporozoite vaccine induces HLA-B8-restricted cytotoxic T lymphocyte responses against two overlapping epitopes of the *Plasmodium falciparum* sporozoite surface protein 2. *J. Exp. Med.* 182 (5): 1435–1445.

Xu, S., Shi, F., and Wu, H. (1991). *Schistosoma japonicum*: some parameters affecting the development of protective immunity induced by a cryopreserved, irradiated schistosomula vaccine in Guinea-pigs. *Parasitology* 102 (1): 45–47.

Xu, L., Liu, Y., Chen, Z. et al. (2012). Surface-engineered gold nanorods: promising DNA vaccine adjuvant for HIV-1 treatment. *Nano Lett.* 12 (4): 2003–2012.

Xue, C., Wang, W., Liu, Q. et al. (2014). Chimeric influenza-virus-like particles containing the porcine reproductive and respiratory syndrome virus GP5 protein and the influenza virus HA and M1 proteins. *Arch. Virol* 159 (11): 3043–3051.

Yin, D., Liang, W., Xing, S. et al. (2013). Hepatitis B DNA vaccine-polycation nano-complexes enhancing immune response by percutaneous administration with microneedle. *Biol. Pharm. Bull.* 36 (8): 1283–1291.

Yole, D.S., Pemberton, R., Reid, G.D., and Wilson, R.A. (1996). Protective immunity to *Schistosoma mansoni* induced in the olive baboon *Papio anubis* by the irradiated cercaria vaccine. *Parasitology* 112 (1): 37–46.

Zecchini, T.A. and Smith, R.J. (1999). Production of high titre disabled infectious single cycle (DISC) HSV from a microcarrier culture. *Cytotechnology* 30: 203–210.

Zevenhoven-Dobbe, J.C., Greve, S., van Tol, H. et al. (2004). Rescue of disabled infectious single-cycle (DISC) equine arteritis virus by using complementing cell lines that express minor structural glycoproteins. *J. Gen. Virol.* 85: 3709–3714.

Zhang, L., Zhang, J., Chen, H.T. et al. (2011). Research in advance for FMD novel vaccines. *Virol. J.* 8: 268.

Zhou, L., Ni, Y.Y., Piñeyro, P. et al. (2012). DNA shuffling of the GP3 genes of porcine reproductive and respiratory syndrome virus (PRRSV) produces a chimeric virus with an improved cross-neutralizing ability against a heterologous PRRSV strain. *Virology* 434 (1): 96–109.

Zou, H.Y., Liu, X.J., Ma, F.Y. et al. (2011). Attenuated *Actinobacillus pleuropneumoniae* as a bacterial vector for expression of *Mycoplasma hyopneumoniae* P36 gene. *J. Gene Med.* 13 (4): 221–229.

Section III

Aspects of Vaccine Production, Quality Control, and Distribution

11

The Manufacture of Veterinary Vaccines: Manufacturing Facilities

Teresa Yeary, Renee Schnurr, Richard Hill, Jr., Mark Pagala, and Douglas Murtle

USDA-APHIS-VS-DB-Center for Veterinary Biologics, Ames, Iowa, USA

11.1 Introduction

The design of manufacturing facilities for veterinary vaccines is guided by the types of vaccines that will be manufactured in them. Essential to the facility design are the types of organisms, antigens or nucleic acids used in the vaccine, the specific technologies and manufacturing processes employed, and the regulatory requirements of the manufacturing facility's locale and the countries where the vaccine will be marketed. Key aspects of production that assure a high-quality finished product are qualification of incoming ingredients and materials, qualified personnel, controlled processes in an appropriate manufacturing facility, proven technology and manufacturing procedures, validated equipment, in-process validation and controls, and testing (Halkjær-Knudsen 2007). Facilities should be designed so that personnel and the environment are protected from harm and the product prepared is protected from the environment. The ultimate design objective is to prepare a pure, safe, potent, and efficacious vaccine product in a facility that is maintained and operated in compliance with all local laws, rules, and regulations of the regulatory authority responsible for the oversight of biologics production (United States Code (USC) 1985; Code of Federal Regulations (CFR) 2020a; USDA Veterinary Services Memorandum 2020).

11.2 Vaccine Production Systems – General Design and Operating Requirements

11.2.1 Facility Arrangement and Construction

Facility design for a manufacturing and testing facility is dependent on the methods of manufacture employed to produce the class of biological products prepared within it, e.g. bacterins or vaccines (live, attenuated, or inactivated), toxoids, subunit virus-like particles, allergens, recombinant DNA, immunoglobulins, immunomodulators, *in vitro* diagnostic test kits, etc. Interior surfaces (floors, walls, ceilings, doors, windows, partitions, etc.) of all rooms and laboratories should be constructed using smooth, solid, impervious materials that can be readily and thoroughly cleaned and disinfected. Aseptic production areas should be arranged to provide adequate and appropriate isolation for each product and prevent cross-contamination from other products and the environment. Segregation of material and personnel flow, unidirectional from clean areas to dirty areas, minimizes the risk of cross-contamination. The degree of air quality should be controlled according to the operations occurring within each production area.

Quality control laboratories pose a risk of contamination to products; thus, testing areas should be isolated from production areas if it is not possible to locate them in a "separate and apart" location (USDA 2019). Manufacturing facilities that also perform research and development or provide ancillary diagnostic testing services should locate these laboratories in "separate and apart" facilities (USDA 2019).

Personnel dressing rooms, toilet facilities, and lavatory accommodations in sufficient number, ample in size, and meeting all requirements as to sanitary construction and equipment must be conveniently located, properly ventilated, and readily accessible to all persons without having to enter or pass through biological preparation areas. These must be separate from rooms or compartments in which biological products are prepared, handled, or stored (CFR 2020g).

11.2.2 Equipment

Equipment used in the preparation of biological products must be in good working order. Preventive maintenance

Veterinary Vaccines: Principles and Applications, First Edition. Edited by Samia Metwally, Gerrit Viljoen, and Ahmed El Idrissi.

plans decrease production deviations due to malfunctioning equipment. Equipment that creates an aerosol should be placed in an appropriate cabinet to minimize cross-contamination and allow appropriate cleaning and sanitation of all equipment. Also, if a product comes in contact with equipment such as continuous flow centrifuges, bioreactors, or fermenters, there must be a validated cleaning, disinfection, and/or sterilization procedure performed between each use (CFR 2020h).

11.2.3 Water Quality – Supply and Effluent

Water supply quality must meet the needs of the production facility to produce the biological products (CFR 2020g) and to clean and sanitize production equipment (CFR 2020h). In most cases, supplemental water treatment systems within the facility are necessary to improve the quality of water used in biologics production. Plumbing systems must include approved traps and vents to prevent backflow of liquid effluents.

The nature of organisms used in the facility, whether live or inactivated, has an impact on disposal methods allowable in compliance with local regulations, especially with regard to liquid effluents. Small quantities of liquids containing viable organisms or agents may be autoclaved sufficiently for discharge into a sanitary sewer system. Larger volumes of effluent may require pretreatment using specialized equipment to effect chemical, thermal, or thermochemical decontamination prior to discharge, thus the composition, volume, and disposal of liquid effluents are additional facility design considerations. Solid waste disposal is also a concern and, depending on the nature of the waste, local, state, and/or national regulations may dictate how these materials will be handled before final disposal (USDA 2008a; CFR 2020j).

11.2.4 Air Handling

A goal of good facility design is to create the cleanest possible manufacturing environment that can be easily maintained (CFR 2020g). All rooms or suites of rooms utilized in the preparation of veterinary vaccines should have a dedicated heating, ventilation, and air conditioning (HVAC) system sufficient to ensure sanitary and hygienic conditions for the protection of product and personnel. The design of the HVAC should provide personnel comfort; protect against airborne materials that could cause hazards to either personnel inside the facility or the environment outside the facility; and control the impact of the environment on the finished product to assure product quality. HVAC systems can maintain temperature, relative humidity, airborne particles, and room pressures and supply fresh air but they cannot clean the surfaces of a contaminated area or compensate for failure to follow appropriate procedures.

Areas where product is directly exposed to the environment should have air supplied from a high efficiency particulate air (HEPA) filtration system that provides clean air. When working with live organisms, especially zoonotic or high consequence/exotic agents ("select agents"), the HEPA filtration of exhaust air is highly recommended (US Department of Health and Human Services 2007; CFR 2020m). HEPA filters should be integrity tested at least annually. There are multiple types of HEPA filters and choosing which to use depends on several factors including but not limited to the organism or agent handled, risk of product contamination due to the nature of the process that is occurring, and the hazard to personnel performing the work. Environmental sampling and monitoring provides greater assurance of the effectiveness of control measures.

The facility should be designed so that air pressure differentials between rooms decrease the chance of cross-contamination. These pressure differentials between critical production rooms should be defined with appropriate alert and alarm settings, and continuously monitored. The use of biosafety cabinets and/or personal protective equipment (PPE) provides another layer of protection especially for product manipulations outside a closed environment. All alarms and deviations from established limits should be investigated (International Society of Pharmaceutical Engineering [ISPE] 2009).

11.3 Biosafety Considerations in the Manufacture of Vaccines

The code of practice for biosafety is the discipline addressing the safe handling and containment of infectious microorganisms and hazardous biological materials. Guidance for the safe use of infectious organisms in laboratories and animal research facilities in the USA is provided in *Biosafety in Microbiological and Biomedical Laboratories* (BMBL), 5th edition (US Department of Health and Human Services 2007).

Although biosafety concerns in laboratory and biological production environments have many commonalities, there are important differences in their environments and desired outcomes. In both situations, personnel safety is a serious concern and risk assessments are required for determining the level of precautions to take for preventing the potential infection of personnel. However, the risk assessments for preventing the escape of infectious microorganisms to the surrounding environment both inside and outside the facility differ somewhat between laboratories and aseptic biologics production facilities (ISPE 2009). The scale and size of a manufacturing facility, the large volumes of live organisms, and the number of different organisms used in making the various products within one facility bring a level of complexity to biosafety considerations beyond that of smaller microbiology laboratories. Whereas research and diagnostic laboratories want to keep infectious agents contained within the facility, the policies and procedures for biologics manufacturing processes also focus on preparing a pure product by preventing cross-contamination and keeping environmental contaminants out of the product.

Aside from liquid and solid waste decontamination considerations, the manner in which air handling systems are designed for aseptic manufacturing facilities can appear to differ from recommendations in the BMBL, but solutions that satisfy both BMBL biosafety guidelines and aseptic manufacturing practices can be forged. From a biosafety viewpoint, air pressure should be negative in areas where high levels of live zoonotic or high consequence/exotic agents are being processed to protect personnel and the environment. The production perspective is to use positive pressure in these areas to protect product. However, both personnel and product protection can be achieved by the use of airlocks that are negative to both the process room and surrounding areas. The use of HEPA filtration, biosafety cabinets, and PPE provide additional protection.

11.4 Registration, Licensing, and Authorization of Vaccine Manufacturing Facilities

Facilities used in the manufacture of veterinary biologics should be registered and/or licensed with the appropriate regulatory authority (USDA 2016e, 2018a; CFR 2020b,c) and should be inspected prior to and throughout the lifetime of the facility for acceptability (USDA 2016d; CFR 2020k). The inspection conducted prior to authorizing the facility is to determine if the conditions, equipment, facilities, processes, and personnel conform to the acceptable requirements as determined by the country's regulatory authority. Any deficiencies noted during this preliminary inspection should be resolved prior to final authorization. The facility must be able to prepare a product that is consistent and meets the quality standards as listed by the regulatory authority (CFR 2020i,j).

11.4.1 Facilities

In order to be able to appropriately evaluate and assess a facility for sufficiency, construction documents describing the facility must be available for review by the regulatory authorities (USDA 2019; CFR 2020g). The facility documents must include an overall site plan and more detailed individual building plans.

The overarching documents include a plot plan that shows the complete layout of all buildings for each particular land area and the use of immediate adjacent properties. An accompanying plot plan legend describes and provides documentation regarding the availability of adequate water, drains, and lighting in all areas used for product preparation. The plot plan legend should fully describe the activities occurring in each building on the plot plan, and describe how all biological materials move between production, testing, and storage locations and outline all precautions taken to maintain proper storage conditions during transport.

Detailed individual building blueprints should be available for all the rooms used in the preparation of biological products. The blueprints should include construction-style line drawings for all production areas in sufficient detail, including the location of all rooms, doors, and important stationary equipment. Corresponding blueprint legends must include a listing of all rooms and a brief description of all activities performed in each room or area and the agents and products handled and prepared in each room. Decontamination procedures and other methods used to prevent cross-contamination in rooms where products are exposed to the surroundings must be described in the legends. A supplemental listing of the stationary equipment and other essential nonstationary equipment maintained in different rooms must be included in sufficient detail to determine if the facility is adequately equipped to conduct the described production for each room or area.

Diagrams describing the flow of materials, personnel, and product are also useful in determining acceptability of the facilities for vaccine production. In summary, this set of facility documents will allow the regulatory authority to determine the fitness of the facilities for the preparation and testing of veterinary vaccines.

11.4.2 Personnel

Veterinary biologics manufacturing facilities must be operated under competent management (CFR 2020b,j). Biographical summaries for key employees having the responsibility for producing biological products should be on file with the appropriate regulatory authority. Personnel conducting day-to-day production and testing functions must also be considered competent, either by education, training, or both (USDA 2016a,b). They must demonstrate fitness to prepare veterinary biological products in accord with quality standards. A regulatory liaison or quality manager should represent each veterinary biologics company and be a point of contact for the regulatory authorities. This liaison person is responsible for and should handle all government submissions and correspondence and will coordinate inspection activities and compliance. Employee training, experience, knowledge, and periodic retraining specific to the products manufactured, including detailed measures to protect product, personnel, and the environment, are evaluated by the regulatory authority during facility inspections and/or product investigations to ensure that manufacturers have proper control of production processes.

11.4.3 Documentation of the Manufacturing Process

Manufacturing directives, reviewed by the regulatory authority and supported by scientific data as to the purity, efficacy, and safety of the product, are the directions on how to consistently prepare a veterinary biological product. These documents should be detailed and accurately reflect all critical and consistent manufacturing procedures such as standard operating procedures and work or manufacturing instructions for all phases of production. Changes in the manufacturing process cannot be made without prior approval by the regulatory authority. Each serial, batch, or production lot must be prepared according to the current version of the manufacturing directive (USDA 2018). Manufacturing directives must be reviewed for accuracy by the manufacturer at least annually (CFR 2020j). A product that has not been prepared in accordance with the manufacturing directive or the regulations may be considered unfit for distribution (USDA 2018d; CFR 2020d,l).

11.5 Internal and External Audits/Inspections

The general goals of an inspection are to determine that the biological products have been produced and tested by competent personnel using acceptable facilities, equipment, and methods; that products being marketed are not worthless, contaminated, dangerous, or harmful (CFR 2020d); and that reports and records of production and testing of products are concurrent, accurate, and complete (CFR 2016). To ensure uniformity and consistency of final product, it is recommended that manufacturers perform internal audits of their own production processes. External audits of suppliers are also advised to assure that only quality materials and supplies adhering to the manufacturer's requirements are used in the preparation of veterinary biological products.

11.5.1 Inspections of Production, Testing, and Distribution Facilities Including Inspections Prior to Registration and/or Licensing

Inspectors utilize a combination of inspection techniques to evaluate whether manufacturers and their facilities are in compliance with the rules and regulations prior to registering a facility or product (USDA 2016d). Throughout the lifetime of such registrations, on-site inspections provide an intermittent review of several aspects related to manufacturing. The state of the facilities and equipment used is observed to ensure they are being maintained appropriately for the purpose of vaccine production. Competency of individuals involved at the different levels of biologics production is observed and appraised. Processes are evaluated and the use of internal controls is reviewed. Well-managed entities have checks and balances built into the methods of operation to minimize or expose errors. This should include a robust quality management system that has well-documented procedures for corrective actions, root cause analysis, risk assessments, and preventive actions.

When a deviation occurs, the first step is to document what happened and then start to determine why the deviation occurred (USDA 2018f). Impact to the product, both immediate and throughout product dating, must be considered prior to distribution of the vaccine. This type of risk assessment may also assist in finding the root cause. Tools, such as a Pareto Diagram and the 5-Why analysis, can be used in determining the root cause of specific issues. Corrective actions may be taken to fix the immediate deviation, but until the root cause is determined, the problem may reoccur. Once the root cause is determined, preventive actions may be implemented. It is important to monitor the effectiveness of the corrective and preventive actions in a meaningful and measurable way.

The on-site inspections include auditing of selected records related to the preparation of product and observations to substantiate the information on file with the regulatory authority. Another technique used during on-site inspections is perambulation. Perambulation is a special class of observations that allows an inspector to unobtrusively watch ongoing operations for a sufficient amount of time to observe unusual or uncharacteristic occurrences, especially regarding manufacturing techniques and procedures.

11.5.2 Record Keeping

Records must be made concurrent with the performance of each successive step in the development and preparation of a biological product (CFR 2020l). Record-keeping requirements apply not only to primary production processes, but also to all ingredients, materials, seeds and cells, supplies and equipment used in production, through post-preparatory steps of keeping accurate inventories, and storing and distributing production serials (USDA 2003a). The records must include such information as the date and time of critical steps, details regarding critical steps, identity and quantity of ingredients added or removed, and initials or signature of the person responsible for the action taken (CFR 2020l). Quality and consistency of the processes must be evaluated by quality control testing throughout the production process and on final product. However, final product testing is only one indicator of product quality (USDA 2016a). Critical steps within the production process should be validated and continuously reviewed to demonstrate that procedures, equipment, systems, and testing are consistent and produce the intended results (USDA 2018b). An ongoing quality assurance program that provides a review of all materials, supplies, equipment, procedures, facilities, and responsible personnel should be integral to all manufacturers.

11.5.3 Ingredients and Materials

Operations within the production facility must be well controlled at all phases in the manufacturing process, including at the supply chain level. Supplies and raw materials should be inspected to a quality standard that ensures all materials will meet the intended purpose and have a high level of traceability and supports consistent production of vaccines. Materials should be stored and handled properly at all times. Accurate inventory records should be maintained. Ingredients of animal origin must be identified as to country of origin to avoid the presence of contaminating or foreign animal disease agents (USDA 2018c). Additionally, animal origin ingredients that have not been subjected to heat sterilization or other acceptable sterilization methods must be tested for extraneous agents and assured to be free of extraneous bacteria, fungi, mycoplasma, and viruses (CFR 2020i,j). *Be aware, there are no acceptable methods of sterilization or heat inactivation to eliminate or neutralize prions that will not destroy the material being treated.* A risk assessment regarding the type of material used and the country of origin can reduce or eliminate issues related to prion contamination.

Use of a certificate of sterility for ingredients and materials that cannot be autoclaved is required and traceability should be ensured by lot, batch, or serial number from the provider. Additional documentation may be required to assure an appropriate level of control, including microbiological quality.

11.5.4 Equipment

The records of operation of major and essential specialized, controlled equipment are reviewed to determine if the equipment is identified, calibrated, maintained and functions properly, and that record keeping is in compliance. It is vitally important that the validation system for automatically controlled equipment is documented and that records are kept by the manufacturer to ensure that it is operating properly (USDA 2017b). Containers, instruments, and other apparatus and equipment which cannot be sterilized by traditional methods, such as steam or dry heat sterilization, must have an approved exemption for an alternative method for sterilization on file with the regulatory authorities (CFR 2020h). This exemption is usually listed as an addendum to the blueprint legend. This also applies to all single-use, disposable systems which are being used more in biologics manufacturing.

11.6 Quality Control and Assurance in the Production of Vaccines

Most countries have laws and regulations that outline appropriate and adequate standards to ensure uniform, consistent, and high-quality veterinary biological products are available to the consumer. The standards meet certain basic principles of performance outcomes and process control (Halkjær-Knudsen 2007; CFR 2020a).

Performance-based standards include the review of data generated by the manufacturer and submitted to the regulatory authority for evaluation prior to registration of a product. This evaluation includes complete characterization and identification of seed material and ingredients, laboratory and host animal safety and efficacy studies, and product stability and monitoring of field performance (CFR 2020i). Performance-based standards are also applied after a product is registered and/or licensed.

Process controls ensure veterinary biologics prepared are pure, safe, potent, and efficacious in accord with the standards defined by the regulatory authorities (CFR 2020i). Under such standards, data must be submitted for review prior to registration of a product or change in the manufacturing process of an already registered and/or licensed product prior to market release. The data, coupled with a standardized process for receipt, review, and feedback, provide consistent expectations independent of the individual manufacturers.

Sound quality control and assurance practices ensure that processes are evaluated and the use of internal controls is required. These processes should include a robust quality management system that has well-documented procedures for risk assessments, root cause analysis, corrective actions, and preventive actions. Unplanned variations in the manufacturing processes that occur prior to submission to the regulatory authority should be addressed by competent personnel of the manufacturer knowledgeable about the product's structure, performance, and life expectation and the manufacturing process. Postmarketing discovery that a product was not prepared in accordance with the manufacturing directives or the regulations necessitates that the manufacturer halt marketing of the product and provides notification to the regulatory authority of the market action to be taken (USDA 2018d; CFR 2020d,l). Analyzing the type of process deviation discovered and when the deviation occurred will allow the firm to determine if the level of impact is at an individual serial, a bulk of antigen used in several serials, or an entire product line. This will inform the decision regarding level and scope of recall, if appropriate.

Whether a deviation is discovered before or after a product has been released to the market, the regulatory authority expects manufacturers of veterinary biologics to perform a systematic or process-oriented approach to dealing with deviations from the manufacturing directive or the regulations. Any deviation must undergo the same detailed and documented product marketing risk evaluation. All incidents where manufacturing was not performed in accordance with the outline of production or regulations must undergo a root cause analysis along with corrective and preventive action. The investigation and final quality risk assessment must be documented and detailed so that an external source, such as the regulatory authority, can adequately evaluate the appropriateness and conclusion of the investigation.

Process control does not just include on-site inspections, it also allows for product inspection prior to the marketing of serial/batches prepared. The market release process requires data for each batch of product prepared (USDA 2016a; CFR 2020i,l). The data include the unique identification of the serial, the expiry date, the test summary and inventory prepared for market. It includes an attestation from the manufacturer that the process on file with the regulatory authority has been followed without deviations. This information is reviewed and a marketing determination is made, either by a qualified person within the manufacturing facility or by a competent regulatory authority.

Quality and consistency of processes can be evaluated by quality control testing throughout the production process and on final product. This final product testing is only one indicator of product quality. Other factors that contribute to product quality can be evaluated through a quality assurance program that provides a review of all procedures, equipment, personnel, and facilities.

Feedback from users of veterinary biologics provides valuable information used by manufacturers and regulatory authorities to ensure that the products they market perform safely and effectively in the field. Internationally harmonized guidelines have been established for such pharmacovigilance programs used for veterinary medicinal products, including veterinary biological products.

11.7 Commercial, Parastatal, and Governmental Vaccine Production Systems

In some cases, veterinary biological products may be prepared by or under the supervision of the local, state, or national regulatory authority (CFR 2020e). This is usually done in response to an official control or eradication program for a specific animal disease. It may also be used for emergency disease situations.

Another consideration for preparing vaccines at a local level are cost saving (per dose and delivery) and the commercial viability of a vaccine. If the disease is limited to a specific geographic area and/or to a specific animal species, there may not be any vaccines available (CFR 2020f). Autologous/autogenous vaccines can bridge this gap. Disease-causing organisms can be isolated from sick or dead animals in a herd (USDA 2016c). These isolates are tested for identity and purity and then used as seed material to prepare a vaccine. The antigen is grown, inactivated, and blended with an adjuvant. Purity and safety testing is conducted on the final product (CFR 2020i). A measurement for efficacy is also determined to ensure there is value in vaccinating with the autologous vaccine (USDA 2017a).

Regardless of why vaccines are prepared under local authority, the standards, as described in this chapter, do not change. Locally prepared vaccines would not be exempted from national laws that require purity, safety, and efficacy (USDA 2003b, 2006; CFR 2020m,n). The requirements applied to vaccines made under a national authority would apply to vaccines made at a local level. The facilities, equipment, personnel, ingredients, and processes are the pillars of good manufacturing methods, ensuring a pure, safe, and efficacious product.

Preparation of inactivated vaccines or bacterins under local jurisdiction reduces the risk of manufacturing a harmful or dangerous product. The inactivation process lowers the possibility of unintentionally introducing other disease-causing agents from the starting ingredients, such as the seed or cell material, serums, or egg substrates. Using prequalified and tested raw materials, especially ingredients of animal origin, in conjunction with a validated inactivation process, decreases the chances of preparing a contaminated or harmful product.

When preparing modified live or live vaccines at the local level, there are additional risks not seen with inactivated vaccines (USDA 2018e). Therefore, added controls must be in place. The most important control is backpassage studies in animals to provide assurance that the master seed material does not revert to virulence (International Cooperation on Harmonization of Technical Requirements of Veterinary Medicinal Products 2007). The route of vaccination, use of susceptible animals, and a validated virus recovery process are key when conducting a reversion to virulence study in target animal species. The data from these studies may also be used to understand if the modified live vaccine is shed and spread by vaccinated animals to unvaccinated animals. In some cases, this may be a useful tool but in other cases in which there is no testing available to determine if the animal is naturally infected or infected due to vaccination of cohorts, it may be problematic if the animals must move to another area and could possibly adversely impact trade with other countries.

The preparation of recombinant vaccines at the local level has similar issues to those noted above regarding modified live vaccines (USDA 2003b). The use of recombinant vaccines must be in compliance with national environmental laws. The level of risk when using a recombinant vaccine is related to the category of biological product. This can range from a biotechnology-derived and inactivated vaccine (USDA 2018h), which may be considered low risk, to a biotechnology-derived, live vector for a foreign gene insert, which may be considered a higher risk. Genetically modified organisms must go through an external biological risk assessment to determine impact to the environment regarding the use of the vaccine. This risk assessment may require additional, carefully controlled studies to be executed in determining the risk of inadvertent recombination, impact to the environment, and effect on nontarget animal species.

Local preparation of vaccines can facilitate interaction between the veterinarian making medical judgments regarding the affected herds and the manufacturing of the vaccine to be used. Rapid adjustments may be made to the vaccine formulation to better address the disease condition. Also, the cost and time required to transport locally made vaccines to the herds in need are decreased and may help in slowing the spread of the disease

Campaign production of vaccine involves the manufacturing of one agent, in a specific sequence for a finite period of time, which can mitigate cross-contamination issues when vaccine is prepared locally in a facility that may also be used for other purposes. Sanitation procedures between campaign productions are also important. Surfaces and equipment must be adequately disinfected and sterilized between each use to lessen the possibility of accidental contamination with a dangerous organism.

Local manufacturing of vaccines can be done within the parameters of fully controlled and validated processes, by competent employees, in an acceptable facility, with equipment in good working order and using qualified ingredients. Implementation of performance-based standards and process controls at the local level provides consistency in the manufacturing of vaccines. But in already high-stress, complicated situations, the lack of external oversight may lead to removing some of the process controls in order to speed up the manufacturing of products. This could lead to the manufacturing of worthless or dangerous vaccines.

External oversight based on accepted processes gives a layer of scientific review that can provide unbiased and valuable information, leading to manufacturing of a consistent product that works as intended (CFR 2020e,k).

11.8 Summary

The process for manufacturing veterinary vaccines is complex and requires a solid foundation of facilities, equipment, processes, and personnel for a successful outcome. It starts with designing a well-arranged facility, allowing the flow of material and people from clean areas to dirty areas to minimize the risk of cross-contamination. The construction materials used in production and testing rooms must be such that surfaces are easily cleaned and disinfected. Air-handling systems must provide an adequate supply of clean air to areas in which the product is exposed to the environment and filtering abilities to contain live organisms within a room or area, especially for zoonotic or highly infectious diseases. Pressure differentials between rooms and areas provide a barrier that assists in ensuring the integrity of the product.

Equipment must be in good working order and, when required, validated to ensure consistency in the production process. Changes in equipment may change the intended outcome of the vaccine. When equipment is upgraded, ensure the final product has not changed. This can be accomplished by in-process testing at critical control points.

The ingredients and materials used to manufacture a veterinary vaccine must meet a preset quality standard. This includes water, ingredients of animal origin, chemicals, and other components required. Once it is determined that the incoming raw materials and ingredients meet the quality standard, they must be stored and maintained in optimal conditions to ensure the reliability of the material.

Accurate and complete inventories allow traceability for these materials.

Concurrent record keeping of all steps in the production process, from receipt of incoming raw materials, to preparation of media and seed inoculation, through harvest and downstream processing to the final batching, filling, packaging and testing of product, documents that the qualified processes were followed and quality ingredients were used. An ongoing quality assurance program that provides a review of these documents is integral to process control and performance outcomes.

The most important requirement when preparing veterinary vaccines is well-trained and competent personnel. Employees need to understand the science underlying the many production and testing processes in order to solve problems when they occur. They must also recognize why regulations are in place and how they support the manufacturing of a pure, safe, potent, and efficacious product for use in animal health.

The information and processes reviewed above provide a regulatory framework and outline general quality requirements for registration/licensing of all manufacturing sites and veterinary biological products. These regulatory processes provide the oversight necessary to assure that only quality biologics are available for the consumer.

References

Code of Federal Regulations (CFR). (2020a). Title 9, Animals and animal products. Subchapter E – Viruses, serums, toxins and analogous products; organisms and vectors, parts 101–124. https://www.govinfo.gov/content/pkg/CFR-2020-title9-vol1/pdf/CFR-2020-title9-vol1-chapI-subchapE.pdf

Code of Federal Regulations (CFR). (2020b). Title 9, Animals and animal products, part 102. Licenses for biological products.

Code of Federal Regulations (CFR). (2020c). Title 9, Animals and animal products, part 104. Permits for biological products.

Code of Federal Regulations (CFR). (2020d). Title 9, Animals and animal products, part 105. Suspension, revocation, or termination of biological licenses or permits.

Code of Federal Regulations (CFR). (2020e). Title 9, Animals and animal products, part 106. Exemption for biological products used in department programs or under department control or supervision.

Code of Federal Regulations (CFR). (2020f). Title 9, Animals and animal products, part 107. Exemptions from preparation pursuant to an unsuspended and unrevoked license.

Code of Federal Regulations (CFR). (2020g). Title 9, Animals and animal products, part 108. Facility requirements for licensed establishments.

Code of Federal Regulations (CFR). (2020h). Title 9, Animals and animal products, part 109. Sterilization and pasteurization at licensed establishments.

Code of Federal Regulations (CFR). (2020i). Title 9, Animals and animal products, part 113. Standard requirements.

Code of Federal Regulations (CFR). (2020j). Title 9, Animals and animal products, part 114. Production requirements for biological products.

Code of Federal Regulations (CFR). (2020k). Title 9, Animals and animal products, part 115. Inspections.

Code of Federal regulations (CFR). (2020l). Title 9, Animals and animal products, part 116. Records and reports.

Code of Federal Regulations (CFR). (2020m). Title 9, Animals and animal products, part 121. Possession, use, and transfer of select agents and toxins.

Code of Federal Regulations (CFR). (2020n). Title 9, Animals and animal products, part 122. Organisms and vectors.

Halkjær-Knudsen, V. (2007). Designing a facility with both good manufacturing practice (GMP) and biosafety in mind. *Applied Biosafety* 12 (1): 7–16.

International Cooperation on Harmonisation of Technical Requirements of Veterinary Medicinal Products (VICH). (2007). VICH Guideline 41 (VICH GL41): Target Animal Safety: Examination of Live Veterinary Vaccines in Target Animals for Absence of Reversion to Virulence. www.ema.europa.eu/en/documents/scientific-guideline/vich-gl41-target-animal-safety-examination-live-veterinary-vaccines-target-animals-absence-reversion_en.pdf

International Society of Pharmaceutical Engineering. (2009). ISPE Good practice guide: heating, ventilation and air conditioning (HVAC). www.ispe.org

US Department of Health and Human Services (2007). *Biosafety in Microbiological and Biomedical Laboratories*, 5e. Washington D.C: US Government Printing Office. www.cdc.gov/biosafety/publications/bmbl5/bmbl.pdf

United States Code (USC). (1985, as amended). Title 21, chapter 5, parts 151–159. Viruses, Serums, Toxins, Antitoxins, and Analogous Products. www.aphis.usda.gov/aphis/ourfocus/animalhealth/veterinary-biologics/biologics-regulations-and-guidance/ct_regs_guidance

USDA. (2003a). VSM No. 800.108. Inventory and Disposition Records.

USDA. (2003b). VSM No. 800.205. General Licensing Considerations: Biotechnology-derived Veterinary Biologics Categories I, II, and III.

USDA. (2006). VSM No. 800.85. Avian Influenza Vaccines.

USDA. (2008). VSM No. 800.56. Disposal of Unsatisfactory and Undesirable Materials.

USDA. (2016a). VSM No. 800.53. Release of Biological Products.

USDA. (2016b). VSM No. 800.63. Personnel at Licensed Establishments.

USDA. (2016c). VSM No. 800.69. Guidelines for Autogenous Biologics.

USDA. (2016d). VSM No. 800.91. Categories of Inspection for Licensed Veterinary Biologics Establishments.

USDA. (2016e). VSM No. 800.101. U.S. Veterinary Biological Product Permits for Distribution and Sale.

USDA. (2017a). VSM No. 800.121. Autologous Therapeutic Biologics.

USDA. (2017b). VSM No. 800.122. Electronic Recordkeeping and Compliance with 9 CFR, Part 116.

USDA. (2018a). VSM No. 800.50. Basic License Requirements and Guidelines for Submission of Materials in Support of Licensure.

USDA. (2018b). VSM No. 800.206. General Licensing Considerations: Preparing Outlines of Production for Vaccines, Bacterins, Antigens, and Toxoids and Diagnostic Test Kits.

USDA. (2018c). VSM No. 800.51. Additives in Administered Animal Biological Products.

USDA. (2018d). VSM No. 800.57. Market Suspensions.

USDA. (2018e). VSM No. 800.201. General Licensing Considerations: Backpassage Studies.

USDA. (2018f). VSM No. 800.210. Manufacturing Deviations Identified Prior to Marketing Release.

USDA. (2018g). VSM No. 800.213. Licensing Guidelines for Production Platform-Based, Non-Replicating, Nonviable Products.

USDA. (2018h). VSM No. 800.214. Prescription Platform Product Biologics.

USDA. (2019). VSM No. 800.78. Preparation and Submission of Facilities Documents.

USDA. (2020). Veterinary Services Memoranda (VSM) 800.50 through 800.301. www.aphis.usda.gov/aphis/ourfocus/animalhealth/veterinary-biologics/biologics-regulations-and-guidance/ct_vb_vs_memos

12

The Manufacture of Veterinary Vaccines: Quality Control of the Manufacturing Process

Mehdi El Harrak, Imane Belkourati, Zineb Boumart, Fatima Fakri, and Jihane Hamdi

MCI Santé Animale, Mohammedia, Morocco

12.1 Introduction

Veterinary vaccines are crucial for animal health, animal welfare, food production, and public health. They are a safe, cost-effective, and efficient way to prevent animal disease, enhance the efficiency of food production, and reduce or prevent transmission of zoonotic and food-borne diseases to humans. Producing safe and effective animal vaccines is essential to ensure good public health (Roth 2011). All veterinary vaccines should be manufactured under controlled and monitored conditions. The quality of veterinary vaccines depends on the starting materials, manufacturing process, building/facilities, equipment, and involved staff. Therefore, during the manufacturing of veterinary vaccines, many controls are essential to ensure the production of a high-quality vaccine.

The control of veterinary vaccine production involves specific considerations arising from the nature of the starting materials and the process. Thus, many precautions are necessary during production.

Manufacturers should apply acceptable approaches in providing a good level of assurance that starting materials used to manufacture vaccine are procured from a reliable source and are of appropriate quality (FAO 1997). Moreover, starting material should be controlled to verify compliance with the required quality.

In-process control is vital to ensure the consistency of vaccine quality. Many controls must be performed at different steps of the production process to verify that all operations are following Good Manufacturing Practices (GMP) requirements and production specifications (WHO 2015).

In this chapter, an overview of batch tests utilized for the control of starting materials and production process of veterinary vaccines will be detailed (Figure 12.1).

12.2 General Principles

The majority of vaccine controls are biological tests. The reliability of the results depends on the correct execution of the tests by adequately trained staff, with correctly calibrated equipment, suitably adapted facilities, and validated control methods. Each element is detailed in the paragraphs below.

12.2.1 Facilities and Equipment

Equipment used during the handling of live organisms and cells, including that used for sampling, should be designed to prevent any contamination during the procedure. There should be a schedule for periodic testing of primary containment in order to ensure the prevention of introduction of any biological agents into the immediate working environment.

Regular qualification and calibration of the premises and equipment should be carried out to minimize the risk of errors and cross-contamination that may affect the quality of results. Effective cleaning and maintenance are needed to avoid cross-contamination, the build-up of dust or dirt and any other adverse effect on the quality of controls and on the health of the staff.

12.2.2 Staff

Laboratory staff must be experienced and thoroughly trained for the task. Training must be updated at regular intervals to insure maintenance of competence for carrying out specific tests.

The staff (including those concerned with cleaning and maintenance) should receive specific training concerning microbiological technique and hygiene in order to perform

Veterinary Vaccines: Principles and Applications, First Edition. Edited by Samia Metwally, Gerrit Viljoen, and Ahmed El Idrissi.

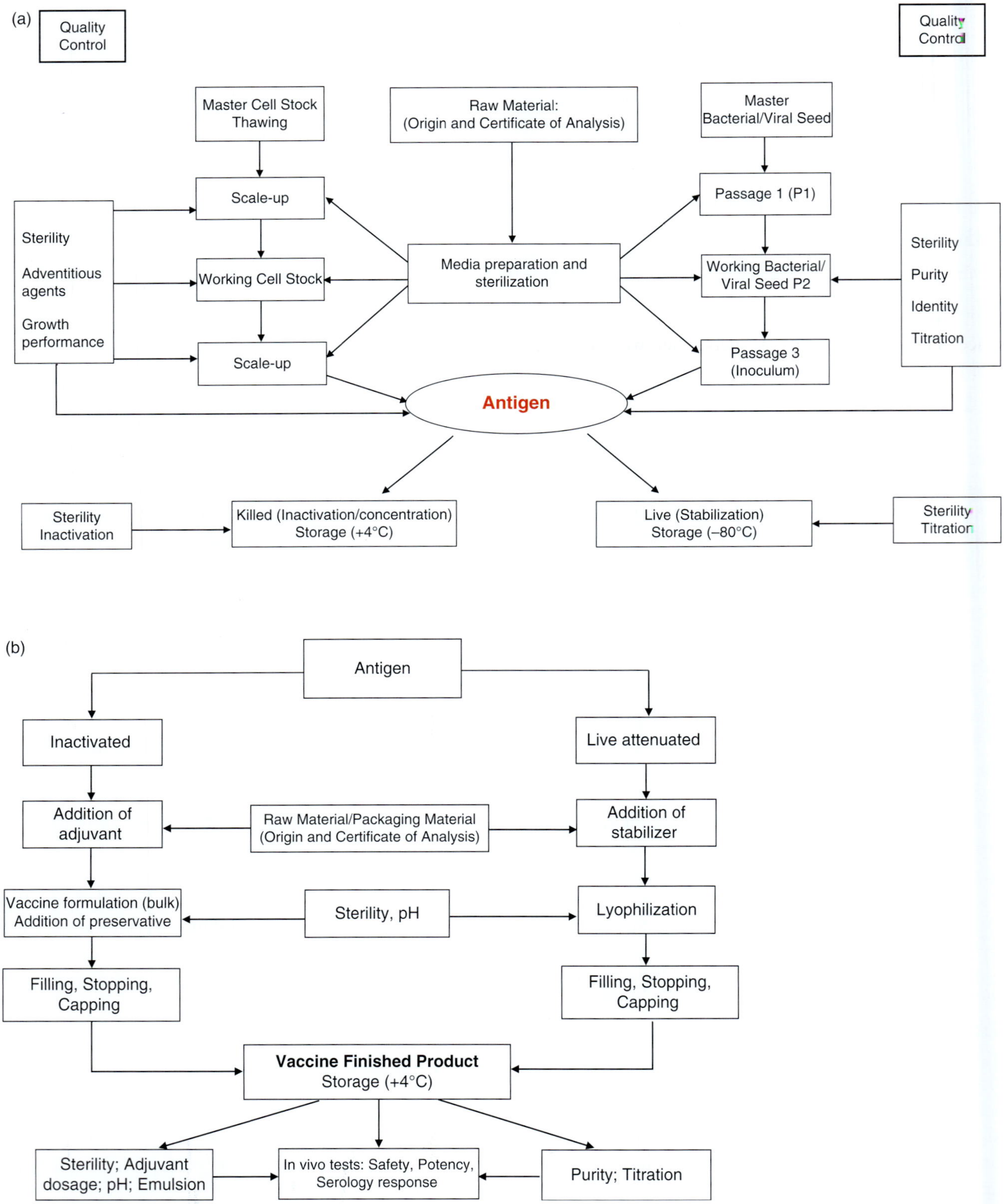

Figure 12.1 (a) Overview of quality controls required for the production of live or inactivated vaccine antigens. (b) Overview of quality controls required for the production and release of live or inactivated vaccines.

the assigned tasks. Persons responsible for production and quality control must have an adequate background in relevant scientific disciplines, such as bacteriology, biology, biometry, chemistry, medicine, pharmacy, pharmacology, virology, immunology, and veterinary medicine (Barakat 2012).

The training records and the efficacy of training should be verified in a documented manner for all staff.

The health status of personnel should also be taken into consideration for product safety. Where necessary, personnel engaged in testing and animal care (and inspections) should be vaccinated with appropriate specific vaccines and undergo regular health checks. Health monitoring of staff should be commensurate with the risk and medical advice should be sought for personnel working with hazardous organisms.

12.2.3 Documentation

The specifications for starting materials should include details of their sources, origin, manufacturing method and the control applied to ensure their suitability for use. All starting and raw material suppliers should be initially qualified based on documented criteria and a risk-based approach, including regular assessments of their status.

The health status of animals from which some starting materials are derived and of those used for quality control and safety testing should be monitored and recorded. The source of cells (laboratory or culture collection) from which the cell substrate derives has to be stated, and relevant references from the scientific literature cited. Information obtained directly from the source laboratory is preferred. When this is not available, literature references may be utilized (Barakat 2012).

Test samples must be received, recorded, handled, and stored according to standardized procedures to ensure that the quality of information gathered from them is accurate and truly representative (WHO 1997).

Control and test details of the starting materials and production process must be done according to appropriate Standard Operating Procedures (SOP) and recorded according to good laboratory practices to ensure traceability of results (WHO 2009).

A procedure should be in place to describe the measures to be taken where out of specification test results are obtained. Such events should be fully investigated and the relevant corrective and preventive actions taken to prevent recurrence documented.

12.2.4 Methods

Methods must be appropriate for their intended use and compatible with the nature of the samples to be tested. These methods must be available in a methods manual and written in the form of an SOP in a clear and unambiguous manner. Noncompendial methods will require validation to verify and confirm the suitability of the test for its intended purpose. The validation is defined as the collection and evaluation of data giving scientific evidence that the control is able to deliver good results meeting the required specifications.

12.3 Control of Starting and Raw Materials

12.3.1 Requirements

For biological medicinal products, "Starting materials shall mean any substance of biological origin such as microorganisms, organs, and tissues of either plant or animal origin, cells or fluids (including blood or plasma) of human or animal origin, and biotechnological cell constructs (cell substrates, whether they are recombinant or not, including primary cells)" (Directive 2001/83/EC 2001). Any other substances such as serum, culture media, reagents, and buffers used in manufacturing of the active substance, but from which this active substance is not directly derived, are defined as raw materials.

12.3.1.1 Sampling

As part of quality control testing, to ensure that testing carried out is representative of the process, the sampling procedure for biological materials must include special consideration of the nature of the materials sampled (WHO 2015).

Products that need to be sampled include starting materials, intermediate products, and final product. Utilities that have to be sampled include water systems, steam systems, and the compressed air system. Parts of premises that must be monitored are those where the product is in direct contact with the environment (surfaces, air).

For at least 1 year after the expiry date of the corresponding finished product, samples of active starting materials should be retained. Samples of other starting materials, as well as intermediates with critical parameters that cannot be tested in the finished product, should be retained for at least 2 years after the release of the product, if their stability allows this storage period (WHO 2015).

12.3.1.2 Reference Standard Materials

Laboratories carrying out analytical testing use reference standards to determine quantitative or qualitative data, performance standards, and calibrators. The quality and purity of reference standards are critical to obtain scientifically valid results.

12.3.1.3 Extraneous Microbial Contaminants

Starting materials and processing conditions used for culture can provide conditions for the growth of specific cells, microorganisms, and extraneous microbial contaminants. Another critical aspect of GMP, for biological products, is to prevent or reduce the risk of contamination by adventitious agents arising from starting materials, facility-derived microorganisms, and from contamination of product materials by operators.

To prevent such contamination events, the design of processes, equipment, facilities, utilities, sampling, and training of operators are key considerations (FDA 2010).

12.3.1.4 Recommendations

The source and origin of starting and raw materials must be clearly defined. All starting and raw material suppliers must be initially qualified, based on documented criteria with regular assessments of their status. Incoming starting and raw materials must be sampled under appropriate conditions and tested by pharmacopoeia or validated approved methods. When sterilization of starting and raw materials is required, heat treatment is recommended, but other appropriate validated methods can be used for this purpose (WHO 2015).

Biological and physicochemical testing should be conducted before and during the manufacturing process. The performed tests serve to verify that the controls on the production procedures have remained valid and that the marketed product meets the specifications agreed by the authorities.

12.3.1.4.1 Physicochemical Tests Depending on the nature of the material, controlled specific testing and methods to check the quality and stability of raw materials should be undertaken, for example to test the emulsion and viscosity for an oily adjuvant, or color evaluation. The pH of liquid products must be checked. Different parameters should be measured and shown to be within the limits set for the product. Concentrations of appropriate substances used in the preparation of the vaccine must also be checked, such as aluminum gel, phenol, and formaldehyde.

12.3.1.4.2 Biological Testing Biological tests allow detection of extraneous viruses, bacteria, mycoplasma, and viable fungi, using different tests and techniques depending on the nature of the biological product. Polymerase chain reaction (PCR), cell culture, inoculation of embryonated eggs or chickens, enzyme-linked immunosorbent assay, neutralization, hemadsorption, or indirect immunofluorescence may be used to demonstrate purity. The techniques used must be listed in the product monograph and other documentations related to the manufacturing process.

For *bacterial and fungal sterility*, the test is carried out by microscopic examination and inoculation of suitable media, in order to check the absence of live microorganisms other than the vaccine strain. In the case of avian live viral vaccines, for nonparenteral use, sterility testing is usually replaced by requirements for the absence of pathogenic microorganisms and for a maximum of nonpathogenic microorganisms per vaccine dose. Samples taken for sterility testing should be representative of the whole batch but should include samples taken from parts of the batch considered to be most at risk of contamination (WHO 2011).

For *mycoplasma detection*, the culture method should be performed to validate the detection limit of a laboratory's mycoplasma detection method, on a low level of the following five strains of mycoplasmas: *Acholeplasma laidlawii*, *Mycoplasma hyorhinis*, *M. orale*, *M. synoviae*, *M. fermentans* (VICH 2014). After validation, molecular biological methods can also be used. Several detection kits based on PCR or immuno-enzymatic tests are available to ensure the absence of mycoplasma.

12.3.2 Raw Material of Nonbiological Origin

The quality of the excipients used in the product formulation, as well as that of the container/closure systems and secondary packaging, should meet pharmacopoeia standards, where available and appropriate; otherwise, suitable acceptance criteria should be established.

12.3.2.1 Antibiotics

Antibiotics used during production are under the restriction of the European Pharmacopoeia Vaccines for Veterinary Use (2017e). The level of remaining antibiotic concentration in the finished product should be indicated in the dossier (EMA CVMP 2013).

12.3.2.2 Preservatives

The test procedures employed for demonstrating preservative efficacy should follow the European Pharmacopoeia Monograph 5.1.3. Efficacy of Antimicrobial Preservation (2017d). The microorganisms chosen for testing should reflect the potential risk.

Other methods should be validated by the applicant to "ensure that any residual antimicrobial activity of the product is eliminated by dilution, filtration, or by the use of a specific inactivator" in the recovery operation. For vaccine preservatives such as formaldehyde or merthiolate, it is important to determine the residual level of formaldehyde within inactivated vaccines to ensure product safety, and assure that the product will not inactivate other products used in combination, and that it remains active throughout its shelf-life (VICH 2002).

The maintenance of the quantity of preservative during the period of the immunological veterinary medicinal product shelf-life should be demonstrated (EMA CVMP 2013).

12.3.2.3 Diluents

Annex I of Directive 2001/82/EC, Title II, Part 1. A states that: "Information on diluents needed for making the final vaccine preparation shall be included in the dossier" (Directive 2001/82/EC 2001). The diluent should not contain any active substance (EMA CVMP 2013).

12.3.3 Starting and Raw Material of Biological Origin

The quality of the raw materials used in the production should meet standards appropriate for their intended use (Figure 12.1a). Biological raw materials or reagents may require careful evaluation to establish the presence or absence of endogenous or adventitious agents.

12.3.3.1 Active Ingredient

Quality control for bacterial seed is focused on the purity, gram stain, biochemical profile (active pharmaceutical ingredient [API] sticks, e.g. growth rates), morphology (shape/size, margin, elevation, color, and texture), identity by serological methods, e.g. by western blot, and control of the bacterial concentration.

Quality control for viral seed is based on propagation (conducted on cells, with biological materials used free from extraneous agents); the identity check is performed by a virus neutralization test, using a specific antiserum (for positive identification, a neutralization index must be at least 2). The identity test can also be performed using reverse transcriptase (RT)-PCR.

Also, the viral seed must be free from bacteria, fungi (European Pharmacopoeia 2017a), mycoplasma (European Pharmacopoeia 2017c) and extraneous viruses (European Pharmacopoeia 2017e) and must be screened for specific extraneous agents (on cells or by RT-PCR).

The viral seed must have a high titer, able to provide satisfactory production of the active ingredient. The titration must be validated according to the "Guideline on validation of analytical procedures: definition and terminology" (VICH 1998a) and "Validation of analytical procedures: methodology" (VICH 1998b). The vaccine virus is titrated by inoculation into embryonated chickens, specific pathogen-free (SPF) eggs or appropriate cell cultures. For live bacteria, the titer is determined by colony counting on suitable solid medium. The API complies with standards if it contains not less than the minimum acceptable number of virus particles or bacteria determined during development studies and indicated on the vaccine label.

12.3.3.2 Raw Material

Raw materials derived from animals should be free from adventitious agents of the species from which they are derived, including bacterial and fungal agents. Appropriate records must be kept for all biological raw materials used for vaccine production (CFR 2004).

Steps in the process used to remove or inactivate potential infectious contaminants from biological raw materials must be validated. The use of qualified raw materials can then reduce the risk of introducing adventitious agents. Inactivation of serum by specific treatment, such as irradiation or heat, could provide additional assurance regarding the purity of the finished product (FDA 2010).

12.3.3.2.1 Cell Lines Cell cultures used for the production of vaccines must comply with the requirement of the current pharmacopeia regarding bacterial, fungal, and mycoplasma sterility, and viral purity.

Viral contamination could come from the original source of the cell lines. An important part of qualifying a cell line for use in the production of a biotechnology product is appropriate testing for the presence of viruses. For a detailed description of cell banking, see the ICH guidance (ICH 1997).

Minimizing the risks of cell bank contamination is based on the use of cell lines (primary cells are used only if essential); their characterization and identification; and sterility (free from bacteria, fungi [European Pharmacopoeia 2017a], mycoplasma [European Pharmacopoeia 2017c] and extraneous viruses [European Pharmacopoeia 2017f]).

12.3.3.2.2 Serum The serum used in vaccine production or stabilization and culture medium has to be tested and certified. Bovine serum should be free of adventitious agents, including bacterial and fungal agents, mycoplasma, mycobacteria, and bovine viruses.

12.3.3.2.3 Minimizing Risk of Transmissible Spongiform Encephalopathy The risk of contamination of starting and raw materials during their passage must be evaluated, including for transmissible spongiform encephalopathy (TSE). Controlled origin/source is a very important criterion to evaluate the safety of the product, due to the resistance of TSE agents to most inactivation methods. The recommended source of materials must be from countries without any reported case of TSE. Producers have to keep the necessary documents to verify the source and as proof that they are free from the risk of TSE. Certificates of suitability for some animal-derived materials can be obtained from the European Directorate for the Quality of Medicines (EDQM). Users could use these certificates to support the safe use of their products (EMEA 2002).

12.3.3.2.4 Other Biological Reagents The species of origin for the trypsin used in vaccine production should be identified. The source of the amino acids used should also be documented. The producer has to evaluate the potential risk for introduction of adventitious agents via other biological reagents used during manufacturing such as insulin or other growth factors used in growth medium.

12.3.3.2.5 Recommended Viral Detection and Identification Assays For the detection of endogenous and adventitious viruses, different types of tests can be used. Assays should include appropriate controls for sensitivity and specificity. The likelihood of specific viruses being present can be predicted from the species of origin of the cell substrate, and specific tests and/or approaches may then be necessary. PCR can be used for detection of specific viruses (EMEA 1997).

- *In vitro assays*: *in vitro* tests are carried out by inoculation of a sample into various susceptible/permissive cell cultures to detect a wide range of viruses. The choice of cells used depends on the species origin of the sample to be tested. Screening should be performed for cytopathic and hemadsorbing viruses.
- *In vivo assays*: a sample should be inoculated into animals and embryonated eggs to identify viruses that cannot grow in cell cultures. Specific animal species may be used depending on the nature and source of the sample being tested.
- *Antibody production tests*: species-specific viruses present in rodent cell lines may be detected by inoculating samples into virus-free animals, and examining the serum antibody level after a specified period.

12.3.4 Sterilization

Products such as growth media or other components are terminally sterilized by heat; otherwise, an alternative method of terminal sterilization following filtration and/or aseptic processing can be used. Moreover, sterilization can be performed by the use of moist or dry heat, by irradiation with ionizing radiation, ethylene oxide (or other suitable gaseous sterilizing agents), or by filtration with aseptic filling of sterile containers. However, heat sterilization remains the method of choice. If possible, growth media should be sterilized, *in situ*, by heat and in-line sterilizing filters for routine addition to fermenters. The microbial contamination of starting materials should be minimal and their bioburden should be monitored before sterilization. It is not possible for some biological ingredients, such as live attenuated bacteria and viruses, to be terminally sterilized. In such circumstances, aseptic processing and purification procedures are required throughout the manufacturing process (WHO 2011, 2015).

12.4 Establishment of the Seed Lot Systems for Both Master and Working Seeds

For the proper use of a vaccine, developed by conventional or biotechnological methods, the manufacturer must evaluate efficacy and safety (FAO 1997). In addition, repeated subcultures or multiple generations can result in unwanted drift of properties (Barakat 2012; OIE 2018). That is why, whenever possible, production of vaccine should be based on a seed lot system (Directive 2001/82/EC 2001). A seed lot system provides a guarantee of continuous production, a safe and pure final product, and offers the advantage that safety and efficacy tests on each batch of vaccine can be limited (FAO 1997).

12.4.1 Definitions

For routine production, the manufacturing of biological products should be based on a system of master and working seed lots and cell banks (Directive 2001/82/EC 2001).

According to the European pharmacopoeia, a seed lot system is “a system according to which successive batches of a product are derived from the same master seed lot.” The master seed (MS) is a culture of a microorganism (it may be a bacterium, virus, or recombinant organism) used in the production of a vaccine. It serves as a source of seed for inoculation of all production cultures in such a manner to ensure vaccine consistency and stability and prevent contamination. On the other hand, the working seed (WS) is a culture of a microorganism derived from the master seed lot by subculturing and intended for use in production (European Pharmacopoeia 2017b).

Regarding cell cultures, a cell bank system is one in which the cells used in the final product are derived from the same master cell seed. It provides characterized cells for production over the expected lifetime of the product. The master cell seed is made first, usually derived from a single source, prepared under defined culture conditions. It is generally developed to generate sufficient quantity of cells to prepare the working cell seed which is intended to prepare the production cell cultures (EMEA 1997).

12.4.2 Requirements

The source of cells from which the cell substrate was derived should be stated. Primary cells should come from animals that are pathogen free or animals which had been quarantined and screened serologically for appropriate adventitious agents (FDA 2010). Embryonated chicken eggs used for the propagation of viral vaccines should be derived from certified SPF flocks (FDA 2010). It is important to provide documentation which describes the history of the cell substrate or microorganism used in the manufacture, in order to show that they are free of adventitious agents (WHO 2006).

Furthermore, cell banks should be stored at temperatures that ensure long-term stability (ultra-low temperature, freezer, or liquid nitrogen) (EMA 1998) after making sure that storage conditions are validated using cell recovery or viability data (FDA 2010). The master cell bank (MCB) and working cell bank (WCB) should be stored in two or more separate areas with controlled access, to avoid loss of cell substrate in case of equipment malfunction (Barakat 2012). The location, identity, and inventory of individual cell vials should be recorded and maintained (ICH 1997).

Seed lots and cell banks used for vaccine production should be stored separately from other materials, in containers hermetically sealed, labeled, and kept at an appropriate temperature. Access should be restricted to authorized persons and handling should be done under the supervision of the responsible person (Barakat 2012). Regarding temperature storage, virus master and working seed lots in liquid form should be stored at a minimum temperature of −70 °C. Freeze-dried seed lots are stored at temperatures known to ensure stability, in such a way as to minimize the risk of contamination or alteration (European Pharmacopoeia 2017b).

On the other hand, seed lots should be prepared using the same type of cells as those used for production of the final vaccine (WHO 2006) and the number of passages between the seed lot or cell bank and the finished product should be established in a way to not exceed a limited number of passages to maintain uniformity and consistency in production (OIE 2018). The number of passages should be consistent with the marketing authorization dossier (Barakat 2012).

For genetically modified microorganisms, the source of the genes and the vector microorganism should be identified and the gene sequences should be known and provided during construction of the modified seed (OIE 2018).

Finally, seed lots and cell banks should be adequately characterized and tested for contaminants as described in the following section (Barakat 2012).

12.4.3 Quality Control

12.4.3.1 Cell Bank

The choice of test for quality control of the cell bank should be based on assessment of risk that the cells could represent for the finished product. The working seed cell is derived from the master cell seed, which is well known and characterized, having been tested for adventitious agents to which it could have been exposed during passages from the MCB.

Master and working cell banks should be tested for freedom from bacteria, fungi, mycoplasma, and viruses (OIE 2018), and the karyotype of the master cell seed should be established (EMEA CVMP 2009). The characterization of the master cell seed should include checks for tumorigenic phenotype, expression of endogenous viruses, growth characteristics, and genetic stability of the cells (FDA 2010).

Regarding the reagents to which the MCB may be exposed, they should be tested for adventitious agents primarily when reagents are animal derived. If bovine-derived materials are used, the risk of TSE contamination should be addressed (FDA 2010), and freedom from oncogenicity or tumorogenicity should be demonstrated by *in vivo* studies in appropriate species, using the highest cell passage that may be used for production (OIE 2018).

12.4.3.2 Seed Lot

12.4.3.2.1 Virus Seed Lot Working virus and cell bank seeds can be subject to less rigorous characterization than the master virus seed. The level of characterization of a working virus seed should be based on the extent of characterization of the master virus seed from which it was derived.

Master virus seed should be characterized and tested free from bacteria, fungi, mycoplasma, and adventitious agents (FDA 2010). Furthermore, it should be shown that it contains only the virus stated (which could necessitate sequencing the entire vaccine strain) (EMA 1998). A risk assessment for TSE should also be carried out for the seed materials (WHO 2006). Finally, the stability of the genotype and phenotype should be demonstrated. Genotypic characterization of a viral seed includes determining its sequence and genetic stability (susceptibility to reversion) (FDA 2010). Phenotypic characterization of viral seed includes evaluation of tissue tropism, temperature sensitivity, and attenuation properties (WHO 2006).

12.4.3.2.2 Bacterial Seed Lot The bacterial seed lot should be subjected to identity and purity control. It must be shown to contain only the species and strain of bacterium stated (Anonymous 1992).

12.4.3.2.3 Recombinant DNA Technology When a seed lot is derived from recombinant DNA technology, mutations responsible for the attenuation should be identified along with mutations that can lead to reversion to partial or full virulence phenotype. The genetic stability of the strain derived by recombinant DNA technology should be confirmed at the passage level used to prepare the vaccine (or beyond) (WHO 2014).

12.5 In-Process Testing

12.5.1 Requirements

The use of raw materials (media, buffer, components) increases the potential for growth of microbiological contaminants. Depending on their origin, process of fabrication, and the use of the API or intermediate, it is necessary to control the bioburden, viral contamination, and/or endotoxin production during manufacturing and monitoring of the process at appropriate stages. Therefore, appropriate controls should be established at all stages of manufacturing to ensure intermediate and/or API quality (Figure 12.1a).

To minimize the risk of contamination, appropriate equipment and environmental controls must be used. The frequency of monitoring and the acceptance criteria for determining environmental quality depend on the production steps and conditions.

In general, in-process controls take into account: (i) the maintenance of the WCB (where appropriate), (ii) proper inoculation and expansion of the culture, (iii) control of the critical operating parameters during fermentation/cell culture, (iv) monitoring of the process for cell growth, (v) viability (for most cell culture processes) and productivity (where appropriate), (vi) harvest and purification procedures that remove cells, cellular debris, and media components with the protection of the intermediate or API from contamination and from loss of quality, (vii) monitoring of bioburden and, where needed, endotoxin levels at appropriate stages of production and also viral safety concerns as described in ICH guidance Q5A Quality of Biotechnological Products: Viral Safety Evaluation of Biotechnology Products Derived from Cell Lines of Human or Animal Origin.

Where appropriate, the removal of media components, host cell proteins, other process-related impurities, product-related impurities, and contaminants should be demonstrated (ICH Expert Working Group 2000).

In-process tests are performed to confirm consistency of the process during the production. The results of in-process testing may be recorded as action limits or reported as acceptance criteria. Data obtained during development and validation runs provide the basis for provisional action limits to be set for the manufacturing process (VICH 2005).

12.5.2 Cell Culture/Fermentation

Closed or contained systems are recommended when cell substrates, media, buffers, and gases are added under aseptic conditions. If inoculation, transfers, or additions are performed in open vessels, then it is mandatory to follow procedures and settle controls in order to minimize the risk of contamination.

Manipulations using open vessels are performed in a biosafety cabinet when the API is at risk of being affected by microbial contamination. Critical operating parameters (such as temperature, pH, etc.) are monitored to ensure consistency with the established process. Cell growth, viability, and productivity have to be monitored (ICH Expert Working Group 2000).

12.5.3 Testing for Viruses in Unprocessed Bulk

The unprocessed bulk constitutes harvests of cells and culture media. When cells are not easily accessible, the unprocessed bulk would constitute fluids harvested from the fermenter. Appropriate testing for viruses is performed at the unprocessed bulk level, unless virus testing is made more sensitive by initial partial processing.

The extent and frequency of virus testing are determined according to the nature of the cell lines used, the virus test results performed during qualification of the cell lines, the cultivation method and the sources of the raw materials. *In vitro* screening tests, using one or several cell lines, are generally employed to test unprocessed bulk. If appropriate, a PCR test or other suitable methods may be used (EMEA 1997).

12.5.4 Harvesting, Isolation, and Purification

Harvesting must be performed in equipment and areas designed to minimize the risk of contamination. Harvest and purification procedures should ensure that the intermediate or API is recovered with consistent quality. Additional controls may be appropriate if equipment is to be used for multiple products (ICH Expert Working Group 2000).

Before inactivation, different controls are carried out: identity, morphological, and culture characterization corresponding to those of the master seed (could be performed by RT-PCR), purity (identical to those performed on seed lots), and antigen concentration by titration.

12.5.5 Purity of Antigen Harvest for Inactivated Vaccines Produced in Eggs

For viruses grown in eggs, each harvested virus should be controlled for the amount of bacteria present. In general, the production process has to ensure that the bioburden is as low as possible. Reduction of the bioburden and validation of the inactivation procedure should also be considered for the bulk antigen prior to inactivation. The maximum bioburden level should be defined by the applicant and has to be controlled in each harvest or bulk as an in-process control (EMA CVMP 2013).

12.5.6 Sterility

Sterility is assured by validation of the sterilization cycle in the case of terminally sterilized products, and by "media simulation" or "media fill" runs for aseptically processed products. The results of the sterility tests should be examined along with batch-processing records and environmental quality records (in the case of aseptic processing). Pharmacopoeial methods should be used for validation and performance of the sterility test.

12.5.7 Inactivation

Viral inactivation is a critical step for some processes and has to be performed within validated parameters. Precautions must be taken to prevent potential viral contamination from pre- to postviral inactivation steps. Open processing must be done in separated areas with independent air handling units (ICH Expert Working Group 2000).

Annex I of the Directive 2001/82/EC, Part 2, D. Control tests during the manufacturing process (Directive 2001/82/EC 2001) states that: "For inactivated or detoxified vaccines, inactivation or detoxification shall be tested during each production run as soon as possible after the end of the inactivation or detoxification process and after neutralization if this occurs, but before the next step of production."

For products that are inactivated by the addition of a reagent, the process has to guarantee the complete inactivation of all live organisms. The inactivant agent must be mixed with culture to allow contact of all product-contact surfaces exposed to live culture and, if required, the transfer to a second vessel (EU Commission 2012).

Validation of the inactivation process is correlated to data showing complete inactivation of the vaccine microorganism. According to European Pharmacopoeia monograph 0062, Vaccines for veterinary use (2017e), data on inactivation kinetics should be obtained using the selected method of inactivation (EMA CVMP 2013).

After inactivation, the control must include sterility checking and total inactivation testing with the antigen concentration determination when possible (titration).

A test for complete inactivation and/or detoxification is performed immediately after the inactivation and/or detoxification procedure and, if applicable, the neutralization or removal of the inactivating or detoxifying agent. The inactivation and/or detoxification test is carried out during preparation of the final bulk, after combination of different batches of antigens but before addition of auxiliary substances that could interfere with the test. For bacterial vaccines, testing consists of at least two passages in a suitable solid or liquid medium and control of abnormal toxicity in animals. For viral vaccines, testing consists of at least two passages in cells, embryonated eggs, or in animals. The vaccine complies with the test if no evidence of any live microorganism is detected (European Pharmacopoeia 2017e).

12.5.8 Stability

Stability studies have to include testing of the vaccine components that are susceptible to change during storage and are likely to influence quality, safety, and/or efficacy. The testing should cover physical, chemical, biological, and microbiological parameters (VICH 2007).

Primary stability studies should demonstrate that the active substance will remain within specification during the retest period, if stored under recommended storage conditions in the proposed bulk storage container. The retest period is based on the results of long-term stability studies performed by the active ingredient manufacturer or the applicant. Testing under defined conditions will normally be every 3 months over the first year, every 6 months over the second year and then annually (EMEA CVMP 2008).

12.5.8.1 Bulk Material

If bulk material needs to be stored before formulation, stability data should be obtained on at least three batches representative of the scale of production used in manufacture. The overall quality of the batches undergoing formal stability studies should be representative of the quality of the material used in preclinical and clinical studies and of the quality of the material to be made at manufacturing scale (VICH 2000).

12.5.8.2 Intermediates

During manufacture of biotechnological/biological products, the quality and control of certain intermediates may be critical to the final product quality. In general, the manufacturer identifies intermediates and generates in-house data and process limits that assure their stability within the bounds of the developed process (VICH 2000).

12.5.9 Storage Conditions

12.5.9.1 Warehousing

Facilities should be available for the storage of all materials under appropriate conditions such as controlled temperature and humidity. Records must be maintained of these conditions if they are critical for the maintenance of material characteristics (ICH Expert Working Group 2000). Storage containers should be hermetically sealed, clearly labeled, and kept at an appropriate temperature (Barakat 2012).

12.5.9.2 Temperature

Because biotechnological/biological products need precisely defined storage temperatures, the storage conditions for real-time/real-temperature stability studies may be confined to the proposed storage temperature (VICH 2000). Storage temperature must be recorded continuously for freezers and properly monitored for liquid nitrogen (Barakat 2012). Sample temperature-controlled storage could be ultra low-temperature storage (−70 and − 80 °C), cold storage (−20 and 5 °C), or controlled room temperature (15–27 °C).

Most active viral ingredients, in liquid form, are kept at −80 °C for long-term storage; some of them, like bluetongue virus, do not survive well at this low temperature and should be stored for as short a period as possible at +4 °C. After conducting stability studies on particularly sensitive active ingredients, manufacturers may prefer to avoid storage of active ingredients and recommend a continuous production process.

12.5.9.3 Humidity

Biotechnological/biological products are generally distributed in containers protecting them against humidity. Therefore, where it can be demonstrated that the proposed containers (and conditions of storage) afford sufficient protection against high and low humidity, stability tests at different relative humidity rates can be omitted. Where humidity-protecting containers are not used, appropriate stability data should be provided (VICH 2000).

12.5.9.4 Light

Applicants have to consult the appropriate regulatory authorities on a case-by-case basis to determine guidance for testing (VICH 2000).

12.6 Internal and External Proficiency Testing

12.6.1 Proficiency Tests

Proficiency tests (PTs) are an important way of meeting the requirement of ISO/IEC 17025 in quality assurance of laboratory results and allow the laboratory to demonstrate its ability to confirm performance and verify the accuracy and reliability of its testing. It also reveals problems in training programs and problems with SOPs, methods, and equipment (ISO 2010, 2017).

12.6.2 External and Internal Proficiency Test

Each laboratory performing nonwaived testing (testing of moderate or high complexity) must participate in an external proficiency test (PT) scheme. The samples for this testing are obtained from a provider outside the laboratory's quality assurance system and the results are reported back to and analyzed by the external provider. The system ensures that different analysts can report the same result for the same test on the same sample and reproduce the same results as obtained by similar laboratories.

External PT or sample exchanges are not always available or feasible. In such cases, the laboratory must implement an internal PT program, reported within the laboratory's quality assurance system, for at least one method, at least twice a year. The internal PT allows assessment of the laboratory's analytical and postanalytical phases of the testing service. It serves to evaluate the ability of the technical staff to process samples, perform testing, and report results.

All PTs have to be performed using routine testing methods. Samples must be tested by the analyst who routinely performs the technique (ISO 2005; SWGANTH 2012).

12.6.3 Results and Corrective Actions

The PT is considered valid when either the defined results are obtained by the analyst or after completing corrective actions in accordance with laboratory policy. Acceptable results are defined as at least 80% correct test performance or better on each attempt, in two consecutive testing events, or two out of three consecutive testing events. If the PT score is less than 80%, the possible reasons for error must be determined by reviewing the procedure and quality control guidelines and discussing the test results with the analyst. Retraining of technical staff could also be considered. The corrective action reports have to be documented and filed with the PT report.

Completion of testing and reporting of results must be performed within the time frame specified in the instructions enclosed with the PT (ISO 2017).

12.6.4 Test Materials and Documents

The documentation related to the PT program should include: (i) the test identification number, (ii) the identity of the individual administering the test and the analyst performing the test, (iii) the date of analysis and completion, (iv) any discrepancies noted, (v) test results, and (vi) when necessary, details of corrective actions. All equipment used must be in good condition and all reagents in date and of the same type as used for routine testing (ISO 2005; IFM 2012).

12.7 Summary

Veterinary vaccine manufacturing is a complex process, performed in a protected environment and following general rules of GMP. In addition, very often, dealing with pathogens requires high containment facilities to protect the product and employees and to prevent release into the environment.

Vaccine quality has always relied on three components: the starting materials, the production process, and the final product testing, all managed under a quality assurance system. Several tests are carried out to demonstrate the quality of the starting materials that should comply with pharmacopoeia requirements. Raw materials can be of biological or nonbiological origin and testing is required for purity and performance.

During the manufacturing process, sampling at the critical steps of antigen production, downstream process, and product formulation is of high importance to guarantee final vaccine quality.

This chapter provides an overview of the starting material and in-process controls with special attention to some requirements that ensure the purity, safety, and efficacy of veterinary vaccines.

References

Anonymous. (1992). General requirements for the production and control of inactivated mammalian bacterial and viral vaccines. https://fdokumen.com/document/7blm2aen.html

Barakat, N.S. (2012). Biological products: manufacturing, handling, packaging and storage. In: *Promising Pharmaceuticals* (ed. D.P. Basnet). InTech. www.intechopen.com/books/promising-pharmaceuticals/biological-products-manufacturing-handling-packaging-and-storage

CFR. (2004). General Biological Products Standards: Cultures. 21 CFR 610.18, US Regulatory Information, Chapter I, Part 610 Subpart B General Provisions. www.gpo.gov/fdsys/pkg/CFR-2004-title21-vol7/pdf/CFR-2004-title21-vol7-part610.pdf

Directive 2001/82/EC. (2001). Directive on the Community code relating to veterinary medicinal products. *Off. J. Eur. Communities* 1–60. https://ec.europa.eu/health/sites/health/files/files/eudralex/vol-5/dir_2001_82_cons2009/dir_2001_82_cons2009_en.pdf

Directive 2001/83/EC. (2001). Directive on the Community code relating to medicinal products for human use 1–173. http://academy.gmp-compliance.org/guidemgr/files/DIR_2001_83_CONS_2012_EN.PDF

EMEA. (1997). Note for guidance on quality of biotechnological products: viral safety evaluation of biotechnology products derived from cell lines of human or animal origin. ICH Top. Q 5 A 1–29. https://www.ema.europa.eu/documents/scientific-guideline/ich-q-5-r1-viral-safety-evaluation-biotechnology-products-derived-cell-lines-human-animal-origin_en.pdf (Accessed October 2018)

EMA. (1998). ICH Topic Q 5 D Quality of Biotechnological Products: Derivation and Characterisation of Cell Substrates Used for Production of Biotechnological/Biological Products. www.ema.europa.eu/documents/scientific-guideline/ich-q-5-d-derivation-characterisation-cell-substrates-used-production-biotechnological/biological-products-step-5_en.pdf

EMEA. (2002). Note for guidance on minimising the risk of transmitting animal spongiform encephalopathies via human and veterinary medicinal products 0–17. https://eur-lex.europa.eu/LexUriServ/LexUriServ.do?uri=OJ:C:2011:073:0001:0018:EN:PDF

EMEA CVMP. (2008). Guideline on stability testing: stability testing of existing active substances and related finished products. EMEA/CVMP/846/99-Rev.1 6, 140586. www.ema.europa.eu/documents/scientific-guideline/guideline-stability-testing-stability-testing-existing-active-substances-related-finished-products_en-0.pdf

EMEA CVMP. (2009). Guideline on data requirements for the replacement of established Master Seed (MS) already used in authorised Immunological Veterinary Medicinal Products (IVMPs) by new master seed of the same origin draft. www.ema.europa.eu/documents/scientific-guideline/guideline-data-requirements-replacement-established-master-seeds-ms-already-used-authorised_en.pdf

EMEA CVMP. (2013). Guideline on requirements for the production and control of immunological veterinary medicinal products. EMA/CVMP/IWP/206555/2010 44. Available at: www.ema.europa.eu/documents/scientific-guideline/guideline-requirements-production-control-immunological-veterinary-medicinal-products_en-0.pdf

EU Commission. (2012). EU Guidelines for Good Manufacturing Practice for Medicinal Products for Human and Veterinary Use Annex 2 Manufacture of Biological Active Substances and Medicinal Products for Human Use. https://ec.europa.eu/health/sites/health/files/files/eudralex/vol-4/vol4-an2__2012-06_en.pdf

European Pharmacopoeia. (2017a). 9 Ed. Sterility (2.6.1.), Biological Tests (2.6.). *European Pharmacopoeia* 04/2011: 20601.

European Pharmacopoeia. (2017b). 9 Ed. General Texts on Biological Products. *European Pharmacopoeia* 01/2008:50201.

European Pharmacopoeia. (2017c). 9 Ed. Mycoplasma (2.6.7), Biological Tests (2.6.). *European Pharmacopoeia* 01/2008: 20607 corrected 6.1.

European Pharmacopoeia. (2017d). 9 Ed. Efficacy of Antimicrobial Preservation (5.1.3). *European Pharmacopoeia* 01/2011: 50103.

European Pharmacopoeia. (2017e). 9 Ed. Vaccines for Veterinary Use. *European Pharmacopoeia* 01/2017: 0062.

European Pharmacopoeia. (2017f). 9 Ed. Cell Cultures for the Production of Veterinary Vaccines. *European Pharmacopoeia* 01/2016: 50204.

FAO. (1997). Vaccine Manual. The production and quality control of veterinary vaccines for use in developing countries. FAO Animal Production and Health Series No.35. www.fao.org/docrep/015/an381e/an381e00.pdf

FDA. (2010). Guidance for Industry. Characterization and Qualification of Cell Substrates and Other Biological Materials Used in the Production of Viral Vaccines for Infectious Disease Indications. www.fda.gov/downloads/biologicsbloodvaccines/guidancecomplianceregulatory information/guidances/vaccines/ucm202439.pdf

ICH. (1997). International Conference on Harmonisation of Technical Requirements for Registration of Pharmaceuticals for Human Use (ICH). Quality of Biotechnological Products Q5D: Derivation and Characterization of Cell Substrates Used for Production of Biotechnological/Biological Products. http://academy.gmp-compliance.org/guidemgr/files/3-1-15.PDF

ICH Expert Working Group. (2000). Good Manufacturing Practice Guide for Active Pharmaceutical Ingredients Q7. ICH Harmonised Tripartite Guideline. https://database.ich.org/sites/default/files/Q7_Guideline.pdf

IFM. (2012). What is proficiency testing? www.ifmqs.com.au/what_is_PT.htm

ISO. (2005). ISO International Standards 9000:2005, 9001:2000; 9004:2000. Quality management and quality assurance.

ISO. (2010). ISO/IEC 17043:2010 Conformity assessment – general requirements for proficiency testing.

ISO. (2017). ISO/IEC 17025 General requirements for the competence of testing and calibration laboratories.

OIE (2018). Vaccine recommendations. Minimum requirements for the production and quality control of vaccines. In: *Manual of Diagnostic Tests and Vaccines for Terrestrial Animals*. www.oie.int/en/international-standard-setting/terrestrial-manual/access-online/

Roth, J.A. (2011). Veterinary vaccines and their importance to animal health and public health. *Procedia Vaccinol* 5: 127–136.

SWGANTH. (2012). Proficiency testing. www.nist.gov/system/files/documents/2018/03/13/swganth_proficiency_testing.pdf

VICH. (1998a). International Cooperation on Harmonisation of Technical Requirements for Registration of Veterinary Medicinal Products (VICH). Validation of Analytical Procedures: Definition and Terminology. VICH GL1. www.ema.europa.eu/documents/scientific-guideline/vich-gl1-validation-analytical-procedures-definition-terminology-step-7-consensus-guideline_en.pdf

VICH. (1998b). Validation of Analytical Procedures: Methodology. VICH GL2. www.ema.europa.eu/documents/scientific-guideline/vich-gl2-validation-analytical-procedures-methodology-step-7-consensus-guideline_en.pdf

VICH. (2000). Veterinary Medicinal Products Stability Testing of Biotechnological/Biological Veterinary Medicinal Products. VICH GL17 17 d. www.ema.europa.eu/documents/scientific-guideline/vich-gl17-stability-testing-biotechnological/biological-veterinary-medicinal-products-step-7_en.pdf

VICH. (2002). Testing of Residual Formaldehyde. VICH GL25 25. www.ema.europa.eu/en/vich-gl25-biologicals-testing-residual-formaldehyde

VICH. (2005). Specifications: Test Procedures/Acceptance Criteria for New Biotechnological/Biological Veterinary Medicinal Products. VICH Harmonized Tripartite Guideline GL40. www.fda.gov/downloads/AnimalVeterinary/GuidanceComplianceEnforcement/GuidanceforIndustry/ucm052475.pdf

VICH. (2007). Stability Testing of New Veterinary Drug Substances and Medicinal Products (Revision). VICH GL3 3, 21. www.fda.gov/downloads/AnimalVeterinary/GuidanceComplianceEnforcement/GuidanceforIndustry/ucm052387.pdf

VICH. (2014). Testing for the Detection of Mycoplasma Contamination. VICH GL34 34. www.ema.europa.eu/documents/scientific-guideline/international-cooperation-harmonisation-technical-requirements-registration-veterinary-medicinal_en.pdf

WHO. (1997). Vaccine Supply and Quality Unit. Manual of laboratory methods for testing of vaccines used in the WHO Expanded Programme on Immunization. www.who.int/iris/handle/10665/63576

WHO. (2006). Annex 1 Guidelines for the production and quality control of candidate tetravalent dengue virus vaccines (live). WHO Technical Report Series No. 932. www.who.int/biologicals/publications/trs/areas/vaccines/dengue/TRS932Annex%201_Dengue%20virus%20vacc%20live.pdf

WHO. (2009). WHO GLP Quality practices for regulated non-clinical research and development. www.who.int/tdr/publications/documents/glp-handbook.pdf

WHO. (2011). WHO good manufacturing practices for sterile pharmaceutical products. WHO Technical Report Series No. 961. www.who.int/medicines/areas/quality_safety/quality_assurance/GMPSterilePharmaceuticalProductsTRS961Annex6.pdf

WHO. (2014). Recommendations to assure the quality, safety and efficacy of poliomyelitis vaccine (inactivated). www.who.int/biologicals/IPV_FINAL_for_BS2233_07072014(2).pdf

WHO. (2015). WHO GMP for Biological Products. www.who.int/biologicals/BS2253_GMP_For_Biologicals_clean.pdf

13

The Manufacture of Veterinary Vaccines: Control of Final Product

Carol Gibbs, Patricia Foley, Monica Reising, Amy Gill, David Siev, and Melisse Schilling

Policy, Evaluation, and Licensing, Center for Veterinary Biologics, USDA APHIS, Ames, Iowa, USA

13.1 Introduction

In the standard licensing process, the full spectrum of evaluation and review of a veterinary vaccine includes: (i) the identification, characterization, and demonstration of the purity of seed materials, product ingredients, and purity of the final product; (ii) determination of environmental, human, and animal safety; (iii) vaccine efficacy, potency, and stability; and (iv) monitoring of field performance both before and after licensure (Hill et al. 2013). In addition to the seed materials and ingredients used in the manufacture of a vaccine, the manufacturing process should be standardized, using an acceptable facility, validated equipment, and well-trained personnel. Ideally, these processes are well established and well controlled, resulting in a consistent product that is pure, safe, and potent. While in-process testing can provide assurance that critical steps in the manufacturing process have been conducted properly, quality control testing of final product is an essential step of the process because this provides the final assurance that the standards in place throughout the manufacturing process met the intended production outcome.

Most countries have laws and regulations that outline appropriate and adequate standard tests to ensure uniform, quality veterinary biological products are available to the consumer (e.g. US Code of Federal Regulations, European Pharmacopoeia, etc.). These standards ensure that the product meets certain basic principles of performance outcome and process control. Because the manufacture of veterinary vaccines involves complex biological procedures, the propagation and harvesting of biological materials (viruses, bacteria, and parasites), even in well-controlled situations, often has an inherent variability. Downstream processing of antigens, blending, filling, and lyophilization or freezing add complexity to an already intricate system, contributing to the variability of the product.

Although agencies and regulations differ, all strive to ensure that products offered to the end-user conform to basic standards. Some regulatory agencies rely on Good Manufacturing Practice (GMP), which includes specifications of materials and validated production methods; in the USA, acceptable manufacturing processes are detailed in the Outline of Production. An approved Outline, along with facilities inspections and confirmatory testing of the final product, serve the same purpose as GMP. Under either approach, a commercial batch of vaccine must undergo testing for purity, safety, and potency before the manufacturer may release it for marketing. A robust batch release process provides transparency and oversight to ensure that each batch of vaccine is pure, safe, and potent.

Sample selection and maintenance is an important facet of final product testing. Samples should be selected in such a way as to be representative of the entire production process. To ensure authenticity of the samples that will be used for testing, for retention samples, and for the samples that will be submitted to regulatory authorities or authorized laboratories for testing, a documented chain of custody and suitable storage and shipping conditions are essential. Well-managed testing laboratories require complete accountability of samples and processes, from receipt of the test sample through reporting the test results.

To ensure accurate results, the testing facilities should be appropriately maintained, standard protocols should be followed, and the personnel conducting the tests should be trained in the specific test. The test documentation should capture all steps in the assay as well as the specific reagents and equipment used. Test protocols, reviewed by the regulatory authority as part of the assay validation process, are specific instructions describing how the product is tested;

Veterinary Vaccines: Principles and Applications, First Edition. Edited by Samia Metwally, Gerrit Viljoen, and Ahmed El Idrissi.

the protocol ensures that products are tested consistently and that the test results are reliable. The protocols should be detailed and accurately reflect all critical steps in the testing process. Equipment should be validated and in good working order to ensure precise and reliable test results are obtained. Changes in the testing process should not be made without submitting data supporting the change to the appropriate regulatory authority for review.

Test records must be made concurrently with the steps performed in testing. The records must include critical information such as the date and time of each test step, identity of the sample and reagents used (including animal identifications, if applicable), equipment used, results, and initials or signature of the person responsible for the action taken.

Many regulatory authorities implement a product inspection process for vaccines prior to allowing individual batches to be marketed or used in animals. This can be carried out by a Qualified Person or can be a process implemented by the regulatory authorities. A Qualified Person is an employee of the manufacturer who is registered with the regulatory authority and is responsible for assuring the product was manufactured within GMP. In cases where regulatory oversight is provided by a competent regulatory authority, the manufacturer or testing laboratory provides a summary of the testing conducted on each batch of a final product and samples of that batch to the regulatory agency. The agency reviews the test results and has an opportunity to test the product for purity, safety, or potency prior to granting market release of the individual batch.

Implementation of controlled procedures and performance-based processes provides the assurance that pure, safe, and potent vaccines are released to the marketplace. Examples of test procedures and processes are provided below.

13.2 Control Tests on the Finished Product

13.2.1 Identity

Identity testing is necessary to ensure that the harvested microorganism is a pure culture, with no introduction of contamination. In addition, where possible, tests should be done to confirm that the culture consists of the correct strain, serotype, or serovar. Testing can be conducted at the time of harvest and/or during downstream processing as well as on final product. The test used would depend on the organism; typical tests would be immunofluorescence, reaction with specific monoclonal antibodies, polymerase chain reaction (PCR), or bacterial colonial morphology and biochemical tests. For recombinant vectored vaccines, the identity of both the vector and the insert should be confirmed. In the case of subunit vaccines, the identity of the subunit must be confirmed; in the case of nucleic acid vaccines, the RNA or DNA sequence must be confirmed.

13.2.2 Chemical or Physical Tests

General chemical tests that may be conducted on the final product include: (i) determination of the pH; (ii) residual moisture content and vacuum (lyophilized products); and (iii) determination of the residual free formaldehyde content (products in which formaldehyde was used to inactivate the microorganism). Other tests that are frequently used include optical density and visual examination of the color, clarity, and emulsion (emulsified products) or cake (lyophilized products). For a nucleic acid vaccine, an evaluation of the quality of the nucleic acid (presence of genomic DNA and/or RNA, plasmid supercoiling, etc.) is often required.

13.2.3 Sterility

Vaccines are routinely tested for the presence of contaminating bacteria, fungi, and mycoplasma; the test procedures are usually culture methods or nucleic acid detection by PCR. The procedures are specified by the regulatory agency and must be followed precisely. The culture media should not support the growth of common contaminants; in cases where antibiotics or other inhibitors of microbial growth are used in a product, the culture volumes must be sufficient to dilute the inhibitor. For nucleic acid detection of mycoplasm by PCR, the primers must be able to detect a broad range of mycoplasma species and related organisms. While in-process testing for these contaminants is encouraged, contaminants can be introduced at any step in the manufacturing process, so testing of final product for these contaminants is essential.

13.2.4 Extraneous Agents

Tests for the presence of extraneous agents are essential for assessing the purity of the final product. The specific tests required for a given product are determined by the regulatory authority and are generally based on a risk assessment for the specific product, which takes into account the host species used to propagate the microorganism, the source of the ingredients of animal origin used in the manufacture, and the species in which the vaccine will be used. For imported vaccines, tests for the presence of agents causing foreign animal diseases may be required as well.

Products in which the microorganism is propagated in an approved, established cell line, thoroughly tested for species-specific extraneous agents, may not require additional testing of the final product provided the risk of extraneous agents being introduced into the cell line during propagation is negligible. Likewise, products manufactured using ingredients of animal origin that have been tested for extraneous agents may not require additional testing of final product.

Products in which the microorganism is propagated in embryonated eggs, in primary chicken embryo cells, or in live birds must be tested for extraneous avian pathogens, including testing for the presence of *Salmonella*, avian lymphoid leukosis virus, and hemagglutinating viruses. Some regulatory agencies require a general test for avian pathogens to be conducted by inoculation of the vaccine in embryonated eggs or in chickens. In some circumstances, additional tests may be required; an example is a test for extraneous chicken anemia virus or reticuloendotheliosis virus.

The suitability of tests for extraneous agents needs to be constantly monitored by the regulatory authorities. As new and emerging diseases appear (for example, transmissible spongiform encephalitis or senecavirus), existing tests should be evaluated to determine whether the procedures will detect those agents or whether new tests must be developed. Likewise, the emergence of new serovars or serotypes that are not detected by existing procedures is of concern.

Many of the tests for extraneous agents are general, able to detect a variety of agents, while others are used to detect specific agents. Examples of general tests include inoculation of the product on cell lines and evaluation of the development of cytopathic effects, or inoculation of the product into embryonated chicken eggs and subsequent evaluation of lesions on the chorioallantoic membrane, internal organs, and embryo death. Examples of specific tests include immunofluorescence assays for defined agents or a test for the detection of avian lymphoid leukosis. Microarray assays and sequencing may be used in some instances to identify contaminants.

13.2.5 Inactivation

During the licensure process for inactivated vaccines, defined inactivation procedures are developed and the method is shown to be effective for inactivating the microorganism. The inactivation process is typically evaluated in a kinetics study in which the presence and/or titer of the microorganism is measured during exposure to the inactivating agent. This study is limited by the ability to detect very low concentrations of the microorganism, and typically requires a direct titer at early time points with concentration of the material at later time points when low titers of the viable microorganism are present. This type of sensitive two-stage test capable of detection of the live agent at very low concentrations is performed on each vaccine lot to confirm that the inactivation was satisfactory; testing can be performed on bulk antigen or on the final product.

In the case of inactivated rabies vaccines, a residual live virus test is required to confirm the completeness of inactivation. The World Organization for Animal Health (OIE) guidelines include the use of an *in vitro* cell culture test, as well as the *in vivo* mouse test (OIE 2013).

13.2.6 Residual Toxicity

Although controlled manufacturing processes minimize toxicity of veterinary vaccines, residual toxicity testing is important for some veterinary vaccines.

In-process testing for clostridial vaccines relies on a variety of analytical techniques and animal tests for measuring the toxicity of the toxin, and the residual toxicity of the toxoid (de Mattia et al. 2015). In-process animal tests typically use mice as indicators of toxicity for clostridial toxoids, but validated cell line-based assays may be used. A validated enzyme-linked immunosorbent assay (ELISA) to measure toxin neutralization for *Clostridium chauvoei* is available (USDA 2015a). Toxin neutralization tests using cell cultures are available for potency testing of *Clostridium perfringens* types C and D, *C. septicum*, and *C. novyi*.

Endotoxin (lipopolysaccharide) is a component of the cell walls of gram-negative bacteria and therefore of vaccines prepared from such bacteria. High levels of endotoxin cause a range of adverse reactions due to endotoxin content and adverse reactions may be seen in animals following vaccination. The maximum content of endotoxin is limited in some countries for certain vaccines. Endotoxin content may be determined by the rabbit pyrogen test or the bacterial endotoxin test using the limulus amebocyte lysate (LAL) test according to the European Pharmacopoeia (European Pharmacopoeia Commission 2013). LAL is an aqueous extract of blood cells from the horseshoe crab, *Limulus polyphemus*. It reacts with bacterial endotoxin or lipopolysaccharide.

13.2.7 Safety

Safety testing is conducted on each batch of vaccine to determine that the batch does not cause an unexpected local or systemic reaction when used as indicated on the label. Because *in vivo* safety testing is limited to a few animals, the safety test can detect major problems with the vaccine batch, but more subtle safety problems may not be detected. Inactivated products may be tested as a single dose, repeated single dose, or overdose, and live vaccines may be tested as an overdose. Tests may be conducted using laboratory animals (mice, guinea pigs), the target animal, or a combination of both. Multispecies vaccines should be tested in the species most sensitive to the antigenic fraction. In cases where there is a consistent, documented manufacturing process and a history of satisfactory safety testing and a robust pharmacovigilance system is in place, final products may be exempted from safety testing in accordance with internationally harmonized guidelines (USDA 2016, 2017; VICH 2017a, 2017b, 2019).

13.2.8 Potency/Titer

Potency is a quantitative measure of the activity of a vaccine lot as indicated in a validated potency assay. Potency is related to the efficacy of the product that was determined in vaccination challenge studies in the target animal. Internationally harmonized guidelines (VICH 2006) state that the specifications for a potency assay should be linked to clinical studies, analytical procedures, manufacturing process, and stability of the product. Potency tests should be developed and validated during the registration or licensure of a product. The design of the host animal vaccine efficacy studies must include specifications for a potency test. The potency test must provide relevant, reliable, and reproducible results that are scientifically sound. A potency assay is required for each antigenic fraction in a vaccine for which there is a label claim. Each potency test must be validated prior to implementation for batch release, with the accuracy, precision, and ruggedness determined.

13.2.8.1 Live Vaccines

The potency test for live vaccines is typically a direct count or titer determination. The minimum titer per dose is based on the titer used in the efficacy study plus an increment to account for assay variability and degradation of the product during the shelf-life.

13.2.8.2 Inactivated Vaccines, Including Subunit Vaccines

The potency test for inactivated vaccines is frequently an *in vitro* assay, but in some instances a vaccination serology or vaccination challenge assay is used. The *in vitro* assay should measure a protective antigen or antigens, and can be a direct or an indirect measurement (relative potency) by comparing the antigenic content in the vaccine to that of a reference that was qualified by a vaccination challenge study.

13.2.8.3 Nucleic Acid Vaccines

The potency test typically includes determination of the nucleic acid concentration along with evaluation of the expression of the gene of interest.

13.3 Key Aspects and Types of Efficacy/Potency Testing Either *In Vivo* or *In Vitro*

There should be a clear correlation between the potency assay and efficacy, and the relationship between the two should be established during the pivotal efficacy study. Efficacy is a measure of the direct effect of the vaccine in a vaccinated individual of the target species to elicit an immune response that provides protection or treatment of the disease listed on the vaccine label, as measured in a clinical study. The potency test should provide an assurance that each batch of vaccine is expected to be efficacious and remain efficacious throughout the shelf-life.

For each fraction in a vaccine, the specific potency test used depends on the type of product, what methods are available for measuring that antigenic fraction, and how robust the method is. The development of a vaccine potency test is the culmination of a long sequence that begins with vaccine development in the prelicensing stage, continues through manufacturing, and has impacts during postmarketing use. Random or systematic uncertainty may be introduced at many points in this sequence, all of which contribute to the uncertainty in the potency test result. The importance of considering uncertainty in measurements or regulatory decisions has been widely discussed (ISO 2011). However, potency testing does provide a measure of consistency in production of a vaccine, given the variations that may be introduced during manufacture and assembly of batches. The critical element is that the potency assay should be validated according to accepted validation principles (USDA 2015b, 2016). A validated potency test provides a method to track antigen content across different batches and lots that may correlate to a specific challenge or clinical model, where required antigen amounts differ on specific vaccination route, on a live or inactivated agent, on age or breeding status of the intended vaccinates, or other differences.

13.3.1 Aspects of *In Vivo* Testing

In vivo potency tests use animals, either the vaccine target animals or laboratory animals, to determine the immunogenic strength of the vaccine. Potency testing *in vivo* may include vaccination challenge or vaccination serology, such as serum neutralization, hemagglutination inhibition, or serum ELISA testing, using serum collected from animals inoculated with the vaccine lot in question.

In a vaccination challenge test, animals are vaccinated either with the newly prepared batch or a placebo. After a specified amount of time to allow for the immunological response to develop, the vaccinated animals are then challenged by exposure to a known standard reference of the pathogen against which the vaccine is purported to protect. If the vaccine protects a prescribed number of animals against disease, it is considered potent. The placebo control group is essential to demonstrate that the challenge was adequate.

In a serological test, the vaccine is inoculated into target animals or laboratory animals according to the label recommendations and regulatory requirements. After a specified time period, most often 3 weeks, the animals are bled and serum prepared and used for the subsequent *in vitro* phase of the test.

Serum neutralization testing entails using the serum obtained from the vaccinated animals to neutralize virus grown in cell culture or embryonated chicken eggs. Hemagglutination inhibition tests can be used to measure antibodies that prevent red blood cells from agglutinating in the presence of a pathogen containing a hemagglutinin protein. By using serial dilutions of the serum with a fixed concentration of red blood cells, a hemagglutination inhibition titer can be determined. This test is performed routinely for influenza vaccines because they induce antibodies to hemagglutinin, which then inhibit agglutination of the red blood cells. Other agglutination tests use sensitized latex beads coated with protein or antibody to measure either protective antibody or viral protein. ELISA testing involves testing serum from vaccinated animals for the presence of antibodies specific to the pathogen against which the vaccine should protect.

13.3.2 Aspects of *In Vitro* Testing

In vitro potency tests are desirable because they avoid the use of animals, but it is critical that the test measures an immunogenic antigen or agent and actually correlates with vaccine efficacy. Typical *in vitro* tests include direct counts or titrations of live vaccines, and relative potency assays for inactivated vaccines, although other types of assays may be used depending on the vaccine.

For live vaccines, titers can be determined using cell culture, embryonated eggs, or direct bacterial counts. The acceptable minimum titer is based on the pivotal efficacy study where a specific titer was shown to be efficacious, with an additional increment to ensure that the vaccine maintains an efficacious level of antigen throughout the shelf-life. For live recombinant viral vaccines, the titer of the vector should be determined and the expression of the foreign antigen evaluated.

Inactivated vaccines are frequently tested using an *in vitro* ELISA assay to measure the amount of a given antigen in the vaccine, provided the ELISA recognizes an immunogenic antigen relevant to efficacy. This type of assay, referred to as a relative potency assay, usually incorporates a validated reference that is tested in parallel with the vaccine so the results obtained with the vaccine can be directly compared with the results of the reference. It is critical to have a robust, validated reference; without a reliable reference, an *in vitro* relative potency test would be meaningless. Inactivated vaccines with complex formulations present a challenge because ingredients such as adjuvants can hinder the recognition of the antigen of interest; likewise, cross-reaction with another fraction or component of the vaccine can be problematic.

In the case of nucleic acid vaccines, the potency assay is often a quantitative measure of the nucleic acid concentration by optical density or PCR, along with another test that measures the expression of the encoded protein of interest.

No matter what type of assay is used, common standards should be in place for the validation of the potency assay. In assays that include a validated reference, the reference must be relatively stable and monitored over time to ensure that it has not degraded.

13.4 Key Aspects and Types of Safety Testing

All products are tested extensively for safety during the licensure process, including numerous tests conducted using the final product. Although prelicense safety studies are a critical component of the registration/licensing process, they do not replace animal safety testing requirements for each batch of vaccines, or an ongoing postmarketing surveillance program. Batch release animal safety test requirements, as mentioned previously, may be waived with appropriate justification, including consideration of consistency in formulation, equipment, location, and method of production. If manufacturing processes are well documented, have parameters set to control process variation, and there is a history of safe use in the field, such products may be considered for animal safety testing exemptions. This is consistent with international recommendations and the principles of reducing, refining, and replacing the use of animals in testing (VICH 2017a, 2017b, 2019).

13.5 Summary

Quality control testing of the final product is the final step in the manufacture of safe and efficacious veterinary vaccines. Confirmation of the identity of the microorganism(s) and demonstration of the lack of detectable extraneous bacteria, fungi, mycoplasma, and viral agents ensure that the vaccine contains the agent of interest without contamination with other microorganisms. Chemical and physical tests, confirmation of the inactivation, and tests for residual toxicity, along with safety testing, provide assurance that the product should be safe in the target animal. For all types of vaccines, potency testing, whether *in vivo* or *in vitro*, provides assurance that each batch of vaccine is efficacious.

References

De Mattia, F., Hendriksen, C., Buchheit, K.H. et al. (2015). The vaccines consistency approach project: an EPAA initiative. *Pharmeur. Bio. Sci. Notes* 2015: 30–56.

European Pharmacopoeia Commission (2013). *European Pharmacopoeia*, 8e. Sainte-Ruffine, France: Maisonneuve.

Hill, R.E., Foley, P.L., Clough, N.E. et al. (2013). Translating research into licensed vaccines and validated and licensed diagnostic tests. In: *Vaccines and Diagnostics for Transboundary Animal Diseases* (eds. J.A. Roth, J.A. Richt and I.A. Morozov), 53–58. Basel: Karger.

ISO. (2011). Uncertainty of measurement – Part 3: Guide to the expression of uncertainty in measurement. www.iso.org/standard/50461.html

OIE (2013). Rabies (infection with rabies virus). In: *Manual of Diagnostic Tests and Vaccines for Terrestrial Animals*. www.oie.int/international-standard-setting/terrestrial-manual/access-online

USDA. (2015a). Potency Testing of Clostridium chauvoei Bacterins using an ELISA Procedure, Testing Protocol BBPRO0220.03. Center for Veterinary Biologics, Animal and Plant Health Inspection Service, United States Department of Agriculture.

USDA. (2015b). Guidelines for Validation of In vitro Potency Assays, Veterinary Services Memorandum No. 800.112. Animal and Plant Health Inspection Service, United States Department of Agriculture.

USDA. (2016). Viruses, serums, toxins and analogous products; organisms and vectors. In: Animals and Animal Products, Code of Federal Regulations, Title 9. United States Department of Agriculture.

VICH. (2006). Specifications: test procedures and acceptance criteria for new biotechnological/biological veterinary medicine products, GL40. www.ema.europa.eu/ en/ vich- gl40-test-procedures-acceptance-criteria- new-biotechnologicalbiological-veterinary-medicinal

USDA. (2017). Target Animal Safety Testing Exemption, Veterinary Services Memorandum No. 800.116. Animal and Plant Health Inspection Service, United States Department of Agriculture.

VICH. (2017b). Harmonisation of criteria to waive laboratory animal batch safetytesting for live vaccines for veterinary use, GL55. www.ema.europa.eu/en/documents/scientific-guideline/vich-gl55-harmonization-criteria-waive-target-animal-batch-safety-testing-live-vaccines-veterinary_en.pdf

VICH. (2017a). Harsmonisation of criteria to waive target animal batch safety testing for inactivated vaccines for veterinary use, GL50. www.ema.europa.eu/en/documents/scientific-guideline/vich-gl50-harmonisation-criteria-waive-target-animal-batch-safety-testing-inactivated-vaccines_en-0.pdf

VICH. (2019). Harmonisation of criteria to waive laboratory animal batch safety testing for vaccines for veterinary use, GL59. www.ema.europa.eu/en/documents/scientific-guideline/draft-vich-gl59-harmonisation-criteria-waive-laboratory-animal-batch-safety-testing-vaccines_en.pdf

14

Registration of Veterinary Vaccines with Respect to Consistency, Safety, and Efficacy

Esther Werner, Babett Kobe, and Veronika von Messling

Veterinary Medicine Division, Paul Ehrlich Institut, Langen, Germany

14.1 Introduction

Veterinary vaccines undergo an approval process to ensure that the products are safe and effective as well as of consistent quality. There are different legal bases upon which a marketing authorization may be applied for, reflecting the type and content of the data submitted in support of the application. The requirements for licensing of vaccines differ throughout the world. To obtain a marketing authorization, veterinary vaccines are subjected to safety, immunogenicity, and efficacy studies in a limited number of individuals of the target species. Their protective potential is assessed by *in vivo* challenge or occasionally by seroconversion studies. Field studies with veterinary vaccines are often limited and typically used to evaluate safety rather than efficacy. The criteria for veterinary vaccines can differ depending on the animal groups under consideration. For livestock vaccines, the key objective is to improve overall production as well as the cost–benefit resulting from vaccination. For companion animal vaccines, the health and welfare of the individual animal are of primary concern. Reduction or elimination of the risk for the consumer is the main goal of vaccination against zoonotic or food-borne infections. Vaccination of wildlife is generally considered with respect to infections that are transmissible to humans (zoonotic diseases) or livestock, although concerns for the welfare of wildlife are of increasing importance.

This chapter provides an overview of the general requirements for the licensing of veterinary vaccines and describes the criteria evaluated during the regulatory assessment process in the European Union (EU). The unique aspects of live vaccines, maternally derived antibodies (MDAs), cross-reactivity with other drugs, and combined products are also discussed.

14.2 Legislative Mechanisms/Systems Including Marketing Authorization Procedures

The regulation and licensing of veterinary vaccines lie within the responsibility of the control authorities in the country or region concerned. The individual countries/authorities are responsible for defining the application process and the outline of the dossier content. A marketing authorization, also referred to as "registration" or "licence," for a veterinary vaccine will be granted after quality, safety, and efficacy of the product have been assessed in accordance with defined legal standards.

The European system was introduced with the objective to ensure that safe, effective, and high-quality veterinary medicines can be made available across the EU (European Commission 2001b; European Parliament 2004). It offers several routes for the authorization of medicinal products for animal use. The centralized procedure is compulsory for products produced with biotechnological methods. The mutual recognition procedure is based on the principle of recognition of an already existing national marketing authorization by one or more member states. The decentralized procedure is used when no national marketing authorization has been issued in any of the member states. Then an application for the marketing authorization of a product can be submitted simultaneously in several member states, one of them being chosen as the "reference member state." Purely national authorizations are also still available for products to be marketed in one member state only.

In the USA, regulatory jurisdiction is established by the Virus-Serum-Toxin Act of 1913 (VST Act 1913), which requires that all veterinary vaccines available within the

Veterinary Vaccines: Principles and Applications, First Edition. Edited by Samia Metwally, Gerrit Viljoen, and Ahmed El Idrissi.

USA are pure, safe, potent, and effective, not worthless, dangerous, contaminated, or harmful. Specific regulations are codified annually in the US Code of Federal Regulations (CFR 2016). The Japanese system is based on granting a marketing approval for veterinary vaccines after examination and evaluation of applications for approval, which guarantees the quality, safety, and efficacy claimed in the application (regulated under the Act on Securing Quality, Efficacy and Safety of Pharmaceuticals, Medical Devices, Regenerative and Cellular Therapy Products, Gene Therapy Products, and Cosmetics in Japan). In other regions of the world, registration and regulation of veterinary vaccines are already part of the national legislation or are under development.

14.3 Requirements for Registration and Authorization Including Quality, Safety, and Efficacy Assessment

A veterinary vaccine can only be marketed after it has been licensed by a relevant competent authority. During the licensing process, quality, safety, and efficacy of the product are evaluated. Toward this, the pharmaceutical company interested in marketing the product submits the documents necessary for this evaluation. In addition to administrative information, the dossier has to contain all the scientific documentation supporting the quality, safety, and efficacy claims. The requirements are outlined in the relevant legal framework (i.e. for the EU: Directive 2001/82/EC, Annex I, European Commission 2001b). This includes detailed descriptions of product composition and development, the manufacturing process, and the origin of source materials, in-process and final product controls, stability results, and information regarding intended use. Furthermore, the results of safety studies in the target species have to be presented to illustrate potential risks associated with the vaccine in the context of its intended use. For live attenuated vaccines, the results of additional tests evaluating transmissibility, spread, and possible shedding of the vaccine strain by the vaccinated animal as well as the risk for reversion to virulence have to be provided. Furthermore, information regarding user safety, potential residues, cross-reactivity with other drugs, and environmental safety are required.

All claims regarding the characteristics, effects, and application of the vaccine have to be supported by results from specific efficacy studies included in the dossier. The potential risks emerging from these studies have to be determined in relation to the benefit expected from the vaccine.

14.4 Batch-to-Batch Consistency Assessment Through In-Process and Final Product Testing

The consistency approach for the routine release of vaccines is based on the principle that the quality of vaccines is a consequence of a quality control system and of consistent production of lots with characteristics similar to those lots that have been shown to be safe and effective in the target species (Hendriksen et al. 2008). A panel of parameters is used to generate a product profile mirroring that of a batch with proven clinical efficacy and safety. This profile has to cover all critical production steps and has to be controlled by suitable test methods and analytical tools, which then become part of the implemented quality system. The concept of consistency of production is state of the art for new-generation vaccines, where batch release, especially in terms of potency testing, is mainly based on non-animal testing methods (de Mattia et al. 2011). For registration purposes, at least three consecutive antigen batches, as well as three final product batches at development and production scales have to be provided in order to demonstrate both consistent antigen production and consistent composition of the finished product in a quantitative and qualitative manner.

14.5 Stability Testing

For licensing purposes, real-time stability studies shall be carried out on no less than three representative consecutive vaccine batches kept at the recommended storage conditions (European Pharmacopoeia, Monograph 0062). The three consecutive production runs may be carried out on a pilot scale as long as the production process reproduces the full-scale production described in the application. Whenever possible, these stability results should be confirmed by data generated from commercial batches. The impact of the container and closure system on vaccine stability and quality has to be tested. Appropriate parameters indicating the stability of the product shall be chosen and the analytical methods used for general monitoring as well as their specifications need to be justified and validated (WHO Technical Report Series No. 962, 201, Annex 3, http://www.who.int/biologicals/vaccines/Annex_3_WHO_TRS_962-3.pdf). Stability studies for veterinary vaccines should encompass both the largest and the smallest container sizes proposed, also referred to as the bracketing concept (VICH 2010).

Where the production process involves storage of bulk material before formulation and final manufacturing, data have to be provided demonstrating that the stability of the finished product is not affected when the vaccine is manufactured with aged antigens. Data generated in accelerated stability studies may be used in addition to real-time stability data to determine the impact of temperature increase over a short time during handling and shipping (WHO Technical Report Series No. 962, 201, Annex 3). Where applicable, an in-use stability testing process needs to be established to support the period of time during which a multidose preparation can be used while retaining quality within an accepted specification once the container has been opened (EMA 2010c). If an antimicrobial preservative is included in the vaccine, the efficacy of the preservative under in-use conditions shall be demonstrated using a batch at the end of the claimed shelf-life (European Pharmacopoeia, Monograph 5.1.3).

14.6 Demonstrating Safety

14.6.1 General Safety Requirements

Target animal safety is of high importance for veterinary vaccines and a basic requirement for the registration or authorization of vaccines in different regions of the world, including the EU, Japan, USA, and Canada. Target animal safety is influenced by factors such as proposed application regimen and dose, type of product, nature of adjuvants, excipients, claims, previous use history of similar products, species, class, and breed. Furthermore, safety studies have to assess the risk to consumers of food derived from treated animals and individuals who come in contact with the product, and also have to evaluate the impact on the environment.

Key safety studies include the analysis of systemic and local reactions, impact on reproductive performance, and immunological functions (European Commission 2001a; VICH 2008; European Pharmacopoeia, Monograph 5.2.6; USDA 2010; CFIA: Veterinary Biologics Guideline 3.29E: www.inspection.gc.ca/animals/veterinary-biologics/guidelines-forms/3-29e/eng/1328625354619/1328625860618). These studies are usually performed as laboratory studies to evaluate target animal safety under controlled conditions. They should be executed and managed based on a detailed study protocol, whenever possible, in accordance with the principles of Good Laboratory Practice (GLP). Safety trials should be conducted with the dosage that is recommended for use. Either a pilot or a production batch containing the maximum release potency or a justified multiple of the minimum release potency should be used. For live vaccines, the vaccine agents should be at the lowest attenuated passage level that will be present in the vaccine to be registered.

Evaluation of safety after vaccination with a single dose should be conducted in the most sensitive category, such as certain breeds or age groups, of each target species proposed, and studies involving the administration of the product by all foreseen routes are recommended. If veterinary vaccines have to be administered more than once as part of the basic vaccination scheme, a study of the repeated administration is required. In the case of overdose testing, which is only required for live vaccines, indicators for disease-specific signs or lesions may be included in the evaluation criteria as part of the risk analysis for the acceptability of the vaccine strain. For this scenario, the general principles of one-dose testing using a 10-fold dose based on the maximum release titer should be considered. For mammals and poultry, the use of eight animals per group is recommended unless otherwise justified, and the serological status of the animals before immunization should be known.

The animals have to be observed for overall clinical health and signs of systemic (body temperature, weight, and other performance measurements) and local reactions (examination of the injection sites by inspection and palpation). The animals should be observed every day for at least 14 days after each administration, and all observations should be documented for the entire period. The observation period should be extended until clinically acceptable resolution of the lesion has occurred or, if appropriate, until the animal is euthanized and examined histopathologically. Detailed postmortem macroscopic and microscopic examinations of the injection site should be performed, where appropriate.

Examination of reproductive performance of breeding animals has also to be considered. Reproductive performance of males and non-pregnant as well as pregnant females, and harmful effects during gestation or on the progeny, including teratogenic and abortifacient effects, should be investigated for each of the recommended routes of administration. Laboratory and field safety studies are suitable to support use in breeding animals. Additional studies may be required to determine the effect of a product on semen, including the shedding of a live vaccine strain. Where the product might adversely affect the immune response by immunosuppression, autoimmunity, or hypersensitivity, immunological functions have to be evaluated in the animal to be treated as well as its progeny, if applicable. Generally, the data from safety tests on combined vaccines may be used to demonstrate the safety of vaccines containing fewer antigens and/or adjuvant components provided the remaining components are identical in each case and it is only the number of antigens and/or adjuvant components that has decreased.

14.6.2 Special Safety Requirements for Live Vaccines

Live vaccines may be capable of replicating in the target animal, thereby stimulating a diverse immune response. Because they cannot be completely characterized by chemical and physical tests alone, the assessment of live vaccines involves additional investigations. Data should be provided on the mode, rate, and duration of shedding. Spread of the vaccine strain from vaccinated to naïve target animals should be evaluated using the recommended route of administration most likely to result in spread. Moreover, it may be necessary to investigate the extent of spread to non-target species that could be susceptible to the live vaccine strain. An assessment has to be made of how many animal-to-animal passages are likely to occur under normal circumstances together with an assessment of the likely consequences. Dissemination of the vaccine strain in vaccinated animals has also to be examined. Feces, urine, milk, eggs, oral, nasal, and other secretions as well as internal organs should be tested for the presence of the vaccine strain. Moreover, systemic dissemination studies may be required, with particular attention being paid to the predilection sites for replication of the organism. In the case of live vaccines for well-established zoonotic diseases in food-producing animals, these studies are obligatory.

Furthermore, the absence of reversion to or increase in virulence, also referred to as backpassage studies, has to be demonstrated to evaluate the genetic stability of the vaccine and to provide assurance that the product will not revert to virulence when passaged in the most sensitive class of each target animal (VICH 2007; European Pharmacopoeia, Monograph 5.2.6; USDA 2018a; CFIA: Veterinary Biologics Guideline 3.29E). These studies consist of successive propagation of the vaccine microorganisms through a series of passages *in vivo*. A recommended route of administration or a natural route of infection that is most likely to lead to reversion to or increase in virulence and results in recovery of the microorganism following replication in the animal should be chosen for the initial administration and subsequent passages. Toward this, the lowest passage of the tested microorganism used for production containing the maximum release titer expected in the recommended dose is administered to a group of susceptible host animals. In cases where no maximum release titer is specified, a justifiable multiple of the minimum release titer should be used. After an appropriate incubation time, the microorganism is then recovered from these animals and administered to a second group of susceptible hosts. Passage inocula should be collected and prepared from the most likely source of spread of the organism. Generally, a minimum of five such successive passages should be performed with a minimum of two animals for the first four groups and of eight animals for the fifth group. The time interval between inoculation of the animal and harvest for each passage must be justified based upon the characteristics of the tested microorganism. In order to confirm the presence and determine the number of test organisms at each passage, appropriate methods, preferably *in vitro* propagation, should be used. In general, *in vitro* propagation may not be used to multiply the passage inoculum.

During the study, general clinical health of the animals has to be observed, including all relevant parameters typical for the disease, which could indicate reversion to or increase in virulence. Animals in the last group should be observed for at least 21 days. If the last group of animals shows no evidence of an increase in virulence during the observation period, further testing is not required. If signs consistent with the target disease are observed, the causality needs to be investigated. The microorganism isolated from the last passage should be characterized genotypically and/or phenotypically, and compared with the master seed to evaluate genetic stability and reversion to virulence. If reversion to or increase in virulence of the tested microorganism is observed after passaging in the target animal, this organism will be considered to be unsuitable for use as a live vaccine strain. In addition, the probability of recombination or genomic reassortment with field or other strains has to be considered.

14.6.3 Special Requirements for Genetically Modified Organisms

In the case of veterinary medicinal products containing or consisting of genetically modified organisms (GMOs), an environmental risk assessment (ERA) in addition to the evaluation of the quality, safety, and efficacy is required (European Commission 2001a). An ERA should be performed in order to identify the potential risks for public health and the environment that may arise due to the use and release of GMOs. On a case-by-case basis, potentially harmful effects of a GMO for humans, domestic and wildlife animals, plants, microorganisms, and the environment at large have to be identified and assessed. Potential adverse effects should be considered irrespective of whether or not they are direct or indirect and whether or not the evolving effects appear immediately or are delayed. Appropriate measures for reduction or elimination of such identified effects have to be defined.

14.6.4 Additional Aspects

14.6.4.1 User Safety

This section has to include a discussion of the effects described in the preceding sections, relating those effects to the type and extent of human exposure to the veterinary vaccine with a view to formulating appropriate user warnings and other risk management measures (EMEA 2007a).

14.6.4.2 Study of Residues

Usually, a study of residues for veterinary vaccines is not necessary. However, where adjuvants and/or preservatives are used in the manufacturing process, consideration has to be given to the possibility of any residues remaining in the foodstuffs. If necessary, the effects of such residues have to be investigated. A withdrawal period should be proposed and its adequacy discussed in relation to any residue studies that have been undertaken.

14.6.4.3 Interactions

If there is a compatibility statement with other veterinary vaccines, the safety of the association has to be investigated. Any other known interactions with veterinary medicinal products have to be described.

14.6.4.4 Environmental Risk Assessment

An ERA has to be provided to evaluate the potential harmful effects which the use of the veterinary vaccine may cause to the environment, and to identify any precautionary measures which may be necessary to reduce such risks. The assessment has to indicate the potential exposure of the environment to the concerned vaccine and the level of risk associated with any such exposure, taking into account in particular the target animal species and the proposed pattern of use, method of administration, possible excretion of the vaccine and its active substances into the environment by treated animals, disposal of unused or waste product, and the risk to humans in case of live vaccine strains which may be zoonotic (EMEA 1996).

14.6.5 Field Study Support

Results from laboratory studies have to be supplemented with data from field studies using batches according to the described manufacturing process (EMEA 2001; USDA 2018b). Safety and efficacy may be investigated in the same field studies. Field studies should be conducted under animal housing and husbandry conditions representative of those regions in which authorization is sought and conform to local animal welfare regulations. More than one geographical site is recommended. The involved animals should represent the age range/class proposed for treatment. The serological status should also be considered. Whenever possible, either a negative or positive control group should be included. All included animals should be managed similarly. The recommended dosage(s) and route(s) for vaccination as well as representative batch(es) of the tested product should be used.

14.7 Demonstrating Efficacy to Confirm Claims Made for the Product

14.7.1 Key Demonstration of Efficacy by Challenge and in Consideration of the Relevance of the Challenge Strain Used

All claims made with regard to the properties, effects, and use of a veterinary vaccine have to be fully supported by results of specific trials included in the application for marketing authorization (Directive 2001/18/EC; USDA 2016). During development of the product, studies are carried out to demonstrate that the product is efficacious when administered by each of the recommended routes and methods of administration and using the recommended schedule to animals of each species and category, considering the minimum age for which the use of the product is to be recommended. Efficacy trials should include untreated or placebo control animals unless this is not otherwise justified for animal welfare reasons (European Pharmacopoeia, Monograph 5.2.7).

In principle, demonstration of efficacy has to be undertaken under well-controlled laboratory conditions by challenge after administration of the veterinary vaccine to the target animal under the recommended conditions of use. As far as possible, the conditions under which the challenge is carried out shall mimic the natural conditions for infection, especially with regard to the amount of challenge organisms and the route of administration of the challenge. An experimental challenge has to be strong enough to generate significant differences between the challenged animals and the controls, whereby the observed differences must be related to clinically relevant efficacy parameters. The primary outcome needs to be defined by the investigator at the time the study is designed and should not be changed after the study is completed. Unless otherwise justified, the challenge should be carried out using a strain different from the one used in the production of the vaccine

(European Pharmacopoeia, Monograph 0062). Details of the challenge strain and its epidemiological relevance have to be provided. The choice of antigens or vaccine strains shall also be justified on the basis of epizoological data.

For live vaccines, batches containing the minimum titer or potency of virus/bacteria at the most attenuated passage level have to be used. For other products, batches containing the minimum active content shall be used, unless otherwise justified (European Pharmacopoeia, Monograph 5.2.7). The batches used for efficacy studies have to be produced according to the manufacturing process described in the Quality Part of the dossier. The dose to be used has to match the volume of the product recommended for use and contain the minimum titer or potency expected at the end of the period of validity (European Commission 2001a). The injection volume must be proportionate and relative to the size of the animal.

Particulars of the study protocols and reports have to be sufficiently detailed to enable an objective judgment. All results obtained, whether favorable or unfavorable, have to be reported. Whenever possible, the immune mechanisms, including cell mediated and humoral, as well as local and general classes of immunoglobulins, induced after the administration of the vaccine to target animals by the recommended route of administration shall be specified and documented. For marker vaccines intended to allow a distinction between vaccinated and infected animals, where the efficacy claim is reliant on *in vitro* diagnostic tests, sufficient data on the diagnostic tests have to be provided to allow adequate assessment of the claims related to the marker properties (European Commission 2001a).

14.7.2 Demonstrating Onset and Duration of Immunity as Well as Efficacy of a Booster Dose

Any claims, stated or implied, regarding onset and duration of protection shall be supported by data from trials. The onset of immunity (OOI) is defined as the period between the final vaccination and the point in time when the challenge is performed in supporting laboratory efficacy studies. The duration of immunity (DOI) that can be claimed is the longest interval between the administration of a vaccine to target animals and the observed protection against the required challenge. Preferably, the vaccine batches used for demonstration of OOI and DOI contain the minimum active content, unless otherwise justified. In general, the duration of protection has to be justified in relation to the length of time for which an animal is likely to be at risk (EMEA 2000).

Where there is no recommendation for repeated administration, a life-long protection is implied. However, for most infectious animal diseases, one administration of a vaccine does not provide protection that will last for the natural or economic life of the animals. Therefore, vaccination regimens are usually necessary. As the natural or economic lifespan of animals differs between species, categories, and regions, the claimed duration of protection has to be specified and supported by sufficient data. The studies required to generate the supporting data shall be conducted under well-controlled conditions. If the necessary studies are difficult to conduct under laboratory conditions, field trials alone may be carried out. However, it has to be ensured that the vaccinated target animals are not exposed to intercurrent field infections, which could boost the immunity. Therefore, it is usually necessary to include unvaccinated target animals as sentinels in laboratory or field studies. Unless otherwise justified, the results from vaccination challenge trials conducted under laboratory conditions shall be supplemented with sufficient data from well-controlled field studies. In these field studies, target animals undergo a natural challenge or a subsequent experimental challenge under laboratory conditions.

If active immunity is induced after the initial vaccination scheme, the duration of protection usually has to be demonstrated by challenge of the vaccinated animals just before the recommended time for revaccination. If passive immunity is induced, the duration of protection of the progeny has to be demonstrated by challenge at the time of natural susceptibility of the offspring of females that have been vaccinated at the maximum interval recommended between vaccination and parturition or lay. In addition, data shall be presented to support the duration of protection claimed for the offspring. After revaccination according to the immunization scheme, a protection that is quantitatively and qualitatively at least equivalent to the response after the initial vaccination schedule has to be shown. Ideally, this is demonstrated by challenge trials performed at suitable times between the end of the revaccination scheme and the end of the claimed period of protection thereafter. However, in order to limit the number of challenge studies necessary to demonstrate the duration of protection, challenge of a more limited number of immunized animals, or quantification of suitable indicators for protection other than challenge may be considered. For an indicator to be acceptable as a correlate of vaccine efficacy, evidence has to be provided that it plays a substantial role in the protection of the target species, and that there is a sufficient qualitative and quantitative relationship between the indicator and the protection of the target species against the disease concerned.

14.7.3 The Influence of Maternally Derived Antibodies

If vaccination is recommended in animals at an age at which maternally acquired immunity may still be present and may interfere with active immunity development, studies should be performed to determine whether or not such interference occurs (European Commission 2001a). Depending on the nature and properties of the vaccine, such as dose and strain of live vaccines, and/or on specific circumstances related to the immunization schedule or the method of administration, such as *in ovo* vaccination or vaccination against ubiquitous pathogens, laboratory and/or field studies are necessary to demonstrate the efficacy of the vaccine administered in the presence of MDAs. In general, the extent and duration of passively acquired immunity should be determined. However, such data can generally be gathered from scientific publications, from field trials, or from the populations on the premises where animals are selected for performing MDA interference studies. The MDA titer investigated should be representative of the titer in animals of the minimum age to be vaccinated under field circumstances. Possible reference made to varying degrees of MDAs should be justified.

To verify the presence or absence of interference by MDAs with vaccine efficacy, the recommended vaccination schedule should be applied. For live vaccines, batches containing the minimum titer or potency have to be used for vaccination, unless otherwise justified. For other products, batches containing the minimum active content shall be used, unless otherwise justified. The study design depends on the particular circumstances associated with the respective product. In any case, a nonvaccinated group of animals with MDAs should be included and should be monitored to follow the decay of MDAs. This group serves as a control to define the endpoint for examining the protection-related parameters in vaccinated animals with representative MDA titers or the time of challenge in all the groups, to control for the absence of intercurrent infection, and to validate the challenge. If the results indicate that the MDAs interfere with vaccine efficacy, this point should be stated in the product literature, and the applicant should define a schedule of vaccination that will ensure protection of animals vaccinated in the presence of MDAs (EMA 2010b).

14.7.4 Field Study Support

In general, results from laboratory trials shall be supplemented with data from field trials carried out with unvaccinated or placebo control groups (EMEA 2001). Where laboratory trials cannot be supportive of efficacy, the performance of field trials alone may be acceptable (EMEA 2001). Field trials should be conducted in accordance with established principles of good clinical practice, unless otherwise justified. The vaccine batches used for field trials should be representative of the manufacturing process described in the marketing authorization application. The use of standard batches is accepted, which allows the investigation of safety and efficacy in the same field studies.

The parameters to be measured have to be clearly defined and justified in relation to the indications and specific claims for the vaccine. There are two types of parameters: main parameters such as mortality, morbidity, clinical signs, weight gain, and epizootic impact, and indicators such as serological responses. As already detailed for the determination of the duration of protection, for such an indicator to be acceptable as a correlate of vaccine efficacy, evidence has to be provided showing that there is a sufficient qualitative and quantitative relationship between the indicator and the protection of the target species against the disease concerned.

14.7.5 Demonstrating Efficacy of Multivalent and Combined Vaccines

The efficacy of each of the components of multivalent or combined vaccines has to be demonstrated (European Commission 2001a; USDA 2007). A multivalent vaccine is defined as vaccine prepared from cultures of two or more strains of the same species or microorganism, whereas a combined vaccine is a product intended for immunization against more than one disease, pathogen, and/or antigen. The combined vaccine can be supplied in a single primary container or in several primary containers, the contents of which are mixed prior to use for administration (EMA 2013). In general, the efficacy requirements for multivalent or combined vaccines are the same as those for vaccines containing one active substance. The tests should be conducted in each target species after administration of the vaccine according to the proposed schedule of administration containing the relevant active substance(s) at the minimum antigen content/minimum titer proposed for the vaccine. The OOI and DOI should be established for the combined vaccine. DOI may be supported by field trial data in place of laboratory studies. If appropriate, the influence of passively acquired and MDAs on the immunity should be adequately evaluated. The data from monovalent vaccines may be suitable to address this point.

In order to avoid unnecessary challenge studies, efficacy data from a vaccine of a larger combination of active substances may be used to support the efficacy of the smaller combination, provided that:

- the components, i.e. antigens, composition of excipients and/or adjuvants, are identical and it is only the number of active substances which is different. Minor differences between the larger and smaller combined products could be accepted if suitable justification is provided, and
- potential interactions of the active substances in the larger combination with the induction of protection in the vaccinated animal are taken into account.

Similarly, the results from challenge studies with a vaccine containing fewer active substances may be used to support the efficacy of the larger combination, provided that:

- the components which have already been tested for efficacy (antigens, composition of excipients and/or adjuvants) are identical, and it is only the number of active substances which is different. Minor differences between the larger and smaller combined products could be accepted if suitable justification is provided, and
- for one or more of the active substance(s) in the smaller combination, a threshold has been defined for a marker parameter (i.e. a specific response to a vaccination which can quantitatively be assessed) that correlates with protection.

In such cases, where a challenge is not performed for the active substance(s) in the larger combined vaccine, it must be demonstrated that the results obtained for the marker parameter with the larger combination are at least equal to the threshold established for this active substance in the smaller combination. Field data for a combined vaccine of a larger combination may be used to support field use of a combined vaccine of a smaller combination provided it can be demonstrated that the active substance(s) which are present in the larger combination but not present in the smaller combination has/have no enhancing effects. The results obtained with a vaccine containing fewer active substances than the combined vaccine can also be taken into account to demonstrate the efficacy, if the conditions mentioned above are fulfilled (EMA 2013).

14.7.6 Considerations on Compatibility with Other Veterinary Medicinal Products

If there is a compatibility statement with other immunological products, the efficacy of the association has to be investigated. In this sense, association is defined as use of two or more vaccines or other immunological veterinary medicinal products (IVMPs), each of which has its own marketing authorization. Usually, the following associations are possible:

- mixing of two or more IVMPs prior to use for administration at one site
- administration of two or more IVMPs at the same time but at different administration sites
- administration of two or more IVMPs at separate times.

The absence of negative interactions after mixing of the individual IVMPs, such as virucidal effect and physico-chemical interactions, should be demonstrated. The associated administration of two or more IVMPs may cause an interaction leading to either a diminished or increased immunological response to individual components compared with the individual administration of each IVMP (EMA 2013). Generally, the protection for all components of the mixed IVMPs should be demonstrated by challenge. In most cases, the batches being mixed should contain the minimum antigen content and the mixture should be administered such that a single dose of each of the individual vaccines is administered to each category of each target species by all the recommended routes of administration. However, if scientific rationale suggests that the various components might interfere with one another, the relative antigen content of the batches to be used might need to be considered on a case-by-case basis.

Special attention should be given to the following aspects:

- If a threshold for an immune response to vaccination recognized as a correlate of protection has been established for one or more of the active substances of the individual vaccine components, the challenge against these active substances can be omitted and the follow-up of these marker parameters after administration of the mixed vaccines is acceptable to support the claim for these active substances.
- If different minimum ages are approved for the individual components, the efficacy of the association should be established for the oldest of the minimum recommended ages for the individual components.
- Follow-up investigations should be similar to those performed when the individual vaccines are given alone.
- Comparison of the results with those obtained when the vaccines are given alone in compliance with data already available in the marketing authorization of each vaccine should be performed.
- Where no validated correlates of protection are available, challenge studies are carried out and the results must be similar and support all the efficacy claims of the individual vaccine components (some level of interference between antigens may be allowed, if justified).

- If a follow-up with validated correlates of protection has been used, it should be demonstrated that the results obtained with the mixed vaccines are at least equal to the threshold established for each individual vaccine component.
- It should be demonstrated that the mixing of vaccines does not negatively affect the OOI and DOI as established for the individual vaccine components.

Administration of two or more vaccines at the same time but at separate administration sites or administration of two or more vaccines at separate times is also referred to as association. Generally, the protection provided by the associated vaccines has to be demonstrated by challenge studies. Standard batches can be used, and a single dose of each of the individual vaccines is administered under conditions most likely to result in interference by using the most sensitive category of each target species and most sensitive route of administration for the study.

The special aspects listed for the mixing prior to use are also valid for associated use at the same time but at different administration sites. Where adequate justification is given, the compatibility may be supported by data from field trials alone. If a correlate of protection has been established, it can be followed during field trials and the results obtained should be at least equal to the threshold established for each individual vaccine.

14.8 Special Licensing Considerations

For certain vaccines such as those against foot and mouth disease, avian influenza, or bluetongue, the concept of a multistrain dossier has been developed (EMA 2010a). This involves a single dossier that includes data for different possible combinations of strains or antigens and thus allows adjusting the vaccine composition according to the respective epidemiological situation. In addition, new strains can be added to the dossier using a simplified licensing process, which shortens the reaction time in the case of outbreaks caused by new serotypes.

There are also special regulations regarding the licensing of vaccines for minor species or minor use (MUMS) limited market to improve the vaccine availability for such species and indications or to provide incentives for the development of products with lesser market shares (EMA 2017).

In exceptional circumstances, provisions may apply in order to facilitate rapid authorization of vaccines in advance of generation of data to meet the full requirements described above. Guidance on minimum requirements on quality, safety, and efficacy data for authorization of these vaccines will be given by competent authorities, e.g. for avian influenza and bluetongue vaccines (EMEA 2007b, 2008). With respect to veterinary vaccines of major interest, particularly from the viewpoint of animal health and therapeutic innovation, an accelerated assessment procedure is possible.

14.9 Minimum Requirements for Monitoring Systems (Legislation)

After licensing, robust safety and efficacy constitute the basis for a successful application in the field. Despite extensive laboratory and field studies during the licensing process, unwanted side effects cannot be completely excluded. Suspected adverse events have to be reported directly to the respective competent authority or to the pharmaceutical company, which then communicates the information to the competent authority. Such adverse events include adverse reactions in the target animal, suspected insufficient efficacy as well as side effects in humans or non-target species. This direct communication from clinical veterinarians in the field is the most important source for the continuous recording and assessment of the safety and efficacy of licensed vaccines and constitutes the basis for corrective measures.

14.10 Summary

Veterinary vaccines play an essential role in improving the health and welfare of animals, increasing the availability of products of animal origin, and preventing animal-to-human transmission of infection from both domestic animals and wildlife. Ensuring the quality, safety, and efficacy of these vaccines is the heart of the regulatory licensing process. While each country or region has its unique legal framework, the underlying objective remains the same. Veterinary vaccine licensing requires the submission of a dossier demonstrating a manufacturing process that ensures consistent quality as well as stability during the proposed shelf-life, including stability of the used antigens. The safety for the target animal as well as the risk for the user and the environment has to be assessed. Furthermore, all claims regarding the immunogenicity and efficacy of the vaccine have to be supported by results from specific investigations. The EU requirements for demonstrating consistency, safety, and efficacy of veterinary vaccines are described in this chapter.

References

Code of Federal Regulations (CFR). (2016). Title 9, Animals and animal products. www.ecfr.gov/cgi-bin/text-idx?gp=&SID=ae72fa9c71ecacce063bcc90893a8b2e&mc=true&tpl=/ecfrbrowse/Title09/9CIsubchapE.tpl

De Mattia, F., Chapsal, J.M., Descamps, J. et al. (2011). The consistency approach for quality control of vaccines – a strategy to improve quality control and implement 3Rs. *Biologicals* 39 (1): 59–65.

EMA. (2010a). EMA/CVMP/IWP/105506/2007: Guideline on data requirements for multi-strain dossiers for inactivated vaccines against avian influenza (AI), bluetongue (BT) and foot-and-mouth disease (FMD). www.ema.europa.eu/en/documents/scientific-guideline/guideline-data-requirements-multistrain-dossiers-inactivated-vaccines-against-avian-influenza_en.pdf

EMA. (2010b). EMA/CVMP/IWP/439467/2007: Reflection paper on the demonstration of a possible impact of maternally derived antibodies on vaccine efficacy in young animals. www.ema.europa.eu/en/documents/scientific-guideline/reflection-paper-demonstration-possible-impact-maternally-derived-antibodies-vaccine-efficacy-young_en.pdf

EMA. (2010c). EMA/CVMP/IWP/250147/2008: Guideline on data requirements to support in-use stability claims for veterinary vaccines. www.ema.europa.eu/en/documents/scientific-guideline/guideline-data-requirements-support-use-stability-claims-veterinary-vaccines_en.pdf

EMA. (2013). EMA/CVMP/IWP/594618/2010: Guideline on the requirements for combined vaccines and associations of immunological veterinary medicinal products (IVMPs). www.ema.europa.eu/en/documents/scientific-guideline/guideline-requirements-combined-vaccines-associations-immunological-veterinary-medicinal-products_en.pdf

EMA. (2017). EMA/CVMP/IWP/123243/2006: Guideline on data requirements for immunological veterinary medicinal products intended for minor use or minor species (MUMS)/limited market. www.ema.europa.eu/en/documents/scientific-guideline/guideline-data-requirements-immunological-veterinary-medicinal-products-intended-minor-use-minor/limited-market-revision-3_en.pdf

EMEA. (1996). EMA/CVMP/074/95: Note for guidance: Environmental risk assessment for immunological veterinary medicinal products. www.ema.europa.eu/en/documents/scientific-guideline/note-guidance-environmental-risk-assessment-immunological-veterinary-medicinal-products_en.pdf

EMEA. (2000). EMA/CVMP/682/99: Note for guidance: Duration of protection achieved by veterinary vaccines. www.ema.europa.eu/en/documents/scientific-guideline/note-guidance-duration-protection-achieved-veterinary-vaccines_en.pdf

EMEA. (2001). EMA/CVMP/852/99: Note for guidance: Field trials with veterinary vaccines. www.ema.europa.eu/en/documents/scientific-guideline/note-guidance-field-trials-veterinary-vaccines_en.pdf

EMEA. (2007a). EMA/CVMP/IWP/54533/2006: Guideline on user safety for immunological veterinary medicinal products. www.ema.europa.eu/en/documents/scientific-guideline/guideline-user-safety-immunological-veterinary-medicinal-products_en.pdf

EMEA. (2007b). EMA/CVMP/IWP/222624/2006: Requirements for an authorisation under exceptional circumstances for vaccines for use in birds against avian influenza. www.ema.europa.eu/en/documents/scientific-guideline/guideline-requirements-authorisation-under-exceptional-circumstances-vaccines-use-birds-against_en.pdf

EMEA.(2008). EMA/CVMP/IWP/220193/2008: Requirements for an authorisation under exceptional circumstances for vaccines for emergency use against bluetongue. www.ema.europa.eu/en/documents/scientific-guideline/guideline-requirements-authorisation-under-exceptional-circumstances-vaccines-emergency-use-against_en.pdf

European Commission. (2001a). Directive 2001/18/EC of the European Parliament and of the Council of 12 March 2001 on the deliberate release into the environment of genetically modified organisms and repealing Council Directive 90/220/EEC. https://ec.europa.eu/health/sites/health/files/files/eudralex/vol-1/dir_2001_18/dir_2001_18_en.pdf

European Commission. (2001b). Directive 2001/82/EC of the European Parliament and of the Council of 6 November 2001 on the Community code relating to veterinary medicinal products, as amended. https://ec.europa.eu/health/sites/health/files/files/eudralex/vol-5/dir_2001_82_cons2009/dir_2001_82_cons2009_en.pdf

European Parliament. (2004). Regulation (EC) No 726/2004 of the European Parliament and of the Council of 31 March 2004 laying down Community procedures for the authorisation and supervision of medicinal products for human and veterinary use and establishing a European Medicines Agency, as amended. https://ec.europa.eu/health/sites/health/files/files/eudralex/vol-1/reg_2004_726/reg_2004_726_en.pdf

Hendriksen, C., Arciniega, J.L., Bruckner, L. et al. (2008). The consistency approach for the quality control of vaccines. *Biologicals* 36 (1): 73–77.

USDA. (2007). VSM No. 800.203: General Licensing Considerations: Compatibility of Components. www.aphis.usda.gov/animal_health/vet_biologics/publications/memo_800_203.pdf

USDA. (2010). VSM No. 800.207: General Licensing Considerations: Target Animal Safety (TAS) Studies Prior to Product Licensure – VICH Guideline 44. www.aphis.usda.gov/animal_health/vet_biologics/publications/memo_800_207.pdf

USDA. (2016). VSM No. 800.202: General Licensing Considerations: Efficacy Studies for Prophylactic and Therapeutic Biologics. www.aphis.usda.gov/animal_health/vet_biologics/publications/memo_800_202.pdf

USDA. (2018a). VSM No. 800.201. General Licensing Considerations: Backpassage Studies. www.aphis.usda.gov/animal_health/vet_biologics/publications/memo_800_201.pdf

USDA. (2018b). VSM No. 800.204: General Licensing Considerations: Field Safety Studies. www.aphis.usda.gov/animal_health/vet_biologics/publications/memo_800_204.pdf

VICH. (2007). International Cooperation on Harmonisation of Technical Requirements of Veterinary Medicinal Products VICH Guideline 41 (VICH GL41): Target Animal Safety: Examination of Live Veterinary Vaccines in Target Animals for Absence of Reversion to Virulence. www.ema.europa.eu/en/documents/scientific-guideline/vich-gl41-target-animal-safety-examination-live-veterinary-vaccines-target-animals-absence-reversion_en.pdf

VICH. (2008). International Cooperation on Harmonisation of Technical Requirements of Veterinary Medicinal Products. VICH GL 44: Target animal safety for veterinary live and inactivated vaccines. www.ema.europa.eu/en/documents/scientific-guideline/vich-gl44-target-animal-safety-veterinary-live-inactived-vaccines-step-7_en.pdf

VICH. (2010). International Cooperation on Harmonisation of Technical Requirements of Veterinary Medicinal Products VICH GL 45 quality: bracketing and matrixing designs for stability testing of new veterinary drug substances and medicinal products. www.ema.europa.eu/en/documents/scientific-guideline/vich-gl-45-quality-bracketing-matrixing-designs-stability-testing-new-veterinary-drug-substances_en.pdf

VST Act. (1913). The Virus-Serum-Toxin Act of 1913. Chapter 5 Viruses, serums, toxins, antitoxins and analagous products. www.aphis.usda.gov/animal_health/vet_biologics/publications/vsta.pdf

15

Aspects of Vaccine Accessibility and Commercialization

Alasdair King[1] *and John Atkinson*[2]

[1] *Merck Animal Health, Madison, New Jersey, USA*
[2] *MSD Animal Health, Milton Keynes, Buckinghamshire, UK*

15.1 Introduction

As countries focus on taking a preventive approach to disease control and strive to reduce the use of antimicrobial treatments, vaccines are increasingly important. Over the last 30 years great strides have been taken in making vaccines accessible for use in animals throughout the world. In the USA alone, there are over 1900 biological products covering more than 200 different diseases (Roth 2011). Despite this, vaccines comprise only around a quarter of the total animal health product market (Meeusun et al. 2007).

While the technology and knowledge exist to produce vaccines to help protect against a wide range of diseases affecting many different species globally, not all of these have moved from the research stage to commercial availability.

Although the range of hosts and pathogens is greater in animal health than human health, market prices are lower and the market size is smaller so that the individual value of vaccines is less. This reduced market value is countered to a degree by the comparatively lower costs of research which result from a slightly simpler regulatory process in the animal health field. Despite this, research driven by the pharmaceutical industry tends to focus on key species and diseases that can have a global market. Public institutes, donor organizations, or government requirements may lead to research in more niche areas but at some stage, to make the vaccine widely available, the research needs to be taken to final production which normally requires a demonstrable commercial market. In veterinary medicine, vaccine accessibility and commercialization are strongly linked and, in the majority of cases, if a vaccine does not have a sustainable commercial market then it is unlikely to be made accessible.

It is also noteworthy that availability is not distributed equally, with North America and Western Europe accounting for over half of the overall global revenue from veterinary vaccines (fmi 2016) (Figure 15.1). Even in regions where a vaccine is commercialized, there may be limitations to packaging sizes available or the species on a license may vary from country to country depending on local registration requirements. There are many factors that dictate if a vaccine should be commercialized and, if so, in which countries and which presentations.

In order for a product to become available in a country, it has to go through a number of stages, from research and development through to commercialization, including proof of principle followed by proof of concept (Figure 15.2). At each point, go/no-go decisions have to be made and these are reflected in a business case that must support the process, even for a vaccine funded through donor organizations or government research. Taking into consideration all the factors above, including the difficulty of discovering a product with the correct characteristics to survive in the market, the probability of a product successfully transitioning from the discovery phase all the way through to global commercialization is around 20–30% (percentage derived from discussion with discovery and R&D experts).

There are four main reasons for the development of veterinary vaccines. First, vaccines for companion animals focus on improving health and welfare; second, vaccines for livestock are developed to increase production while being cost-effective; and third, a small number look to reduce and prevent disease transmission for animals to humans. The fourth and final reason, food security for the future, has recently become an additional concern. However, the unsolved issue with the third and fourth categories is who should pay, veterinary health or human

Veterinary Vaccines: Principles and Applications, First Edition. Edited by Samia Metwally, Gerrit Viljoen, and Ahmed El Idrissi.

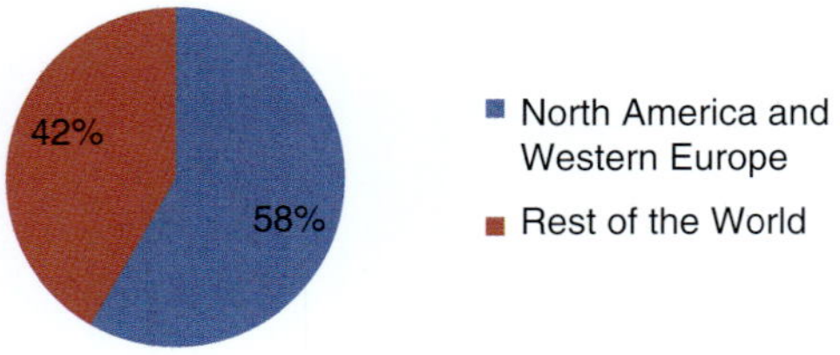

Figure 15.1 Veterinary vaccines market, 2015, by revenue. Source: Future Market Insights (fmi 2016).

health, and until this is solved then the value of the markets will remain relatively low.

Nonetheless, all these reasons have a direct influence on the commercialization and accessibility of veterinary vaccines. Veterinary pharmaceutical companies have commercial interests, generally with shareholders, and have to make a profit so there must be a value to any product and any market. Donor organizations want to see a return on their investment, often in the form of sustainable usage models, and governments need to balance the risk of a disease against the cost of developing a vaccine.

15.2 Development

15.2.1 Research and Development

Typically, the research-driven animal health companies (as opposed to generics) invest around 8–12% of their sales income back into R&D (IP Pragmatics n.d.). It has been estimated that, in normal situations, the R&D component of a new biological (vaccine) will take between 5 and 7 years (IFAH 2008). While there have been a few notable exceptions in response to emerging diseases, for instance vaccines to protect against Schmallenberg virus and bluetongue serotype 8 virus in Europe were granted provisional licences (Animal Research Info n.d.) within 2 years of the disease emerging, in these cases the R&D continued even after the product was available on the market in order to complete the necessary research for a full licence.

As well as deciding on the best scientific approach to a vaccine, scalability is also important. Vaccines that can be produced at laboratory level are not always stable when scaled up to commercial level.

15.2.2 Registration and Legislation

Regulatory processes take between 1.5 and 3 years (IFAH 2008) after R&D is completed. There is evidence that over the last 15 years, the overall time to market has increased within the European Union (EU) (EMA 2016), and this is probably true for other regional markets as well.

Markets must be identified at this stage to allow submissions to regulatory departments. National policies and legislation can play a large part in the commercialization of a product. As it is not possible to get one "global" license, companies must select the key markets in which to introduce a new product. With new technologies, early discussions with the authorities to address concerns can be beneficial for all parties involved.

Generally, veterinary vaccines must be proven to be safe and, to a lesser extent, efficacious. The emphasis on these two factors varies between countries and regional organizations. In some countries, it is considered that market forces will address any lack of efficacy, although often the very low price of poor-quality vaccines may unfortunately mean that there remains a place for them.

In the USA, vaccines can fall under the jurisdiction of either the FDA or the USDA, both with its own

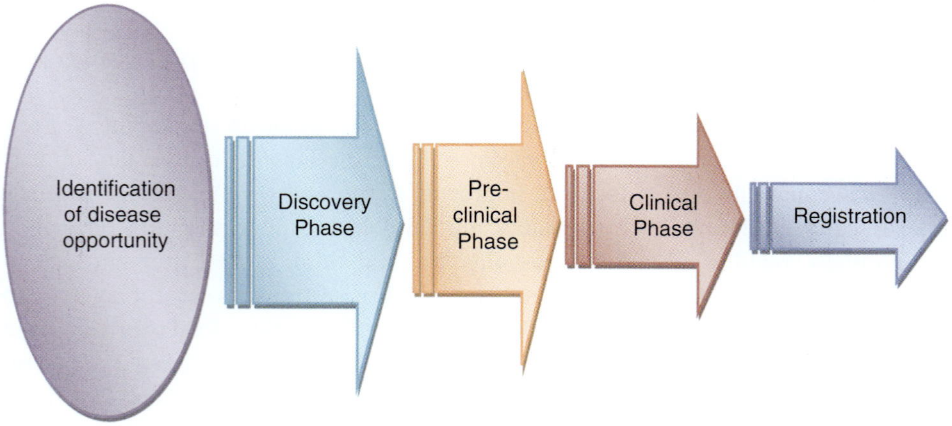

Figure 15.2 Stages in vaccine development.

requirements, depending on whether the vaccine is considered to be to improve production and reproduction or to control infectious disease respectively.

In the EU, vaccines may be licensed under one of three procedures, centralized, mutual recognition or decentralized, each with its own advantages and disadvantages. Some procedures can be simpler, or open up more opportunities than others. For instance, the centralized authorization procedure in the EU, while complex, provides a marketing authorization for all EU countries (EMA n.d.).

The many variations in legislation make the process potentially burdensome and deciding on the best route is a key skill within a company.

15.2.3 Market Size

While R&D work is taking place on the initial development of a product, the commercial department will be assessing the overall market size. Establishing a good market potential is essential to any decision to continue development. This becomes an issue when considering emerging diseases; with no historical data to support future markets, it can be difficult to justify the development of vaccines when compared with high-priority products with known market value. Hence products aimed at the major animal species and large, well-developed countries are more likely to see realization.

The commercial department also needs to determine likely pack sizes and minimum product requirements. Stability data need to be submitted to licensing authorities for each pack size and as these studies are, by nature, over long time periods they must be initiated as soon as possible. By setting minimum product requirements, based on understanding what is required in the market, then a product has more chance of success or can be stopped if those minima cannot be reached, thus avoiding extensive but useless investment.

15.2.4 Manufacturing Site

An important component of development is the decision on where the product will be manufactured. This is partly dictated by the potential market. For instance, products for the EU must be produced in an EU Good Manufacturing Practice-approved site, unless in exceptional circumstances such as an outbreak of a new disease, so an appropriately licensed site must be selected. Companies need to consider whether they can utilize a current site through accessing spare capacity or expansion, or whether a new site is required. Sites are often specialized toward the production of one or two types of vaccine, so a new vaccine with a different production method may not fit.

15.3 Commercialization

During the development cycle, as described above, it is important to hold regular meetings to ensure all these factors are on track. "Go/no-go" points are established. Assumptions must be challenged and checked. Only once all this is achieved may the product be commercialized. Cost, priority markets, and packaging must be considered. This is important to set the end price and to forecast initial volumes.

15.3.1 Manufacturing Site Costs

There are fixed costs associated with running a manufacturing plant. Staff, utilities, and routine maintenance represent ongoing costs that are, in large part, independent of how many doses are produced a year. In addition, different techniques and processes, depending on the type of vaccine, require different facilities. For instance, the current technology for foot and mouth disease (FMD) vaccines requires the handling of live virus and therefore any FMD plant must be built as biosecurity level 3 (BSL3), which requires a wide range of special control measures, including filters, negative pressure, and inactivation (CDC 2009). Maintaining such facilities, even before a dose of vaccine is produced, demands considerable investment.

The running costs of a plant have to be covered by the sales of the vaccine. As the costs are shared across the entire volume of vaccine produced, if the plant is running at near 100% capacity then the cost per dose is significantly lower (Figure 15.3). The drawback of running at high utilization is that there is little chance for the plant to suddenly respond to an increase in demand. If only a small proportion of the plant capacity is being utilized then there is greater ability to respond to market demand but the cost per dose is higher. For instance, if a vaccine is produced in a 100 million dose capacity plant costing US$10 million to operate then at 100% capacity, the fixed cost to the company is US$0.10 per dose but if the same plant actually only produces 10 million doses in the year then the fixed cost to the company is US$1.

15.3.2 Vaccine Costs

In addition to the fixed costs of running a manufacturing site, there are variable costs that are dependent on the type of vaccine. Adjuvants, stabilizers, and freeze-drying all add to the cost on top of the antigen production. There are costs for both upstream (handling of live organisms) and downstream (purification) processes. As the downstream process is responsible for ensuring no contaminants are found in the vaccine, this is usually the more expensive part of manufacture.

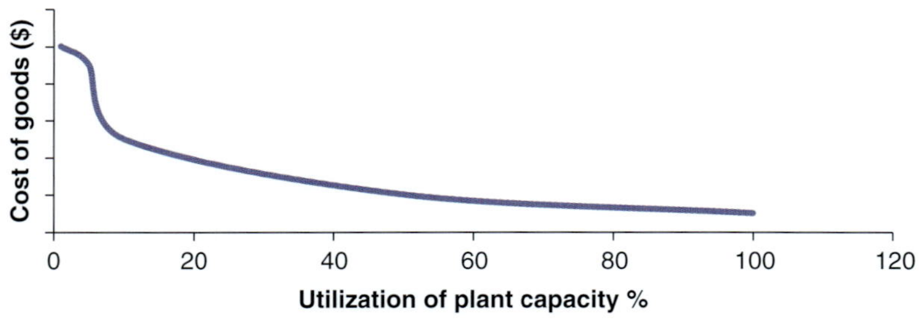

Figure 15.3 Impact of plant utilization on cost of goods.

15.3.3 Needs and Feasibility

While the initial commercial assessment is decided by establishing the overall potential for a product, once it is ready for production then each market has to be looked at individually. It is unlikely that manufacturing will be able to go into full-scale production immediately, so decisions have to be made as to the first markets to approach.

How a disease presents in each country may influence the need and therefore whether a vaccine is made available. For example, a vaccine may be available against a particular disease in one country, but if that disease presents differently elsewhere (e.g. strain variations, clinical impact) then the vaccine may not be licensed in other countries.

15.3.4 Basic Infrastructure

The infrastructure of a country as well as the company organization must also be considered. If the airports cannot handle large cargo planes, or the transport and warehouse system is not capable of maintaining a cold chain, then there may be little point in licensing a product in a particular country.

The logistical infrastructure of the manufacturer is important for how and where a product can be commercialized. For smaller companies, it can be difficult to manage the complex shipping requirements in order to deliver a product to another country. This can limit their options for where they can commercialize a product.

15.3.5 Packaging

For large animals, because of the wide variation in individual herd numbers, it is common for the manufacturing company to receive complaints from end-users regarding a lack of variety in packing sizes. Vaccines generally do not contain long-term preservatives and therefore any unused product should be discarded on the day of opening. This means that large vials can lead to a lot of wastage, with owners of smaller herds/flocks usually wanting to source smaller pack sizes.

However, there is little difference in fixed costs between processing a 100-dose vial and a five-dose vial. The necessary increase in price per dose to absorb these fixed costs can be prohibitive. For instance, if the costs for processing a vial are US$25 and the costs of the vaccine US$0.50 per dose then in a 50-dose vial the final cost of goods is US$50 or US$1 per dose. To produce the same vaccine in a five-dose vial then the cost of goods is US$27.50 or US$5.50 per dose (Figure 15.4).

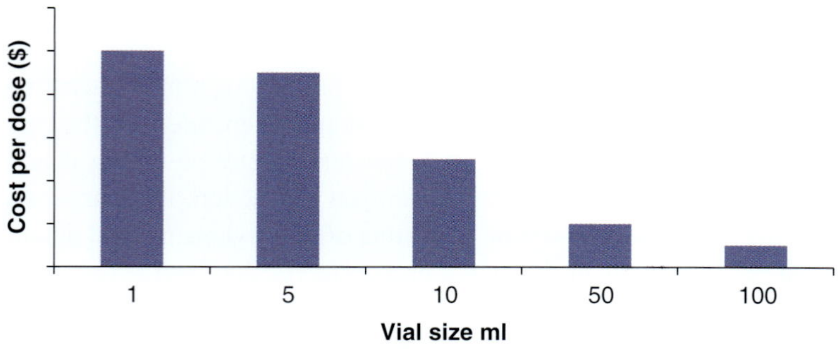

Figure 15.4 Impact of vial size on cost per dose.

15.4 Accessibility

15.4.1 Presales Support (Marketing)

Once the decision to commercialize in a country has been made, then it is up to the marketing and technical departments to properly prepare the potential prescribers and users. Exactly what can be said, and to whom, is often controlled by legislation in the individual country. Veterinary marketing is generally subject to very tight controls and is much more restricted than nonpharmaceutical markets. In many countries, direct comparisons with other products may not be made, exaggerated claims are not allowed, and certain words such as "safe" are closely controlled (NOAH 2015). The regulations may be self-governed through an industry body – for instance, the National Office of Animal Health in the UK publishes a Code of Practice for the Promotion of Animal Medicines.

It is important that veterinary surgeons and animal owners are properly educated and understand how the vaccine should be used, including the dose volume, frequency of dosing, and route of administration. Expectations need to be established so that prescribers and end-users understand any safety considerations, as well as what level of protection is afforded (e.g. prevention of infection, reduction of clinical signs, and/or reduction of shedding of the pathogen).

15.4.2 Distribution

Distribution networks vary considerably between countries. In some cases, products will go direct to the veterinary surgeon or trade retailer. In other countries, a wholesaler may act as a distributor from the pharmaceutical company to the end-user (Figure 15.5). Many products must be kept at strictly controlled temperatures, e.g. 2–8 °C, and there has long been suspicion that the lack of a cold chain in some countries has lead to vaccination failures in the field. There has been little robust research in animal health to support this but there are publications in the human health field confirming that the cold chain has an impact on field efficacy (Fowotade et al. 2015).

15.4.3 Final Vaccine Cost

The price of a vaccine to the end-user can vary considerably because, while vaccine manufacturers need to set a Notional List Price (NLP), they are not allowed to set the final price, which is decided by each prescriber and affected by market forces. The number of people in the distribution chain has a direct impact on cost as all require a margin of profit.

Exceptions to this include when governments and other bodies put out tenders for vaccines, such as FMD vaccines, and secure large volumes of a vaccine that is then made available at a set cost, or no cost.

In addition to the cost of the vaccine, there may be a cost attached to the vaccination equipment (e.g. automatic vaccinator, needles) and the time/labor needed to handle the animals and administer the vaccine. These latter costs may be less obvious, and can be reduced if vaccines have additional claims for concurrent or simultaneous use, which enable more than one vaccine to be administered to the same animal on the same day, thus reducing the number of handlings.

15.4.4 Postsales Support (Technical)

Especially in the case of new vaccines, significant training of veterinary surgeons and end-users may be necessary. Technical staff will arrange training and, in some cases, independent key opinion leaders may be used. Many companies provide dedicated support systems, including call centers and field representatives, to help respond to technical queries that veterinary surgeons and end-users may have about the products that have been purchased and used.

15.4.5 Pharmacovigilance

The need for pharmacovigilance was established after McBride wrote to the *Lancet* in 1961 and drew the connection between thalidomide and birth defects. Before this, there was no requirement for continued evidence of safety and efficacy (Emanuel et al. 2012).

Pharmaceutical companies now have a legal responsibility to monitor their products in the field. This is to help ensure that products are safe and efficacious. Any reports received should be investigated and then submitted to the authorities. While the vast majority of investigations indicate that the medicine is not the issue, in a few cases important facts have been learnt that have led to improved usage and safety.

15.4.6 Forecasting

Production of most vaccines takes 6–8 months (IFAH 2008). To maintain supply requires good forecasting to allow planning in manufacturing sites. As most veterinary sites produce more than one vaccine, scheduling is normally planned a year in advance. Sudden increases in demand can be difficult to accommodate as an increase in one vaccine would normally impact on the production of another vaccine. Emerging and reemerging diseases pose a particular forecasting problem, with demand in individual countries being hard to estimate with any degree of accuracy if the disease has not yet reached that country but is

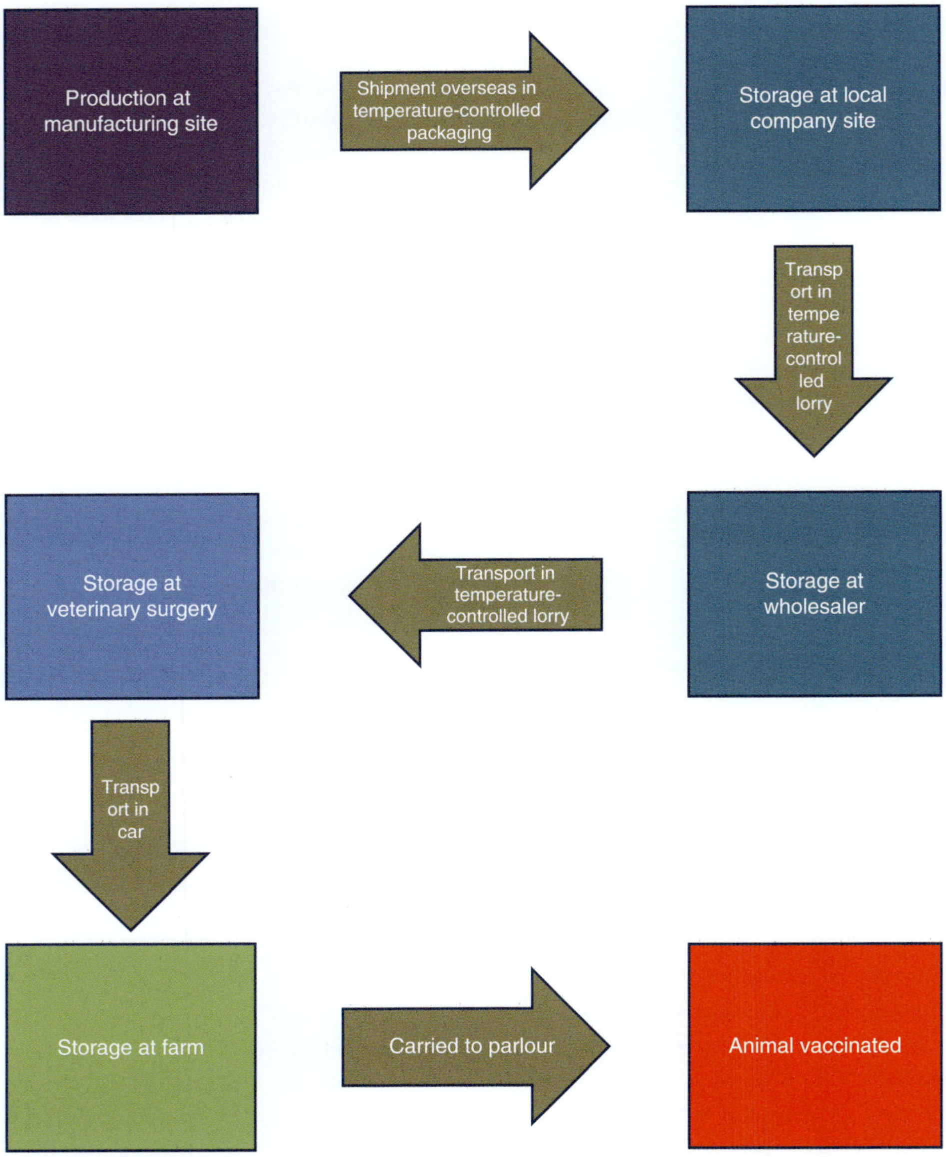

Figure 15.5 Possible distribution route for vaccine.

threatening to reach it. Veterinary surgeons and end-users may only want to vaccinate once the disease has been confirmed in the country, but then suddenly want access to large volumes. Companies will forecast what they expect is reasonable and, where possible, have a plan to upscale production in the event it is needed. For this reason, stable markets are more attractive to companies as they allow planning.

15.4.7 Subsidization and Cooperative Programs

There are a number of donor and nongovernment organizations working to improve vaccine accessibility in developing countries. These may provide funding for further research, for local manufacturing, or even supply product direct. In many cases, pharmaceutical companies may be involved with these as corporate social responsibility (CSR) projects. Because of the time lines and costs involved, it is unlikely that products will be specifically developed for these "low-value" markets but when the products exist, there is a great willingness in the animal health sector to support the use. These programs usually focus either on agriculture, e.g. FMD, or on "One Health," e.g. rabies.

The difficulty with this approach remains how to develop sustainable models. Models have shifted from the adoption of better farming practices to being people centered, then focusing on sustainable livelihoods, and finally the pro-poor livestock development paradigm (Heffernan 2012). Throughout, while vaccines are being subsidized then it is possible to increase the uptake but when the funding is withdrawn, the use of vaccines decline. For this reason, the focus for many organizations, such as the Global Alliance for Livestock Veterinary Medicine, has shifted toward the development and establishment of markets.

15.5 Challenges of Producing Vaccine in the Country

There is a place for both local companies addressing the needs for a single market and multinational companies addressing global requirements. While local production for a single country reduces the logistic demands of a product, it loses out on the efficiencies of scale when producing for a global market.

Although regulations and licensing requirements may be simpler in some developing countries, making the process of commercialization less expensive, the markets are also usually smaller than in developed countries. Ease of licensing versus size of market becomes a trade-off. In recent years, developing countries have started to adopt regulatory processes from Europe or America and this has the effect of making the overall process too burdensome. This increases the risk that levels of accessibility to medicines in poorer countries may become lower as companies concentrate on the large markets.

For small vaccine producers, the knowledge and skill levels available become a greater challenge. Large companies have departments and divisions specifically tasked with the upscale of production, bringing in global expertise where needed to tackle difficulties in the manufacturing process. Local companies do not have this knowledge base to draw upon, although they may be able to bring in consultants.

15.6 Antigen or Vaccine Bank Systems

In some cases, although a disease is not present in a country, the disease itself may still represent a significant threat to a national economy should there be an outbreak. This is particularly true of those diseases that are declared notifiable by the OIE. In these cases, an epidemic may mean that international trade is stopped.

Often the vaccines against these diseases are not commercially available and the government may actually prohibit general sale. In order to mitigate the risk, governments may consider establishing an antigen or vaccine bank. The concept behind a bank is that a certain number of doses are held, normally by the manufacturing company, in stock. In the case of an outbreak then the vaccine is quickly released by order of the government and distributed according to a predetermined plan.

The bank may be held as formulated vaccine or antigen, each with its own advantages and disadvantages. Antigen banks often cost less as the product only goes through final manufacturing if there is an outbreak and the bank is drawn on. In addition, antigen often has a longer shelf-life than final product. Vaccine banks can sometimes be run as rolling stock, so there is no risk of product expiring and, as the product is already packed, then it is ready to ship, leading to quicker delivery times.

15.7 Improving Accessibility

Despite the fact that vaccines represent the most cost-effective approach to improving animal health, for many diseases there are no vaccines or vaccines that are inadequate, especially in livestock. This can be because there is a lack of critical mass of researchers and a lack of funding (ILVAC 2014). This lack typically has the biggest impact on smallholder farmers in the poorest countries. In response to this, new business models are required, and organizations such as GALVmed and ILVAC are specifically trying to address this need.

Time to market remains a crucial barrier in many cases. There are two key approaches to reducing this. The first is to prioritize the necessary data required for a marketing authorization, setting a minimum standard which can be added to as time progresses, thus allowing an early phase vaccine on to the market. This is especially applicable if the vaccine is using older and well-understood technologies. The second is to develop a global standard so that one license allows access to a large number of markets, rather than needing to repeatedly move through the authorization process in different countries.

15.8 Summary

While the technology exists to produce a wide range of veterinary vaccines, commercialization and accessibility are governed by complex decisions made by animal health companies with reference to market sizes, disease profiles, logistics, and regulatory conditions in specific countries. This dictates in which countries products may be available, or even if they are available at all.

The steps from first concept to a product being accessible in a market involve many processes and people (Figure 15.6). Companies have to consider all the factors

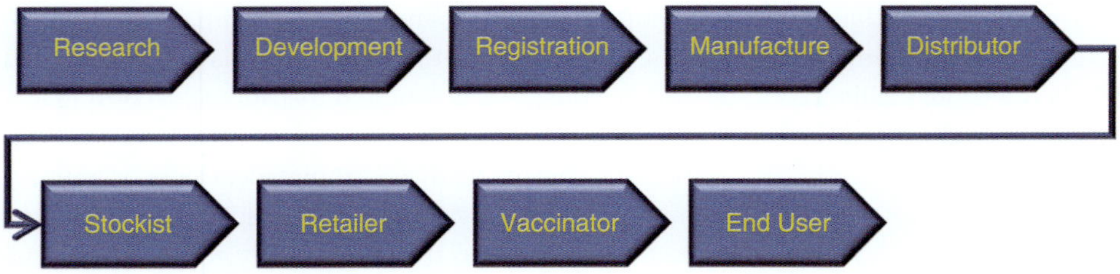

Figure 15.6 Possible steps to accessibility.

in order to establish the viability of a future vaccine. Marketers will examine the potential market and determine a possible price for selling the product. If the cost of goods is too high, or the vaccine cannot meet other market requirements such as duration of immunity, then the product may never reach a point of commercialization.

Once the decision is made to enter a market then the vaccine is supported through marketing and technical activities, as well as legal requirements to ensure efficacy and safety.

Emerging and transboundary diseases require special attention because the markets are less predictable and may fluctuate with changes in the disease. Being able to respond quickly to demands is an additional challenge.

In certain situations subsidized programs, funded by donor organizations or by governments recognizing a specific risk, may allow less commercial products to reach the market. However, without a sustainable model to drive the use of the product then such injections of money can be short-lived and not result in long-term control of disease. For this reason, public funding has limited effect on a company deciding whether to invest, although it may alter when a company decides to invest (IP Pragmatics n.d.). In addition, they can run the risk of supporting low-quality vaccines that can have a negative impact on public perceptions when they are accompanied by reactions or lack of efficacy.

In the long term, improved accessibility to medicines requires a new business model that allows high-quality producers to have a reliable and predictable market while supplying vaccines at an affordable cost to smallholders and developing countries.

References

Animal Research Info. (n.d.) Schmallenberg virus (SBV) and vaccine. www.animalresearch.info/en/medical-advances/veterinary-medicine/schmallenberg-virus-sbv-and-vaccine

Centers for Disease Control and Prevention (CDC) (2009). Section IV – Laboratory biosafety level criteria. In: *Biosafety in Microbiology and Biomedical Laboratories*. www.cdc.gov/labs/pdf/CDC-BiosafetyMicrobiological Biomedical Laboratories-2009-P.PDF

EMA (2016). Increasing the availability of veterinary vaccines in the EU. www.ema.europa.eu/ema/index.jsp?curl=pages/news_and_events/news/2016/08/news_detail_002584.jsp&mid=WC0b01ac058004d5c1

EMA. (n.d.). Authorisation of medicines. www.ema.europa.eu/ema/index.jsp?curl=pages/about_us/general/general_content_000109.jsp

Emanuel, M., Rawlins, M., Duff, G., and Breckenridge, A. (2012). Thalidomide and its sequelae. *Lancet* 380 (9844): 781–783.

fmi (Future Market Insights). (2016). Veterinary Vaccines Market: Faster Innovation and Better Relationship Management Key to Garner Higher Market Shares 2016–2026. www.marketwatch.com/press-release/veterinary-vaccines-market-faster-innovation-and-better-relationship-management-key-to-garner-higher-market-shares-2016-2026-2019-12-11?mod=mw_quote_news

Fowotade, A., Okonko, I.O., Nwabuisi, C. et al. (2015). Measles vaccine potency and sero-conversion rates among infants receiving measles immunization in Ilorin, Kwara State, Nigeria. *J. Immunoassay Immunochem.* 36 (2): 195–209.

Heffernan, C. (2012). Whatever happened to the pro-poor livestock development paradigm? Backcasting to a sustainable future for Africa's livestock keepers. https://assets.publishing.service.gov.uk/media/5aa6613ce5274a3e3603a61b/12_Abstract_paper_3__Heffernan_Final_18June13.pdf

IFAH. (2008). IFAH Europe Factsheet: Animal Vaccines: Development, Registration and Production. www.bft-online.de/fileadmin/bft/aktuelles/IEvaccstate_final__2_.pdf

ILVAC (2014). Planting the orchard – an ILRI livestock vaccine initiative (ILVAC). https://cgspace.cgiar.org/handle/10568/43795

IP Pragmatics. (n.d.). Commercialisation of veterinary pharmaceuticals and vaccines technology. www.ip-pragmatics.com/

Meeusen, E.N.T., Walker, J., Peters, A. et al. (2007). Current status of veterinary vaccines. *Clin. Microbiol. Rev.* 20 (3): 489–510.

NOAH. (2015). Code of Practice for the Promotion of Animal Medicines. www.noah.co.uk/wp-content/uploads/2016/04/Code-of-Practice-Booklet-26-effective-December-2015.pdf

Roth, J.A. (2011). Veterinary vaccines and their importance to animal health and public health. *Procedia Vaccinol.* 5: 127–136.

16

Vaccine Strategic Reserves

Paul Barnett[1] *and Alf-Eckbert Füssel*[2]

[1] *Veterinary Medicine Directorate, Addlestone, Surrey, UK*
[2] *Animal Health and Welfare Unit, European Commission, Brussels, Belgium*

16.1 Introduction

Agriculture is continually subjected to the threats and economic consequences of a variety of livestock diseases. Under certain circumstances, where it is considered that vaccination can provide an effective disease control tool, particularly for emergency outbreak management, successful implementation of a vaccination program may depend upon the accessibility and amounts of vaccine available. The need to have a reliable and rapid supply of large quantities of a vaccine, particularly one which might not normally be readily available, has led to many countries establishing strategic vaccine reserves.

Strategic vaccine reserves, or banks, as an adjunct to the control of important veterinary diseases go back to the late 1960s and early 1970s in their development and the best examples are those established for control of the highly contagious foot and mouth disease (FMD). The severe impact on livestock productivity, and international trade resulting from FMD has led to many countries, and in particular those which are disease free, having contingency plans in place which, depending on circumstance, may include so-called emergency vaccination as a control measure. "Emergency vaccine" and "emergency vaccination" can have different connotations, but the terms are usually applied to make a distinction from routine prophylactic (preventive) vaccination (OIE 2016b).

Foot and mouth disease has seven serotypes and within each serotype a number of strains that exhibit varying degrees of antigenic diversity. This has led to the availability of a wide range of different vaccine strains and the continual need to monitor vaccine suitability and performance and, when required, develop new vaccine strains. In an emergency situation, the vaccine must protect as rapidly as possible and it was the recognition that an appropriate vaccine of sufficient potency and quantity may not be immediately available commercially which highlighted the need to have instantaneous access to vaccines to support contingency plans.

Indeed, the report from the Northumberland Commission, set up to review the circumstances of the 1967–1968 UK FMD outbreak, recommended a routinely maintained, bulk reserve of formulated vaccine for emergency use (Northumberland 1969). Though this recommendation was implemented, it was quickly recognized that an alternative approach was required, given the financial burden of constantly needing to replace the vaccines because of their limited shelf-life and changing strain requirements to meet new threats. Such an alternative approach was developed in Denmark and the practice of storing concentrated FMD antigens over liquid nitrogen for use after subsequent formulation (Lei and McKercher 1979) predisposed the USA to establish its own emergency reserve using this principle. Canada and Mexico later subscribed to the US bank, which became the first international strategic reserve, namely, the North American vaccine bank. There are now a considerable number of reserves established globally, which are organized in different ways.

Strategic reserves have not only supported their members (Muroga et al. 2012) but have provided vaccines to countries not directly associated to them. The European Union (EU) vaccine bank, also referred to as the European Commission vaccine bank, which was formally established in 1991 by Council Decision 91/666/EEC (European Communities 1991), has, for example, provided emergency vaccine to Albania and the former Yugoslav Republic of Macedonia in 1996, Morocco and Algeria in 1999, the Far East in 2000, Turkey in 2000, 2006, and 2007, Iran, Lebanon, and Iraq in 2009, Zambia in 2010, Tunisia and Algeria in

Veterinary Vaccines: Principles and Applications, First Edition. Edited by Samia Metwally, Gerrit Viljoen, and Ahmed El Idrissi.

2014, and more recently Mauritius in 2016. However, the administration of FMD vaccine from EU antigen banks has not, to date, been used in EU member states, partly as a result of old trade rules that encompassed a lengthy delay in regaining FMD-free trading status after using vaccine as well as the absence of reliable DIVA (differentiating infected from vaccinated animals) testing strategies (Lombard and Füssel 2007). The trade rules are now considered more favorable for implementing emergency vaccination, and there have been significant developments in the available DIVA tests.

It is accepted that strategic vaccine reserves have an important supporting role in the control of a number of other veterinary diseases. The World Organization for Animal Health (OIE) has developed global experience in the management of vaccine banks and delivery of vaccines against avian influenza (AI), rabies (vaccination of dogs), and peste des petits ruminants (PPR), through the financial support of many countries or charitable institutions. These OIE vaccine banks have been established through international calls for tender and selection procedures that encompass autonomous committees of appropriate experts and representatives of the donor bodies, and have played a key part in disease control (http://www.oie.int/support-to-oie-members/vaccine-bank). For example, both the regional and global AI vaccine banks, which were set up by the OIE in 2006 and 2007 respectively, facilitated the delivery of 62017 million H5N2 doses of vaccines to Mauritania, Senegal, Egypt, Mauritius, Ghana, Togo, and Vietnam. The establishment of a PPR vaccine bank for the provision of high-quality PPR vaccines to eligible African countries in 2013 not only ensured the timely supply of high-quality vaccines that complied with international standards, but also facilitated the harmonization of PPR control methods in Africa. Through this bank, the OIE delivered 8 million doses of PPR vaccine to three African countries up until July 2014.

The efficiency with which the OIE procured its vaccines for such reserves did not go unnoticed and led to the World Health Organization (WHO) placing all of its orders for rabies vaccines for dogs through the OIE Rabies vaccine bank in 2014, which, as of March 2016, facilitated the WHO in the delivery of 7.85 million doses of rabies vaccines. This bank is principally a rolling stock of vaccines produced as and when required and supplied by the manufacturer, selected through an international call for tender to beneficiary countries, upon official request from their veterinary services (www.oie.int/fileadmin/Home/eng/Media_Center/docs/pdf/Rabies_portal/EN_BrochRVB.pdf). The OIE has also established a regional FMD vaccine bank for Asia with the aim of supporting targeted immunization in buffer zones around FMD-free zones, well-defined areas at risk of FMD resurgence, hotspots where vaccination should contribute in reducing the risks of disease and areas where exceptional circumstances exist that merit the consideration of vaccine supplies (www.oie.int/en/support-to-oie-members/vaccine-bank/).

Overall, it is perceived that the supply of vaccines from these OIE regional and global vaccine banks for different diseases provides benefits in quality, supply, cost, and coordination, (OIE 2014), with priority given to developing countries with the lowest GDP that have no immediate access to high-quality vaccines. However, in order to be eligible, such countries must provide justification of their need, as well as information on the epidemiological, logistical, and administrative frameworks that would encompass their use. For example, in the case of the need for rabies vaccine, the applicant country, beside submitting a "Specific Request for Rabies Vaccine Delivery" to the OIE Director-General, through the OIE sub-regional office (that includes a commitment that veterinary services of the country will facilitate the importation of the vaccines), must in particular:

- prove that there is an increase in biting rates and human mortality; that the location of the outbreak(s) increases the risk of spread to people and/or animals; and that further spread of the disease could occur
- provide a statement that the national veterinary services are engaged and will have the authority to implement or supervise the vaccination of dogs
- submit a specific vaccination control strategy
- specify the nature and quantities of vaccines required
- agree to international transportation conditions.

Notably, relevant nongovernmental organizations (NGOs) can have access to the rabies vaccine bank if they implement dog vaccination campaigns under the supervision of official veterinary services and they inform the beneficiaries on the origin of the vaccines (www.oie.int/for-the-media/press-releases/detail/article/oie-regional-vaccine-bank-for-asia-provides-50000-rabies-vaccines-to-lao-pdr).

The Global Alliance for Livestock Veterinary Medicines (GALVmed) is a not-for-profit, public-private partnership and registered charity that also supports developing countries by working with its partners to make a sustainable difference in the access to animal health products for poor livestock keepers (see Chapter 3). Its focus is on key diseases under four categories, namely cattle, small ruminant, swine, and avian diseases that are most relevant to poverty reduction and improved livelihoods. GALVmed is working on contagious bovine pleuropneumonia (CBPP) which is one of the most serious transboundary diseases in Africa, as well as contagious caprine pleuropneumonia

(CCPP), a disease capable of killing 60–100% of affected goats. Both CBPP and CCPP are highly contagious diseases caused by members of the *Mycoplasma* genus. Though successfully eradicated from Australia, North America, and Europe by slaughter in the 1960s, CBPP remains endemic in eastern Africa and parts of western, central, and southern Africa. Through three interrelated programs of study, GALVmed is evaluating the use of antimicrobials as well as improved production processes for an existing T1/44 vaccine and the so-called BEN-1 vaccine that has been developed in China, with a potential view to future development.

Though at this stage it is unclear whether an improved vaccine for CBPP will lead to the establishment of its own vaccine bank, GALVmed has previously supported such an approach for another disease, Rift Valley fever (RVF). At the invitation of GALVmed, 15 experts from a range of public and private sector organizations assembled in Pretoria in 2011 to discuss the technical feasibility of a strategic stock of RVF vaccine consisting of bulk preformulated vaccine antigen or bottled vaccine. The experts agreed that it was feasible to consider a strategic reserve based on the RVF clone 13 vaccine (RVF C13), for use in RVF-endemic areas. Such a reserve might consist of 50 million doses, with capacity to promptly manufacture a further 20 million doses during a confirmed outbreak. A number of other practicalities were considered including alternative storage sites, where the bulk antigen, already quality controlled by the producer, could be stored at ultra-low temperature, and be ready for rapid bottling, freeze-drying, and despatch when required and use of the OIE guidelines for setting up and operating such a bank (www.galvmed.org/wp-content/uploads/2016/07/GALVmed-newsletter-April-2012.pdf). The implementation of a RVF bank has also been under discussion.

GALVmed is one of the members of the Steering Committee of the African Union Pan African Veterinary Vaccine Centre (AU/PANVAC) established in 2004 to promote the use of good-quality vaccines and reagents for the control and eradication of animal diseases in Africa (see Chapter 3).

In the European Union, Council Directive 82/894/EEC of 21 December 1982 on the notification of animal diseases in the Community (European Communities 1982) lists, in Part A of Annex I, 24 diseases of terrestrial animals which are subject to notification, all of which are traditionally considered to have a major impact on animal health and trade, and in some cases are also zoonotic. Regulation (EU) 2016/429 ("Animal Health Law") (European Union 2016) provides a list of diseases of Union concern and procedures to list, prioritize, and categorize such diseases. While FMD, African and classic swine fever (CSF), highly pathogenic AI, and African horse sickness (AHS) are specifically mentioned in Article 5 of that Regulation, other diseases are listed in Annex II to that Regulation and are subject to review with a view to amend that Annex where necessary. Listed diseases are to be categorized according to the criteria set out in Annex IV to that Regulation and disease prevention and control measures shall be defined. One of the four categories of diseases defined in that Regulation is transmissible diseases that normally do not occur in the EU and which are subject to immediate eradication. For the control and eradication of those diseases, the EU Commission may establish antigen and vaccine banks.

However, only some of these diseases have been identified as justifying, in principle, the establishment of strategic reserves of emergency vaccine and these are AI, CSF, AHS, and bluetongue (European Commission 2010). More recently, the EU Commission established a vaccine bank for lumpy skin disease (European Commission 2015), which, in the case of incursion, is solely intended to provide a first line of defense through the supply of a limited number of vaccine doses necessary to contain the disease until the affected EU member states or neighboring non-EU countries have made their own arrangements to procure further vaccine for the continued control of the disease. Nevertheless, it is often the perceived low market demand for such vaccines and the consequential low return on investment that have hindered manufacturers in developing strategies for storing these other vaccines in reserves.

A good example was the manufacture of a number of batches of inactivated AHS serotype 4 and vesicular stomatitis antigen (House et al. 1992, 2003; Sanchez Vizcaino 2004) for freezing and subsequent reformulation in the early 1990s, by a commercial producer. In consideration of the establishment of a reserve of vaccines against AHS, the EU, with a total equid population of about 7 million animals, estimated the immediate need of monovalent live attenuated freeze-dried vaccines against AHS at 100 000 doses for each of the serotypes 1, 2, 3, 4, 6, 7, and 8 of the vaccine described in Section 2.5.1. of the *Manual of Diagnostic Tests and Vaccines for Terrestrial Animals* 2012, in the version adopted by the World Assembly of Delegates of the OIE in May 2017 (European Commission 2009; OIE 2017). The procurement was, however, not accomplished for contractual reasons.

However, the OIE in cooperation with the Fédération Equestre Internationale and the International Federation of Horseracing Authorities commissioned a study into the availability and efficacy of AHS vaccines and vaccine candidates and into the economics of the use of modern vaccines against AHS (OIE 2016a).

With respect to CSF, significant successes, such as that seen following oral vaccination of wild boar in certain parts of the EU, created enough interest to establish a reserve which has been used before the end of its shelf-life in the successful vaccination of large-scale pig herds in Romania in the last decade (European Commission 2010).

While the approach of relying on strategic reserves for a number of other important veterinary diseases has seen greater momentum in recent years, the associated use of diagnostic tests to support vaccines from such reserves in an emergency has become a hugely important issue (European Commission 2010). Indeed, the credibility of emergency vaccination is now seen by some to be directly linked to the availability of effective diagnostic tools that can be used to substantiate that vaccinated animals, or the meat and meat products obtained from them, are free from infection and can be safely used for trade (European Commission 2010). To this end, establishing a strategic reserve for many diseases today will go hand in hand with establishing the necessary diagnostics to support the use of vaccines and may in turn lead to so-called diagnostic banks.

Where animals vaccinated in an emergency are kept alive and eventually slaughtered for human consumption (so-called "vaccination to live"), an assurance is required that the vaccines to be administered have a marketing authorization for use in food-producing animals, which includes not only consideration of maximum residue limits of key components but also the indicated shelf-life of the antigens and the vaccines reconstituted from them. This in turn has a significant effect on the storage time of antigens and the need to organize the timely turnover and replacement of antigens in banks.

The question of whether vaccine stockpiles are still required, or are a liability, after a disease has been eradicated globally became pressing after the world was declared officially free from rinderpest infection at the OIE General Session in May 2011. Rinderpest virus stocks, vaccines, and associated biological samples are still stored in over 40 different laboratories worldwide. There is now concerted effort by the OIE and the Food and Agriculture Organization of the United Nations (FAO) to safely destroy or transfer such potential sources of infection to a minimum number of approved high-containment laboratories in order to minimize accidental release or potential for a deliberate act of bioterrorism. To this end, all OIE and FAO member countries agreed to destroy remaining virus samples or to safely store them in a minimum number of approved high-containment laboratories, to remain vigilant to reoccurrences of the disease, and to cease all unapproved research activities. The OIE has designated a small number of facilities as approved for holding rinderpest virus-containing material, which will be subject to reevaluation every 3 years (www.oie.int/for-the-media/rinderpest).

16.2 Types of Strategic Reserves or Banks

Strategic reserves are recognized as being essentially of two types: those that hold the final end-product, a ready-to-use fully formulated vaccine, and a reserve, which principally holds the active component for subsequent formulation (OIE 2016b). In the latter case, the active components are stored under conditions which maintain their integrity for a considerable period of time and in excess of the normal shelf-life of the final formulated product. This is the approach that has been usually adopted for FMD, because of the economic benefits, particularly in relation to the continual need for replacing formulated FMD vaccines that exceed their shelf-life (OIE 2016b).

However, the availability of a fully formulated product provides almost instantaneous access in an emergency situation, in contrast to any delay that might result from the need to subsequently formulate the active component, and for this reason there are some reserves that hold both types.

Beside a bank being classified based on the type of holding component, reserves can also be categorized in accordance with their governance and/or location. There are essentially four types:

- National, government-administered and -financed vaccine banks.
- International, government-administered and -financed vaccine banks.
- Commercially maintained vaccine banks.
- Vaccine banks organized by international organizations based on contracts with commercial producers, e.g. the vaccine bank for rabies, PPR, and FMD established by the OIE (2016b).

Apart from those FMD strategic reserves already maintained within a commercial environment, all the other FMD reserves are essentially holding facilities located at a different site which, during an emergency, would require the active ingredient to be returned to the original manufacture for formulation. Though this may delay the acquisition and administration of these vaccines in the field, it may be necessary for legal reasons in some countries, and during any delay, the time can be used constructively in preparation for the vaccination campaign.

In contrast, the former International FMD Vaccine Bank (IVB), based at Pirbright in the UK, was the only example of a strategic reserve that had its own blending facility which could independently formulate its emergency vaccines. Following a request, it successfully formulated and dispatched 500 000 doses of vaccine during the UK's 2001 outbreak, although the vaccine was not subsequently used. However, after 16 years' existence, it became increasingly clear that a significant financial investment would be required for it to continue formulating products with marketing authorization from the Veterinary Medicines Directorate, which subsequently led to the IVB being officially dissolved in 2003.

Having vaccine banks maintained by the commercial vaccine manufacturer itself has become more attractive in recent years, as the co-locality of antigen component in a strategic reserve with manufacturing facilities has obvious benefits and maintains the Good Manufacturing Practice (GMP) conditions throughout the production chain under the responsibility of the holder of the marketing authorization. As a result, there has been a significant shift by both national governments and international organizations to follow this route in the administration and financing of reserves of antigens or vaccines. Nevertheless, a certain delay of at least 48–72 hours is usually built into contractual arrangements, for example, to allow the manufacturer to complete other ongoing formulation commitments.

16.3 Requirements for Strategic Reserves or Banks

Foremost in the establishment of a strategic reserve is the need to set up a managerial system to run and maintain it and this can be complicated depending on the number of member countries involved. Formal agreements are required between members of the reserve, not only in relation to the financial commitments associated with establishing and maintaining such a facility, but also specific to the drawing rights for each individual member. For example, some smaller member countries may consider that they do not require access to all the quantities of a specific vaccine that may be in the reserve. A good example of the managerial organization of a reserve was that set up originally for the IVB. Its executive body was a commission, comprising the Chief Veterinary Officers (CVOs) of all the member countries, which was chaired by the UK CVO and empowered to take decisions relating to the activities of the IVB. According to the agreement it established between the member countries, the administering authority of the IVB was the UK Ministry of Agriculture, Fisheries and Food (MAFF), which later became the Department for Environment, Food and Rural Affairs (DEFRA), and provided a Secretariat. Scientific staff at the Institute for Animal Health, Pirbright, managed and maintained the IVB facility and the Director of the IVB was the Head of the Pirbright Laboratory. Advice upon the selection of foot and mouth disease virus (FMDV) antigens held by this reserve and other technical matters was provided by a technical advisory group consisting of FMD world experts.

According to Council Directive 2003/85/EC, the EU grants access to the stocks of antigens in its FMD antigen bank to all member states of the EU regardless of whether they maintain their own national bank or not, and whether vaccination is initiated by the member state itself or based on a decision taken by all member states (European Union 2003).

The regulatory requirements for any veterinary medicinal product must be uppermost in the decision process of countries who wish to establish and utilize vaccine from a strategic reserve. As an example, all veterinary medicinal products that are placed on the EU market must hold a marketing authorization addressing the EU requirements for such authorizations. This provides assurance on the quality, safety, and efficacy of the product and in doing so conveys a degree of confidence to the authorities tasked with the decision to use these products. Moreover, Council Directive 2003/85/EC, in regard to policy on the control of FMD, places more emphasis on the use of vaccines as part of a vaccinate-to-live policy (European Union 2003). This makes the issue of using an authorized product even more important, particularly where there is intention to use these vaccinated animals subsequently in the food chain with the support of authorities responsible for human health. The specific requirements for the authorization of vaccines against FMD has been summarized by the European Medicines Agency, and this position paper may serve as a template for the evaluation of vaccines used against pathogens characterized by genetic and antigenic diversity (EMA 2002).

When authorizing vaccines, including those against FMD, account should be taken of the risks of transmitting animal spongiform encephalopathy agents via medicinal products (European Commission 2001a,b) including guidelines to be considered to minimize those risks (European Commission 2011).

The importance of a licensed product cannot be overemphasized. The EU requires that the antigens held in the EU antigen bank, and the vaccines reconstituted from them, have a marketing authorization in at least one of the member states (European Union 2003) and Article 7 of Directive 2001/82/EC allows member states, in particular, to administer to animals veterinary medicinal products which have been authorized by another member state in accordance with that Directive. Nevertheless, Article 8 of Directive 2001/82/EC (European Union 2001) permits, in the event of serious epizootic diseases, the provisional use of immunological veterinary medicinal products (IVMPs) without a marketing authorization, in the absence of a suitable authorized medicinal product and after informing the Commission of the detailed conditions of use. While this provision would be applicable in case of vaccination with a particular vaccine not available in the EU, such as vaccines against bluetongue in 2000 or lumpy skin disease in 2015, in the EU, it would not apply to antigens stored in the EU FMD antigen bank.

A number of immunological products are covered by individual monographs in official pharmacopeias to which the standards for safety, efficacy, sterility, and quality are detailed (see Chapter 13). Indeed, they may also provide guidance that is specific to products destined for strategic reserves. Even in the absence of a specific monograph, referral can be made to the introductory chapters of the OIE *Manual of Diagnostic Tests and Vaccines for Terrestrial Animals* (OIE 2018) where minimum standards are set and would still apply (Chapters 2.3.3, 2.3.4, and 2.3.5). Reserves should comply with requirements for stockpiling and formulation in premises that follow GMP and are officially quality assured. Such facilities and their activities should be guided by standard operating procedures (SOPs) which are routinely reviewed. Strategic reserves also benefit from being officiated by a suitable Qualified Person (QP) and certified as holding an appropriate manufacturing license.

It is also well to remember that, beside the antigen component/s, any adjuvant or other pharmacologically active ingredient used in the formulation of the vaccine must also conform to the necessary guideline requirements, not least those relating to residues in food-producing species.

The primary containers, outer containers, labeling, holding vessels or equipment, and storage areas within a building must comply with the required national or internationally accepted standards of GMP. Though this should be the case when a reserve is located in a "licensed" vaccine plant that is scrutinized under routine inspection by the licensing authority, those outside such jurisdiction will need to seek guidance from such authorities on what the required standards should be. This is particularly true of a reserve that is co-located or associated with a laboratory or other facility that handles live pathogens, where adequate separation and, where necessary, quarantining of personnel associated to this bank must be assured.

Outside the strategic storage facilities themselves, countries should recognize the importance of good contingency planning to ensure stored vaccine or active component is distributed and administered in an efficient and speedy manner. In this regard, managers of such banks should be fully aware of the steps in a decision tree and the processes by which the appropriate authority can call a given reserve into action to supply vaccine to requesting countries. Steps should also be put into place for guaranteed accessibility to storage and transportation facilities, including those that allow a suitable uninterrupted cold chain that maintains the integrity of the product.

How emergency vaccine is applied strategically in the field is a governmental decision, though it should be administered in line with the veterinary product literature that accompanies the vaccine. Vaccination protocols, the establishment of well-trained vaccination teams, as well as all the other necessary documentation, equipment, reagents, and clothing which need to be sufficiently stockpiled to support any required vaccination campaign, although highly important, are also considered to be the responsibility of appropriate governmental bodies and outside the remit of any given strategic reserve. Managers and technical staff of strategic reserves can, however, support these additional contingency steps in an advisory capacity. For assurance that all the necessary steps are in place to effectively instigate an emergency vaccination campaign from reserve to the field, it is recommended that periodic outbreak simulations and exercises are carried out by all parties that would be involved in the implementation of emergency vaccination.

16.4 What and How Much Vaccine Should Be Stored in a Strategic Reserve?

The types, strains, and quantities of vaccines that should be stored in strategic reserves are dependent on a number of factors. For example, there are five types of AI vaccines available, namely inactivated, live, subunit, recombinant vectors expressing AI genes, and DNA vaccines, and each has its advantages and disadvantages. There may, of course, be other better AI vaccines being developed, some of which may improve the logistics of vaccination coverage by route of application. However, only a minority will be licensed for use in some countries and this is likely to be an overriding factor in the choice of vaccine type stored.

OFFLU, the joint network of expertise on animal influenza between the FAO and OIE (www.offlu.net/), recommends that countries should ensure the availability of a sufficient amount of quality-controlled vaccine to support contingency plans, through the establishment of vaccine banks and/or strategic stockpiling of vaccines and/or specific arrangements with vaccine producers. It also promotes the introduction of systems for fast-track registration of vaccines containing updated seed strains, investment in quality vaccine production, and the timely withdrawal from the market of poorly matched vaccines (OFFLU 2013).

Ultimately, though, such vaccines must be safe and of high quality in respect of international standards and guidelines in order to achieve a high degree of protection against clinical signs and a significant reduction in excretion and transmission of the pathogen target itself. To this end, both onset and duration of immunity following vaccination in the intended target host should, if possible, be well defined, with onset being as rapid as possible, considering use under emergency conditions. In this context, the potency of the vaccine is considered to be an important issue and higher potency FMD vaccines, principally by use of a higher antigen dose payload, have normally been the choice for emergency reserves, the benefits of which, including a more rapid onset and antigenically broader protection, are well documented (Barnett et al. 2013). Indeed, it has been shown that such higher potency FMD vaccines can confer protection against strains that serologically would not have been considered antigenically related enough for the vaccine to be effective (Barnett et al. 2013); these findings were supported in practice during the control of FMD serotype O in Tunisia and Algeria in 2014 and 2015, where a vaccine was used which scored low in the respective *in vitro* vaccine matching test but effectively protected the vaccinated animals. The benefits of increasing the antigen payload in a vaccine have to be balanced against the resultant reduction in the number of doses that can be formulated.

Aside from choosing the type of vaccine to be stored, a number of diseases have the added complication of antigenic diversity. Indeed, some diseases are constantly evolving antigenically, requiring continuous monitoring of the antigenic characteristics of circulating strains through surveillance and regular review of which strains to include in vaccine reserves. Recommendations on which vaccine strains are most likely to be required for emergency use should be sought from the necessary experts, such as those based in national or international reference laboratories. For FMD, the FAO World Reference Laboratory based at the Pirbright Institute publishes an annual list of high- medium- and low-priority vaccine strains which should be considered for FMD vaccine reserves (www.wrlfmd.org/sites/world/files/quick_media/OIE-FAO%20FMD%20Ref%20Lab). The methodology of deciding about priority antigens for FMD antigen banks has been further developed by the European Commission for the Control of FMD (EuFMD) at the FAO, in close cooperation with the FAO World Reference Laboratory for FMD, Pirbright, by including risk factors such as geographical dominance of certain serotypes and strains of the virus (virus pools) and trade-related factors in the assessment (EUFMD 2015; McLaws et al. 2016).

The report of the Scientific Committee on Animal Health and Animal Welfare in April 2003 on 'Diagnostic techniques and vaccines for FMD, CSF, AI, and some other important OIE diseases' (European Commission 2003) recommended support for the validation of appropriate tests such as those based on real-time polymerase chain reaction (RT-PCR) assays, marker immunoassays or enzyme-linked immunosorbent assays (ELISAs) as well as appropriately designed vaccines so that virus or antibody detection methods can identify infected animals in vaccinated herds (DIVA strategy). Literature is available which provides different strategies that can be used toward this goal (European Commission 2010) as well as guidance on the necessary surveillance (OIE 2018).

The minimum number of vaccine doses required in a strategic reserve will depend on many factors, not least the contingency planning that exists for each disease and the vaccination policy that is likely to be applied. This will not only relate to what the intended target species are and their population sizes and densities, but how vaccination will be applied, since this might encompass zonal, barrier, or ring vaccination or indeed a combination of these, as well as a possible requirement for boosters. Vaccine wastage is also an important consideration which will be affected by the bottle sizes used, the amounts issued to vaccination teams, and how the vaccine is ultimately administered. While some countries might only plan to vaccinate a single species, for other diseases, the vaccination of all susceptible individuals may be a requirement since this may lead to better results. As found in the past, the quantities stockpiled by a bank may also need to take into account the possibility of supplying vaccine to neighboring countries that pose a risk to the disease-free status of bank members.

Clearly, there is no easy route to determining exactly how much vaccine should be stored for emergency use, but while data analyses and use of computational modeling can assist in addressing this specific question, there will always be limitations to the knowledge we have over events that may or may not take place, following a disease incursion (Dekker and Barnett 2007). Ultimately, a well-considered and balanced approach will be required from experts that consider the most likely scenarios based on current epidemiological knowledge and past experience.

16.5 Selecting and Sourcing Candidate Vaccines for a Reserve

The acquisition of the appropriate antigen/s or vaccine/s will be reliant on whether they are available commercially, from government institutions, or can be produced in house.

Of principal importance when considering the sourcing of vaccines or vaccine components for a reserve are the quality of such products and the suitability of the manufacturing facilities in which they are produced.

Regulatory concerns over current or new IVMPs and the recommendation to use approved authorized products should predispose a reserve bank to acquire and manage its stocks selectively. Appropriately licensed manufacturers which have the necessary marketing authorization and internationally accepted standards of GMP, with modern quality assurance and a QP for product release, should therefore be used for source materials (OIE 2016a).

In addition, it is important to consider whether or not the adjuvant and formulation are compatible with use in the chosen target species, since some adjuvants may be less suitable for certain targets, or alternatively may provide an option to vaccinate many different susceptible species. A good example is the mineral oil formulations used in the manufacture of FMD vaccines, which are efficacious in large and small ruminants as well as pigs, which is in contrast to the FMD vaccines adjuvanted with aluminum hydroxide that are much less effective in pigs. A decision on what vaccines should be held in the reserve and how they should be stored (i.e. ready formulated or as a separate antigen component for subsequent formulation) must be made by disease control authorities in consultation with the vaccine bank administrators. The value of any given vaccine reserve is wholly reliant on the suitability of the vaccine strains it holds for field application, particularly for those diseases that are made up of a number of serotypes and have wide strain diversity.

Globally, we are a more interdependent community where the rapid and extensive movement of people, animals, and animal products and potential to deliberately introduce disease through bioterrorism heighten the risk of an incursion and make prediction of specific disease threat difficult. However, the process by which vaccine strain candidates are selected can be improved by a continuous exchange of information and increased cooperation and collaboration between the many different international, regional and national authorities, vaccine manufacturers, and vaccine reserve authorities. Regular genetic and antigenic characterization of isolates is an essential precondition in mapping the evolution of new strains and to assess the need for the development of new or better adapted vaccines. Unfortunately, without financial support, the least developed countries, where many diseases occur, may not have the resources to submit outbreak samples to reference laboratories.

16.6 Acceptance Testing – Ensuring Safety, Efficacy, and Quality of Strategic Vaccines

Where possible, strategic reserve managers should request tenders from various suppliers for the vaccines or antigens required in a reserve. It is particularly important to find out about the safety, efficacy, and quality of the product. Those seeking such products may wish to gain advice from appropriate licensing authorities on the necessary standards required. Making a request for tender helps ensure both a competitive price and a veterinary medicinal product manufactured to the required level of quality. It is also important to ascertain that candidate suppliers can produce the desired product and amounts within a required time interval that allows both necessary and mandatory tests of compliance, including safety and efficacy.

Regardless of whether such antigen/s or vaccine/s are to be held at the principal site of manufacture or at a suitable storage site elsewhere, disease control authorities should consider only accepting such products after they have been shown to have passed the necessary acceptance testing procedures. Notably, if the antigen/vaccine has to be located in a bank prior to completion of any acceptance testing, this material should be stored separately and labeled as quarantined until, following acceptance testing, the product has shown full compliance to the requirements of the strategic reserve. This should go hand in hand with the necessary regulatory requirements for any given veterinary medicinal product and should be considered carefully by any country linked to a strategic reserve wishing to have the necessary authorization to use such vaccines in the field (OIE 2016b).

For many veterinary medicinal products, the standards for safety, efficacy, and quality will be described by individual monographs in official pharmacopeias which provide a good template for disease control authorities to use in qualifying products for a strategic reserve by acceptance testing. In cases where no specific monograph is available, the disease control authorities can consider the general section on vaccines for veterinary use where the minimum standards are prescribed, though authorities may wish to add further individual requirements. Strategic reserve managers and the associated disease control authorities should also consider the value of having the product independently tested, particularly for efficacy/potency (www.oie.int/doc/ged/D7709.PDF). In the case of the EU FMD Vaccine Bank, the European Community Reference Laboratory has carried out heterologous potency tests when there has been doubt as to the cross-protection that can be afforded by bank vaccines against newly emerged viral threats (Li et al. 2012).

Finally, and as discussed earlier in this chapter, differentiating between animals that have been vaccinated and those that have either recovered from infection or have acquired subclinical infection may be important post vaccination. If the veterinary medicinal product and any associated diagnostic assay/s are capable of supporting a DIVA approach then this should be an important aspect that must be considered for inclusion in any acceptance testing regime (OIE 2016b).

16.7 Storage and Monitoring of Strategic Vaccines

It is important that the areas of storage to hold emergency antigens/vaccines meet national or international standards of GMP. This is usually covered when a bank is held in a "licensed" and routinely inspected commercial vaccine plant. However, if the reserve is located outside a nominated vaccine formulation facility, disease control authorities may wish to seek advice from appropriate licensing authorities on the standards required.

Storage facilities and procedures therein should ensure the security of the stored antigen and prevent tampering, contamination, or damage. The EUFMD provides minimum biorisk management standards for laboratories working with FMDV (EUFMD 2013) that may be consulted for more detail.

How the antigens/vaccines are stored in an emergency reserve will depend on the nature of the product, which may be a chemically inactivated or killed virus or a live attenuated vaccine. The antigens themselves may be concentrated and held at ultra-low temperature, such as those held over liquid nitrogen, or it may be a freeze-dried commodity where low temperature may be less important. Whatever the method of storage, it is vital that the materials are optimally maintained and routinely monitored in order to have assurance that they will be efficacious when required and that a back-up facility is also available in the event of technical issues (Lombard and Füssel 2007).

To facilitate the monitoring and testing of stored antigen/vaccine and to identify any deterioration in quality, depositories should include an appropriate number of small samples that are representative of the larger batches of stock and which should be stored alongside the batches they correspond to. Where possible, these should be in a primary container made of the same material/s as that holding the main bulk of the stored product. Indeed, managers of vaccine reserves should ensure that the necessary arrangements are in place to monitor their reserves on a routine basis and to include where necessary, and at appropriate time intervals, a testing regime to ensure stability/integrity of the antigen or active component or acceptable potency of the final product. This may, however, not be necessary where the antigens or vaccines are replaced at the end of a guarantee period provided by the manufacturer in the technical specification of the marketing authorization. To this end, a timetable of tests is given in Table 16.1, as an example of that followed by the IVB, in order to monitor the stability/integrity of the FMD antigen component stored at ultra-low temperature.

The type of container used to hold antigen concentrate is important not only in the context of suitability for a pharmaceutical component but because it may well be stored under ultra-low temperature conditions. Such containers

Table 16.1 Procedures followed by the International Vaccine Bank in order to monitor the stability/integrity of the FMD antigen component stored at ultra-low temperature.

Time	Test
On receipt of the concentrated vaccine antigen (year 0) and every 5 years thereafter	Measure intact virion content by 146S quantification using ultracentrifugation and sucrose density gradient analysis[a] Potency test in cattle: this may rely on serological techniques where potency has been adequately correlated with immunogenicity for the antigen component concerned or, at the discretion of the bank holder, may be performed as a "truncated" test[b] to demonstrate that the minimum potency of the vaccine remains greater than the minimum requirement; however, a truncation approach could still underestimate actual vaccine potency
Years 2 and 4, and immediately before formulation if the need arises	146S quantification by ultracentrifugation and sucrose density gradient analysis
Every 5 years	Ongoing evaluation of all relevant potency test results and 146S quantification data from the preceding 5 years to assess whether there is a need to replace the concentrated antigen component

[a] Other physicochemical tests for FMD virus such as SDS-PAGE have been used to evaluate integrity of the VP1 virion protein but are not sufficiently validated for routine use.

[b] In a truncated test, all the animals that would have been used in the next reduced vaccine volume or vaccine dilution group but are deliberately not incorporated in the actual test are assumed to have not been protected. The test therefore may result in a lower PD_{50} value than actual but reduces the number of animals used in line with the principles of the 3Rs (Replacement, Reduction, and Refinement) (www.nc3rs.org.uk/the-3rs).

should be made from materials that do not become brittle or fragile at a temperature range that allows both heat sterilization and ultra-low storage. Nevertheless, periodic inspection of these containers for cracks or leakage is still advised.

Although there are national and international guidelines on the required labeling of veterinary medical products, there are no such guidelines for emergency stored materials such as the antigen component of a vaccine, as these are essentially regarded in regulatory terms as "in process" materials. However, it is important to label batches of antigen, particularly when several different strains or batches are held in the same freezer storage facility. Under ultra-low temperature conditions, the method of labeling must of course be of a durable nature. In such cases, wire tagging the bottles is an advised option using a metal tag sizeable enough to accommodate the information required. Such information should include the antigen/vaccine strain, batch number, and date received and should also include an individual container or stock number. This information should be clear to read and marked on the tag using an indelible marker pen. Aluminum metal tags have been used for such a purpose and these can be obtained with different color coatings to allow better identification and accessibility. Metal tags also allow information to be permanently engraved.

Finally, it would be advisable for member countries of a reserve to monitor the literature published for any important advances that are made in the areas relating to vaccine banks and vaccine storage. Ongoing research does lead to improvements of product, equipment, manufacture, and distribution and therein more efficient and practical use of the reserves themselves.

16.8 Future Developments for Strategic Vaccine Banks

Worldwide, it is unclear exactly how many vaccine banks currently exist, or indeed what, and how many, stocks of different vaccines are held overall. This in part is the result of a considered need for confidentiality, particularly in case of a deliberate disease introduction through bioterrorism. The location of any reserve is a key issue and for those considering setting up a reserve within the commercial sector, there is a need to consider the impact that could follow from any potential demise of the chosen commercial producer, particularly given the ever reducing options in terms of choice of pharmaceutical manufacturers. A good but small example for a (temporary) incapacitation is the lack of vaccines against equine viral arteritis, with huge consequences for shuttle stallions in the EU (www.thetba.co.uk/wp-content/uploads/2017/08/TBA-EVA-Advice-290817.pdf). Furthermore, if some producers were to cease production of specific vaccines for whatever reason, it is very unlikely that other manufacturers would take over the responsibility of formulating from an established reserve because of the legal implications and access to strains. Therefore, the placement of an independent formulation/blending facility still has merit if only in a supportive capacity.

However, in recent years there have been developments in the FMD vaccine field which have seen the real possibility of freezing fully formulated oil vaccines (Goovaerts et al. 2010) of known efficacy and quality, even without the need to stratify the separate components (Barnett and Statham 2002). This not only allows more immediate availability of a fully quality tested vaccine with a long vaccine shelf-life, but also increases the options on where such vaccines could be stored. More recently, it has become possible to efficiently express recombinant empty FMDV capsids in eukaryotic cells at yields seen as attractive to industry (Porta et al. 2013). Using both vaccinia virus- and baculovirus-driven expression, enhanced capsid stability has been achieved by rationally designed mutation. This offers several potential advantages, but in the context of an emergency vaccine reserve, an enhanced temperature stability of the product may make way in the future for alternative and better storage options.

The biggest investment in a reserve is the stockpiling of adequate and relevant vaccine strains, the choice of which, depending on disease, has to be assessed on the basis of probable risk as well as dose level requirements. This certainly has been something that has been considered in depth for the EU FMD vaccine reserve (Dekker and Barnett 2007). It is well documented that for FMD, there is no cross-serotype protection observed from any FMD vaccine strain and limited cross-protection within serotypes. This is particularly true for the A serotype which has often led to the costly stockpiling of a number of different A serotype strains in reserves. However, it has been shown that potency can compensate for poor antigenic match in a higher potency A serotype vaccine against heterologous strains *in vivo* (Brehm et al. 2008). More recent work using higher potency O1 Manisa vaccine against challenge with O/Vietnam/2010 (O Mya98 topotype) in pigs also concluded that higher potency vaccines protect pigs against heterologous virus when vaccination is effective (Vosloo et al. 2012). Another new study using a high-potency Asia Shamir vaccine also conferred good protection against a heterologous challenge virus, despite poor antigenic match (Li et al. 2012). Remarkably, against certain heterologous strains some vaccines were still of sufficient potency to merit a PD_{50} potency value in excess of 6, which would automatically qualify them for acceptance into a reserve.

Given that the breadth of cross-protection shown *in vivo* was not confirmed by serological relatedness, this brings into question the value of some of the data resulting from the use of the current serological tests. More importantly, for FMD, it questions the need to hold so many different strains in a strategic reserve, though some caution needs to be exercised given that another study, using the vaccine strain O Manisa against challenge to a more serologically related O Campos strain, only gave rise to 25% protection (Srinivasan et al. 2006), even though this could be improved by substantially increasing the antigen payload (Nagendrakumar et al. 2011). Furthermore, for some serotypes of FMD, such as those of the Southern African Territories, it is difficult to make vaccines of very high potency due to lower *in vitro* yields and poorer antigen stability. Overall, these observations merit further study since vaccines with sufficient potency may potentially give rise to the holding of just a few "key" strains in a reserve to improve logistics and reduce some of the economic implications associated with it.

Finally, the concept of spreading the risk and financial burden among a large number of customers is well established in the insurance industry. A strategic vaccine reserve is an insurance policy for countries that may, or may not, require specific vaccines to control important veterinary diseases in the future. It is, therefore, sensible for such countries with similar concerns to work closely, as a network of individual banks, in order to facilitate an exchange of information, materials, and reagents. This, in theory, could make available a comprehensive reserve of vaccine strains in sufficient quantities and potency to satisfy any perceived risk. Toward such an accomplishment, a network of FMD vaccines banks has been initiated, in order to realize a system of resource sharing that has both practical and economic benefits to all parties concerned (Barnett et al. 2010). This type of networking approach would have similar benefits for countries which establish reserves for many other veterinary diseases. Further progress in FMD vaccine cooperation was reported in 2016, after Australia, Canada, Mexico, New Zealand, and the USA signed a vaccine-sharing arrangement.

In practice, the EU, in accordance with Article 83 of Council Directive 2003/85/EC, granted temporary access to its antigen and vaccine bank to Australia and New Zealand during the period of transformation of their antigen reserves (European Commission 2004).

16.9 Summary

Strategic vaccine reserves are an extremely valuable adjunct in the control of important veterinary diseases and increasingly go hand in hand with DIVA diagnostic tests to support vaccination and its monitoring in emergency situations. For exotic diseases, vaccination can reduce preventive animal culling, which is costly and is usually associated with considerable public concern regarding animal welfare.

The type of strategic reserve is largely defined by how the end-product is stored and formulated, but also takes account of governance and location. Key requirements for the establishment of a strategic reserve (Table 16.2) include a sound managerial system that facilitates decision making and takes into account appropriate and up-to-date regulatory requirements.

The types and quantities of vaccine that should be stored in a reserve are largely dictated by the disease itself. However, aspects such as safety, efficacy, quality, and the suitability of the vaccine for field use are generically important. This can be substantiated through product licensing. Where applicable, the ability to support differentiation between infected and vaccinated animals is of key importance. Both contingency planning and vaccination policy will influence the minimum number of doses required in a reserve, taking account of disease, target species, population densities, and how vaccine is applied.

Acquisition of the appropriate antigen/s or vaccine/s depends on availability, commercially, from government institutions or from in-house production. Product quality should be uppermost in this decision process, as well as the suitability of the formulation in respect of the intended target species. Requests for vaccines intended for reserves should be instigated, ideally, by tender, as this ensures both a competitive price and a veterinary medicinal product manufactured to the desired level of quality. Such product should only be accepted if it has passed the necessary acceptance testing procedures.

The areas used for storage of emergency antigens/vaccines should be suitable in the context of the required nationally or internationally accepted standards of GMP and should be optimally maintained and routinely monitored. Procedures should be in place to ensure the security of these stored commodities.

Independent strategic reserves have also supported many research achievements relating to this field. There is also benefit in networking between individual reserves in order to facilitate an exchange of information, materials, and reagents so as to reduce some of the financial burden associated with these facilities.

Table 16.2 Key elements in the establishment and management of vaccine banks.

Requirement for a bank	Consider justification of need, as well as information on the epidemiological, logistical, and administrative framework for their use
Type of bank	Holding fully formulated vaccine, active component only, or both. Dependent on type of vaccine and associated stability, as well as disease and need for timely access
Membership	Spread the risk and financial burden by membership with countries with similar concerns to either work closely as a single bank or as a network of individual banks in order to facilitate exchange of information, materials, and reagents
Managerial system	Foremost in the establishment of a strategic reserve in order to run and maintain it
Governance	National, government-administered and -financed vaccine banks
	International, government-administered and -financed banks
	Commercially maintained vaccine banks
	Vaccine banks organized by international organizations based on contracts with commercial producers
Formal agreement	To establish relationship and/or financial commitment of member countries, as well as potential drawing rights
Acquisition of vaccines	Regulatory concerns and the recommendation to use approved authorized products should predispose a reserve to acquire and manage its stocks selectively
	Where possible, use appropriately licensed manufacturers which have the necessary marketing authorization and internationally accepted standards of Good Manufacturing Practice (GMP)
	Request vaccine/antigen supplies by tender from each supplier
	Incorporate acceptance testing criteria ensuring safety, efficacy, and the quality of strategic vaccines
	Consider suitability of adjuvant to species target
Regulatory requirements	Where possible, use an authorized licensed product ensuring quality, safety, and efficacy
	Many immunological products are covered by individual monographs in official pharmacopeias to which the standards for safety, efficacy, sterility, and quality are detailed
	Referral should be made to the introductory chapters of the OIE *Manual of Diagnostic Tests and Vaccines for Terrestrial Animals* where minimum standards are set and would still apply
	Ensure conformity on the type of adjuvant or other pharmacologically active ingredient used in the vaccine formulation
	Disease control authorities may seek other additional requirements such as standards relating to strain identity, freedom from adventitious agents, innocuity, absence of toxicity, antigen dose payload, and potency
	Stockpiling and manufacture in premises should follow GMP and be officially quality assured. These should be guided by standard operating procedures
	Strategic reserves would benefit from being officiated by a suitable Qualified Person and certified as holding an appropriate manufacturing license
	Primary containers, outer containers, labeling, the holding vessels or equipment, and storage areas within a building should be in line with the required national or internationally accepted standards of GMP
Storage monitoring	Optimally maintained and routinely monitored to assure efficacy
	For routine replacement at the end of the guarantee period
	Should include container integrity
	Need for appropriate detailed labeling
Locality	Within or outside member countries
How much to hold	Dependent on disease
	Vaccine targets
	How it is applied in the field
	Whether available for use in neighboring countries
	Can be considered by use of computational modeling
	Wastage considerations associated with use of the vaccine
Requirement of different strains	Seek guidance from OIE/FAO network of reference laboratories and/or the national and European Union reference laboratories respectively
Use of DIVA vaccines	Consider need to differentiate infected from vaccinated animals
Diagnostic tests	Associated use of diagnostic tests to support the use of vaccine from a reserve
Contingency planning	Ensure efficient distribution and strategic application in the field through the appropriate availability of trained staff and equipment
	Use of simulation exercises

References

Barnett, P.V. and Statham, R.J. (2002). Stratified and cryogenically stored (SACS) vaccines, a new concept in emergency foot-and-mouth disease vaccine formulation and storage. *Vaccine* 20: 2060–2064.

Barnett, P.V., Bashiruddin, J.B., Hammond, J.M. et al. (2010). Toward a global foot-and-mouth disease vaccine bank. *Rev. Sci. Tech. Off. Int. Epiz.* 29 (3): 593–602.

Barnett, P.V., Geale, D.W., Clarke, G. et al. (2013). A review of OIE country status recovery using vaccinate-to-live versus vaccinate-to-die foot-and-mouth disease response policies I: benefits of higher potency vaccines and associated NSP DIVA test systems in post-outbreak surveillance. *Transbound. Emerg. Dis.* 62: 367–387.

Brehm, K.E., Kumar, N., Thulke, H.-H., and Haas, B. (2008). High potency vaccines induce protection against heterologous challenge with foot-and-mouth disease virus. *Vaccine* 26 (13): 1681–1697.

Dekker, A. and Barnett, P. (2007). Minimum size of antigen stocks in the EU vaccine bank. Report of the 37th Session of the European Commission for the Control of Foot and Mouth Disease. 18–20 April, Rome, Food and Agriculture Organization of the United Nations, Appendix 24, pp. 183–187.

EMA. (2002). Position Paper on Requirements for Vaccines against Foot-and-Mouth Disease, EMEA/CVMP/775/02-Final. www.ema.europa.eu/docs/en_GB/document_library/Scientific_guideline/2009/10/WC500004592.pdf

EUFMD. (2013). European Commission for the Control of Foot and Mouth Disease. Minimum Standards for Laboratories Working with Foot-and-Mouth Disease Virus. Report of 40th General Session of EUFMD, 22–24 April, Rome, Italy, Appendix 7. www.fao.org/fileadmin/user_upload/eufmd/Lab_guidelines/FMD_Minimumstandards_2013_Final_version.pdf

EUFMD. (2015). Report of the 41st General Session of the European Commission for the Control of Foot and Mouth Disease, FAO, Rome, 23–24 April. www.fao.org/fileadmin/user_upload/eufmd/41st_General_Session/4.Technical_progress_VB-Ryan.pdf

European Commission. (2001a). Position paper on risk assessment of the use of starting materials of ruminant origin in veterinary medicinal products intended for use in ruminant species (EMEA/CVMP/121/01) adopted by the Committee for Veterinary Medicinal Products (CVMP) – July 2001. Official Journal, C 286, 12.10.2001, pp. 10–11.

European Commission. (2001b). Position paper on the assessment of the risk of transmission of animal spongiform encephalopathy agents by master seed materials used in the production of veterinary vaccines (EMEA/CVMP/019/01) adopted by the Committee for Veterinary Medicinal Products (CVMP) – July 2001. Official Journal, C 286, 12.10.2001, pp. 12–14.

European Commission. (2003). Diagnostic techniques and vaccines for foot-and-mouth disease, classical swine fever, avian influenza and some other important OIE list A diseases. Report of the Scientific Committee on Animal Health and Welfare. http://ec.europa.eu/food/fs/sc/scah/out93_en.pdf

European Commission. (2004). Commission Decision 2004/288/EC of 26 March 2004 granting Australia and New Zealand temporary access to the Community reserves of foot-and-mouth disease virus antigens. Official Journal, L91, 30.3.2004, pp. 58–59. http://eur-lex.europa.eu/legal-content/en/ALL/?uri=CELEX%3A32005D0209

European Commission. (2009). Commission Decision 2009/3/EC of 18 December 2008 establishing Community reserves of vaccines against African horse sickness. Official Journal, L2, 6.1.2009, pp. 9–10. http://eur-lex.europa.eu/legal-content/EN/TXT/?qid=1467098122069&uri=CELEX:32009D0003

European Commission. (2010). Expert opinion on vaccine and/or diagnostic banks for major animal disease – strategic planning options for emergency situations or major crises. Health & Consumers Directorate-General, Directorate D –Animal Health and Welfare. D1-Animal Health and Standing Committees, SANCO/7070/2010; 1–75. http://ec.europa.eu/food/animal/diseases/strategy/pillars/docs/7070-vaccine-bank-summary_en.pdf

European Commission. (2011). Note for guidance on minimising the risk of transmitting animal spongiform encephalopathy agents via human and veterinary medicinal products (EMA/410/01 rev.3). Official Journal, C 73, 5.3.2011, pp. 1–18. www.ema.europa.eu/docs/en_GB/document_library/Scientific_guideline/2009/09/WC500003700.pdf

European Commission. (2015). Commission Implementing Decision of 18.12.2015 on the adoption of a financing decision regarding the Union financial contribution to emergency measures to combat lumpy skin disease in Greece in 2015 and establishing a stock of vaccines against lumpy skin disease. C(2015) 9573 final. http://ec.europa.eu/dgs/health_food-safety/funding/cff/docs/animal_emergency-measures_eu-decision_2015-9573_greece_en.pdf

European Communities. (1982). Council of the European Communities (1982). Council Directive 82/894/EEC of 21 December 1982 on the notification of animal diseases within the Community. Official Journal, L 378, 31.12.1982, pp. 58–62.

European Communities. (1991). Council of the European Communities (1991). Council Decision 91/666/EEC of 11 December 1991 establishing Community reserves of foot-and-mouth disease vaccines. Official Journal, L 368, 31.12.1991, pp. 21–25.

European Union. (2001). European Parliament and Council of the European Union (2001). Council Directive 2001/82/EC of the European Parliament and of the Council of 6 November 2001 on the Community code relating to veterinary medicinal products. Official Journal, L 311, 28.11.2001, pp. 1–66.

European Union. (2003). Council of the European Union (2003). Council Directive 2003/85/EC of 29 September 2003 establishing Community measures for the control of foot-and-mouth disease repealing Directive 85/511/EEC and Decisions 89/531/EEC and 91/665/EEC and amending Directive 92/46/EEC. Official Journal, L 306, 22.11.2003, pp. 1–87.

European Union. (2016). European Parliament and of the Council (2016). Regulation (EU) 2016/429 of the European Parliament and of the Council of 9 March 2016 on transmissible animal diseases and amending and repealing certain acts in the area of animal health ('Animal Health Law'). Official Journal, L 84, 31.3.1016, pp. 1–208.

Goovaerts, D., Visser, N., Janssen, P., et al. (2010). Freezing of formulated FMDV vaccines and vaccines banks: potential for a faster response in emergency situations. Report, Session of the Research Group of the Standing Technical Committee of the European Commission for the Control of Foot-and-Mouth Disease and the Foot-and-Mouth Disease Subgroup of the Scientific Veterinary Committee of the Commission of the European Community, Vienna.

House, J., Lombard, M., House, C. et al. (1992). Efficacy of an inactivated vaccine for African horse sickness serotype 4. In: *Bluetongue, African Horse Sickness and Related Orbiviruses* (eds. T.E. Walton and B.I. Osburn), 891–895. Boca Raton: CRC Press.

House, J., House, C., Dubourget, P., and Lombard, M. (2003). Protective immunity in cattle vaccinated with a commercial scale inactivated bivalent vesicular stomatitis vaccine. *Vaccine* 21 (17–18): 1932–1937.

Lei, J.C. and McKercher, P.D. (1979). Report, Session of the Research Group of the Standing Technical Committee of the European Commission for the Control of Foot-and-Mouth Disease and the Foot-and-Mouth Disease Subgroup of the Scientific Veterinary Committee of the Commission of the European Community, 12–14 June, Lindholm, Denmark, Rome, Food and Agriculture Organization, Appendix B1: 24.

Li, Y., Statham, B., Armson, B. et al. (2012). Cross protection against current Asia 1 isolates provided by a high potency Asia Shamir vaccine. Open Sessions of the Standing and Technical Committees of the EUFMD Commission, Appliance of science in the progressive control of FMD, 29–31 October, Jerez de la Frontera, Spain, Appendix 27. 128.

Lombard, M. and Füssel, A.-E. (2007). Antigen and vaccine banks: technical requirements and the role of the European antigen bank in emergency foot and mouth disease vaccination. *Rev. Sci. Tech. Off. Int. Epiz.* 26 (1): 117–134.

McLaws, M., King, D., Hickey, K., et al. (2016). Which vaccines are most important? PRAGMATIST: a decision support tool for FMD vaccine bank managers. Open Session of the European Commission for the Control of FMD, Cascais, Portugal. www.ipcinfo.org/fileadmin/user_upload/eufmd/Open_Session2016/Pragmatist_McLaws.pdf

Muroga, N., Hayama, Y., Yamamoto, T. et al. (2012). The 2010 foot-and-mouth disease epidemic in Japan. *J. Vet. Med. Sci.* 74 (4): 399–404.

Nagendrakumar, S.B., Srinivasan, V.A., Madhanmohan, M. et al. (2011). Evaluation of cross-protection between O(1) Manisa and O(1) Campos in cattle vaccinated with foot-and-mouth disease virus vaccine incorporating different payloads of inactivated O (1) Manisa antigen. *Vaccine* 29: 1906–1912.

Northumberland. (1969). Report of the Committee of Inquiry on Foot-and-Mouth Disease. Presented to Parliament by the Minister of Agriculture, Fisheries and. Food. By Command of Her Majesty. Cmnd. 3999 & 4225. December. London: Her Majesty's Stationery Office.

OFFLU. (2013). Developing guidance on vaccines and vaccination against HPAI from lessons learned, Report of technical meeting 4–6 December, Beijing, PR China. www.offlu.net/fileadmin/home/en/meeting-reports/pdf/OFFLU_Beijing_2013/OFFLU_Recommendations_Beijing_Dec_2013_final.pdf

OIE. (2014). Vaccine Banks. www.oie.int/doc/ged/D14110.PDF

OIE (2016a). Transboundary competition horse movement: the HHP concept as an option to improve global access to equestrian sport. *OIE Bull.* 2016 (1): 51–54. www.oie.int/fileadmin/Home/eng/Publications_%26_Documentation/docs/pdf/bulletin/Bull_2016-1-ENG.pdf.

OIE. (2016b). Vaccine Banks. Chapter 1.1.10. *Manual of Diagnostic Tests and Vaccines for Terrestrial Animals*, 7th edn. Paris: OIE.

OIE. (2017). African horse sickness. Chapter 2.5.1. *Manual of Diagnostic Tests and Vaccines for Terrestrial Animals*, 7th edn. Paris: OIE.

OIE. (2018). Principles of vaccine production. Chapter 1.1.8. *Manual of Diagnostic Tests and Vaccines for Terrestrial Animals*, 8th edn. Paris: OIE.

Porta, C., Kotecha, A., Burman, A. et al. (2013). Rational engineering of recombinant Picornavirus capsids to produce safe, protective vaccine antigen. *PLoS Pathog.* 9 (3): 1–8.

Sanchez Vizcaino, J.M. (2004). Control and eradication of African horse sickness with vaccine. In: *Control of Infectious Animal Diseases by Vaccination* (eds. A. Schudel and M. Lombard), 255–258. Basel: Karger.

Srinivasan, V.A., Nagendra Kumar, S.B., Madhan, M., et al. (2006). Preliminary results to evaluate cross-protection between O1 Manisa and O1 Campos in cattle. Report, Session of the Research Group of the Standing Technical Committee of the European Commission for the Control of Foot-and-Mouth Disease, Paphos, Cyprus. Rome: Food and Agriculture Organization of the United Nations, Appendix 30, 207–214.

Vosloo, W., Morris, J., Nguyen, T.T.H., et al. (2012). Testing the efficacy of O1 Manisa High Potency vaccine against challenge with O/Vietnam/2010 (O Mya 98 Topotype) in pigs. Open Sessions of the Standing and Technical Committees of the EUFMD Commission, Appliance of science in the progressive control of FMD, 29–31 October, Jerez de la Frontera, Spain, Appendix 28. 130.

Section IV

Veterinary Vaccines for Selected Animal Diseases

17

Foot and Mouth Disease

Samia Metwally[1], Bryan Charleston[2], and Nicholas Lyons[2]

[1] Animal Production and Health Division, Food and Agriculture Organization of the United Nations, Rome, Italy
[2] The Pirbright Institute, Pirbright, Surrey, UK

17.1 Introduction

Foot and mouth disease (FMD) is a highly contagious and economically important viral disease of domestic cloven-hoofed animals including cattle, buffaloes, goats, sheep, pigs, and more than 100 wildlife species (Grubman and Baxt 2004; Weaver et al. 2013). FMD is still widespread throughout the world and occurs in large parts of Africa, the Middle East, and Asia. Countries that are free of FMD today remain under constant threat of an incursion. The disease is well known for its ability to severely affect and indeed disrupt regional and international trade in animals and animal products and is notorious for the enormous financial damage it can cause in FMD-free countries hit by an outbreak. In FMD-endemic countries, usually low- and middle-income countries, the disease threatens food security and the livelihoods of smallholders and prevents animal husbandry sectors from developing their economic potential. However, the magnitude of the burden involving the loss of livestock biodiversity and the lowering of production efficiency is generally much less well known or is underestimated.

Foot and mouth disease is caused by a single-stranded positive-sense RNA virus belonging to the genus *Aphthovirus* in the family Picornaviridae. FMD virus (FMDV) has a high mutation rate and exists as seven distinct serotypes (O, A, C, Asia 1, South African territories [SAT] 1, SAT2, and SAT3), with three pools covering east Asia, south Asia, west Asia, and the Middle East, three pools covering Africa, and one pool covering South America (Figure 17.1). The concept of "regional virus pools" provides an organizing principle for coordinating laboratory and epidemiology activities toward diagnostics, vaccination, and disease surveillance.

In the past decade, multiple unexplained jumps of FMDV infection have occurred, resulting in regional epidemics affecting millions of animals (Paton et al. 2017). It was shown that three FMD viral lineages (O/SEA/Mya-98, O/ME-SA/PanAsia, and A/ASIA/Sea-97) have spread northwards from southeast Asia into countries in east Asia (2009–2010). Furthermore, samples collected during 2015 from outbreaks in Israel and the Palestinian Autonomous Territories showed that they are also closely related to those from southeast and east Asia within the O/ME-SA/PanAsia lineage. The O/ME-SA/Ind-2001 lineage found in the Indian subcontinent has been detected in the United Arab Emirates, Saudi Arabia, and Bahrain, and has also spread in a westerly direction across North Africa from Libya into Tunisia, Algeria, and Morocco (2013–2015). More recently, this lineage has also spread into mainland southeast and east Asian countries. During 2015, the A/ASIA/G-VII [G-18] viral lineage also emerged from the Indian subcontinent and has been spreading rapidly in the Middle East (Saudi Arabia, Iran, Armenia, Turkey, and Israel). Importantly, vaccine-matching data using *in vitro* tests indicate that field isolates of this lineage are not well matched against commercially available vaccines and those held in vaccine banks.

Serotype SAT 2 (topotype VII) has expanded from sub-Saharan into North Africa and the Middle East since 2012, causing extensive FMD outbreaks in Egypt with separate introduction to Libya. Similar long-distance movements of O/EA-3 lineage occurred from East Africa into Egypt, Palestine, and Israel as well as into a number of West and Central African countries during 2018 (including Burkina Faso, the Gambia, Guinea, Mauritania, Senegal, and Sierra Leone). Recent FMD cases in the Maghreb countries of North Africa (Algeria, Tunisia, and Morocco) have epidemiological connections to these cases in West Africa.

Clinical signs of FMD are fever, lameness, salivation, vesicular lesions in the mouth, tongue, lips, feet and udder,

Veterinary Vaccines: Principles and Applications, First Edition. Edited by Samia Metwally, Gerrit Viljoen, and Ahmed El Idrissi.

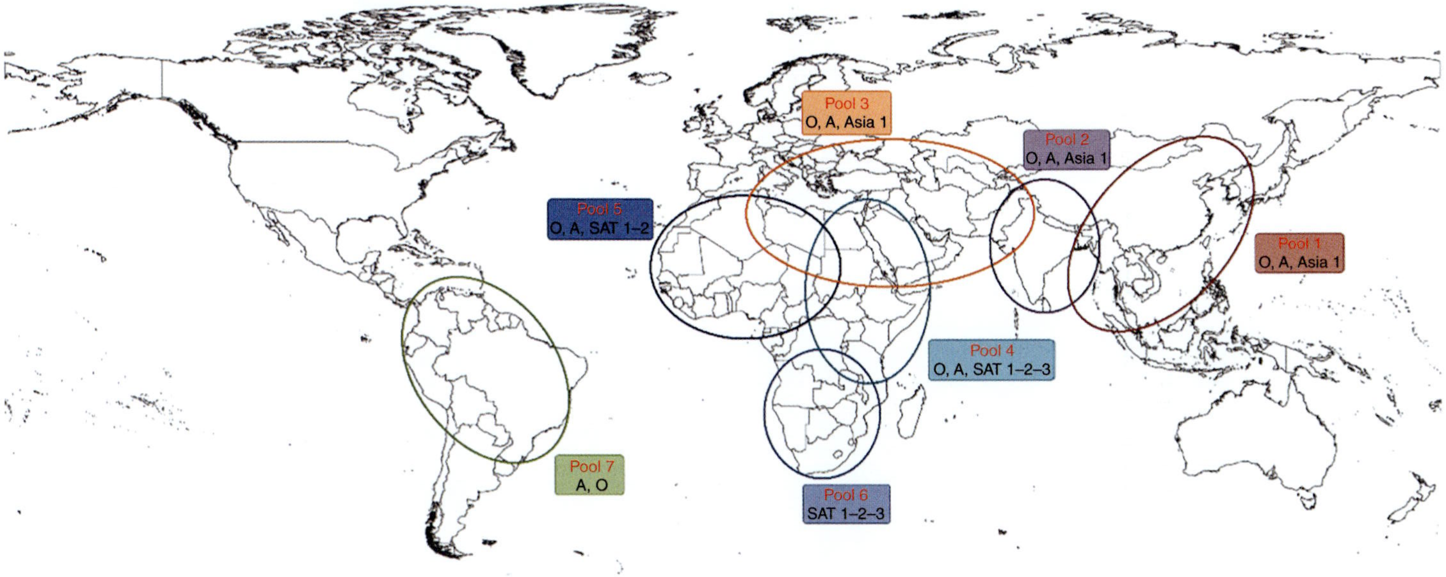

Figure 17.1 Global map with distribution of FMD serotypes among the seven virus pools. Pool 1, southeast Asia spillover into east Asia; pool 2, southern Asia; pool 3, Eurasia including the Middle East; pool 4, east Africa; pool 5, western Africa; pool 6, southern Africa; pool 7, South America.

weight loss, and drop in milk production. The morbidity of FMD is often high in exposed adult animals but mortality is uncommon. In contrast, high mortality can occur in young animals due to myocarditis, and in some cases as a result of dehydration/starvation because the affected dams were not able to feed their offspring due to mastitis (personal field observation during O/EA-3 outbreaks in West Africa – Metwally 2019).

On recovery from FMD, at least 50% of ruminants may become "carriers" with a persistent subclinical infection. A carrier is defined as an animal with an unapparent infection, where a virus can be isolated from the oropharynx beyond 28 days of the initial virus infection. Persistent FMDV infection occurs in both vaccinated and naïve cattle, regardless of the occurrence of clinical disease. The African buffalo is the only species demonstrated to transmit FMDV to naïve buffalo during the carrier state (Vosloo et al. 1996; Perez-Martin et al. 2016; Tekleghiorghis et al. 2016). A recent study suggested that the duration of FMDV persistent infection in cattle may be longer than previously documented, while supporting earlier conclusions that the risk of virus transmission from carriers to contact cattle under field conditions is low (Bertram et al. 2018). In contrast, swine do not appear to become carriers even if some contrary evidence has been published (Mohamed et al. 2011).

The past decade has been an exciting period for efforts for FMD control and elimination, as a result of a novel stepwise methodology for a risk-based and cost-effective control approach, referred to as the Progressive Control Pathway (PCP) which was followed by development of the FAO-OIE Global FMD Control Strategy in 2012 (www.fao.org/3/an390e/an390e.pdf).The PCP for FMD was designed to assist endemic countries to develop sustainable national FMD control policies appropriate to their livestock sectors, and medium- to long-term national strategies for progressive reduction of the disease impact.

Foot and mouth disease outbreaks are usually controlled by vaccination, quarantines and movement restrictions, euthanasia of affected and in-contact animals, and cleaning and disinfection of affected premises, equipment, and vehicles. Good biosecurity measures should be practiced on uninfected farms to prevent entry of the virus. Vaccines have a crucial role in the control, prevention, and eradication of the disease as demonstrated by eradication of FMD from Europe and the control and progressive elimination of FMD in South America since the 1940s. Effective vaccination programs have been shown to reduce virus shedding and transmission from vaccinated to susceptible naïve animals and decrease virus persistence (Mahy 2004; Orsel et al. 2007a,b). An effective vaccination program depends on the quality of the vaccine and the match to the circulating virus, among other important factors (Metwally and Münstermann 2016).

The main objective of this chapter is to provide a review on FMD vaccines, vaccination strategy, application, and effectiveness of vaccination programs.

17.2 Types of Vaccines

Attempts to develop FMD vaccines were started in the early twentieth century by Belin who succeeded in the attenuation of the virus (Belin 1927). In the 1960s, intensive studies on attenuated FMD vaccines were conducted, but faced major problems with unpredictable virulence in the field. This led to the development of inactivated vaccines (Waldmann et al. 1937) using virus from the epithelium and vesicular fluid of tongues of deliberately infected cattle and inactivation of the virus with formaldehyde in the presence of aluminum hydroxide gel. Clearly, the need to deliberately infect cattle was undesirable and production of Waldmann-type vaccines was greatly assisted by the work of Frenkel (1947) who used suspensions of epithelial tissues obtained from the tongues of recently slaughtered healthy cattle to propagate the virus.

The Frenkel procedure became the cornerstone of vaccine production for many years. The disadvantages with the use of bovine tongue epithelium included the logistics of collecting sufficient material as well as maintaining sterility throughout the process, which prompted research to find a cell line more appropriate to production needs. Mowat and Chapman (1962) adapted the baby hamster kidney (BHK-21) monolayer cell line for industrial-scale virus and vaccine production. The most significant industrial developments in this area were made by Capstick (Capstick et al. 1962), who adapted BHK monolayer cells to growth in suspension, and by Telling and Elsworth (1965) who produced the suspension cells in large-scale fermenters. Almost all current FMD vaccines are now produced in this way.

While formaldehyde inactivation proved to be an acceptable process for many years, it became increasingly apparent that its use carried a slight risk of residual contamination of inactivated vaccines with live virus. From a regulatory standpoint, binary ethyleneimine (BEI) inactivation was invariably demanded by national and international authorities, and formaldehyde inactivation was no longer acceptable. Additionally, the use of adjuvants with inactivated FMD antigen preparations was essential for satisfactory potency such as aluminum hydroxide with a second adjuvant, saponin. Both adjuvants are still routinely used in aqueous vaccines for ruminants but in pigs they induce poor antibody responses.

17.2.1 Killed Vaccines

Conventional, killed FMD vaccines have been used effectively for many years, providing good immunity if used correctly. The virus is usually propagated in BHK cells and the virus suspension is clarified by filtration or centrifugation to remove cell debris. The clarified virus is then inactivated by BEI followed by virus concentration by precipitation, ultrafiltration, or a combination of both. The use of viral antigen purified of nonstructural proteins (NSP) allows the differentiation of infected from vaccinated animals (DIVA) (Cao et al. 2017). Based on the type of adjuvant, the vaccines can be in aqueous or oil form. Aqueous vaccines are formulated with aluminum hydroxide and saponin and the oil vaccines come in single and double emulsion. Vaccines containing aluminum hydroxide and saponin as adjuvants have several deficiencies such as the induction of short-lived antibody responses which require relatively frequent revaccinations at intervals of 6 or even 4 months. In contrast, oil-based vaccines appear to have several advantages such as the induction of high titers and long-lived antibody responses for more effective protection which can also overcome interference by maternal antibodies in neonates (Iyer et al. 2000). Aqueous vaccines are used in cattle, sheep, goats, and buffalo, and oil vaccines used in all species.

Killed vaccines only confer protection against the serotype(s) in the vaccine, and in some cases do not provide intraserotype protection given the antigenic variation existing among strains within a serotype (Doel 1996). Vaccination with multiple serotypes or strains broadens the protection conferred overall, if not by each vaccine strain individually (Lyons et al. 2017; Waters et al. 2018). Increasing the potency can also increase the range of protection among strains within a serotype (Brehm et al. 2008). It is important to note that the instability of some serotypes, such as SAT, affects the quality of vaccines and therefore the duration of immunity. As a consequence, many countries in Africa have to rely on a triple or quadruple annual vaccination schedule.

The killed vaccines present other shortcomings, such as expense, possible incomplete virus inactivation, need for biosafety level 3 laboratories meeting the Good Manufacturing Practice (GMP) or Good Laboratory Practice (GLP) international standards for production and requirement for a cold chain to preserve antigen stability. Several areas of improvements are needed in longevity of the immune response, ease of differentiation between vaccinated and infected animals, prevention of carrier animals, route of inoculation, and elimination of the need for maintenance of a cold chain (Barnett et al. 2002). Additionally, quality assurance and quality control testing of finished products by independent vaccine quality control centers should be the common practice prior to the batch release.

In recent years, "vaccine banks" have been developed containing purified antigen concentrates which may be used to produce high-potency emergency vaccines at short notice. More information on vaccine banks can be found in Chapter 16.

17.2.1.1 Vaccination Schedule

According to the European Pharmacopoeia (Council of Europe 2013), the minimum protective level of an FMD vaccine cannot be less than $3PD_{50}$ (50% protective dose). In addition, vaccines with a $6PD_{50}$ protective level can be used in emergency situations. It was reported that vaccination with a $6PD_{50}$ vaccine as a primary dose followed by a secondary dose, 2–8 weeks apart, should be used to overcome maternal immunity (Cokcaliskan et al. 2017). Then subsequent booster vaccination every 4–6 months (Doel 2003) should be followed for prolonged protection. Once animals have reached an age of 2 years, only annual booster doses may be necessary to maintain protective immunity.

17.2.2 Live Attenuated Vaccine

Live vaccines have been used historically. Virus strains attenuation was attempted by passage in mice, rabbits, guinea pigs, chick embryos, and later tissue culture. Their use ceased due to the following problems:

- Difficult to achieve a balance between loss of virulence and maintenance of capability to induce protection against challenge.
- Strains which appeared to have been successfully modified under laboratory conditions may be pathogenic under some field conditions.
- Vaccine adverse reactions.
- Incomplete protection.
- Attenuation for one species does not guarantee attenuation for other species.
- Time taken to develop correct degree of attenuation is disadvantageous when faced with an outbreak involving a new virus subtype requiring the development of a new vaccine.
- Restriction of meat and animal products importation from areas where live modified vaccines were used.
- Risk of contamination with other viruses.

17.2.3 Novel Vaccines in the Pipeline

Though inactivated vaccines are widely applied for control of FMD, they have certain limitations, including safety concerns during manufacture and the consequent costs of high-containment vaccine manufacturing facilities. There has also been considerable interest in the development of novel vaccines which would, for example, not need to be kept refrigerated during storage. There are as yet no fully developed thermostable vaccines, although some promising candidates have been made by mutating residues at the capsid interface using predictive modeling (Scott et al. 2017).

17.2.3.1 Recombinant Vaccines

Recombinant vaccines have been considered as they are safe to produce, noninfectious, DIVA compliant, and can be produced in a BSL2 facility (Grubman et al. 2010). Among the newer vaccine candidates with promising potential are the human replication-defective adenovirus 5 (Ad5) vectored FMD vaccines that have been demonstrated to be effective for protection against FMDV (Grubman et al. 2010; Moraes et al. 2011). Ad5-FMD vaccines have so far been developed against A24, O1 Campos, O1 Manisa, and O/China/99 with varying degrees of success. Ad5-A24 is by far the most successful recombinant vaccine, conferring complete protection from challenge in swine and cattle as early as 7 days post vaccination and the vaccine has been granted a conditional license in the USA for use in cattle in an emergency situation (Grubman et al. 2012). Recent studies suggested that while the recombinant Ad5-FMD vaccine has potential use in a monovalent form, its application in multivalent form is not currently encouraging (Sreenivasa et al. 2017).

17.2.3.2 Peptide Vaccines

Peptide vaccines are an attractive alternative strategy to the inactivated vaccines that rely on the use of short peptide fragments to induce a highly targeted immune response, consequently avoiding allergenic and/or reactogenic sequences (Li et al. 2014). Various synthetic peptide or recombinant protein vaccines based on the FMDV VP1 G-H loop have been shown to be effective in pigs (Shao et al. 2011), but they have shown limited efficacy in cattle (Zhang et al. 2015), pointing to the limitations of these vaccines in eliciting broad protective responses in different hosts. Synthetic peptides are particularly attractive vaccine candidates as they are highly pure, defined, stable, and safe, and due to their modular approach, they can incorporate different B and T cell peptides (Blanco et al. 2016). A recent study showed that two dendrimeric peptides, B2T and B4T, can elicit specific humoral responses in cattle and confer partial protection against challenge with a heterologous type O virus (O1/Campos/Bra/58) (Soria et al. 2018).

17.2.3.3 DNA Vaccines

DNA vaccines have not been completely evaluated in livestock despite promising preliminary data in mice and pigs. A study in pigs showed that plasmid vaccine encoding two FMDV VP1 epitopes (amino acid residues 141–160 and 200–213) provided protection against the development of clinical signs such as increased body temperature, foot lesions, or mouth lesions when challenged with FMDV (Wong et al. 2000). A plasmid DNA vaccine administered intramuscularly in pigs was found to produce an enhanced immune response when co-administered with interleukin-2 (Wong et al. 2002). A DNA vaccine expressing single FMDV B and T cell epitopes was able to protect mice, despite the mice not having detectable antibodies at the time of challenge.

17.3 Immune Response and Duration of Immunity

Immune responses can be subdivided broadly into two parts: innate and adaptive immunity. Innate immunity provides a rapid and broad response to challenge by pathogens, the adaptive response is characterized by antigen specificity and, under certain circumstances, the development of immunological memory.

Passive immunity studies in cattle have shown that protection from FMDV infection can be mediated by antibody. Also, studies performed in cattle demonstrated that calves born to dams regularly vaccinated against multiple FMDV serotypes had protective levels of FMDV-specific maternal antibodies and this protection declined in parallel with the reduction in maternal antibody titers (Auge de Mello et al. 1989).

Cattle that have recovered from FMDV challenge remain protected from further rechallenge with the same FMDV strain for many years (Cunliffe 1964). This suggests that FMDV challenge results in the development of a long-lasting antibody response that is able to protect the animal from rechallenge. Indeed, Pega et al. (2013) have shown that FMDV infection results in the rapid induction of plasma cells at the site of viral replication. Thus, it is proposed that the sustained antibody response seen in cattle recovered from FMDV challenge is the result of continuous stimulation of the immune system and prolonged duration of immunity. Pega et al. (2013) have also demonstrated that rapid induction of FMDV-specific plasma cells in local lymphoid tissue, following live virus challenge, is consistent with induction of a rapid protective antibody response.

Foot and mouth disease virus vaccines are inactivated virus formulated in adjuvant and predominantly comprise structural proteins assembled into capsids (Doel 1996). There are several different conformations of the FMDV structural proteins: the whole virus particle (146S), empty virus particles (75S), and a pentameric cluster formed of VP1, 2, and 3 (12S) (Doel 1996). The immunogenicity of each of these virion structures differs, with 146S being the most immunogenic and 12S the least (Doel and Baccarini 1981; Doel and Chong 1982). FMDV capsids are inherently unstable structures which are sensitive to both heat and pH. There is a correlation between the thermal stability of the FMDV virion and its immunogenicity. Thus, stability of the 146S structure is essential for promoting good vaccine efficacy and the poor thermal stability exhibited by the FMDV capsid may account for the lack of long-term immunity derived from FMDV vaccination (Doel 1996).

There are five antigenic sites on the FMDV capsid, including the GH-loop, which is regarded as being highly immunogenic (Crowther et al. 1993). The GH-loop is used by FMDV as the integrin cell attachment site (Acharya et al. 1989). The GH-loop is located within the VP1 protein (135–156) and is a fully exposed, highly disordered, and mobile structure (Acharya et al. 1989). These structural features are likely acting as a T-dependent (T-D) epitope. Indeed, $CD4^+$ T cell depletion in cattle resulted in the reduction of G-H loop (VP1 135–156) specific antibodies, which indicates that the antibody response to this epitope is dependent upon the presence of specific $CD4^+$ T cells (Juleff et al. 2009).

During FMDV live virus challenge, $CD4^+$ T cell depletion also resulted in the loss of antibody responses to NSPs, which again indicates the T-dependency of the NSP-specific antibody response (Juleff et al. 2009). Carr et al. have also shown that stimulating $CD4^+$ T cell response during FMDV vaccination is important for generating an optimum protective antibody titer in cattle (Carr et al. 2013).

Empty FMDV capsid antigens that are structurally indistinguishable from FMDV virions (Porta et al. 2013) were also able to induce FMDV protective specific antibody responses after primary immunization. Therefore, FMDV vaccines based on the intact capsid structure can rapidly induce protective antibody responses because T cell help is not required for them to induce antibody.

17.4 Vaccine Selection

Because immunity to FMDV is serotype specific, and in some cases strain specific, the aim is to select a vaccine that incorporates one or more vaccine strains that are able to induce protective immunity against high-risk virus strains. The levels of protective immunity that can be induced depend upon three main factors: (i) the potency of the vaccine, (ii) the antigenic match between the vaccine strain and the field strain, and (iii) the vaccination schedule (Nicholls et al. 1984). For example, a highly potent vaccine may cross-protect against a wide range of divergent strains and give relatively long-lasting immunity after a single dose. In contrast, a vaccine with a low potency will induce an antigenically narrow and short-lived protection, but if a second round of vaccination, 1 month after the first dose, has been given, the boost in antibodies will contribute to broader and longer-lasting protection (Metwally and Münstermann 2016).

When selecting viruses for matching to inform vaccine selection in an endemic scenario, it is important to ensure that several isolates are included and that they are representative of different geographical areas, matching to the currently circulating strains (considering that long-distance virus spread can occur – see Introduction), species affected, and time periods. The serological relationship between a field isolate and a vaccine virus ("r" value) can be determined by virus neutralization test (VNT) or enzyme-linked immunosorbent assay (ELISA). A list of recommended vaccine strains for each region is regularly updated and published in the annual report of the OIE-FAO FMD reference laboratory network (www.wrlfmd.org; www.foot-and-mouth.org/Ref-Lab-Network).

17.5 Desired Specifications When Ordering Vaccine

Purchasing vaccines in most cases follows tendering procedures with information provided by the tenderer and manufacturers. These procedures are fully described in the FMD vaccination and postvaccination monitoring guidelines (Metwally and Münstermann 2016).

The vaccine manufacturer should meet the following requirements:

- The vaccine must be produced in facilities which can prove to be in compliance with GMP, have a valid GMP certificate and have been inspected in the last 2 years.
- The vaccine production and quality control testing of the final batch and the finished product must be conducted in accordance with OIE standards – Chapters 1.1.8 and 3.1.8 of the *Manual of Diagnostic Tests and Vaccines*.
- Licensing: the vaccine must be registered and licensed or otherwise, a special permission should be arranged by the recipient government.

- Vaccines must be transported in insulated containers, accompanied by cold chain monitors during transportation and in transit warehouses, and should be kept at the temperature prescribed by manufacturer. For the cold chain monitoring, each individual package should contain a temperature control card, type UNICEF/UNIPACK 1183. 050 (WHO, EPI/CC/15/81.8) or equivalent.

The procurement of vaccines should include the following information from the tenderers to enable the manufacturer to provide a satisfactory vaccine along with the necessary documentation:

- Vaccine type: specify the vaccine serotypes and virus strains (i.e. polyvalent vaccine).
- Species: the FMD vaccine must be approved for use in the target animals.
- Quantity: specify number of doses and doses per vial.
- Route of administration.
- Adjuvant: specify type of adjuvant (single oil emulsion, double oil emulsion, or aluminum hydroxide and saponin).
- Potency: specify vaccine potency in PD_{50} (usually >3 PD_{50}), specify the onset (usually 2 weeks) and duration of immunity (usually 6 months or longer).
- Stability: the shelf-life of the vaccine (finished product or batch) must be stated (usually a period of at least 12 months).
- Reference sera: indicate if sera for homologous vaccine strains to use as reference standards in serological tests for postvaccination monitoring (PVM) can be made available to the tenderer.
- Recommended vaccination schedule: normally requires a two-dose primary course to achieve 6 months of protection.
- Special requirements concerning the label (e.g. size, language, warnings).

17.5.1 Information to Be Provided by the Manufacturer with the Vaccines

Each batch of FMD vaccine should be accompanied by documentation specific to the batch, signed by an authorized, suitably qualified expert of the manufacturer, containing all the product information:

- Manufacturer's name, contacts, and provision of production schedule.
- Manufacturer's authorization.
- Certificate of GMP.
- Vaccine quality control certificate.
- Quality control test results of the vaccine batch(s) with associated standard operating procedures to demonstrate compliance with OIE standards including sterility, safety, innocuity, and potency tests.
- Type of vaccine, name of strains, date of batch production, batch identification, volume of contents, dose per species, storage recommendations, and expiry date. Package insert may be in English with instructions on recommended dose per species and vaccination protocol and scheme.
- Tenders should be accompanied by full details concerning the tenderer's legal status. Proof should be given of the GMP and quality assurance (QA) system that is applied and of recent audits by the international or national accreditation body.
- When appropriate, provide data showing that the vaccine does not induce antibodies to the 3ABC NSP. The data should also provide evidence of the duration of immunity following a single vaccination and after a booster given 1–3 months after primo-vaccination.
- Provide available data on the expected onset and duration of immunity of each serotype/strain.
- Provide available correlation data between protection and antibody titer, and specify test used for such correlation (type of ELISA and virus neutralization test). These data will be valuable in determining level of postvaccination herd immunity and the evaluation of the vaccination program.
- The tender dossier should be submitted in the desired language and must provide documentation/proof on all the points listed above, as well as the date and port of delivery, the storage recommendations, and the expiry date.

17.6 Quality Assurance and Control Testing

17.6.1 In-Process Control

Virus inactivation and follow-up safety tests are the most critical steps in the preparation of inactivated FMD vaccines. Vaccines must be quantified for their antigen content.

- Biological test systems may be used such as cell culture tests.
- Complement fixation tests may be used to give a quantitative estimate of total antigenic mass or of just the major 140S immunogen. An ELISA is used to estimate 140S particles.
- Sucrose density gradient analysis is a quantitative test, estimating the 140 S antigen in μg/mL. Now accepted internationally as a standard test.

17.6.2 Final Product Batch Tests

The vaccine batch of the final product should be testing by the manufacturer as described in Chapters 1.1.8 and 3.1.8 of the *Manual of Diagnostic Tests and Vaccines* for safety, sterility, identity, innocuity, purity, and potency.

17.7 Vaccine Application for Disease Control

Vaccination strategies for the control of FMD depend on the objectives of the control program and the epidemiology of infection. Three strategy scenarios can be described.

17.7.1 Risk-Based Vaccination

Risk is a combination of the probability of a hazard occurring and the magnitude of the consequences. In the context of risk-based control of livestock diseases, this involves an understanding of risk factors for disease or infection, or risk hotspots for transmission along the value chain, and the impact they have on different production sectors. There are many examples of risk factor studies for FMD in the scientific literature (for example: Bronsvoort et al. 2004; Allepuz et al. 2015; Elnekave et al. 2015; Emami et al. 2015; Elnekave et al. 2016; Abdela 2017), and factors vary in different settings. The impact of disease can be thought of in terms of effects on production (e.g. milk yield, weight gains, mortality) although these data are less commonly reported (Knight-Jones and Rushton 2013; Knight-Jones et al. 2017). The combination of risk factor analysis and impact can be used to highlight areas where control measures like vaccination could be applied to give the maximum benefit from available resources. Risk-based vaccination has been used for numerous other transmissible infections including avian (Swayne et al. 2011) and human influenza (Blank and Szucs 2009).

Risk-based vaccination is most likely to be appropriate in settings where resources are limited. A risk-based approach to control and vaccination is a fundamental feature of the PCP-FMD (FAO and OIE 2018). Decisions on vaccinating small ruminants for FMD are one example of risk-based vaccination since both their role in the epidemiology of FMD and the consequences of disease in this population need to be considered. Because their role will vary in different settings depending on factors including population density and management systems, field data should be collected to justify their inclusion within the objectives of the overall control strategy.

17.7.2 Reactive Vaccination

Reactive vaccination uses vaccine in response to the suspected or confirmed presence of a target pathogen. It can be considered a type of risk-based vaccination in that it is responding to a heightened risk based on confirmed presence of disease or infection although other types of risk-based vaccination involve planned campaigns.

This type of vaccination can be described as suppressive (to reduce the spread of infection by vaccinating in known infected areas) or protective (to protect animals beyond the immediate surroundings of an infected area that are at risk of potential exposure) (Animal Health Australia 2014). For the latter, vaccine is normally applied over a defined area outside a nonvaccinated buffer zone (Figure 17.2). This nonvaccinated buffer zone is needed to reduce the risk of vaccinating animals that are incubating infection that would render vaccination ineffective, and also to reduce the risk of vaccinators carrying virus from infectious to susceptible farms and contributing to onward transmission. It is often referred to as "ring" vaccination due to the hypothetical circular shape of the vaccination zone around an outbreak, although often these shapes are not uniform, making the term "reactive" more appropriate and consistent with language used in the literature (Tildesley et al. 2006).

A reactive vaccination strategy for FMD is commonly considered in free countries in the event of an incursion. There are many examples in the literature of simulation models that predict the impact of reactive vaccination if outbreaks occurred in free countries. These models are useful in developing contingency plans and may consider a range of conditions, including the size of the vaccination zone that typically varies from 3 to 10 km (Roche et al. 2015). In countries already using mass vaccination (see next section), it may also be used as an additional strategy to contain an outbreak. Reactive vaccination is also commonly applied in low-resource endemic settings due to low availability of vaccines and other resources. In either context, the size and shape of the zones are likely to vary depending on the livestock density, geographical distribution of outbreaks, vaccine availability, and vaccination capacity.

For a reactive strategy to be effective, there are fundamental requirements related to surveillance, vaccines, vaccination, and other control measures (Box 17.1). If these conditions cannot be satisfied, then the rationale of this approach should be questioned. In endemic settings with low vaccine availability, a nonreactive, risk-based approach should be considered the primary vaccination strategy.

In countries wishing to gain or regain official disease-free status from the OIE, reactive vaccination may or may

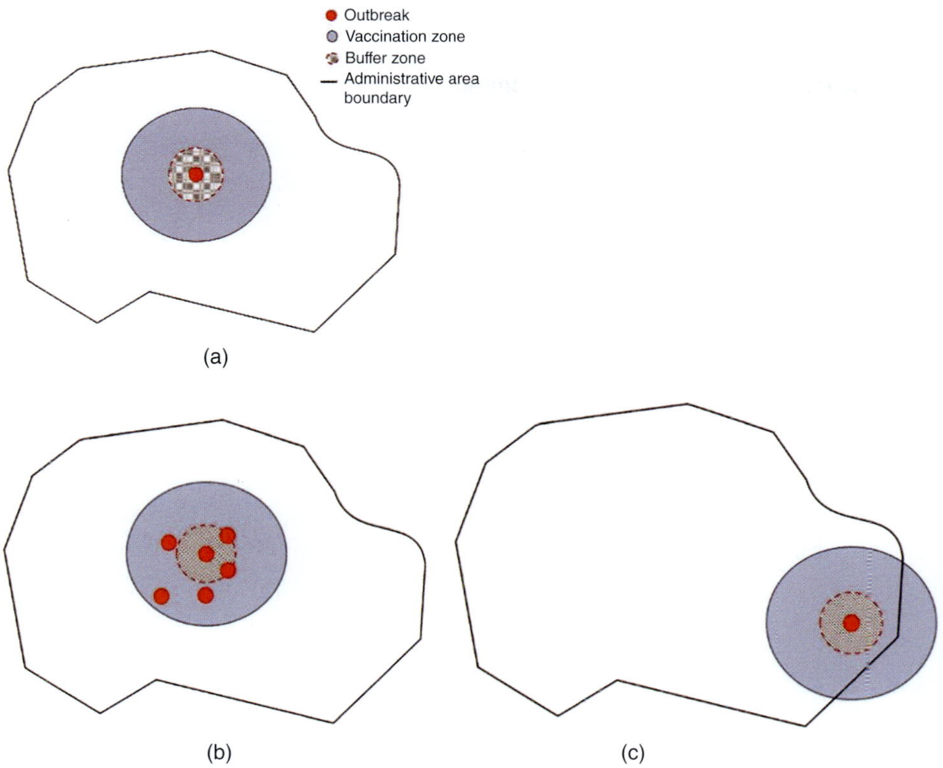

Figure 17.2 Schematic representation of reactive vaccination and associated problems with the approach. (a) Buffer and vaccination zones around a single outbreak location. (b) Possibility of unknown infections within the buffer and vaccination zones. (c) Zones overlapping administrative boundaries.

Box 17.1 Conditions required for successful implementation of reactive vaccination for FMD surveillance

An efficient early-warning surveillance system with rapid reporting of outbreaks: effective targeted surveillance to give confidence in the location of infected farms and the required size of the buffer and vaccination zones

Livestock movement controls

- strict animal and product movement restrictions within the buffer and vaccination zones

Vaccine

- Use of a high-potency vaccine with a minimum $6PD_{50}$ (although higher [$>10PD_{50}$] is preferred)
- Good match between the field and vaccine virus strains
- NSP purified vaccines to allow post outbreak sero-surveillance (essential in free settings with objective to regain FMD free status; less important in endemic settings)

Vaccination

- Rapid mobilization of vaccines and capacity to vaccinate
- Optimum biosecurity practices of the vaccination teams
- High vaccine coverage targeting all FMD-susceptible livestock in the vaccination zone

not be followed by culling of vaccinated animals as specified in the OIE Terrestrial Code (OIE 2018). The need for culling comes from the possibility that vaccinated animals may be infected and become carriers of FMD virus with imperfect tests to detect these animals. A "vaccinate to die" strategy involves culling these animals and can lead to a disease-free status being regained 3 months after the slaughter of all vaccinated animals and serological surveillance. A "vaccinate to live" strategy does not cull vaccinated animals and lengthens the time before free status can be regained to 6 months. A review of the scientific rationale behind these prolonged restrictions with vaccination suggests it is feasible to have similar restriction periods with or without culling of vaccinated animals if sufficient evidence can be provided of the effectiveness of vaccination and the absence of infection (Geale et al. 2015).

In endemic settings, reactive vaccination is sometimes applied directly to epidemiological units (e.g. individual farms, villages) that already have evidence of active disease. This practice is likely to increase the risk of within-farm transmission through mixing animals, using communal facilities, sharing equipment, and movements of personnel. It is very challenging to apply adequate biosecurity to prevent transmission on infected farms except in certain circumstances where the infected group is located far from the main herd. Moreover, vaccination is unlikely to be effective if animals are exposed within a few days of vaccination or have already been exposed when vaccine has been applied. Despite these theoretical risks and lack of beneficial evidence in the literature, anecdotally many people believe this strategy reduces the overall incidence and severity of disease on an infected unit. There is a need to generate epidemiological and economic data to test this approach, for example through a cluster-randomized trial, although these studies are challenging to perform.

17.7.3 Mass Vaccination

Mass vaccination aims to achieve a high coverage of a target susceptible species in a defined area. For FMD, it is typically used in high-resource settings with the objective of eliminating circulation of virus from the target population. Due to the short duration of immunity and high population turnover of livestock, mass vaccination must be repeated regularly (Knight-Jones et al. 2016), requiring a high level of commitment that can take decades to reach the required objectives (Naranjo and Cosivi 2013).

A key consideration when implementing mass vaccination is the target coverage that must be achieved to meet the program objectives. For any transmissible infection, this can be estimated from an understanding of the basic reproduction number (R_0), which is the average number of secondary cases for each primary case in an immunologically naïve population (Figure 17.3). The net reproduction number (R_n) is the same measure, but in a population with some level of immunity through natural exposure or vaccination. If the R_n is less than 1, the circulation of the pathogen will ultimately cease in that population. Reproduction numbers are in part dependent on the effective contact rate between infectious and susceptible individuals (Vynnycky and White 2010). Although classically considered to be a measure for individuals, for livestock, this is often considered at the epidemiological unit level (for example farms).

The "herd immunity threshold" is the percentage of a population that must be immune in order for the R_n to be equal to 1 (Figure 17.4). Population-level immunity in excess of this threshold means the number of secondary cases for each primary case is less than 1 and infection will

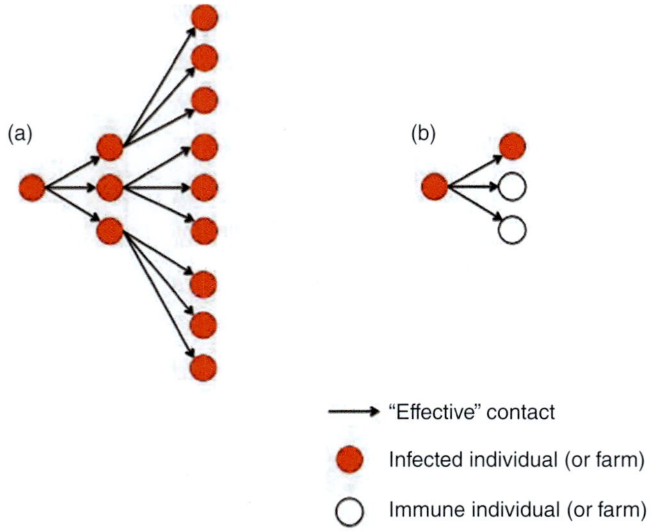

Figure 17.3 Reproduction number. (a) The basic reproduction number (R_0) is the average number of secondary cases for each primary case of disease in an immunologically naïve population. In this example the R_0 is 3. (b) The net reproduction number (R_n) is the same measure but in a population with some level of immunity such as through natural exposure or vaccination. In this example, of the three effective contacts, two were with immune individuals so the R_n is 1, meaning the infection remains at a steady endemic level in the population. On average, the R_n must be below 1 in order for the infection to be eliminated from a population.

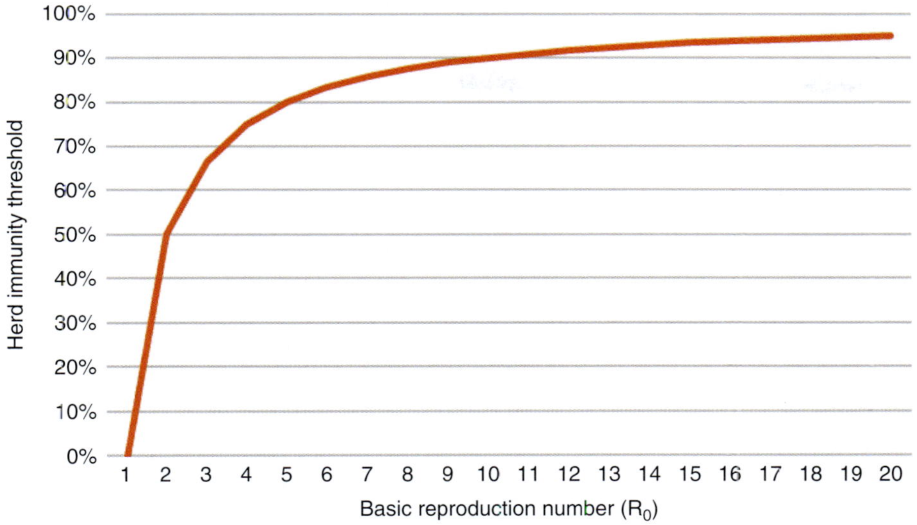

Figure 17.4 Relationship between the basic reproduction number (R_0) and the herd immunity threshold. R_0 is the average number of secondary cases for each primary case in an immunologically naïve population. The net reproduction number (R_n) is the same measure but in a population with some level of immunity through natural exposure or vaccination. The herd immunity threshold is the level of immunity in a population required to bring the R_n to 1.0 so that population-level immunity in excess of this value should result in a R_n less than 1 and infection dying out from the population. R_0 values are typically based on individual animals although where farms are well-defined epidemiological units with infection risk highly clustered at the farm level, whole farms can be considered in the R_0 calculation.

die out from the population. It can be shown that the herd immunity threshold can be related to R_0 through the following equation:

$$Herd\ immunity\ threshold = 1 - \frac{1}{R_0}$$

Estimates of the R_0 for FMD based on individual animals in the literature are scarce but have been estimated to vary between 2 and over 70 (Woolhouse et al. 1996), which require vaccine coverages of 50.0–98.6% respectively to reduce the R_0 to 1. However, in actual FMD control programs, the target coverage is almost always between 80% and 85% with the origin of this recommendation unclear and the target unproven (Lombard and Schermbrucker 1994). Based on our knowledge of the reproduction number and herd immunity threshold, the required target will vary depending on the level of transmission within the population. This is reflected in the R_0 estimate that should be based on data collected from the field. Where farms are in well-defined epidemiological units, and disease risk is likely to be highly clustered at the farm level, it may be more appropriate to consider whole farms for the R_0 rather than individual animals (Thornley and France 2009), and coverage as the percentage of farms.

It is also important to appreciate that vaccinated is not the same as immunized, and there are numerous reasons why vaccinated animals may not be rendered immune from infection. It is therefore important to use rigorous, repeatable epidemiological methods to measure coverage and population-level immunity. These are described in the FAO-OIE postvaccination monitoring guidelines (Metwally and Münstermann 2016). For a high-resource strategy like mass vaccination, it is essential that an appropriate monitoring and evaluation system be implemented to ensure targets are being achieved and resources are being appropriately allocated.

17.8 Combination with Other Vaccines

Due to the high frequency of FMD vaccination, it is often desirable to vaccinate livestock concurrently with other vaccines for the diseases of priority. Currently available FMD vaccines are killed, and it is often the case that co-administration with a live vaccine is desired (e.g. lumpy skin disease, peste des petits ruminants [PPR]). Interactions between the immune responses that the different vaccine types induce is possible and could be enhanced or reduced (Fletcher et al. 2004). The evidence in the literature for co-vaccination with FMD vaccines is limited. One study in goats demonstrated that combining a live attenuated PPR vaccine with a killed FMD vaccine led to a higher antibody response to FMD virus compared with administering the FMD vaccine alone (Mansoor et al. 2018). Similar studies with different vaccines of interest in target species are necessary and multiple immunizations should be evaluated to avoid immune system dysfunction prior to implementing co-vaccination programs.

17.9 Postvaccination Monitoring

Foot and mouth disease vaccines elicit an antibody response against the structural proteins of the virus which can be measured by serological tests to determine the level of immunity. Based on challenge studies, there is a correlation between the level of structural protein antibodies and protection. This correlation can be established for a particular vaccine with serological tests (ELISA and virus neutralization test), and compared with the vaccine-induced serological responses measured in the field.

There are two general approaches to assessing the immune status of a population.

- Assessing the population immunity at individual animal level. This method is recommended whenever vaccination is carried out in countries at PCP stage 2 or 3 (when FMD virus is still circulating).
- Assessing the population immunity at herd level. This method is recommended at higher stages of PCP (stages 3 and 4) when the virus circulation is low and a country is achieving official status of freedom with or without vaccination.

Details on the methodological computation and interpretation of results are provided in the PVM guidelines (Metwally and Münstermann 2016).

17.10 Outbreaks in Vaccinated Animals

Investigation of outbreaks in vaccinated animals is an important aspect of monitoring the effectiveness of vaccination. A systematic approach is recommended to assess if the vaccination performance is below target and requires further follow-up to assess the underlying reasons. This should include an assessment of all the steps where the problem could potentially have occurred from initial vaccine quality, suitability, through vaccine storage, delivery and vaccination, vaccine coverage, etc. The timing of outbreaks in relation to vaccination is a key consideration as immunity takes time to develop and then wanes (Figure 17.5).

17.11 Vaccine Adverse Reactions

Administration of a dose of some FMD vaccine strains may produce swellings at the injection site in many animals. These local reactions normally resolve over a period of 4 weeks postvaccination, but may persist for longer in a small number of animals. It is common to observe a slight increase of rectal temperature of up to 0.7 °C for 4 days postvaccination in the absence of other generalized clinical signs.

In Brazil, it was reported in 2016 that in some cases the intramuscular administration of vaccines containing saponin may cause anaphylactic shock or formation of abscesses in the forehead and neck. Such lesions should be removed after slaughter. This causes great damage to both the farmers and the slaughterhouses because of the disposal of that part of the meat. Estimates indicate that the producers lose an average of 2 kg of meat per animal due to vaccine reaction at the site of injection. Additionally, it was reported in 2016 that approximately 30 million head were processed through abattoirs and about 70 000 tons of meat were discarded (www.beefpoint.com.br/nota-tecnica-cna-reacoes-adversas-a-vacina-contra-febre-aftosa). Similarly, the issue of injection site granulomas postvaccination has been documented in the Republic of Korea (Lyons et al. 2016) and has been proposed as an important factor that has contributed to a reduced uptake of vaccination that has compromised coverage and reduced the value of the carcases.

One study reported a case of adverse postvaccination allergic reactions, which occurred in a dairy cattle herd 8 days after the annual FMD vaccination (Yeruham et al. 2001). The dermatological lesions observed in these cattle included urticaria, exudative and necrotic dermatitis, along with edema and vesicles on the teats. These reactions occurred in 11.3% of the heifers, in 10% of the first-lactating cows, and in 14.6% of the adult cows. The average loss of milk production for an affected cow on this farm was 21.5% per day, for 7 consecutive days. The extent of the lesions was apparently related to concurrent diseases such as bovine virus diarrhea–mucosal disease complex and Johne's disease and, to a lesser degree, correlated with the age or breed (Yeruham et al. 2001).

17.12 List of Manufacturers

Please see Table 17.1.

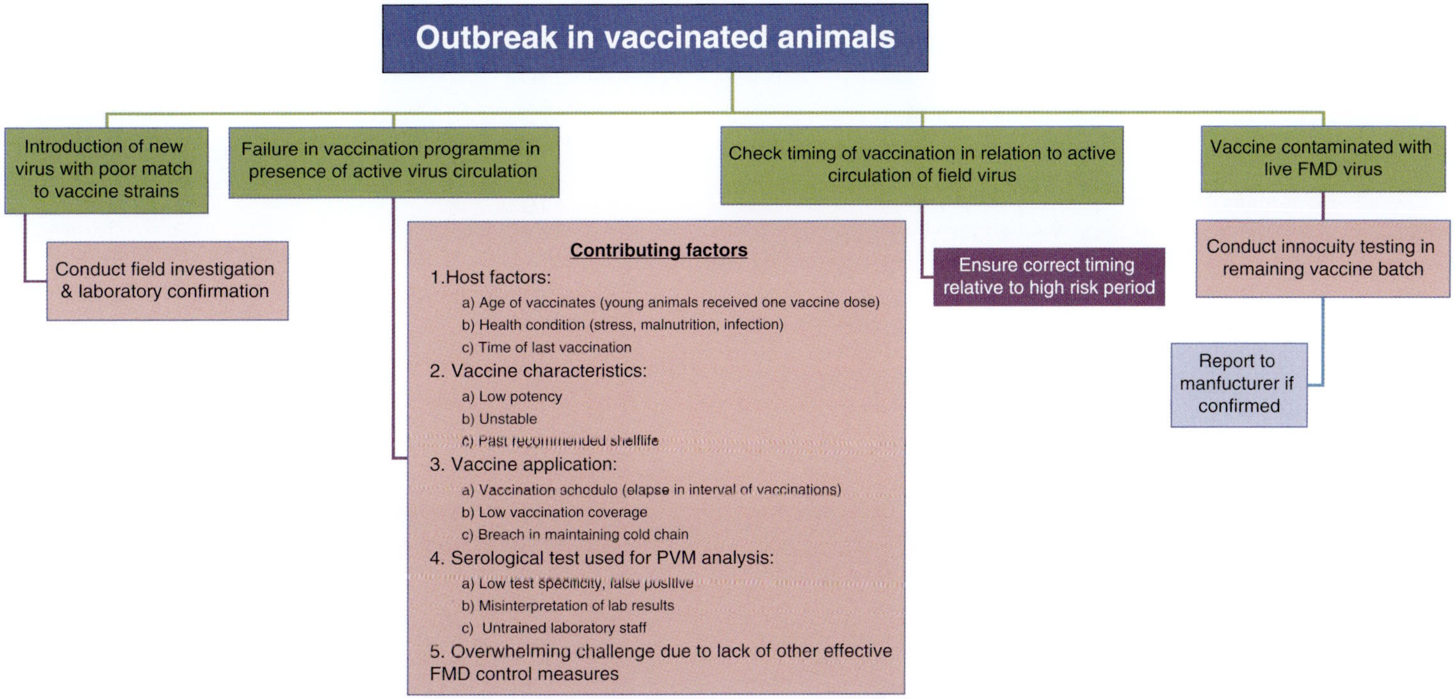

Figure 17.5 Factors contributing to vaccine and vaccination failures.

Table 17.1 List of FMD vaccine manufacturers.

Company Name	Product Name	Strain/Subtype	Adjuvant	Composition	Animal Species
Agrovet http://www.agrovet.ru/index.eng.htm	Bivalent FMD vaccine	A22, O1	Not Available	Inactivated vaccine composed of A22, O1.	Cloven-hoofed animals
Agrovet http://www.agrovet.ru/index.eng.htm	FMD (A), BHK-21 culture	Type A	Not Available	Inactivated vaccine composed of Type A.	Cloven-hoofed animals
Agrovet http://www.agrovet.ru/index.eng.htm	FMD (Asia-1), BHK-21 culture	Type Asia-1	Not Available	Inactivated vaccine composed of Type Asia-1.	Cloven-hoofed animals
Agrovet http://www.agrovet.ru/index.eng.htm	FMD (O), BHK-21 culture	Type O	Not Available	Inactivated vaccine composed of Type O.	Cloven-hoofed animals
Agrovet http://www.agrovet.ru/index.eng.htm	FMD (C), BHK-21 culture	Type C	Not Available	Inactivated vaccine composed of Type C.	Cloven-hoofed animals
Agrovet http://www.agrovet.ru/index.eng.htm	Trivalent FMD, BHK-21 culture	O, A, Asia-1	Not Available	Inactivated vaccine composed of O, A, Asia-1.	Cloven-hoofed animals
Agrovet http://www.agrovet.ru/index.eng.htm	Trivalent FMD, epithelial culture	O, A, C	Not Available	Inactivated vaccine composed of Type O, A, C.	Cloven-hoofed animals
Agrovet http://www.agrovet.ru/index.eng.htm	FMD (A), epithelial culture	Type A	Not Available	Inactivated vaccine composed of Type A.	Cloven-hoofed animals
Agrovet http://www.agrovet.ru/index.eng.htm	FMD (O), epithelial culture	Type O	Not Available	Inactivated vaccine composed of Type O.	Cloven-hoofed animals
Agrovet http://www.agrovet.ru/index.eng.htm	FMD (C), epithelial culture	Type C	Not Available	Inactivated vaccine composed of Type C.	Cloven-hoofed animals
Biogénesis-Bagó S.A. http://www.biogenesisbago.com/en/	Bioaftogen®	A24 Cruzeiro, A2001 Argentina, O1 Campos, C3 Indaial	Oil	Inactivated vaccine. Oily vaccine with FMD virus type O1 Campos, A24 Cruzeiro, A2001 and C3 Indaial, obtained in BHK cell culture, inactivated with BEI	Cattle, Swine,. Sheep and goats
Biogénesis-Bagó S.A. http://www.biogenesisbago.com/en/	Aftosan® 3	A24 Cruzeiro, O1 Campos, O1 Campos	Oil	Oil-inactivated bivalent vaccine against foot-and-mouth disease in cattle.	Cattle
Biogénesis-Bagó S.A. http://www.biogenesisbago.com/en/	Aftosan®	O1 Campos, A24 Cruzeiro, C3 Indaial	Oil	Inactivated vaccine composed of Type O1 Campos, A24 Cruzeiro, C3 Indaial.	Cloven-hoofed animals
Biogénesis-Bagó S.A. http://www.biogenesisbago.com/en/	Aftogen® Oil	O1 Campos, A24 Cruzeiro, C3 Indaial	Mineral oil, saponin	Oily vaccine. Bivalent oil vaccine with FMD virus types O1 Campos and A24 Cruzeiro obtained in cultured BHK cells and inactivated with BEI.	Cattle
Biopharma(Production Biological Society, Pharmaceutical and Veterinary) https://www.biopharma.ma/index.php/en/	Aftovax	Type O (Algeria 99)	Aluminum hydroxide, saponin	Monovalent foot-and-mouth disease vaccine type O, Algeria 99 prototype, concentrated and purified antigen, inactivated and adjuvanted with aluminum hydroxide and saponin, from multiplied viral suspensions on BHK cell cultures, ensuring protection of 3 DP50 at minimum per bovine dose.	Cattle/Sheep

Biovet https://www.biovet.com.br/	Bio-Afto-Vet	O1 Campos, A24 Cruzeiro, C3 Indaial	Mineral oil, saponin	Inactivated vaccine composed of Type O1 Campos, A24 Cruzeiro, C3 Indaial.	Cloven-hoofed animals
Boehringer Ingelheim International GmbH https://www.boehringer-ingelheim.com/locations/south-america	Aftopor® Foot-and-Mouth Inactivated Vaccine	O-Type Strains	Water in oil	Inactivated vaccine composed of O-Type Strains.	Cloven-hoofed animals
Botswana Vaccine Institute https://bvi-bw.com/	Aftovax™	O, A, SAT-1, SAT-2, SAT-3	Aluminum hydroxide, saponin	Inactivated Foot and Mouth Disease Virus containing any type of 5 serotypes appropriate to the region.	cattle, buffalo, sheep and goats
Botswana Vaccine Institute https://bvi-bw.com/	Aftovaxpur™	O, A, SAT-1, SAT-2, SAT-3	Aluminum hydroxide, saponin	Purified Inactivated Foot and Mouth Disease Virus containing any type of 5 serotypes appropriate to the region.	cattle, buffalo, sheep and goats
Brilliant Bio Pharma Ltd. https://brilliantbiopharma.com/	FUTVAC™	Types O (strain IND/O/R2/75), A (strain IND/A/40/2000), Asia-1 (strain IND/Asia1/63/72)	Oil	The viruses are propagated on BHK-21 cell culture, inactivated with aziridine compound before purification and concentration. Mineral oil (ISAMontanide 206 from Seppic, France) is added as an adjuvant and Thimerosal (0.01%w/v) as a preservative.	cattle, buffaloes, sheep and goats
Bureau of Veterinary Biologics https://brilliantbiopharma.com/	Foot and Mouth Disease Vaccine	O, A, Asia-1	Aqueous	Inactivated vaccine composed of O, A, Asia-1.	Cloven-hoofed animals
Bureau of Veterinary Biologics https://brilliantbiopharma.com/	Foot and Mouth Disease Vaccine for Swine	O, A, Asia-1	Oil	Inactivated vaccine composed of O, A, Asia-1.	Cloven-hoofed animals
Centro Diagnóstico Veterinario https://www.centrodiagnosticoveterinario.it/centro-diagnostico-veterinario/centro-diagnostico-veterinario-napoli/	Viral Aftosa Vaccine	O1 Campos, A24 Cruzeiro, A Argentina 2001, C3 Indaial	Oil	Inactivated vaccine composed of O1 Campos, A24 Cruzeiro, A Argentina 2001, C3 Indaial.	Cloven-hoofed animals
Centro Diagnóstico Veterinario https://www.centrodiagnosticoveterinario.it/centro-diagnostico-veterinario/centro-diagnostico-veterinario-napoli/	Viral Aftosa Trivalent Vaccine	O1 Campos, A24 Cruzeiro, C3 Indaial	Oil	Inactivated vaccine composed of O1 Campos, A24 Cruzeiro, C3 Indaial.	Cloven-hoofed animals
Centro Diagnóstico Veterinario https://www.centrodiagnosticoveterinario.it/centro-diagnostico-veterinario/centro-diagnostico-veterinario-napoli/	CDVac Aftosa Export Bivalent Vaccine	O1 Campos, A24 Cruzeiro	Oil	Inactivated vaccine composed of O1 Campos, A24 Cruzeiro.	Cloven-hoofed animals
China Agricultural Vet. Bio. Science and Technology Co., Ltd http://www.cavetbio.com/a/International_Services/2018/0815/225.html	FMD Trivalent Vaccine, Inactivated	O, A, Aisa-1	Not Available	Inactivated vaccine composed of O, A, Aisa-1.	Pigs

(Continued)

Table 17.1 (Continued)

Company Name	Product Name	Strain/Subtype	Adjuvant	Composition	Animal Species
China Agricultural Vet. Bio. Science and Technology Co., Ltd http://www.cavetbio.com/a/International_Services/2018/0815/225.html	Bovine Foot and Mouth Disease Bivalent Vaccine, Inactivated	Type O, Type A	Not Available	Inactivated vaccine composed of Type O, Type A.	Cloven-hoofed animals
China Agricultural Vet. Bio. Science and Technology Co., Ltd http://www.cavetbio.com/a/International_Services/2018/0815/225.html	Swine Foot and Mouth Disease Vaccine, Inactivated	Type O	Not Available	Inactivated vaccine composed of Type O.	Cloven-hoofed animals
China Agricultural Vet. Bio. Science and Technology Co., Ltd http://www.cavetbio.com/a/International_Services/2018/0815/225.html	Swine Foot and Mouth Disease Type O Synthetic Peptide Vaccine	Type O	Not Available	Inactivated vaccine composed of Type O.	Cloven-hoofed animals
China Animal Husbandry Co., Ltd. (CAHIC) https://www.cahic.com/ABOUT/index.jhtml	Foot and Mouth Disease Vaccine, Inactivated	Type O	Not Available	Inactivated vaccine composed of Type O.	Cloven-hoofed animals
China Animal Husbandry Co., Ltd. (CAHIC) https://www.cahic.com/ABOUT/index.jhtml	Bovine Foot and Mouth Disease Bivalent Peptide Vaccine	Type O, Asia1	Not Available	Inactivated vaccine composed of Type O, Asia1.	Cloven-hoofed animals
China Animal Husbandry Co., Ltd. (CAHIC) https://www.cahic.com/ABOUT/index.jhtml	Swine Foot and Mouth Disease Peptide Vaccine	Type O	Not Available	Inactivated vaccine composed of Type O.	Cloven-hoofed animals
China Animal Husbandry Co., Ltd. (CAHIC) https://www.cahic.com/ABOUT/index.jhtml	Foot and Mouth Disease Bivalent Vaccine, Inactivated	Type O, Strain OS + Asia-1, Strain JSL	Not Available	Inactivated vaccine composed of Type O, Strain OS + Asia-1, Strain JSL.	Cloven-hoofed animals
China Animal Husbandry Co., Ltd. (CAHIC) https://www.cahic.com/ABOUT/index.jhtml	Foot and Mouth Disease Trivalent Vaccine, Inactivated	O, A, Asia-1	Not Available	Inactivated vaccine composed of O, A, Asia-1.	Cloven-hoofed animals
FGBI - Federal Centre for Animal Health http://www.arriah.ru/en	FMD Sorbat Mono and Polyvalent	O, A, C, Asia-1, SAT-1, SAT-2, SAT-3	Not Available	Inactivated vaccine composed of O, A, C, Asia-1, SAT-1, SAT-2, SAT-3.	Cloven-hoofed animals
FGBI - Federal Centre for Animal Health http://www.arriah.ru/en	FMD Mono and Polyvalent Emulsion Vaccine	O, A, C, Asia-1, SAT-1, SAT-2, SAT-3	Oil	Inactivated vaccine composed of O, A, C, Asia-1, SAT-1, SAT-2, SAT-3.	Cloven-hoofed animals
FGBI - Federal Centre for Animal Health http://www.arriah.ru/en	ARRIAH-VAK Mono and Polyvalent FMD Emulsion Vaccine	O, A, C, Asia-1, SAT-1, SAT-2, SAT-3	Oil	Inactivated vaccine composed of O, A, C, Asia-1, SAT-1, SAT-2, SAT-3.	Cloven-hoofed animals

FMD Center	Foot and Mouth Disease Vaccine for Pigs	O, A, Asia-1	Oil	Inactivated vaccine composed of O, A, Asia-1.	Cloven-hoofed animals
FMD Center	Foot and Mouth Disease for Cattle, Sheep, Goats	O, A, Asia-1	Aqueous	Inactivated vaccine composed of O, A, Asia-1.	Cloven-hoofed animals
Green Cross Veterinary Products Co. Ltd. https://www.gcvp.co.kr/	FMD Vaccine	Not Available	Not Available	Inactivated vaccine.	Cloven-hoofed animals
Indian Immunologicals Limited https://www.gcvp.co.kr/	Raksha-Ovac	O, A, Asia-1	Oil	Raksha OVac Contains inactivated tissue culture FMD virus strains O, A, C and Asia-1 adjuvanted with Mineral Oil. Complete inactivation of the virus is ensured by the use of Aziridine compound.	Cattle, Buffaloes, Calves & Pigs, Sheep & Goats
Inner Mongolia Bigvet Biotech Co., Ltd.	Foot and Mouth Disease Tervalence Vaccine, Inactivated	Type O, Strain OHM/02 + TypeA, Strain AKT-III + Type Asia1, Strain Asia 1KZ/03	Not Available	Inactivated vaccine composed of Type O, Strain OHM/02 + TypeA, Strain AKT-III + Type Asia1, Strain Asia 1KZ/03.	Cloven-hoofed animals
Inova Biotecnologia Saúde Animal Ltda. http://www.innovaresaudeanimal.com.br/	AFTOMUNE	O1 Campos, A24 Cruzeiro, C3 Indaial	Oil	Inactivated vaccine composed of O1 Campos, A24 Cruzeiro, C3 Indaial.	Cloven-hoofed animals
Jinyu Bao Ling Biological Pharmaccutical Co., Ltd. http://www.jinyubaoling.com.cn/index.asp	Foot-and-Mouth Disease O-type Inactivated Vaccine	OZK/93, OR/80	Not Available	Inactivated vaccine composed of OZK/93, OR/80.	Cloven-hoofed animals
Jinyu Bao Ling Biological Pharmaceutical Co., Ltd. http://www.jinyubaoling.com.cn/index.asp	Foot-and-Mouth Disease O type, Asian Type I Divalent Inactivated Vaccine	OJMS, JSL	Not Available	Inactivated vaccine composed of OJMS, JSL.	Cloven-hoofed animals
Jinyu Bao Ling Biological Pharmaceutical Co., Ltd. http://www.jinyubaoling.com.cn/index.asp	Foot-and-Mouth Disease O-type, Asia Type 1, Type A Trivalent Inactivated Vaccine	O/MYA98/BY/2010, Asia1/JSL/ZK/06, Re-A/WH/09	Not Available	Inactivated vaccine composed of O/MYA98/BY/2010, Asia1/JSL/ZK/06, Re-A/WH/09.	Cloven-hoofed animals
Kenya Veterinary Vaccines Production Institute (KEVEVAPI) https://kevevapi.or.ke/	FOTIVAX™	A, O, C, SAT-1, SAT-2	Aluminum hydroxide gel, saponin	FOTIVAX TM is a Foot and Mouth Disease vaccine preparation containing chemically inactivated, tissue culture derived FMD virus strains.Each batch undergoes potency tests in live cattle to ensure that each dose contains at least 6.6 PD 50.	cattle, pigs, sheep and goats

(Continued)

Table 17.1 (Continued)

Company Name	Product Name	Strain/Subtype	Adjuvant	Composition	Animal Species
Limor de Colombia https://limordecolombia.godaddysites.com/	Aftolimor	O1 Campos, A24 Cruzeiro	Oil	Injectable oil vaccine against foot-and-mouth disease virus type A24 Cruzeiro and O1 Campos. Each 2ml contains Virus A24 Cruzeiro and O1 Campos 1 mL; Emulsion oil adjuvant 1 mL	Cattle
Merck Animal Health (MSD Animal Health) https://www.msd-animal-health.com/	DECIVAC®-FMD-DOE	O1, A, C, Asia-1, SAT-1, SAT-2, SAT-3(serotype dependent upon location)	Oil	An inactivated oil adjuvanted vaccine for the immunization of pigs, cattle, buffalo, sheep and goats against Foot and Mouth Disease (FMD). FMD strains included in the vaccine are dependent on the local situation where the vaccine is required.	pigs, cattle, buffalo, sheep and goats
Merck Animal Health (MSD Animal Health) https://www.msd-animal-health.com/	Aftovacin® Oleosa	O1 Campos, A24 Cruzeiro, C3 Indaial	Oil	Inactivated vaccine composed of O1 Campos, A24 Cruzeiro, C3 Indaial.	Cloven-hoofed animals
Merck Animal Health (MSD Animal Health) https://www.msd-animal-health.com/	BOVILIS™ Clovax	O, A, Asia-1	Oil	Inactivated vaccine composed of O, A, Asia-1.	Cloven-hoofed animals
Merial Brazil	Aftobov® Oleosa	O1 Campos, A24 Cruzeiro, C3 Indaial	Oil	Inactivated vaccine composed of O1 Campos, A24 Cruzeiro, C3 Indaia.	Cloven-hoofed animals
Merial Philippines https://www.boehringer-ingelheim.com.br/saude-animal/institucional?merial=true	Aftopor Monovalent	O1 Philippines	Oil	Inactivated vaccine composed of O1 Philippines.	Cloven-hoofed animals
Merial Philippines https://www.boehringer-ingelheim.com.br/saude-animal/institucional?merial=true	Aftopor Trivalent	A24 Cruzeiro, C3 Philippines, O1 Philippines	Oil	Inactivated vaccine composed of A24 Cruzeiro, C3 Philippines, O1 Philippines.	Cloven-hoofed animals
Middle East for Veterinary Vaccine (ME VAC) http://www.me-vac.com/	Tri-APHTHOVAC	A, O, SAT 2	Montonide ISA-50	Inactivated vaccine composed of A, O, SAT 2.	Cloven-hoofed animals
Middle East for Veterinary Vaccine (ME VAC) http://www.me-vac.com/	APHTHOVAC	O-PanAsia 2, O-Sudan, O-Manisa, SAT-2, A-African, A-Iran 05	Oil	Inactivated vaccine composed of O-PanAsia 2, O-Sudan, O-Manisa, SAT-2, A-African, A-Iran 05.	Cloven-hoofed animals
Middle East for Veterinary Vaccine (ME VAC) http://www.me-vac.com/	Bi-APHTHOVAC	Not Available	Oil	Inactivated vaccine.	Cloven-hoofed animals
Ourofino Saúde Animal https://www.ourofinosaudeanimal.com/	Ourovac® Aftosa	O1 Campos, A24 Cruzeiro, C3 Indaial	Oil	O1 Campos and A24 Cruzeiro inactivated antigens, emulsifying in mineral oil.	Bovine and bubalus

Shanghai Hile Bio-Pharmaceutical Co., Ltd. http://www.hile-bio.com/	Swine Foot and Mouth Disease Bivalent Synthetic Peptide Vaccine	Type O, Type A (Peptides 2700 + 2800 + MM13)	Oil	Inactivated vaccine composed of Type O, Type A (Peptides 2700 + 2800 + MM13).	Cloven-hoofed animals
Shanghai Hile Bio-Pharmaceutical Co., Ltd. http://www.hile-bio.com/	Swine Foot and Mouth Disease Synthetic Peptide Vaccine	Type O (Peptides 2600 + 2700 + 2800), Type O	Oil	Inactivated vaccine composed of Type O (Peptides 2600 + 2700 + 2800), Type O.	Cloven-hoofed animals
United Biomedical, Inc. http://unitedbiomedical.com/	UBITh® FMDV Vaccine	Not Available	Water in oil	Inactivated vaccine.	Cloven-hoofed animals
Vallée SA https://www.msd-saude-animal.com.br/a-empresa/vallee/	Bovicel	O1 Campos, A24 Cruzeiro, C3 Indaial	Mineral oil, saponin	Inactivated vaccine composed of O1 Campos, A24 Cruzeiro, C3 Indaial.	Cloven-hoofed animals
Vallée SA https://www.msd-saude-animal.com.br/a-empresa/vallee/	AFTOGÁN®	A24 Cruzeiro, O1 Campos	Oil	Inactivated vaccine composed of A24 Cruzeiro, O1 Campos.	Cloven-hoofed animals
Vetal Animal Health Products S.A. https://vetal.com.tr/en/	Aftovac-Oil™	O1, A22, Asia-1	Oil	Inactivated vaccine composed of O1, A22, Asia-1.	Cloven-hoofed animals
Vetal Animal Health Products S.A. https://vetal.com.tr/en/	Aftovac™	O1, A22, Asia-1	Aluminum hydroxide, saponin	Inactivated vaccine composed of O1, A22, Asia-1.	Cloven-hoofed animals
Veterinary Serum and Vaccine Research Institute http://vsvri.com/	Bivalent Inactivated Foot and Mouth Disease Vaccine	O1 93, AEGY/06	Aluminum hydroxide	Inactivated vaccine composed of O1 93, AEGY/06.	Cloven-hoofed animals
Veterinary Serum and Vaccine Research Institute http://vsvri.com/	Polyvalent Inactivated Foot and Mouth Disease Oil Vaccine	O, A, SAT2	Oil	Inactivated vaccine composed of O, A, SAT2.	Cloven-hoofed animals

Disclaimer: It was the authors' intention to list all vaccine producers and are not responsible for the safety, quality, and effectiveness of the vaccines listed in the table.

17.13 Summary

Foot and mouth disease is a highly contagious viral disease of cloven-hoofed animals including large and small ruminants and swine, threatening food security and the livelihoods of smallholders and disrupting the regional and international trade of animals and animal products. The disease occurs in large parts of Africa, the Middle East, and Asia. The FMD virus has a high mutation rate and exists as seven distinct serotypes that do not cross-protect and multiple strains within each serotype, where cross-protection may be reduced. The inactivated vaccines have been available for over 70 years and been critically important in control, prevention, and eradication of the disease, if used in combination with other control measures. The effective vaccination programs depend on the quality of the vaccine, the match to the circulating virus, vaccination schedule, and vaccine applications. Next-generation vaccines have been in development for many years and some appear promising to replace the current inactivated vaccines.

References

Abdela, N. (2017). Sero-prevalence, risk factors and distribution of foot and mouth disease in Ethiopia. *Acta Trop.* 169: 125–132.

Acharya, R., Fry, E., Stuart, D. et al. (1989). The three-dimensional structure of foot-and-mouth disease virus at 2.9 Å resolution. *Nature* 337 (6209): 709.

Allepuz, A., Stevenson, M., Kivaria, F. et al. (2015). Risk factors for foot-and-mouth disease in Tanzania, 2001–2006. *Transbound. Emerg. Dis.* 62 (2): 127–136.

Animal Health Australia. (2014). Australian animal health plan: disease strategy: foot-and-mouth disease. Version 3.4. www.animalhealthaustralia.com.au/download/9810

Auge de Mello, P., Gomes, I., and Bahnemann, H.G. (1989). The vaccination of young cattle with an oil adjuvant foot-and-mouth disease vaccine. *Bol. Centr. Panam. Fiebre Aftosa* 55: 9–14.

Barnett, P., Garland, A.J.M., Kitching, R.P., and Schermbrucker, C.G. (2002). Aspects of emergency vaccination against foot-and-mouth disease. *Comp. Immunol. Microbiol. Infect. Dis* 25 (5–6): 345–364.

Belin, M.L. (1927). *Complexes Vaccino-Aphteux*, 437–446. Norfolk, UK: Horizon Bioscience.

Bertram, M.R., Vu, L.T., Pauszek, S.J. et al. (2018). Lack of transmission of foot-and-mouth disease virus from persistently infected cattle to naïve cattle under field conditions in Vietnam. *Front. Vet. Sci.*: 5.

Blanco, E., Guerra, B., Beatriz, G. et al. (2016). Full protection of swine against foot-and-mouth disease by a bivalent B-cell epitope dendrimer peptide. *Antiviral Res.* 129: 74–80.

Blank, P.R. and Szucs, T.D. (2009). Increasing influenza vaccination coverage in recommended population groups in Europe. *Exp. Rev. Vaccine* 8 (4): 425–433.

Brehm, K.E., Kumar, N., Thulke, H.H., and Haas, B. (2008). High potency vaccines induce protection against heterologous challenge with foot-and-mouth disease virus. *Vaccine* 26 (13): 1681–1687.

Bronsvoort, B.D.C., Nfon, C., Hamman, S.M. et al. (2004). Risk factors for herdsman-reported foot-and-mouth disease in the Adamawa Province of Cameroon. *Prev.Vet. Med.* 66 (1–4): 127–139.

Cao, Y., Li, D., Fu, Y. et al. (2017). Rational design and efficacy of a multi-epitope recombinant protein vaccine against foot-and-mouth disease virus serotype A in pigs. *Antiviral Res.* 140: 133–141.

Capstick, P.B., Telling, R.C., Chapman, W.G., and Stewart, D.L. (1962). Growth of a cloned strain of hamster kidney cells in suspended cultures and their susceptibility to the virus of foot-and-mouth disease. *Nature* 195 (4847): 1163.

Carr, B.V., Lefevre, E.A., Windsor, M.A. et al. (2013). CD4+ T-cell responses to foot-and-mouth disease virus in vaccinated cattle. *J. Gen. Virol.* 94 (Pt 1): 97.

Cokcaliskan, C., Turkoglu, T., Uzunlu, E. et al. (2017). Influence of vaccine potency and booster administration of foot-and-mouth disease vaccines on the antibody response in calves with maternal antibodies. *J. Vet. Sci.* 18: 315–322.

Council of Europe, European Pharmacopoeia Commission. (2013). European Pharmacopoeia. 8th ed. www.edqm.eu/medias/fichiers/index_english.pdf

Crowther, J.R., Farias, S., Carpenter, W.C., and Samuel, A.R. (1993). Identification of a fifth neutralizable site on type O foot-and-mouth disease virus following characterization of single and quintuple monoclonal antibody escape mutants. *J. Gen. Virol.* 74 (8): 1547–1553.

Cunliffe, H.R. (1964). Observations on the duration of immunity in cattle after experimental infection with foot-and-mouth disease virus. *Cornell Vet.* 54: 501–510.

Doel, T.R. (1996). Natural and vaccine-induced immunity to foot and mouth disease: the prospects for improved vaccines. *Rev. Sci. Tech.* 15: 883–991.

Doel, T.R. (2003). FMD vaccines. *Virus Res.* 91 (1): 81–99.

Doel, T.R. and Baccarini, P.J. (1981). Thermal stability of foot-and-mouth disease virus. *Arch. Virol* 70 (1): 21–32.

Doel, T.R. and Chong, W.K.T. (1982). Comparative immunogenicity of 146S, 75S and 12S particles of foot-and-mouth disease virus. *Arch. Virol* 73 (2): 185–191.

Elnekave, E., Zamir, L., Hamd, F. et al. (2015). Risk factors for foot and mouth disease outbreaks in grazing beef cattle herds. *Prev. Vet. Med.* 120 (2): 236–240.

Elnekave, E., van Maanen, K., Shilo, H. et al. (2016). Prevalence and risk factors for foot and mouth disease infection in small ruminants in Israel. *Prev. Vet. Med.* 125: 82–88.

Emami, J., Rasouli, N., McLaws, M., and Bartels, C.J.M. (2015). Risk factors for infection with foot-and-mouth disease virus in a cattle population vaccinated with a non-purified vaccine in Iran. *Prev. Vet. Med.* 119 (3–4): 114–122.

FAO and OIE. (2018). The Progressive Control Pathway for Foot-and-Mouth Disease Control (PCP-FMD): Principles, Stage Descriptions and Standards. www.fao.org/3/CA1331EN/ca1331en.pdf

Fletcher, M.A., Fabre, P., Debois, H., and Saliou, P. (2004). Vaccines administered simultaneously: directions for new combination vaccines based on an historical review of the literature. *Int. J. Infect. Dis.* 8 (6): 328–338.

Frenkel, H.S. (1947). La culture du virus de la fièvre aphteuse sur l'épithelium de la langue des bovidés. *Bull. Off. Int. Epiz.* 28: 155–162.

Geale, D.W., Barnett, P.V., Clarke, G.W. et al. (2015). A review of OIE country status recovery using vaccinate-to-live versus vaccinate-to-die foot-and-mouth disease response policies II: waiting periods after emergency vaccination in FMD free countries. *Transbound. Emerg. Dis.* 62 (4): 388–406.

Grubman, M.J. and Baxt, B. (2004). Foot-and-mouth disease. *Clin. Microbiol. Rev.* 17 (2): 465–493.

Grubman, M.J., Moraes, M.P., Schutta, C. et al. (2010). Adenovirus serotype 5-vectored foot-and-mouth disease subunit vaccines: the first decade. *Future Virol.* 5 (1): 51–64.

Grubman, M.J., Diaz-San Segundo, F., Dias, C.C. et al. (2012). Use of replication-defective adenoviruses to develop vaccines and biotherapeutics against foot-and-mouth disease. *Future Virol.* 7 (8): 767–778.

Iyer, A.V., Ghosh, S., Singh, S.N., and Deshmukh, R.A. (2000). Evaluation of three 'ready to formulate' oil adjuvants for foot-and-mouth disease vaccine production. *Vaccine* 19 (9–10): 1097–1105.

Juleff, N., Windsor, M., Lefevre, E.A. et al. (2009). Foot-and-mouth disease virus can induce a specific and rapid CD4+ T-cell-independent neutralizing and isotype class-switched antibody response in naive cattle. *J. Virol.* 83 (8): 3626–3636.

Knight-Jones, T.J.D. and Rushton, J. (2013). The economic impacts of foot and mouth disease–What are they, how big are they and where do they occur? *Prev. Vet. Med.* 112: 161–173.

Knight-Jones, T.J.D., Gubbins, S., Bulut, A.N. et al. (2016). Mass vaccination, immunity and coverage: modelling population protection against foot-and-mouth disease in Turkish cattle. *Sci. Rep.* 6: 22121.

Knight-Jones, T.J.D., McLaws, M., and Rushton, J. (2017). Foot-and-mouth disease impact on smallholders-what do we know, what don't we know and how can we find out more? *Transbound. Emerg. Dis.* 64 (4): 1079–1094.

Li, W., Joshi, M., Singhania, S. et al. (2014). Peptide vaccine: progress and challenges. *Vaccines* 2 (3): 515–536.

Lombard, M.F. and Schermbrucker, C.G. (1994). Vaccines for control of foot-and-mouth disease worldwide: production, selection and field performance. Workshop paper. ACIAR Proceedings, Australian Centre for International Agricultural Research.

Lyons, N.A., Lyoo, Y.S., King, D.P., and Paton, D.J. (2016). Challenges of generating and maintaining protective vaccine-induced immune responses for foot-and-mouth disease virus in pigs. *Front. Vet. Sci.* 3: 102.

Lyons, N.A., Ludi, A.B., Wilsden, G. et al. (2017). Evaluation of a polyvalent foot-and-mouth disease virus vaccine containing A Saudi-95 against field challenge on large-scale dairy farms in Saudi Arabia with the emerging A/ASIA/G-VII viral lineage. *Vaccine* 35 (49): 6850–6857.

Mahy, B.W. (2004). Overview of foot-and-mouth disease and its impact as a re-emergent viral infection. In: *Foot-and-Mouth Disease. Current Perspectives* (eds. F. Sobrino and E. Domingo), 437–446. Boca Raton: CRC Press.

Mansoor, M.K., Al-Rawahi, A.H., El-Tahir, H.A. et al. (2018). Concurrent vaccination of goats with foot and mouth disease (FMD) and peste des petits ruminants (PPR) booster vaccines. *Trop. Anim. Health Prod.* 50 (1): 1–3.

Metwally, S. and Münstermann, S. (eds). (2016). Foot and mouth disease vaccination and post-vaccination monitoring: guidelines. www.fao.org/3/a-i5975e.pdf

Mohamed, F., Swafford, S., Petrowski, H. et al. (2011). Foot-and-mouth disease in feral swine: susceptibility and transmission. *Transbound. Emerg. Dis.* 58 (4): 358–371.

Moraes, M.P., Diaz-San Segundo, F., Dias, C.C. et al. (2011). Increased efficacy of an adenovirus-vectored foot-and-mouth disease capsid subunit vaccine expressing nonstructural protein 2B is associated with a specific T cell response. *Vaccine* 29 (51): 9431–9440.

Mowat, G.N. and Chapman, W.G. (1962). Growth of foot-and-mouth disease virus in a fibroblastic cell line derived from hamster kidneys. *Nature* 194 (4825): 253.

Naranjo, J. and Cosivi, O. (2013). Elimination of foot-and-mouth disease in South America: lessons and challenges. *Philos. Trans. R. Soc.Lond B Biol. Sci.* 368 (1623): 20120381.

Nicholls, M.J., Black, L., Rweyemamu, M.M. et al. (1984). The effect of maternally derived antibodies on the response of calves to vaccination against foot and mouth disease. *Epidemiol. Infect.* 92 (1): 105–116.

OIE (2018). *Infection with Foot and Mouth Disease Virus*. Paris: OIE. www.oie.int/fileadmin/Home/eng/Health_standards/tahm/3.01.08_FMD.pdf

Orsel, K., de Jong, M.C.M., Bouma, A. et al. (2007a). The effect of vaccination on foot and mouth disease virus transmission among dairy cows. *Vaccine* 25 (2): 327–335.

Orsel, K., Dekker, A., Bouma, A. et al. (2007b). Quantification of foot and mouth disease virus excretion and transmission within groups of lambs with and without vaccination. *Vaccine* 25 (14): 2673–2679.

Paton, D.J., Gubbins, S., and King, D.P. (2017). Understanding the transmission of foot-and-mouth disease virus at different scales. *Curr. Opin. Virol.* 28: 85–91.

Pega, J., Bucafusco, D., di Giacomo, S. et al. (2013). Early adaptive immune responses in the respiratory tract of foot-and-mouth disease virus-infected cattle. *J. Virol.* 87 (5): 2489–2495.

Perez-Martin, E., Zhang, F., Maree, F. et al. (eds.) (2016). FMD virus persistence and transmission in African buffalo. In: *Open Session of the European Commission for the Control of Foot-and-Mouth Disease*. Portugal: Cascais.

Porta, C., Kotecha, A., Burman, A. et al. (2013). Rational engineering of recombinant picornavirus capsids to produce safe, protective vaccine antigen. *PLoS Pathog.* 9 (3): e1003255.

Roche, S.E., Garner, M., Sanson, R. et al. (2015). Evaluating vaccination strategies to control foot-and-mouth disease: a model comparison study. *Epidemiology and Infection* 143: 1256–1275.

Scott, K.A., Kotecha, A., Seago, J. et al. (2017). SAT2 foot-and-mouth disease virus structurally modified for increased thermostability. *J. Virol.* 91 (10): e02312–e02316.

Shao, J.J., Wang, J.F., Chang, H.Y., and Liu, J.X. (2011). Immune potential of a novel multiple-epitope vaccine to FMDV type Asia 1 in guinea pigs and sheep. *Virol. Sin.* 26 (3): 190–197.

Soria, I., Quattrocchi, V., Langellotti, C. et al. (2018). Immune response and partial protection against heterologous foot-and-mouth disease virus induced by dendrimer peptides in cattle. *J. Immunol. Res.* 2018: 349740.

Sreenivasa, B.P., Mohapatra, J.K., Pauszek, S.J. et al. (2017). Recombinant human adenovirus-5 expressing capsid proteins of Indian vaccine strains of foot-and-mouth disease virus elicits effective antibody response in cattle. *Vet. Microbiol.* 203: 196–201.

Swayne, D.E., Pavade, G., Hamilton, K. et al. (2011). Assessment of national strategies for control of high-pathogenicity avian influenza and low-pathogenicity notifiable avian influenza in poultry, with emphasis on vaccines and vaccination. *Rev. Sci. Tech.* 30 (3): 839.

Tekleghiorghis, T., Moormann, R.J., Weerdmeester, K., and Dekker, A. (2016). Foot-and-mouth disease transmission in Africa: implications for control, a review. *Transbound. Emerg. Dis.* 63 (2): 136–151.

Telling, R.C. and Elsworth, R. (1965). Submerged culture of hamster kidney cells in a stainless steel vessel. *Biotechnol. Bioeng.* 7 (3): 417–434.

Thornley, J.H.M. and France, J. (2009). Modelling foot and mouth disease. *Prev. Vet. Med.* 89: 139–154.

Tildesley, M.J., Savill, N.J., Shaw, D.J. et al. (2006). Optimal reactive vaccination strategies for a foot-and-mouth outbreak in the UK. *Nature* 440 (7080): 83.

Vosloo, W., Bastos, A.D., Kirkbride, E. et al. (1996). Persistent infection of African buffalo (Syncerus caffer) with SAT-type foot-and-mouth disease viruses: rate of fixation of mutations, antigenic change and interspecies transmission. *J. Gen. Virol.* 77 (7): 1457–1467.

Vynnycky, E. and White, R. (2010). *An Introduction to Infectious Disease Modelling*. Oxford: OUP. www.scirp.org/(S(i43dyn45teexjx455qlt3d2q))/reference/ReferencesPapers.aspx?ReferenceID=1949661

Waldmann, O., Kobe, K., and Pyl, G. (1937). Die aktive immunisierung des rindes gegen Maul-und Klauenseuche mittels formolimpfstoff. *Zentbl. Bakteriol. Parasitenkd. Infektkhrankh* 138: 401–412.

Waters, R., Ludi, A.B., Fowler, V.L. et al. (2018). Efficacy of a high-potency multivalent foot-and-mouth disease virus vaccine in cattle against heterologous challenge with a field virus from the emerging A/ASIA/G-VII lineage. *Vaccine* 36 (14): 1901–1907.

Weaver, G.V., Domenech, J., Thiermann, A.R., and Karesh, W.B. (2013). Foot and mouth disease: a look from the wild side. *J. Wildlife Dis.* 49 (4): 759–785.

Wong, H.T., Cheng, S.C.S., Chan, E.W.C. et al. (2000). Plasmids encoding foot-and-mouth disease virus VP1 epitopes elicited immune responses in mice and swine and protected swine against viral infection. *Virology* 278 (1): 27–35.

Wong, H.T., Cheng, S.C.S., Sin, F.W.Y. et al. (2002). A DNA vaccine against foot-and-mouth disease elicits an immune response in swine which is enhanced by co-administration with interleukin-2. *Vaccine* 20 (21–22): 2641–2647.

Woolhouse, M.E.J., Haydon, D.T., Pearson, A., and Kitching, R.P. (1996). Failure of vaccination to prevent outbreaks of foot-and-mouth disease. *Epidemiol. Infect.* 116 (3): 363–371.

Yeruham, I., Yadin, H., Haymovich, M., and Perl, S. (2001). Adverse reactions to FMD vaccine. *Vet. Dermatol.* 12 (4): 197–201.

Zhang, Z., Pan, L., Ding, Y. et al. (2015). Efficacy of synthetic peptide candidate vaccines against serotype-A foot-and-mouth disease virus in cattle. *Appl. Microbiol. Biotechnol.* 99 (3): 1389–1398.

18

Avian Influenza

David Swayne[1] and Leslie Sims[2]

[1] Southeast Poultry Research Laboratory, Agricultural Research Service, US Department of Agriculture, Athens, Georgia, USA
[2] Asia Pacific Veterinary Information Services, Montmorency, Victoria, Australia

18.1 Introduction

18.1.1 The Disease and Infections

Avian influenza (AI) is a disease of poultry caused by infection with type A influenza viruses, i.e. avian influenza viruses (AIV)[1] (Swayne and Spackman 2013). All AIV contain eight gene segments, and can be further classified into different subtypes based on the surface glycoproteins, more specifically the 16 hemagglutinin (HA) (H1–16) and nine neuraminidase (NA) (N1–9) subtypes, coded by gene segments 4 and 6, respectively. Therefore, each AIV will have an HA and NA subtype designation, e.g. H5N1, H9N2, etc. In addition, AIVs are further classified into two broad pathotypes, low pathogenicity (LP) and high pathogenicity (HP), based on capacity to produce disease and lethality in chickens (*Gallus gallus domesticus*) using an intravenous pathogenicity test. All naturally occurring HPAIV have been H5 or H7 subtypes while LPAIV have been any of the H1–16 subtypes. The HPAIV arise from mutation of H5 or H7 LPAIV at some point in their history. The A/goose/Guangdong/1/1996 (Gs/GD) lineage AIVs of the H5 subtype have circulated widely as a HPAIV for more than 20 years.

In poultry, LPAIV cause a localized infection of the respiratory and gastrointestinal tracts resulting in variable clinical outcomes ranging from subclinical infection to mild-to-severe respiratory disease (Swayne and Spackman 2013). Subclinical infections are most common in experimental laboratory studies with LPAIV alone, while infections in the field typically, but not always (e.g. influenza A [H7N9]), include accompanying clinical respiratory disease and variable mortality as the result of secondary infections with other pathogens such as Newcastle disease virus, *Mycoplasma gallisepticum*, or *Escherichia coli*. In addition, LPAIV infection in layers and breeders can produce a variable decrease in egg production and temporary appearance of abnormal-shaped eggs with poor-quality eggshells. LPAIV replication is typically limited to epithelial cells of the upper respiratory tract and intestinal epithelium, but in some instances replication can occur within the epithelium of the deep respiratory tract, the epithelium lining the cloacal bursa, kidney epithelium and, rarely, pancreatic epithelium and oviduct epithelium of specific species such as turkeys (*Meleagris gallopavo*).

With HPAIV, infections in most nonvaccinated gallinaceous poultry (chickens, turkeys, quail, pheasants, and partridge) result in severe systemic disease with high mortality and cessation of egg production (Swayne and Spackman 2013). The virus replicates in all cells and is especially prominent in endothelial cells, cardiac myocytes, and neurons of the brain. HPAIV infections of domestic ducks have variable effects ranging from subclinical infection to high mortality depending on the vaccination status, virus strain, age of the birds, challenge dose, and species of duck (Pantin-Jackwood et al. 2013; 2007).

18.1.2 Vaccine Use Within Control Strategies

High-pathogenicity avian influenza (HPAI) and H5/H7 low-pathogenicity avian influenza (LPAI) are listed diseases reportable to the OIE (Swayne 2012a). Historically, HPAI has been controlled by stamping-out programs as immediate

[1] Note that the OIE Terrestrial Code (2014) defines avian influenza for trade purposes as any infection with viruses of the H5 or H7 subtype or any virus with an intravenous pathogenicity index greater than 1.2. This paper uses the broader definition of avian influenza that covers infection with influenza A viruses of all subtypes detected in birds.

Veterinary Vaccines: Principles and Applications, First Edition. Edited by Samia Metwally, Gerrit Viljoen, and Ahmed El Idrissi.

eradication is the goal, but vaccination has been added as a management tool in some outbreaks based on decision by individual countries. The European Commission has pointed out that vaccination can be an effective tool to supplement disease control measures and to avoid massive killing and destruction of poultry or other captive birds. It can also be used as a short-term measure in emergencies and also as a long-term measure to prevent disease in situations of higher risk of introduction of AIVs (European Council 2015). As of 2016, vaccination has been used in five of the 40 HPAI epizootics as an additional control tool: (i) H5N2 in Mexico (1995), (ii) H7N3 in Pakistan (1995–2004), (iii) H7N7 in Democratic People's Republic of Korea (2005), (iv) H5 Gs/GD lineage in 14 countries in Asia/Africa/Europe (1996–present), with the vast majority of vaccine used in China, Vietnam, Indonesia, and Egypt, and (v) H7N3 in Mexico (2012–present) (Swayne et al. 2013; Brown et al. 2016; Swayne 2016). For non-H5/H7 LPAIV, management instead of eradication is usually the goal. Therefore, vaccination has been widely practiced, especially for H9N2, with billions of doses used across the Middle East and Asia (Swayne and Kapczynski 2008; Swayne et al. 2016). To a lesser extent, vaccines have been used to control other LPAIV subtypes. Vaccination has been used to assist in elimination of specific strains of H5/H7 LPAIV from large farms (Halvorson 2009).

Application of vaccination to control AIV is dependent upon many factors, including the species and age of poultry, pathotype, and HA subtypes of AIV, country freedom or endemic status on AIV (including the capacity to eliminate the virus once endemic), the attitudes of veterinary authorities toward vaccination, and in-country availability of vaccine and logistics for vaccination. From an OIE survey covering 2002–2010, 21 countries used vaccines in HPAI control (11 in poultry only, seven in zoological birds and three in both poultry and zoological birds), eight countries for H5 and H7 LPAI control, and 12 for non-H5/H7 LPAI control (Swayne et al. 2011). Unsanctioned use of vaccine for H5 HPAI control has been reported to occur in a number of other countries within Asia (Sims, unpublished data). More doses of vaccine have been used in poultry to control H5/H7 HPAI than H1–16 LPAI (Swayne et al. 2011). Vaccination against HPAI is a relatively recent occurrence, with the first recorded field use during 1995 in Mexico against H5N2 and Pakistan against H7N3 HPAI.

The OIE Terrestrial Animal Health Code recognizes the role vaccination can play in prevention and control of avian influenza, and has provisions for use of vaccination that would not inhibit trade in poultry and poultry products. This is achieved by conducting appropriate surveillance to demonstrate lack of virus circulation in vaccinated flocks and/or lack of antibodies that are the consequence of infection (OIE 2017).

18.2 Types of Vaccines

The ideal AI vaccine should be inexpensive, usable in multiple avian species, provide protection after a single dose, be applied by low-cost mass application methods, allow easy identification of infected birds within the vaccinated population, produce a protective immune response in the presence of maternal antibodies, be applied at one day of age in hatchery or *in ovo*, and be antigenically close to field virus (Table 18.1) (Swayne and Spackman 2013). However, no current vaccine or vaccine technology meets all of these

Table 18.1 Properties of an ideal avian influenza vaccine for poultry.

Desired property	Current situation
Inexpensive	Current cost for inactivated AIV vaccine: \$0.05–0.10/dose plus cost of administration (\$0.05–0.07 per dose for individual handling and injection) (Swayne and Kapczynski 2008)
Use in multiple avian species	Most used in meat, layer, and breeder chickens, but large quantity also used in ducks; minor amounts in turkeys, geese, quail, etc. (Swayne et al. 2011)
Single dose protection	Most situations require minimum of 2 doses; prime-boost scenario is optimal with additional boost in long-lived birds at 6–12 mo intervals (Swayne 2006; Steensels et al. 2009)
Mass application	95.5% is inactivated vaccine administered by handling and injecting individual birds, with 4.5% as vectored vaccine given by mass spray vaccination (0.04%, rNDV-H5 vector) or injection at 1 d of age (0.005%, rFPV-H5) (Swayne et al. 2011)
Identify infected birds in vaccinated population	Serological differentiation tests are available, but only minor use. Most vaccine applied without using a serological DIVA strategy for surveillance (Swayne 2006)
Overcome maternal antibody block	Maternal antibody to AIV hemagglutinin or virus vector inhibits primary immune response. Initial vaccination must be timed for declining maternal antibody titers to allow optimal primary immune response (Maas et al. 2011)
Given at 1 d of age in hatchery or *in ovo*	Inactivated vaccine provides poor protection if given at 1 d of age. Vectored vaccines can be given at 1 d of age, but generally require a boost with inactivated vaccine 10 d or more later
Antigenically close to field virus	The majority of inactivated whole AIV vaccines use reverse genetic generated vaccine seed strains to antigenically match field viruses. The strain of virus used should also be a strong immunogen (Swayne et al. 2011; Swayne 2012b)

Source: Modified from Swayne and Spackman (2013).

eight criteria and the user must select licensed vaccines that provide as many of the ideal features that are relevant to their needs.

18.2.1 Licensed Vaccine Technologies

Licensed poultry AI vaccines are based on five technologies (Figure 18.1): (i) wild-type (wt) or reverse genetic (rg) whole AIV grown in embryonating chicken eggs, chemically inactivated (formalin, β-propiolactone, or binary ethyleneimine), and adjuvanted to enhance the immune response (e.g. mineral oil plus surfactants, or alum) (Schickli et al. 2001; Swayne and Spackman 2013), (ii) HA antigen (or virus-like particles) produced in insect cells by a genetically engineered baculovirus (Crawford et al. 1999; Beato et al. 2013) (iii) HA DNA vaccine with proprietary lipid/polymer matrix adjuvant (Anonymous 2017), (iv) recombinant technologies utilizing live virus vectors to express AI virus HA and in some cases NA gene inserts (recombinant herpes virus turkey [rHVT-AIV], recombinant Newcastle disease virus [rNDV-AIV], or recombinant fowlpox virus [rFPV-AIV]) (Taylor et al. 1988; Nakaya et al. 2001; Rauw et al. 2011), or (v) defective-replicating alphavirus (defective Venezuelan equine encephalitis virus with H5 AI virus gene insert [*dα*-H5]) (Schultz-Cherry et al. 2000; Vander Veen et al. 2013) (Table 18.2).

The inactivated whole AI vaccines use established embryonating chicken egg propagation technology and proprietary mineral oil adjuvant systems, which have been successfully used for over 40 years to produce trillions of doses of potent and efficacious inactivated or live attenuated vaccines for Newcastle disease, infectious bronchitis, infectious bursal disease, and other viral pathogens. These inactivated whole AI vaccines have contained various seed strains, initially based on LPAI outbreak viruses, of the same HA subtype as the field viruses. However, as usage of vaccines to control H5 Gs/GD lineage HPAI outbreaks extended beyond emergency vaccination programs, drift variant field viruses have emerged, necessitating the development and licensing of reverse genetic H5 HPAIV seed strains, rendered LP, that provided a closer antigenic match to field viruses and thus better protection (Swayne 2012a). Rapid antigenic change is rendering these vaccines less effective in some places due to the time taken to introduce new vaccine antigens. This mature technology is still expected to predominate in the market place in the near future. Subunit vaccines and live vectored vaccines for use in the hatchery, or for dual protection against the vector and insert when given at a later age, will continue to grow in use and, potentially, may expand for use in ducks and minor poultry species, especially when these products offer advantages over inactivated vaccines such as early immunity or broader cross-protection. Other adjuvants, such as bursopentene and toll-like receptor agonists, may prove to be useful in enhancing the immune response to killed antigens (Li et al. 2011; Singh et al. 2016).

A *dα*-H5 vaccine containing a Gs/GD-lineage clade 2.3.4.4 H5 HA gene insert was licensed in the USA during 2015 (Bertran et al. 2017). The *dα*-H5, rHVT-H5 (clade 2.2) and rgH5N1 inactivated (clade 2.3.4.4) vaccines were added to the USA emergency poultry vaccine bank.

Other technologies have been used in experimental vaccines, but commercialization of these technologies for poultry has not been achieved (Table 18.3). To be commercially viable, new vaccines must provide better protection and be of equivalent or lower cost than current licensed products or allow mass administration in the field that would facilitate administration and reduce labor costs (Swayne and Spackman 2013).

Emergency vaccination using live virus vectored vaccines is being studied given the difficulties associated with individual injection of poultry, but major barriers need to be overcome before field application is possible, as antibody-mediated maternal or active immunity against the vector, e.g. Newcastle disease virus (NDV) vector, can inhibit replication and prevent a significant active immune response to vaccination. The development of chimeric virus vectors or new virus vector systems that lack immunity in commercially reared poultry may allow spray application of vaccine vectors in emergency situations (Hai et al. 2011). Live AI vaccines have not been promoted as an option in the past due to fears of reversion to virulence. However, vaccines that are engineered to replicate only in the presence of a substance that is not found in animal cells (Si et al. 2016) and vaccines with a truncated nonstructural protein have been tested experimentally (Wang et al. 2008; Chen et al. 2017).

Finally, a vaccine specific for domestic duck production systems is needed. A recombinant duck enteritis virus vectored H5 vaccine (rDEV-H5) based on A/duck/Anhui/1/06 (clade 2.3.4) has been developed in China and is pending registration approval (Liu et al. 2011).

18.2.2 Vaccine Doses Used in the Field

Between 2002 and 2010, ~113 billion doses of H5 and H7 AI vaccines were manufactured and used for HPAI control in poultry, with >99% of the usage in China, Egypt, Indonesia, and Vietnam, i.e. countries with endemic H5 Gs/GD lineage HPAIV (Table 18.4) (Swayne et al. 2011). Of the AIV vaccine used in poultry, 95.5% (108 billion doses) were inactivated whole AIV vaccine (Swayne et al. 2011) and 4.5% (5 billion doses) were live recombinant vectored vaccines (Swayne et al. 2011), either as rFPV-H5 vaccine

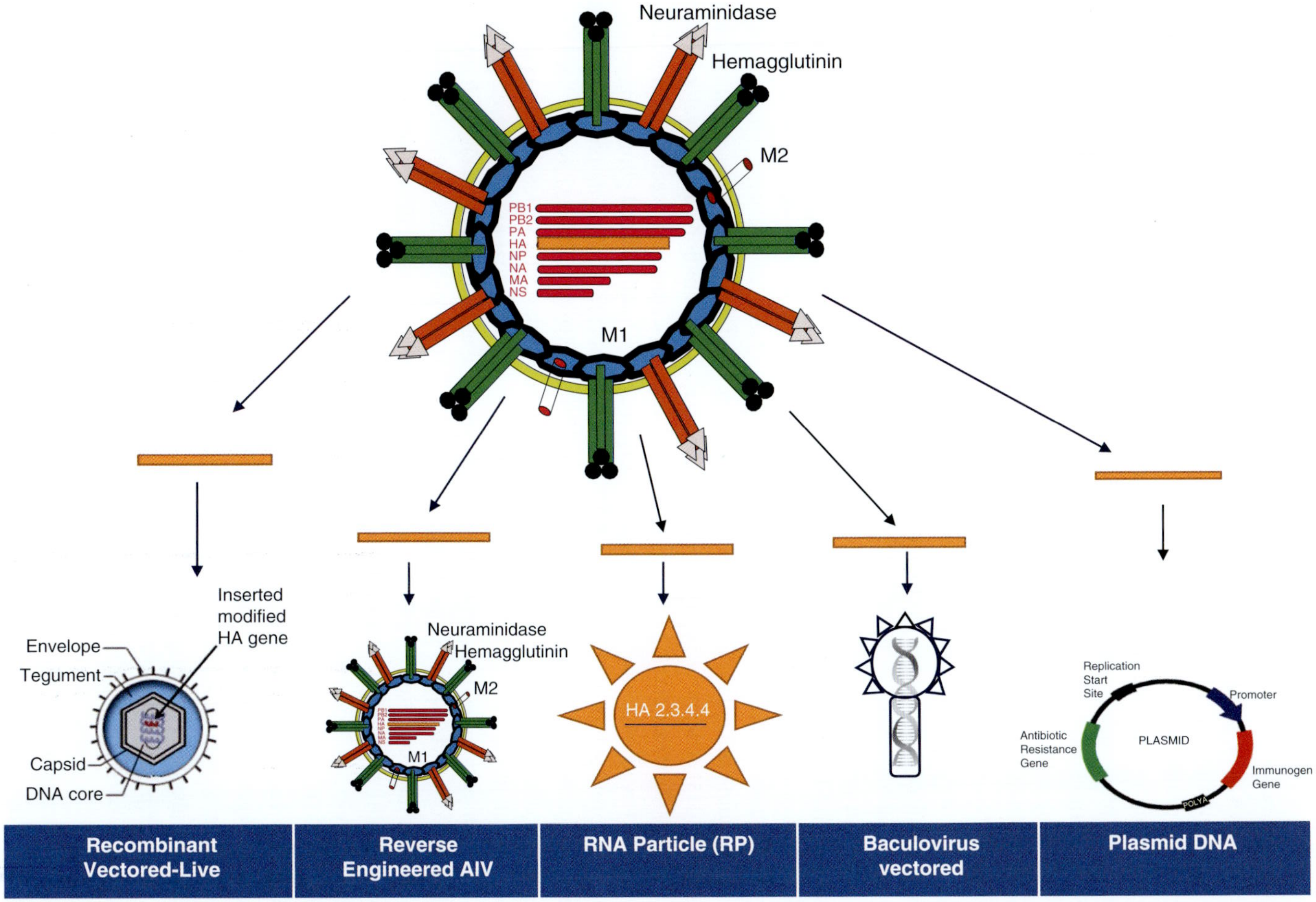

Figure 18.1 Schematic of technologies used for the five registered types of avian influenza vaccines: recombinant live poultry virus vectored (rHVT-H5, rFPV-H5, and rNDV-H5), reverse engineered (H5Nx avian influenza virus for inactivated vaccines), RNA particle, baculovirus-vectored for tissue culture expression of HA and DNA plasmid. Source: Modified from Kapczynski (2015).

Table 18.2 Current vaccine technologies licensed and used in the field for H5 and H7 avian influenza vaccines (compiled from available information: De et al. 1988; Chen 2009; FAO 2009; Spackman and Swayne 2013; Fan et al. 2015; Oliveira et al. 2017; Shi et al. 2018, and personal communications). Information on seed strains for other subtypes was unavailable.

Technology	Current seed strains or subunit source[a]	Previously available seed strains or subunits	Adjuvants	Countries licensed
Inactivated whole AIV	A/chicken/Mansehra/2006 (H5N1); A/duck/Novosibirsk/2/2005 (H5N1, clade 2.2); rgA/chicken/Egypt/18-H/2008 (H5N1, clade 2.2.1); rgA/duck/Guangdong/S1322/2010 (H5N1: Re-6 H5N1, clade 2.3.2.2); rgA/chicken/Guizhou/4/2013 (H5N1: Re-8, clade 2.3.4.4); rgA/bird/China/CG1/2017 (H5N2; rD8, clade 2.3.4.4)[b] rg-HA(H5)-A/Gyrfalcon/Washington/40188-6/2014 plus N1 PR8 (H5N1, clade 2.3.4.4) rgA/chicken/Shanxi/2/2006 (H5N1: Re-4, H5N1, clade 7); rgA/chicken/Liaoning/2011 (H5N1: Re-7, clade 7.2); A/duck/Guangdong/D7/2007 (H5N2; D7, clade 2.3.2); H5N2 strain rSD57: H5N2 strain rFJ56 + H7N9 strain rGD76; rgA/duck/Guizhou/S4184/2017 (H5N1: RE-11); rgA/chicken/Liaoning/SD007/2017 (H5N1: strain RE-12) A/duck/Potsdam/1402/86 (H5N2); A/chicken/Guanajuato/CPA-20966-15-VS/2015 (H5N2); A/turkey/Minnesota/3689-1551/81 (H5N2); A/turkey/California/20902/2002 (H5N2); A/duck/Potsdam/2243/84 (H5N6); A/turkey/Wisconsin/68 (H5N9); A/chicken/Italy/22A/98 (H5N9); rg-HA(H5)-A/chicken/Vietnam/C58/04 plus N3- A/duck/Germany/1215/73; A/chicken/Italy/1067/99 (H7N1); A/chicken/Italy/473/99 (H7N1); A/chicken/New York/273874/03 (H7N2); A/turkey/Oregon/1971 (H7N3); A/turkey/Utah/24721-10/95 (H7N3); A/duck/Potsdam/15/80 (H7N7) rgA/chicken/Guangxi/SD098/2017(H7N9: H7-Re2)	wt & rg A/chicken/Legok/2003 (H5N1); wt & rg A/goose/Guangdong/1996 (Re-1) (H5N1, clade 0); rgA/duck/Anhui/2/2006(Re-5) (H5N1, clade 2.3.4.1); A/turkey/England/N-28/73 (H5N2); A/chicken/Mexico/232/94/CPA (H5N2) rgA/pigeon/Shanghai/S1069/2013 (H7N9; H7-Re1); A/chicken/Durango/1558/2006 (H5N2)	Proprietary mineral oil or alum	Many

(Continued)

Table 18.2 (Continued)

Technology	Current seed strains or subunit source[a]	Previously available seed strains or subunits	Adjuvants	Countries licensed
DNA	HA(H5)-A/Gyrfalcon/Washington/40188-6/2014 (clade 2.3.4.4)		Proprietary lipid/ polymer matrix	USA
dα-AIV	H5-A/Gyrfalcon/Washington/40188-6/2014 (clade 2.3.4.4)		None	USA
rBaculovirus-AIV	H5-A/duck/China/E319-2/2003 (clade 2.3.2)[c]		Proprietary mineral oil	Bangladesh, Egypt, and Mexico
rFPV-AIV	H5-A/turkey/1378/Ireland/1983; H5-A/chicken/Scotland/59	H5 & N1-A/goose/Guangdong/1996 (H5N1, clade 0)	None	China, Mexico, Guatemala, USA
rNDV-AIV	H5-A/duck/Anhui/1/2006 (rLH5-5; clade 2.3.4); H5-A/duck/Guangdong/S1322/2010 (rLH5-6; clade 2.3.2) H5-A/chicken/Mexico/435/2005	H5-A/goose/Guangdong/1996 (rLH5-1; clade 0);	None	China, Mexico
rHVT-AIV	H5-A/swan/Hungary/4999/2006 (clade 2.2)		None	Bangladesh, Egypt, Mexico, Vietnam, USA

AIV, avian influenza virus; rFPV, recombinant fowlpox virus; rg, reverse genetic (uses PR8 internal gene backbone); rHVT, recombinant herpesvirus turkey; rNDV, recombinant Newcastle disease virus; wt, wild type; *dα*, defective alphavirus (Venezuelan equine encephalitis virus).

[a] Some seed strains have veterinary license but are not currently manufactured while status of some is unknown.

[b] The poultry species and province were not available at time of publication. The backbone of the seed strain is D7 virus.

[c] Coding region: several amino acids substitutions (Ser120Asn, Asp155Asn, and Ser223Asp) and one amino acid (328Lys) at the polybasic cleavage site.

Table 18.3 Experimental AIV vaccines using technologies that are not currently licensed for commercial use.

Vaccine category	Vaccine	Route [a]	Comments	Additional references
Live AIV	Live wild-type LPAI virus	IM, IT Spray	Rumors of intentional exposure with LPAIV to protect from HPAIV have been reported in H5N1 and H5N2 HPAI outbreaks in 1990s and 2000s	Alexander and Parsons (1980) and Hunt et al. (1988)
	Attenuated LPAI virus	Spray	Temperature-sensitive mutant or replace HA with ectodomain of NDV HN gene; risk assessment needed for reassortment potential	Park et al. (2006) and Zhang et al. (2012a)
Live vector	rd-Adenovirus	SQ, IN, *in ovo*	rd = Replication defective, only 1 round of replication occurs after injection. SQ and *in ovo* protected	Gao et al. (2006)
	Avian leukosis virus	IM		Hunt et al. (1988)
	Infectious laryngotracheitis virus	Eye	N1 did not protect	Veits et al. (2003) and Pavlova et al. (2009)
	att-*Salmonella typhimurium*	Oral	Attenuated vaccine strain. Failed to protect from HPAIV challenge with single oral immunization	Layton et al. (2009) and Pan et al. (2009)
	Vaccinia	IM, IC	Low to no antibody response	Chambers et al. (1988)
	Duck enteritis virus	IM	Specific vector for domestic ducks	Liu et al. (2011)
In vitro produced hemagglutinin	Eukaryotic systems (plants or cell cultures)	IM or SQ	Tobacco (*Nicotiana* sp.), duckweed (*Lemna minor*)	Kalthoff et al. (2010) and Bertran et al. (2015)
DNA	Naked DNA	IM	Not financially viable. Improvements needed in promoters and adjuvants to decrease quantity of nucleic acid needed and reduce number of doses for protection	Suarez and Schultz-Cherry (2000) and Rao et al. (2008)

[a] Eye, conjunctival sac; IC, intracoelomic; IM, intramuscular; IN, intranasal; IT, intratracheal; SQ, subcutaneous.
Source: Modified from Swayne and Spackman (2013).

(2005, 613 million doses) or rNDV-H5 (2006–2010, 4.4 billion doses) (Chen 2009). The rFPV-H5 was used only in China and is no longer being used in Asia. Since 2010, a rHVT-H5 (Rauw et al. 2011) has been licensed and used in chickens against H5 Gs/GD lineage HPAI in Egypt and Bangladesh, and against H5N2 LPAI in Mexico. Current usage of H5 AI vaccines for poultry is at approximately 25 billion doses per year, thus, an additional estimated 125 billion doses of H5 and H7 vaccine have been used in poultry for HPAI control between 2011 and 2015, mostly as inactivated AIV vaccine in five of the H5 Gs/GD lineage HPAIV endemic countries (Bangladesh, China, Egypt, Indonesia, and Vietnam), and 500 million to 1 billion doses of H7N3 inactivated vaccine in Mexico each year since 2012 (Swayne, unpublished data). Over 91% of vaccine for HPAI was produced in China but only of the H5 subtype.

In contrast to 113 billion doses of AIV vaccine used in poultry, fewer than 300 000 doses of H5 or H7 AI vaccine were used in zoo, hunting, companion, conservation, or endangered birds as a preventive measure against HPAI in 20 European and Asian countries on 292 premises, which equates to 0.000003% of total vaccine used in HPAI programs (Swayne et al. 2011). Vaccine against the zoonotic H7N9 virus (delivered as a bivalent H5/H7 vaccine) was introduced as a compulsory measure for Chinese poultry in 2017 (FAO 2017).

In contrast to HPAI control between 2002 and 2010, 10.1 billion doses of H5 or H7 vaccine were used in control programs against LPAI, mostly in Mexico and Central America (Table 18.4) (Swayne et al. 2011). These vaccines included inactivated AI vaccines (57%, 5.8 billion doses) and rFPV-H5 vaccine (43%, 4.3 billion doses). The rFPV-H5 is used as a priming vaccine in the hatchery for meat chickens followed by inactivated AIV vaccine boost in the field. An estimated total of 9 billion doses of rFPV-H5 was used in Mexico, Guatemala, and El Salvador from 1998 to 2016 (M. Bublot, personal communication) (Table 18.5).

The number of non-H5/H7 LPAI vaccine doses used is not available, since reporting to national veterinary authorities is not required, but H9N2 is the most frequent subtype for which vaccination is used. It is estimated that billions of doses have been used across North Africa, the Middle

Table 18.4 Data on the 113 billion doses of H5/H7 AIV vaccine used in poultry between 2002 and 2010 for HPAI control (Swayne et al. 2011).

Country	HA subtype	Year	Doses (1000s)	Global usage (%)
China	H5	2004–2010	103 715 621	90.9
Cote d'Ivoire	H5	2006	8000	<0.01
Egypt	H5	2006–2010	5 298 926	4.65
France	H5	2006	816	<0.01
Hong Kong	H5	2002–2010	85 573	0.08
Indonesia	H5	2004–2010	2 642 800	2.32
Israel	H5	2006	6	<0.01
Kazakhstan	H5	2006–2010	35 000	0.03
DPR Korea	H7	2005	2202	<0.01
Mongolia	H5	2005–2010	2799	<0.01
Netherlands	H5	2006–2008	68	<0.01
Pakistan	H5, H7	2004–2010	108 800	0.12
Russia	H5	2006–2010	425 327	0.37
Sudan	H5	2006–2007	6326	<0.01
Vietnam	H5	2005–2010	1 626 510	1.43
			113 982 174	100

Table 18.5 Data on the 10.1 billion doses of H5/H7 AIV vaccine used in poultry during 2002 and 2010 for LPAI control (Swayne et al. 2011).

Country	HA subtype	Year	Doses (1000s)	Global usage (%)
El Salvador	H5	2002–2010	639 214	6.4
Guatemala	H5	2002–2010	898 338	8.9
Italy	H5, H7	2002–2008	197 335	2.0
Mexico	H5	2002–2010	8 315 232	82.7
Portugal	H5	2008–2010	27	<0.01
USA	H5	2002–2003	8400	<0.01
			10 058 546	100

East, and Asia (Swayne and Kapczynski 2008). Vaccine use is expanding to countries where H9N2 subtype virus has recently emerged. All commercial, non-H5/H7 AI vaccines have been inactivated whole AIV, but experimental recombinant fowlpox virus vaccines with HA inserts from H9N2 LPAIV (rFPV-H9) have been developed, as have modified live virus H9 vaccines with a truncated NS1 protein (Chen et al. 2017). Between 2002 and 2010, non-H5/H7 commercial inactivated AI vaccines (i.e. H1, H2, H3, H4, H6, and H10) were used on a very limited basis in reporting countries of Canada, Germany, and USA (Swayne et al. 2011), but this is likely an underestimate of countries with use, as these vaccines manage a nonreportable disease.

Historically, targeted LPAI vaccination programs used 22.7 million doses of inactivated AIV vaccine in outdoor-reared turkeys in Minnesota (1979–2000) covering 108 outbreaks, which included 20 H5 or H7 LPAI outbreaks (Halvorson 2002, 2008). As turkey production moved indoors and infections from wild bird LPAIV decreased, AI vaccine use declined to a minimal number of doses by 1998. In comparison, 13.4 million doses of vaccines were used from 2004 to 2010 in targeted vaccination programs of turkey breeders against H1 and H3 swine influenza virus in Minnesota (D. Lauer, personal communication).

It is expected that the use of vaccines against AI will continue to expand given the scale of development of the poultry sector, the threat posed by new strains of virus spreading globally, and the severe economic consequences of repeated infection.

18.3 Immune Response and Duration of Immunity

Immunization with vaccines or field exposure to AIV produces antibodies against various viral proteins, but only antibodies against the HA, NA, and type 2 matrix (M2) surface proteins have shown any degree of protection (Swayne et al. 2013b). The HA elicits antibodies that provide the best protective response indicated by preventing mortality and clinical signs, maintaining egg production, and reducing virus replication, but such protection is only directed against the specific HA subtype, i.e. H5 protects against H5 but not H7, etc., and is mediated by both IgG and IgA class antibodies (Brugh and Stone 1987; van den Berg et al. 2008). Protective hemagglutination inhibiting (HI) antibodies appear as early as 7 days after infection and are similarly produced following immunization (Sá e Silva and Swayne 2012). There is some limited evidence that high levels of antibodies against NA can provide protection against homologous NA subtypes in poultry (Sylte et al. 2007), but such protection is of limited use in the field. In contrast, antibodies to the M2 protein have provided only minimal protection of chickens against HPAIV challenge (Zhang et al. 2011), and antibodies against any of the individual internal proteins do not protect against mortality following HPAIV challenge (Webster et al. 1991). An experimental vaccine containing a multivalent M2e protein attached to the C-terminus of *Mycobacterium tuberculosis* heat shock protein 70 has been shown to reduce viral shedding in chickens experimentally infected with H9N2 LPAIV (Dabaghian et al. 2014). Addition of M2e to inactivated H9N2 vaccine suggested enhancement of immunity and reduction in viral shedding (Park et al. 2014).

In contrast to humoral immunity, cellular immune responses directed against the nucleoprotein or other influenza proteins have reduced virus titers in the late stages of virus replication (Kodihalli et al. 1994). One experimental study suggested that H9N2 LPAIV infection could produce heterotypic cell-mediated protection against H5N1 Gs/GD lineage HPAIV, using low challenge doses (Seo and Webster 2001). The presence of widespread infection by H9N2 LPAIV and vaccination with inactivated H9N2 vaccines in Asian poultry has not prevented the H5N1 Gs/GD-lineage HPAI epizootic, thus raising doubts regarding the value of such heterotypic cell-mediated immunity for complete field protection, but such immunity might provide some protection from mortality for birds infected with H5N1 Gs/GD lineage HPAIV in live poultry markets and farms where co- or sequential infection occurs. In the laboratory, immunization of chickens with inactivated A/turkey/Oregon/1971 (H7N3) vaccine did not prevent mortality against high-dose A/chicken/Queretaro/14588-19/1995 (H5N2) HPAIV challenge, but did provide reduction in initial virus replication in the respiratory tract (Swayne et al. 1999).

The duration of immunity is variable depending on the species of poultry, number of vaccinations, antigen content of the vaccine, and concurrent diseases that affect the immune competence of the birds at the time of vaccination. Immunity under experimental conditions, especially using specific pathogen-free (SPF) chickens, generally lasts longer than that achieved under field conditions. The presence of HI antibodies against the field strain has a positive predictive value for protection with killed antigen vaccines (Swayne et al. 2015). However, the link between HI titers and protection is imperfect as the lack of HI titers in vaccinated birds, i.e. negative predictive value, does not always predict lack of protection (Spackman et al. 2014; Swayne et al. 2015).

In the presence of low HI titers, timing of revaccination should be based on falls in antibody level. For example, if the goal is to minimize virus shedding following infection, revaccination could be conducted when HI titers of 80% of the tested population fall below 1:128. Field experiences in Indonesia with repeated doses of vaccines containing inactivated antigen in older layer chickens suggest that it can sometimes be difficult to maintain titers even with regular revaccination (Sims, unpublished data).

18.4 Desired Specifications when Ordering Vaccine

In writing tender specifications for vaccine, essential information should include: (i) master seed requirements, (ii) information on challenge virus strain and challenge dose for efficacy studies along with parameters to be measured for protection and the minimum level found to be protective (see below), (iii) quantity of HA antigen in each dose and the volume per dose, (iv) number of doses per vial which for inactivated vaccine is typically 500 mL vials or 1000 doses, and the total number of doses needed, (v) host species and age or age range of administration, (vi) route of administration, (vii) withdrawal period, (viii) any special provisions for batch release such as minimal antibody titer production in SPF chickens, and (ix) items to be included on the label.

18.4.1 Master Seed Selection: HA Subtype and Antigenic Matching

The master seed for the inactivated whole AIV vaccine should contain the HA of the same subtype as the field AIV virus, and be a reasonable antigenic match and be well characterized (OIE 2015). Undefined AIV seed strains and even autogenous products may be suboptimal choices for AI vaccination programs even if they appear to be a close antigenic match. It appears that some strains of virus incorporated into killed vaccines are more immunogenic than others and this factor needs to be considered in antigen selection. In part, this can be explained by the presence or absence of glycosylation sites (Zhang et al. 2014).

Historically, for HPAI vaccination, the initial vaccine seed strains have been the same HA subtype as the one causing the outbreak, but obtained from LPAI outbreaks in poultry or from wild waterfowl. This has largely been superseded by use of antigens derived using reverse genetic (rg) technology from HP field strains associated with the outbreak.

In a number of countries where vaccine is used, antigenic variant viruses have emerged, necessitating a change in vaccine seed strains to genetically and antigenically more closely related viruses, e.g. H5N2 LPAIV in Mexico and H9N2 LPAIV and H5 Gs/GD lineage HPAIV in various Middle Eastern and Asian countries. With H5N2 in Mexico and H9N2 in various countries, the vaccine seed strains were updated to a newer field LPAIV. In China, multiple antigenic variants have emerged that were a poor match to existing vaccine strains. This has been seen with a number of viruses. In the case of H9N2 in China, it has been proposed as a factor in the genesis of the zoonotic H7N9 virus that emerged in 2013 (Zhang et al. 2012b; Pu et al. 2014).

Updates for H5 Gs/GD lineage HPAI vaccines have been handled in one of two ways. First, some countries such as Indonesia and Pakistan have updated their H5 and H7 vaccines by using newer HPAIV as seed strains, a practice that is discouraged because of the need to propagate large quantities of HP and potentially zoonotic virus (OIE 2015). Second, in some countries such as China, rg seed strains have been constructed in the laboratory that use the HA gene from a recent field H5 Gs/GD lineage HPAIV, but the HA proteolytic cleavage site has been changed from HP to LP, and the resulting new HA gene plus the avian NA gene are incorporated into a high-growth vaccine backbone to yield a LPAIV seed strain that grows to high titer and antigenically matches the circulating field HPAIV.

By contrast to inactivated AI vaccines, the live recombinant vectored vaccines have not changed HA gene inserts as often and these vaccines seem to provide broader protection within the HA subtype. Some recombinant vaccines such as rFPV-H5 have been used in Mexico since 1998 and shown good laboratory and field protection (Swayne et al. 2000b), and the rHVT-H5 has demonstrated broad H5 HPAI protective properties against diverse Gs/GD lineage HPAI viruses (Rauw et al. 2011; Soejoedono et al. 2012; Kapczynski et al. 2015). However, when there is evidence of reduced vaccine effectiveness, updates of live vectored vaccines may be needed to provide a closer antigenic match of the insert (Richard-Mazet et al. 2014). In some studies, vector vaccines have provided a better immune response and protection when used as a priming vaccine, followed by a boost with an inactivated vaccine that matches the field strain (Kilany et al. 2015; Richard-Mazet et al. 2014).

18.4.2 Efficacy Studies for Licensing

For issuance of the registration or license, the competent veterinary authority should require efficacy testing to show the vaccine protects in the target species of poultry against a recent, relevant HPAIV or LPAIV strain that is circulating within or is threating entry into the country. Results from a single challenge strain can be misleading, even when genetically similar viruses are used, if diverse antigenic strains are circulating, and more than one challenge strain may be required (Spackman et al. 2014). Most testing has used chickens as the target species, but some vaccines have been tested and licensed for use in turkeys or ducks. Off-label usage of the vaccine in other avian species should be carefully evaluated by a qualified veterinarian, in consultation with the licensing veterinary authority. In the efficacy study, there should be sufficient numbers of birds for statistical comparison between the test-vaccinated and sham-vaccinated challenged groups in the parameters of protection. General guidance suggests conducting the challenge at 3 or more weeks postvaccination and challenge with 10^6 mean embryo infectious doses (EID_{50}) (OIE 2015). For a successful efficacy study for a vaccine against a HPAIV, the shams should experience ≥90% mortality and the vaccine test group ≥80% protection.

For both HPAI and LPAI studies, the other important metric of protection is reduction or prevention of replication of challenge virus and shedding from respiratory and gastrointestinal tracts, and, for LPAI, prevention or reduction of drops in egg production. Trials should be conducted blind and by a party independent of the vaccine manufacturer (Sims et al. 2016).

Once licensed, additional efficacy testing is not required until the license expires. The license expiry date should be 2–5 years after issuance, unless evidence of vaccine resistance emerges in the field. Approval of each batch of vaccine should require a release test, usually based on a minimum serological response in vaccinated SPF chickens.

Efficacy testing with *in vivo* challenge for each batch is not necessary (OIE 2015).

18.4.3 Quantity of HA Protein or Infectious Titer

Each batch of inactivated vaccine should contain the minimum amount of HA antigen in each dose that will produce a protective immune response in the target species as specified by the national veterinary vaccine authority. When using a direct assay for HA protein, each dose should contain: (i) a minimum of 3 μg (range 1–5 μg) or, if using an indirect assay, sufficient antigen in each dose to produce a minimum HI serological titer in vaccinated SPF White Leghorn chickens; each dose should produce a minimum titer of 1:32 to protect from mortality or 1:128 to provide best reduction in challenge virus replication and shedding, or (ii) 50 mean protective doses (PD_{50}) of HA (Swayne and Kapczynski 2008; OIE 2015).

For inactivated vaccines, criteria for adjuvant incorporation should be specified, in order to promote an optimal immune response.

For live vectored vaccines, the specifications should require a minimum titer per dose of vaccine which will provide the needed replicating virus to produce the protective immune response.

18.5 Quality Assurance and Control Testing

The master seed for inactivated vaccines should pass tests to assess and assure sterility, safety, potency, and absence of specified extraneous agents (OIE 2015). The master seed and working seeds should be propagated in SPF or specific antibody-negative (SAN) embryonating chicken eggs. The vaccine should have accompanying test results that indicate the minimum quality of HA antigen in each dose based on either direct or indirect tests as specified in the prior section. In multivalent vaccines, the antigen concentration for each individual seed strain must be equal to that of a monovalent vaccine, i.e. simple mixing of aqueous or final product of monovalent vaccine into a multivalent product will reduce antigen concentration of each seed strain to 1/2 in bivalent and 1/3 in trivalent vaccines, which is unacceptable.

The manufacturer must provide assurance that the seed strain used in the vaccine is the specific licensed seed strain and is clearly listed on the label. Two prior studies reported that commercial vaccines sold in Mexico and Indonesia contained seed strains other than those licensed and listed on the label (Eggert et al. 2010; Swayne et al. 2015). The veterinary licensing authority should periodically test final products to confirm that the correct seed strains have been used. Controls to prevent smuggled vaccine also need to be in place. Illegal vaccination has occurred in a number of countries that do not permit vaccination against AI and, in some cases, tests on illegally imported vaccines have demonstrated no detectable antigen in the vaccine. Illegally imported vaccine may have been the source of an H5N2 LPAI outbreak virus in Chinese Taipei (Lee et al. 2014).

Live vaccines should be assessed for sterility, safety, potency, and absence of specified extraneous agents, and should contain viable vaccine virus of the titer specified on the label. Desired quality assurance and control testing are provided in the OIE *Manual of Diagnostic Tests and Vaccines for Terrestrial Animals* (OIE 2015).

18.6 Vaccine Application for Disease Control

18.6.1 Vaccination Strategy

18.6.1.1 Initial Decision Process

Use of vaccination against HPAI raises many ethical and operational questions and issues that need to be considered carefully before vaccination is used (Castellan et al. 2014). If virus elimination is deemed to be unlikely using stamping out, then an assessment should be made as to whether vaccination might be of benefit in reducing the effects of the disease, minimizing zoonotic transmission of virus, and reducing economic losses (Sims et al. 2016).

There are a number of situations where the use of vaccination can be of benefit, but potential complications that can arise from use of vaccination also need to be considered. If eradication is feasible and is the immediate objective of the control program, improper use of vaccines can slow down eradication and complicate surveillance. Vaccination also has the potential to lead to complacency among farmers in maintaining biosecurity practices to exclude entry of the virus on their premises (Swayne and Spackman 2013). Recognition of these issues allows introduction of suitable measures to overcome potential limiting factors if vaccination is used (e.g. changes to surveillance methods, enforcement of biosecurity standards, etc.).

All AI contingency plans should contain regular review time points to assess whether the strategy being used remains appropriate, whether a change in objective is necessary because of the extent of infection (from immediate-to-long term virus elimination), and whether and how vaccination can assist in this process.

The national veterinary authorities should determine whether vaccination will be used as one of the measures for control and prevention of the disease and should exercise overall control of the vaccines administered. Veterinary authorities are responsible for determining the objectives and scope of vaccination programs and for monitoring whether the objectives are being achieved. Vaccination alone (or any measure used in isolation) will not eradicate AI. Vaccination increases resistance to infection, and reduces poultry mortality, infections, and virus production, thus reducing environmental contamination with virus, and specifically decreases virus spread. It can allow disease and infection to be managed until changes can be made in production, transportation, and marketing practices and animal health services that will facilitate eradication.

In countries where H5 Gs/GD lineage HPAIV is endemic, the changes required to these practices are so large that the prospects of eradication in the foreseeable future are low. In such cases, regular reviews of the scope of and need for vaccination should be conducted (OFFLU 2014). This should include assessment of any antigenic variation in field strains and decisions on antigenic or genetic updating of inactivated vaccine seed strains or HA gene inserts within live vectored vaccines. Long-term use of vaccination in places where the virus continues to circulate has been associated with emergence of antigenic variants and systems must be in place for detecting these strains and for rapid updating of vaccine antigens (Lee et al. 2016).

The decision to use vaccination needs to take into account resources required and logistics for vaccination programs. Cooperation with the commercial poultry sector is essential as in most cases they will be responsible for administering the vaccine to their poultry. If vaccination of village poultry or smallholder flocks is included in the vaccination program, resources must be available to deliver and safely administer appropriately stored vaccine at the field level, including taking into account the need for appropriate cold chain to maintain the viability of the vaccine and adequate biosecurity for the vaccination crews to allow safe administration.

It is essential to define the objectives of the vaccination program to enable future assessment against outcomes such as management of disease, reduction in susceptibility and mortality of poultry, reduction in human exposures, maintenance of the livelihoods of the rural poor, or elimination/eradication of the virus (OFFLU 2014; Spackman and Pantin-Jackwood 2014). It has been suggested by a number of authors that vaccination has failed to eliminate H5 Gs/GD lineage HPAIV circulation in places such as China and Vietnam (Sakoda et al. 2012; Capua and Cattoli 2013), but this was not the objective of the programs, given virus elimination was recognized as a long-term objective (FAO 2011). In the countries where the virus is endemic, one of the main objectives of vaccination is to reduce the likelihood of high-level virus shedding by infected poultry, thus allowing management of the disease and reduced spread of the virus. These countries have high concentrations of poultry, reared using a mixture of production systems, from free range grazing ducks to highly intensive production systems, and sale of poultry through live bird markets and traders. Changes are occurring in these systems but some high-risk systems remain. It has been possible to prevent infection in the large commercial sector using a combination of biosecurity and vaccination and this is the first essential step on the road toward virus elimination. Without the initial management to reduce levels of infection through vaccination and other measures, elimination is not possible.

Vaccination is commonly accepted as a management strategy for non-H5/H7 LPAIV, which are economic diseases, and has been used to manage H5/H7 LPAIV in some countries. Experiences with the use of vaccination against H9N2 LPAIV demonstrate the importance of regular updating of vaccine antigens once antigenic variants emerge against which existing vaccines are less effective (Pu et al. 2014; Lee et al. 2016). From a public health perspective, the long-term objective should be to minimize all AIV infections in poultry so as to reduce the likelihood of emergence of novel zoonotic strains with pandemic potential.

18.6.1.2 Application Strategies

Vaccines for HPAI or LPAI prevention or control have been applied in the field utilizing three different approaches, used alone or in combination, depending on the country (OIE 2007):

- Preventive or prophylactic vaccination conducted when a high risk of virus incursion is identified, such as when AIV has been detected in wild birds within the country or in poultry in adjacent countries.
- Emergency vaccination in outbreak areas or outer buffer zones, in the face of an epizootic, after cases have been identified in poultry, as part of an overall management response.
- Routine targeted vaccination, within country or within areas or compartments, performed when AIV has become endemic in poultry.

Vaccines should be applied to the highest risk poultry populations and to sufficient numbers of poultry to produce population immunity; typically, a minimum of between 60% and 80% of the poultry should have a protective immune response in the target population (Bouma et al. 2007; Swayne et al. 2011). This can be achieved relatively easily in intensively reared poultry but is more difficult to achieve in multiage scavenging flocks. When flock immunity is lower than 60–80% there is a high probability of infection transmitting in a flock if exposed to the virus, but the quantities of virus generated will be lower in immune poultry within that flock than in nonimmune birds.

In Vietnam, in 2005, when mass vaccination was first used, the objective of the program was to reduce the risk of human exposures to virus and therefore the number of human zoonotic cases (at the time Vietnam had experienced more human cases than any other country). Levels of flock immunity in small flocks varied and were often below the 60–80% level but the number of human cases fell, suggesting that specific gains can still be made even with imperfect coverage. A controlled trial of vaccination in smallholder and village poultry in Indonesia resulted in significant reductions in events typical of HPAI when two doses of vaccine were administered 3 weeks apart four times in 1 year (Bett et al. 2013). Overall, less than half of the poultry tested (which included both vaccinated and unvaccinated birds) in vaccinated areas seroconverted (McLaws et al. 2014) with the levels of protection influenced by the levels of vaccination coverage.

Regardless of the overall objective of a vaccination program, the goal should always be to maximize the number of vaccinated poultry achieving a suitable titer. In any mass campaign involving smallholder and village poultry with high rates of turnover, overall population immunity is not expected to reach levels required for virus elimination.

The most effective vaccination programs immunize at-risk poultry, although defining the target at-risk population is not always a simple task, complicated in places with multiple types of poultry reared under a range of conditions. The number of vaccinations per birds varies. In most situations, two vaccinations separated by 2 or more weeks is the minimum to achieve field protection. For example, in meat (broiler) chickens in Mexico, priming with rFPV-H5 in the hatchery followed by a booster vaccination with inactivated H5N2 vaccine in the field at 10–14 days of age has been effective against H5N2 LPAIV, but additional booster vaccinations of layers and breeders have been administered to maintain protection, usually boosting at approximately 6-month intervals. Similarly, rHVT-H5 in the hatchery has been shown to provide reasonable protection in Egypt against H5N1 Gs/GD lineage HPAIV challenge (Kilany et al. 2015). Turkeys may need more than two vaccinations to maintain protection through the entire grow-out period. Maternal antibodies, when present, will interfere with development of immunity when vaccines containing killed antigens are used at an early age and may inhibit replication of some recombinant virus vectored vaccines (Swayne et al. 2000a; Beltran et al. 2018).

Most occurrences of "vaccine" failures are actually failures in application (i.e. vaccination program) as the populations of poultry in most vaccinating countries are large, containing many individual owners/farmers, not all of whom will choose to vaccinate their poultry or do so properly. In addition, the short generation time with rapid production of poultry progeny and rapid movement of poultry over considerable distances within a region make it difficult to maintain appropriate levels of immunity in at-risk populations. Generally, vaccination of all at-risk poultry at specific ages, year round, to maintain a resistant population is the ideal preferred strategy. Seasonal vaccination has been used but this means that some poultry receive their first dose of vaccine at an age when the immune response may be poorer. Periods of enhanced poultry vaccination coverage may be effective when centered round times of year when poultry production peaks and poultry movements are enhanced, such as Chinese New Year or other festivals.

18.6.1.3 Best Practices

Specific vaccination programs should be risk based as to application within geographic region, production sector, and/or species. Short-lived meat chickens (broilers) should generally receive a minimum of two vaccinations, separated by 2–3 weeks, in order to provide consistent protection if progeny have maternal antibodies against HA or possibly the vector. For this type of vaccination program to be feasible in short-lived broilers, the first dose of vaccine should be a vector vaccine delivered in the hatchery either *in ovo* or at 1 day of age. In chicks from HA and vector antibody-negative breeders, single vaccination with live vectored vaccines may be sufficient to protect for the short production life. However, either strategy may leave chicks susceptible to infection if exposed during the first 3–4 weeks of life and necessitate boosting breeders, thereby providing longer protection from maternal antibodies.

Initial studies with rHVT-H5 vaccines in broilers with maternal antibody suggested that a single dose may be sufficient to reduce shedding of virus and mortality in infected birds challenged at 4 weeks of age (Rauw et al. 2012). In 2015 USA studies, rHVT-H5 *in ovo* or at 1 day of age, followed by a booster vaccination with *da*-H5 vaccine 3 weeks later, gave 100% protection in both chickens and turkeys, and was compatible with identification of infected animals in vaccinated populations, i.e. differentiating infected from vaccinated animals (DIVA), using existing agar gel immunodiffusion (AGID) and enzyme-linked immunosorbent assay (ELISA) tests for antibodies against M/NP proteins. The feasibility of such DIVA serological testing assumes no other influenza viruses are circulating in the flock, which can be a major impediment in many developing countries. Similarly, priming with rHVT-H5 and boosting with inactivated vaccines provided good protection in chicken and turkeys, but necessitates use of a different NA subtype in the vaccine from the field virus if DIVA surveillance strategies using a NA serology test against the field virus are being applied.

Additional, inactivated vaccine administration may be needed in meat turkeys and long-lived poultry (breeders/layers) to maintain effective immunity throughout production life. In long-lived layers and breeders, booster vaccination every 6 months has been suggested and, in some places, boosters are provided more frequently (OIE 2015; Swayne et al. 2015). Measurement of HI serological titers to detect average flock HI titers below the minimum set by the veterinary authority, e.g. 1:32 or 1:128, in more than 20% of the poultry on the farm, would be cause to administer a booster vaccination.

18.6.1.4 Logistics and Other Issues

The cold chain should be maintained from the manufacturer to the field for any live vectored vaccines and avoidance of high temperatures should be monitored for inactivated vaccines. Live virus vaccines are very susceptible to thermal inactivation and heat can destroy antigenicity of inactivated vaccines, rendering them useless. Finally, the vaccination crew must practice the highest level of biosecurity so they do not spread AIV or even other diseases between farms.

18.6.2 Considering Epidemiological Settings and Objectives

The application of vaccines varies depending on the local conditions, epidemiological situation, and objectives of the vaccination program. The range of vaccination programs undertaken has included: (i) high-value nonpoultry species in zoological parks, (ii) individual poultry farms or premises, (iii) ring vaccination of poultry around and naïve poultry within AI outbreak zones, (iv) targeted vaccination of outdoor poultry at high risk of exposure, (v) targeted vaccination of a specific production sector of poultry, and (vi) routine vaccination of all or most poultry in a country or within a large geographic region (Swayne et al. 2011; Swayne 2012a).

First, following the 2005 spread of H5N1 Gs/GD lineage HPAIV into Europe associated with wild birds and the outbreaks of H7N7 HPAI in Dutch poultry in 2003, vaccination was undertaken in a variety of birds on over 292 zoological parks in 20 countries to protect them from H5 and/or H7 HPAI (Swayne et al. 2011). Second, in another limited situation, during 2006, ostriches were vaccinated on a single farm in Israel against H5N1 Gs/GD lineage HPAI, but within a few months, all the birds were culled, i.e. a strategy of vaccination then elimination of vaccinated poultry. Similarly, during 2002–2003 a single layer company vaccinated chickens in Connecticut, USA, against H7N2 LPAI, ending vaccination after 18 months with demonstration of virus freedom. Third, historically, programs under emergency vaccination orders have used ring vaccination around and within the outbreak zone for susceptible naïve poultry and replacement stocks such as with H7N3 outbreaks in Pakistan after 2003. Both Vietnam and China also practice ring vaccination when outbreaks of H5N1 Gs/GD lineage HPAI are detected. Fourth, during the 2005 H5N1 Gs/GD lineage HPAIV wild bird outbreaks in Europe, targeted vaccination was practiced in high-risk poultry, including outdoor ducks in France and free-range layers in the Netherlands. In addition, poultry reared under conditions of poor biosecurity near wetlands were vaccinated in Siberia, Russia. Hong Kong SAR has been using vaccination since 2002 as an additional measure for disease prevention given the high risk of viral incursion on to farms that biosecurity measures alone could not prevent, and to ensure high-level immunity in poultry sold in live poultry markets. Fifth, focused sector-specific vaccination was practiced over wide geographic areas in northern Italy in turkeys and capons during 2003–2005 against both H5 and H7 LPAI (Marangon et al. 2004). Sixth, mass vaccination of poultry, in whole country or targeted geographic regions, has occurred in some H5 HPAI endemic countries and in places at high risk of virus incursion (i.e. China, Egypt, Vietnam, and Indonesia for H5 Gs/GD lineage) and 10 Middle Eastern and Asian countries for H9N2 LPAI (Swayne et al. 2011).

18.6.3 Possible Combination with Vaccines of Other Diseases

Initially, when AI vaccines were implemented as an emergency control tool in specific countries, only monovalent vaccines matching the field HA subtype were used, and such monovalent vaccines have continued to be used in many countries where only one subtype or only a single lineage, clade, or antigenic group of a single subtype circulates. However, as some AIV became endemic, control programs in some countries shifted from short-term emergency vaccination to longer term routine vaccination strategies with multivalent products introduced to reduce the number of times poultry were handled and vaccinated (FAO 2009). Initial bivalent offerings were combined inactivated Newcastle disease vaccines with inactivated AIV such as H9N2 or H5N1 Gs/GD lineage seed strains, or bivalent vaccines for multiple HA subtypes of AIV such as an inactivated vaccine with H9N2 and H5N1, or H5N1 and H7N3 seed strains (Chen 2009; FAO 2009). As more HA subtypes of AIV have become endemic in some countries, multivalent vaccines have appeared such as H9N2, H5N1, and H7N3 multivalent vaccine in Pakistan. Finally, bivalent vaccines with two clades of H5N1 Gs/GD lineage seed strains have appeared such as in Indonesia with clades 2.1.3 and 2.3.2.1 seed strains, and in China with clades 0 and 7, and 2.3.4 and 2.3.2.1 seed strains (Chen 2009; CFSPH 2012).

In all cases of multivalent vaccines, the concentration of each seed strain should be the same as in the monovalent product, in order to achieve adequate protection for each seed strain. Antigens of other poultry pathogens (e.g. infectious bronchitis virus) can be combined with AI vaccines in multivalent products to reduce the number of vaccinations administered to poultry. There is the potential for a reduced immune response to individual antigens in multivalent vaccines due to antigenic competition and this should be assessed experimentally before any combined vaccine is used in the field.

18.6.4 Use of Vaccine in the Face of an Outbreak

Avian influenza vaccines have been used during AI outbreaks in emergency vaccination programs under two scenarios: (i) LPAI-affected farms during the outbreak, and (ii) naïve poultry in a HPAI outbreak zone. During the outbreak of H7N2 LPAI in a large Connecticut farm in 2003, layers in all houses were vaccinated once to produce uniform protective antibody titers which would not be achieved by natural infection alone (Swayne and Akey 2005). This is because the transmission efficiency drops during the acute infection phase, as the number of naïve birds declines, such that 100% infection never occurs and the virus is maintained in the population at low level between widely dispersed naïve birds. The goal was to stop the slow spread of the LPAIV in the large population of chickens within each house (i.e. 100 000 birds per house) because handling and vaccination of each chicken on the affected farm raised the number of birds with protective immunity to nearly 100% and stopped this slow transmission cycle.

The second scenario is vaccination within an HPAI outbreak zone on known naïve farms to reduce the number of susceptible poultry and thus stop the farm-to-farm spread of virus. However, the maximum level of biosecurity must be practiced to prevent movement of virus as the vaccination crews move on and off farms in the outbreak zones, as was considered to have spread NDV in southern California during outbreaks in 1972–1973 (Utterback and Schwartz 1973). HPAI-affected flocks should not be vaccinated, but instead should be depopulated; however, on a farm basis it may be possible to vaccinate unaffected houses as was done successfully in Hong Kong in the face of an H5N1 Gs/GD lineage HPAI outbreak in 2003 (Ellis et al. 2004). In the future, if a suitable live virus vaccine were to become available, vaccination in the face of an outbreak might prove valuable for very large flocks of caged layers (1 million birds plus) where humane stamping out cannot be conducted rapidly.

18.6.5 When Vaccination is Not Recommended

For HPAIV, eradication is the goal and freedom is most quickly achieved in places where detection is early and completed through a stamping-out program (OIE 2017). The presence of highly competent national, state/provincial, and local veterinary services has been associated with more rapid time to eradication and fewer outbreaks, but higher culling rates (Pavade et al. 2011). In a 2010 survey of chief veterinary officers (CVO) from 69 countries that had experienced HPAI or H5/H7 LPAI, 21 countries had used AI vaccine in poultry, eight in preventive programs, 14 in emergency programs, and eight in routine vaccination programs (Swayne et al. 2011). However, most CVOs favored using stamping out without vaccination in poultry unless rapid eradication was not achieved, or if risk assessments indicated significant and immediate threat of spread within country or from a neighboring country, or if HPAIV was endemic in poultry. Under these scenarios, vaccination would be considered as a supplementary tool for control (Swayne et al. 2011). In these situations, a stockpile of suitable vaccine is usually required.

18.7 Monitoring and Vaccine Effectiveness

18.7.1 Postvaccination Monitoring

To monitor field protection, representative, long-lived poultry should be sampled for HI antibody titer determination. HI tests should be performed using the vaccine virus as antigen (or a very similar strain) to assess whether vaccination has been done correctly through stimulation of an appropriate immune response in vaccinated flocks. The competent veterinary authority should set the minimum desired HI titer and when titers fall below this level, booster vaccination is indicated.

Serological tests should also be undertaken using the circulating strains as the HI test antigen, when the presence of HI antibodies is a positive predictor of protection (Swayne et al. 2015). Although there is imperfect correlation between antibody levels and protection, as a rule, the higher the titer to the field strain, the lower the likelihood of death and shedding of virus. As a guide, White Leghorn chicken flocks with a minimum average titer of 1:32 in 80% of the birds are likely to be protected from mortality. Higher titers of ≥1:128 in 80% of the chickens should be optimal to reduce challenge virus replication and shedding. Nevertheless, chickens with titers below these levels can still be protected from death (Ma et al. 2014) and shed substantially lower quantities of virus than sham-vaccinated infected birds (Spackman et al. 2014).

The minimum protective titer for other chicken breeds or poultry species has not been scientifically established, but recommendations can be made by the competent veterinary authority based on field experience. Postvaccination titers in ducks tend to be lower than those in chickens, yet still offer protection from challenge (Middleton et al. 2007; Pu et al. 2014). Some geese with no apparent titers after vaccination have been protected from death following experimental infection (Rudolf et al. 2009; Pu et al. 2014). With rHVT-H5 vaccines it is possible to monitor vaccine uptake by detecting the vector in feather follicles (Rauw et al. 2015).

18.7.2 Outbreaks in Vaccinated Animals

Poultry that are properly vaccinated with high-potency, antigenically matched vaccines are well protected and such vaccination is associated with increased resistance to infection and reductions in virus transmission (Goot et al. 2003; Swayne et al. 2013). Outbreaks in "vaccinated" poultry have been reported on individual farms in Mexico, Egypt, China, Indonesia, Hong Kong, and Vietnam (Swayne 2012a). These outbreaks have occurred either from: (i) failure of the vaccines, such as low-potency vaccines or the emergence of antigenic variants against which the seed strain in use provides limited or no protection, or (ii) failure from improper administration of vaccine (e.g. vaccinating day-old chickens with a vaccine containing a killed antigen in the face of maternally derived antibody) (Peyre et al. 2009), or inability to vaccinate and produce a protective immune response in at least 60–80% of the at-risk poultry population in the flock (Swayne 2012a). Some countries have applied targeted mass vaccination in the face of endemic infection. Delivery of billions of vaccine doses to poultry owned by millions of people is a huge logistic process and the difficulties associated with these programs need to be recognized (OFFLU 2014).

In addition, the emergence of drift variant field viruses resistant to vaccines emphasizes the need for continual surveillance to detect field virus that have escaped vaccine-induced immunity and to periodically update seed strains when vaccine resistance emerges in the field. This is becoming increasingly difficult for Gs/GD-lineage HPAIVs of the H5 subtype. Circulation of multiple antigenic variant strains can make decisions on antigenic composition extremely difficult and stretches the capacity of vaccine manufacturers, especially given the lead time between detection of an antigenic variant, introduction of a new vaccine strain, and registration of the new vaccine by an individual country's competent veterinary authority. Even when antigenic variants emerge, they do not necessarily persist, as was the case with clade 2.3.2.1b H5N1 Gs/GD lineage viruses in Vietnam and China (Le and Nguyen 2014; Pu et al. 2014), complicating decisions on vaccine antigen selection.

18.8 Vaccine Adverse Reactions

In commercial poultry, because of low individual economic value, adverse reactions from vaccines and vaccination have not been a major issue limiting vaccination as a control tool. Nevertheless, adverse reactions were reported in mass campaigns and were cited as a reason for reluctance by farmers to allow their birds to be vaccinated. These included short-term suppression of lay from handling and reluctance to eat in young chicks vaccinated in the neck (Sims and Dung 2009). In some cases, off-label use of poultry vaccines in valuable zoological birds has produced minor local tissue reactions at the injection sites (Philippa Joost et al. 2005), while the stress of catching and handling these captive wild birds has produced some mortality, necessitating a risk–benefit analysis for determining if the production of low mortality from capture and handling is justified for any real or perceived risk of HPAIV exposure and infection (EFSA 2007).

18.9 Availability and List of Manufacturers

The global availability of AI vaccines is dynamic and there is no continuously updated list of vaccine seed strains and manufacturers, although in 2012, 27 manufacturers were recognized (CFSPH 2012). Because LPAI, except for H5 and H7, is not a reportable disease to the OIE or within most countries, information on the availability and use of vaccines against H1–4, H6, H8, and H10–16 LPAI is largely unavailable. However, vaccines utilizing H9N2 LPAIV vaccines are commonly used in official control programs in industrial poultry in 10 countries across the Middle East and Africa (Swayne et al. 2011). The H5 vaccines have the widest range of manufacturers, number of monovalent and multivalent vaccines, and number of seed strains available, but the availability of H5 and H7 AI vaccines was last updated in 2009 on the Food and Agriculture Organization website (FAO 2009) and in 2012 on the Center for Food Security and Public Health website (CFSPH 2012).

Since 2009, the number of manufacturers of H5 and H7 vaccines has reduced and vaccines made with many of the listed seed strains are no longer available. For example, the A/chicken/Mexico/232/94/CPA (H5N2) LPAIV seed strain widely used in Mexico to control H5N2 LPAI was available from 1995 through 2009, but has been replaced by a newer seed strain, A/chicken/Durango/1558/2006 (H5N2) LPAIV, and a more recent H5N2 seed strain, A/chicken/Guanajuato/CPA-20966-15-VS/2015(H5N2) (Table 18.2). Also, inactivated vaccines with seed strain A/Turkey/England/N-28/73 (H5N2) LPAIV are no longer available, as well as rgA/Goose/Guangdong/1996 (H5N1, clade 0) LPAIV and wild-type A/chicken/Legok/2003 (H5N1) HPAIV seed strains. In addition, the live recombinant fowlpox virus with insert of the H5 and N1 gene from A/Goose/Guangdong/1996 (clade 0) is no longer produced. Multiple new seed strains have been added for H5 both for poultry vaccines and as potential pandemic preparedness vaccines for humans.

18.10 Future Considerations

Vaccination will be used as a control and preventive measure for AI in the foreseeable future. The Gs/GD lineage of H5Nx HPAI will continue to be endemic in multiple developing countries/areas including China, Vietnam, Indonesia, Egypt, and southern Asia (Bangladesh and India) with threats for reintroduction to neighboring countries and additional intercontinental waves of infection. Vaccination will continue to serve as an intermediate strategy to control and prevent HPAI until such time as conditions allow a shift to virus elimination. In some of these places, this prospect appears remote. Vaccination programs should be reassessed regularly and modified in these countries with new vaccine technologies that offer advantages likely to be adopted. The disease in West Africa remains incompletely controlled since 2015. Vaccination has been considered but is not yet being used.

Sporadic incursions of H5/H7 LPAI are likely to occur from the wild bird reservoir into domestic poultry with mutation to HPAI viruses. The vast majority of such incursions will be eradicated through stamping-out programs (Pavade et al. 2011) but the potential for use of vaccination should be included in contingency plans (Sims et al. 2016).

Vaccination should be considered as a preventive measure in places where incursions of avian influenza virus occur regularly. This practice will be facilitated if the system for monitoring infection in vaccinated flocks can be simplified and the associated costs of monitoring reduced. Vaccination in the face of outbreaks will be facilitated if suitable vaccines that can be administered by mass application are developed.

The decision on whether to use vaccines for HPAI control and prevention will be made by each individual country based on consideration of multiple factors: (i) the level of risk of introduction from neighboring countries or from migratory aquatic birds (Castellan et al. 2014) and the cost of previous outbreaks, (ii) the cost of the vaccine and the cost to administer vaccine assessed against the expected benefits, (iii) availability of suitable, well-matched vaccines from in-country and out-of-country vaccine manufacturers, (iv) availability of logistic support to administer the vaccine and the vaccine program, (v) in places where virus elimination is possible, the ability to identify infections within vaccinated populations (e.g. DIVA), and (vi) the extent of infection as well as the prospects of success using other measures (e.g. is the virus endemic and are there any prospects of virus elimination in the next 1–2 years using stamping out?).

Well-managed vaccination programs will continue to provide a public health benefit, as the use of vaccines in poultry results in increased resistance to AIV infection, and reduces replication in and shedding of AI virus from the respiratory and gastrointestinal systems. This translates into reduced environmental contamination and reduced transmission to humans. The positive public health aspects were best demonstrated in Vietnam, which had 93 human H5N1 Gs/GD lineage HPAI cases in the first 3 years of the H5N1 Gs/GD lineage HPAI outbreak (2003–2005), but after full implementation of a national poultry vaccination campaign, no human cases occurred in 2006. Although it is not possible to ascribe all of the gains to vaccination given other measures were also implemented concurrently, it was considered to be an important factor (Sims and Dung 2009; WHO 2011). Vaccination of poultry against H7N9 subtype viruses has been introduced as a compulsory measure in China following the large number of human cases in 2016–2017 and is also expected to reduce the likelihood (and number) of new human cases.

Vaccination against H9N2 virus will continue to be used in places where these viruses are circulating in poultry. It is not expected that these viruses, which are well adapted to chickens, will be eradicated.

18.11 Summary

Based on the information presented and discussed, the following conclusions may be drawn:

1) Vaccines have been used as a management tool for both LPAI and HPAI. Although the preferred goal for HPAI

is immediate eradication achieved through rapid stamping out, perhaps in combination with emergency vaccination, when immediate eradication cannot be achieved some countries have used vaccination as an additional control/preventive tool to protect livelihoods, to reduce zoonotic risk to humans, and to provide time to change production systems to favor eventual elimination. Experiences in Asia with H5 Gs/GD lineage HPAI suggest that elimination will be a long-term goal and may never be achieved. Similarly, vaccination has been used for H5/H7 LPAI as a secondary control tool and as a means of virus elimination from large poultry farms. LPAI caused by other subtypes (e.g. H9N2) are generally seen as economic diseases without international reporting requirements and vaccination has been used as a primary control tool to manage disease. Pressure is likely to build for better control of all zoonotic influenza viruses and this could result in changes to management strategies for these viruses, including the way in which vaccines are used.

2) Vaccination against H5/H7 AI should be overseen by national veterinary authorities and form part of an overall management plan for the disease. This applies even to countries where infection is endemic. Emergency disease management plans should consider conditions under which vaccination might be used and include regular review points to determine if vaccination might have a role to play in disease control and prevention. Every vaccination program should have clear objectives and regular review points to determine if the objectives are being met and to modify the program as required.
3) In the past, most HPAI and LPAI vaccines used were inactivated whole AIV utilizing LPAIV seed strains that matched the field virus HA subtype and were antigenically closely related. For HPAI control, the majority of seed strains are constructed with HA gene sequence of the HPAIV field viruses altered through reverse genetics to be high-growth LPAIV. In some countries, HPAIV seed strains are used in inactivated AI vaccines. A significant amount of live recombinant rFPV-H5 and rNDV-H5 vaccines and recently rHVT-H5 have been used to control H5 HPAI and LPAI with some success.
4) The primary protective immune response has been HA subtype-specific humoral immunity. However, cell-mediated and innate immunity do contribute to protection, especially with vector vaccines.
5) Inactivated vaccines used in the field should contain relevant seed strains that antigenically match the circulating field viruses and an appropriate adjuvant system to produce a protective immune response in the target poultry species. In most situations, a minimum of two doses of vaccine is needed, but for long-lived poultry additional booster vaccinations are usually needed.
6) Inactivated whole virus and subunit vaccines should contain well-characterized and antigenically matched seed strains, and be safe, potent, and free of extraneous agents as determined by appropriate manufacturing standards and quality control testing. Strains of virus that are highly immunogenic should be used as antigens. Vector vaccines and RNA particle vaccines should be assessed regularly for efficacy/efficiency under laboratory and field conditions. If evidence suggests inadequate protection, updating of the insert should be considered. Some vector vaccines produce better results if used as a priming dose.
7) Vaccines should be administered through preventive, emergency, or routine vaccination programs targeted to at-risk poultry, although defining the at-risk population is not always straightforward. Not all species respond in the same way to AI vaccines, and this variation also has to be considered in planning vaccination programs. Maternal antibody may interfere with immunity generated by vaccines if breeder flocks have been vaccinated.
8) The AI vaccine seed strains can be combined with seed strains of other poultry pathogens to produce multivalent vaccines that reduce the number of times poultry are handled for vaccination, thus reducing the overall cost of disease control and improving acceptance by farmers. However, the concentration of each seed strain must be the same in multivalent as in the original monovalent products in order to achieve matching levels of immunity. Multivalent vaccines need to be tested to ensure antigenic competition does not interfere with immunity.
9) Poultry in the field should be monitored for protective HI titers to assess the vaccination program and to determine timing of booster vaccinations in long-lived poultry for maintenance of protective immunity. Correlation between HI titers and levels of protection is imperfect but if appropriate titers are obtained, this provides the best chance of limiting the effect of infection, including reduced viral shedding. Titers in fully vaccinated domestic ducks are often lower than those in chickens.
10) Vaccination is one of the tools that can be used in combination with other measures to assist in control and prevention of AI and in, some situations, elimination of virus. The use of vaccine to prevent AI should not inhibit trade in poultry and poultry products provided adequate surveillance is used to demonstrate avian influenza virus freedom in vaccinated flocks.

References

Alexander, D.J. and Parsons, G. (1980). Protection of chickens against challenge with virulent influenza A viruses of Hav5 subtype conferred by prior infection with influenza A viruses of Hsw1 subtype. *Arch. Virol.* 66: 265–269.

Anonymous (2017). *DNA Influenza Vaccine Licensed for Chickens*. Florence: Zootechnica International http://zootecnicainternational.com/news/dna-influenza-vaccine-licensed-chickens

Beato, M.S., Realpe-Quintero, M., Bonfante, F. et al. (2013). Cross-clade protection against H5N1 HPAI strains recently isolated from commercial poultry in Egypt with a single dose of a baculovirus based vaccine. *Vaccine* 31: 5075–5081.

Bertran, K., Thomas, C., Guo, X. et al. (2015). Expression of H5 hemagglutinin vaccine antigen in common duckweed (Lemna minor) protects against H5N1 high pathogenicity avian influenza virus challenge in immunized chickens. *Vaccine* 33: 3456–3462.

Bertran, K., Balzli, C., Lee, D.H. et al. (2017). Protection of White Leghorn chickens by U.S. emergency H5 vaccination against clade 2.3.4.4 H5N2 high pathogenicity avian influenza virus. *Vaccine* 35: 6336–6344.

Bertran, K., Balzli, C., Lee, D.H. et al. (2018). Maternal antibody inhibition of recombinant Newcastle disease virus vectored vaccine in a primary or booster avian influenza vaccination program of broiler chickens. *Vaccine* 36: 6361–6372.

Bett, B., McLaws, M., Jost, C. et al. (2013). The effectiveness of preventative mass vaccination regimes against the incidence of highly pathogenic avian influenza on Java Island, Indonesia. *Transbound. Emerg. Dis.* 62 (2): 163–173.

Bouma, A., Tiensin, T., Claassen, I. et al. (2007). Estimation of the critical proportion of chickens in a flock to be immunized to prevent major outbreaks of HPAI H5N1. In: *Abstracts of OIE/FAO Conference on Vaccination: A Tool for the Control of Avian Influenza*, 60. Paris: World Organization for Animal Health.

Brown, I.H., Abolnik, C., Garcia-Garcia, J. et al. (2016). High pathogenicity avian influenza outbreaks since 2008 except multi-continental panzootic of H5 goose/Guangdong-lineage viruses. In: *Animal Influenza* (ed. D.E. Swayne), 248–270. Ames: Wiley.

Brugh, M. and Stone, H.D. (1987). Immunization of chickens against influenza with hemagglutinin-specific (H5) oil emulsion vaccine. In: *Proceedings of the Second International Symposium on Avian Influenza* (eds. C.W. Beard and B.C. Easterday), 283–292. Richmond: US Animal Health Association.

Capua, I. and Cattoli, G. (2013). Prevention and control of highly pathogenic avian influenza with particular reference to H5N1. *Virus Res.* 178: 114–120.

Castellan, D.M., Hinrichs, J., Fusheng, G. et al. (2014). Development and application of a vaccination planning tool for avian influenza. *Avian Dis.* 58: 437–452.

CFSPH (2012). *Vaccines: Avian Influenza*. Ames: Center for Food Security and Public Health, Iowa State University.

Chambers, T.M., Kawaoka, Y., and Webster, R.G. (1988). Protection of chickens from lethal influenza infection by vaccine-expressed hemagglutinin. *Virology* 167: 414–421.

Chen, H. (2009). Avian influenza vaccination: the experience in China. *Rev. Sci. Tech. Off. Int. Epiz.* 28: 267–274.

Chen, S., Zhu, Y., Yang, D. et al. (2017). Efficacy of live-attenuated H9N2 influenza vaccine candidates containing NS1 truncations against H9N2 avian influenza viruses. *Front. Microbiol.* 8: 1086.

Crawford, J., Wilkinson, B., Vosnesensky, A. et al. (1999). Baculovirus-derived hemagglutinin vaccines protect against lethal influenza infections by avian H5 and H7 subtypes. *Vaccine* 17: 2265–2274.

Dabaghian, M., Latify, A.M., Tebianian, M. et al. (2014). Vaccination with recombinant 4xM2e.HSP70c fusion protein as a universal vaccine candidate enhances both humoral and cell-mediated immune responses and decreases viral shedding against experimental challenge of H9N2 influenza in chickens. *Vet. Microbiol.* 174: 116–126.

De, B.K., Brownlee, G.G., Kendal, A.P., and Shaw, M.W. (1988). Complete sequence of a cDNA clone of the hemagglutinin gene of influenza A/Chicken/Scotland/59 (H5N1) virus: comparison with contemporary North American and European strains. *Nucleic Acids Res.* 16: 4181–4182.

EFSA. (2007). Opinion of the Scientific Panel on Animal Health and Welfare (AHAW) on a request from the Commission related with the vaccination against avian influenza of H5 and H7 subtypes as a preventive measure carried out in Member States in birds kept in zoos under Community approved programmes. www.efsa.europa.eu/en/efsajournal/pub/450.htm

Eggert, D., Thomas, C., Spackman, E. et al. (2010). Characterization and efficacy determination of commercially available Central American H5N2 avian influenza vaccines for poultry. *Vaccine* 28: 4609–4615.

Ellis, T.M., Leung, C.W., Chow, M.K. et al. (2004). Vaccination of chickens against H5N1 avian influenza in the face of an outbreak interrupts virus transmission. *Avian Pathol.* 33: 405–412.

European Council. (2015). Council Directive 2005/94/EC of 20 December 2005. Community measures for the control of avian influenza and repealing Directive 92/40/EEC. http://eur-lex.europa.eu/legal-content/EN/TXT/HTML/?uri=CELEX:32005L0094&from=EN

Fan, X., Hu, Y., Zhang, G., and Wang, M. (2015). Veterinary influenza vaccines against avian influenza in China. *Future Virol.* 10 (5): 585–595.

FAO. (2009). Avian influenza vaccine producers and suppliers for poultry. www.fao.org/3/a-ai326e.pdf

FAO. (2011). Approaches to controlling, preventing and eliminating H5N1 Highly Pathogenic Avian Influenza in endemic countries. FAO Animal Production and Health Paper 171:1–50. www.fao.org/3/a-i2150e.pdf

FAO (2017). *H7N9 Weekly Situation Update, 24 November 2017*. Rome: Food and Agriculture Organization www.fao.org/ag/againfo/programmes/en/empres/h7n9/wave_6/Situation_update_2017_11_24.html

Gao, W., Soloff, A.C., Lu, X. et al. (2006). Protection of mice and poultry from lethal H5N1 avian influenza virus through adenovirus-based immunization. *J. Virol.* 80: 1959–1964.

Goot, J.A., Koch, G., Jong, M.C., and Boven, M.v. (2003). Transmission dynamics of low- and high-pathogenicity A/Chicken/Pennsylvania/83 avian influenza viruses. *Avian Dis.* 47: 939–941.

Hai, R., Garcia-Sastre, A., Swayne, D.E., and Palese, P. (2011). A reassortment-incompetent live attenuated influenza virus vaccine for protection against pandemic virus strains. *J. Virol.* 85: 6832–6843.

Halvorson, D.A. (2002). Twenty-five years of avian influenza in Minnesota. In: *Proceedings of the 53rd North Central Avian Disease Conference*, 65–69. Minneapolis: North Central Avian Disease Conference.

Halvorson, D.A. (2008). Control of low pathogenicity avian influenza. In: *Avian Influenza* (ed. D.E. Swayne), 513–536. Ames: Blackwell Publishers.

Halvorson, D.A. (2009). Prevention and management of avian influenza outbreaks: experiences from the United States of America. *Rev. Sci. Tech. Off. Int. Epiz.* 28: 359–369.

Hunt, L.A., Brown, D.W., Robinson, H.L. et al. (1988). Retrovirus-expressed hemagglutinin protects against lethal influenza virus infections. *J. Virol.* 62: 3014–3019.

Kalthoff, D., Giritch, A., Geisler, K. et al. (2010). Immunization with plant-expressed hemagglutinin protects chickens from lethal highly pathogenic avian influenza virus H5N1 challenge infection. *J. Virol.* 84: 12002–12010.

Kapczynski, D.R. (2015). Research Update on H5 Highly Pathogenic Avian Influenza in the U.S. Presentation at 87th Northeastern Conference on Avian Diseases. Penn Stater Conference Center and Hotel, State College, Pennsylvania. 16-17 September.

Kapczynski, D.R., Esaki, M., Dorsey, K.M. et al. (2015). Vaccine protection of chickens against antigenically diverse H5 highly pathogenic avian influenza isolates with a live HVT vector vaccine expressing the influenza hemagglutinin gene derived from a clade 2.2 avian influenza virus. *Vaccine* 33: 1197–1205.

Kilany, W.H., Hassan, M.K., Safwat, M. et al. (2015). Comparison of the effectiveness of rHVT-H5, inactivated H5 and rHVT-H5 with inactivated H5 prime/boost vaccination regimes in commercial broiler chickens carrying MDAs against HPAI H5N1 clade 2.2.1 virus. *Avian Pathol.* 44: 333–341.

Kodihalli, S., Sivanandan, V., Nagaraja, K.V. et al. (1994). A type-specific avian influenza virus subunit vaccine for turkeys: induction of protective immunity to challenge infection. *Vaccine* 12: 1467–1472.

Layton, S.L., Kapczynski, D.R., Higgins, S. et al. (2009). Vaccination of chickens with recombinant Salmonella expressing M2e and CD154 epitopes increases protection and decreases viral shedding after low pathogenic avian influenza challenge. *Poult. Sci.* 88: 2244–2252.

Le, T.H. and Nguyen, N.T. (2014). Evolutionary dynamics of highly pathogenic avian influenza A/H5N1 HA clades and vaccine implementation in Vietnam. *Clin. Exp. Vaccine Res.* 3: 117–127.

Lee, C.C., Zhu, H., Huang, P.Y. et al. (2014). Emergence and evolution of avian H5N2 influenza viruses in chickens in Taiwan. *J. Virol.* 88: 5677–5686.

Lee, D.H., Fusaro, A., Song, C.S. et al. (2016). Poultry vaccination directed evolution of H9N2 low pathogenicity avian influenza viruses in Korea. *Virology* 488: 225–231.

Li, D., Xue, M., Wang, C. et al. (2011). Bursopentine as a novel immunoadjuvant enhances both humoral and cell-mediated immune responses to inactivated H9N2 avian influenza virus in chickens. *Clin. Vaccine Immunol.* 18: 1497–1502.

Liu, J., Chen, P., Jiang, Y. et al. (2011). A duck enteritis virus-vectored bivalent live vaccine provides fast and complete protection against H5N1 avian influenza virus infection in ducks. *J. Virol.* 85: 10989–10998.

Ma, Q.X., Jiang, W.M., Liu, S. et al. (2014). Subclinical highly pathogenic avian influenza virus infection among vaccinated chickens, China. *Emerg. Infect. Dis.* 20: 2152–2154.

Maas, R., Rosema, S., Van, Z.D., and Venema, S. (2011). Maternal immunity against avian influenza H5N1 in chickens: limited protection and interference with vaccine efficacy. *Avian Pathol.* 40: 87–92.

Marangon, S., Capua, I., Pozza, G., and Santucci, U. (2004). Field experiences in the control of avian influenza outbreaks in densely populated poultry areas. *Dev. Biol. (Basel)* 119: 155–164.

McLaws, M., Priyono, W., Bett, B. et al. (2014). Antibody response and risk factors for seropositivity in backyard poultry following mass vaccination against highly pathogenic avian influenza and Newcastle disease in Indonesia. *Epidemiol. Infect.* 143: 1632–1642.

Middleton, D., Bingham, J., Selleck, P. et al. (2007). Efficacy of inactivated vaccines against H5N1 avian influenza infection in ducks. *Virology* 359: 66–71.

Nakaya, T., Cros, J., Park, M.S. et al. (2001). Recombinant Newcastle disease virus as a vaccine vector. *J. Virol.* 75: 11868–11873.

OFFLU. (2014). OFFLU technical meeting: Developing guidance on vaccines and vaccination against HPAI from lessons learned. 4–6 December 2013, Beijing, China. www.offlu.net/fileadmin/home/en/meeting-reports/pdf/OFFLU_Beijing_2013/OFFLU_Recommendations_Beijing_Dec_2013_final.pdf

OIE. (2007). Avian influenza vaccination: OIE information document and Verona recommendations. www.oie.int/eng/info_ev/Other%20Files/A_Guidelines%20on%20AI%20vaccination.pdf

OIE (2015). 2.3.4. Avian Influenza. In: *Manual of Diagnostic Tests and Vaccines for Terrestrial Animals*. Paris: World Organization for Animal Health.

OIE (2017). 10.4. Infection with avian influenza viruses. In: *Terrestrial Animal Health Code*. Paris: World Organization for Animal Health www.oie.int/index.php?id=169&L=0&htmfile=chapitre_avian_influenza_viruses.htm

Oliveira, C.M., Vaughn, E., Capua, I. et al. (2017). A genetically engineered H5 protein expressed in insect cells confers protection against different clades of H5N1 highly pathogenic avian influenza viruses in chickens. *Avian Pathol.* 46: 224–233.

Pan, Z., Zhang, X., Geng, S. et al. (2009). Priming with a DNA vaccine delivered by attenuated *Salmonella typhimurium* and boosting with a killed vaccine confers protection of chickens against infection with the H9 subtype of avian influenza virus. *Vaccine* 27: 1018–1023.

Pantin-Jackwood, M.J., Suarez, D.L., Spackman, E., and Swayne, D.E. (2007). Age at infection affects the pathogenicity of Asian highly pathogenic avian influenza H5N1 viruses in ducks. *Virus Res.* 130: 151–161.

Pantin-Jackwood, M., Swayne, D.E., Smith, D., and Shepherd, E. (2013). Effect of species, breed and route of virus inoculation on the pathogenicity of H5N1 highly pathogenic influenza (HPAI) viruses in domestic ducks. *Vet. Res.* 44: e62.

Park, M.S., Steel, J., Garcia-Sastre, A. et al. (2006). Engineered viral vaccine constructs with dual specificity: avian influenza and Newcastle disease. *Proc. Natl. Acad. Sci. U.S.A.* 103: 8203–8208.

Park, J.K., Lee, D.H., Cho, C.H. et al. (2014). Supplementation of oil-based inactivated H9N2 vaccine with M2e antigen enhances resistance against heterologous H9N2 avian influenza virus infection. *Vet. Microbiol.* 169 (3–4): 211–217.

Pavade, G., Awada, L., Hamilton, K., and Swayne, D.E. (2011). Analysis of economic indicators, poultry density and performance of veterinary services for control of high pathogenicity avian influenza in poultry. *Rev. Sci. Tech. Off. Int. Epiz.* 30: 661–671.

Pavlova, S.P., Veits, J., Mettenleiter, T.C., and Fuchs, W. (2009). Live vaccination with an H5-hemagglutinin-expressing infectious laryngotracheitis virus recombinant protects chickens against different highly pathogenic avian influenza viruses of the H5 subtype. *Vaccine* 27: 5085–5090.

Peyre, M., Samaha, H., Makonnen, Y.B. et al. (2009). Avian influenza vaccination in Egypt: limitations of the current strategy. *J. Mol. Genet. Med.* 3: 198–204.

Philippa Joost, D.W., Munster, V.J., Bolhuis, H.v. et al. (2005). Highly pathogenic avian influenza (H7N7): vaccination of zoo birds and transmission to non-poultry species. *Vaccine* 23: 5743–5750.

Pu, J., Wang, S., Yin, Y. et al. (2014). Evolution of the H9N2 influenza genotype that facilitated the genesis of the novel H7N9 virus. *Proc. Natl. Acad. Sci. U.S.A.* 112 (2): 548–553.

Rao, S., Kong, W.P., Wei, C.-J. et al. (2008). Multivalent HA DNA vaccination protects against highly pathogenic H5N1 avian influenza infection in chickens and mice. *PLoS One* 3: e2432.

Rauw, F., Palya, V., Van, B.S. et al. (2011). Further evidence of antigenic drift and protective efficacy afforded by a recombinant HVT-H5 vaccine against challenge with two antigenically divergent Egyptian clade 2.2.1 HPAI H5N1 strains. *Vaccine* 29: 2590–2600.

Rauw, F., Palya, V., Gardin, Y. et al. (2012). Efficacy of rHVT-AI vector vaccine in broilers with passive immunity against challenge with two antigenically divergent Egyptian clade 2.2.1 HPAI H5N1 strains. *Avian Dis.* 56: 913–922.

Rauw, F., Van, B.S., Welby, S. et al. (2015). Quantification of rHVT-F genome load in feather follicles by specific real-time qPCR as an indicator of NDV-specific humoral immunity induced by day-old vaccination in SPF chickens. *Avian Pathol.* 44: 154–161.

Richard-Mazet, A., Goutebroze, S., Le Gros, F.X. et al. (2014). Immunogenicity and efficacy of fowlpox-vectored and inactivated avian influenza vaccines alone or in a prime-boost schedule in chickens with maternal antibodies. *Vet. Res.* 45: e107.

Rudolf, M., Poppel, M., Frohlich, A. et al. (2009). Efficacy of a commercial inactivated H5 influenza vaccine against highly pathogenic avian influenza H5N1 in waterfowl evaluated under field conditions. *Rev. Sci. Tech. Off. Int. Epiz.* 28: 275–291.

Sá e Silva, M. and Swayne, D.E. (2012). Serum and egg yolk antibody detection in chickens infected with low pathogenicity avian influenza virus. *Avian Dis.* 56: 601–604.

Sakoda, Y., Ito, H., Uchida, Y. et al. (2012). Reintroduction of H5N1 highly pathogenic avian influenza virus by migratory water birds, causing poultry outbreaks in the 2010-2011 winter season in Japan. *J. Gen. Virol.* 93: 541–550.

Schickli, J.H., Flandorfer, A., Nakaya, T. et al. (2001). Plasmid-only rescue of influenza A virus vaccine candidates. *Philos. Trans. R. Soc. London B Biol. Sci.* 356: 1965–1973.

Schultz-Cherry, S., Dybing, J.K., Davis, N.L. et al. (2000). Influenza virus (A/HK/156/97) hemagglutinin expressed by an alphavirus replicon system protects chickens against lethal infection with Hong Kong-origin H5N1 viruses. *Virology* 278: 55–59.

Seo, S.H. and Webster, R.G. (2001). Cross-reactive, cell-mediated immunity and protection of chickens from lethal H5N1 influenza virus infection in Hong Kong poultry markets. *J. Virol.* 75: 2516–2525.

Shi, J., Deng, G., Ma, S. et al. (2018). Rapid evolution of H7N9 highly pathogenic viruses that emerged in China in 2017. *Cell Host Microbe*: 24, 558–568. https://doi.org/10.1016/j.chom.2018.08.006

Si, L., Xu, H., Zhou, X. et al. (2016). Generation of influenza A viruses as live but replication-incompetent virus vaccines. *Science* 354: 1170–1173.

Sims, L. and Dung, D.H. (2009). Vaccination of poultry in Vietnam against H5N1 highly pathogenic avian influenza. 1–50. Montmorency, Australia, Asia Pacific Veterinary Information Services Pty Ltd.

Sims, L.D., Tripodi, A., von Dobschuetz, S., Gardner, E., and Aguanno, R. (2016). Rational use of vaccination for prevention and control of H5 highly pathogenic avian influenza. *FOCUS ON* 10:1–12. Rome, FAO. www.fao.org/3/a-i5625e.pdf

Singh, S.M., Alkie, T.N., Nagy, E. et al. (2016). Delivery of an inactivated avian influenza virus vaccine adjuvanted with poly(D,L-lactic-co-glycolic acid) encapsulated CpG ODN induces protective immune responses in chickens. *Vaccine* 34: 4807–4813.

Soejoedono, R.D., Murtini, S., Palya, V. et al. (2012). Efficacy of a recombinant HVT-H5 vaccine against challenge with two genetically divergent Indonesian HPAI H5N1 strains. *Avian Dis.* 56: 923–927.

Spackman, E. and Pantin-Jackwood, M.J. (2014). Practical aspects of vaccination of poultry against avian influenza virus. *Vet. J.* 202: 408–415.

Spackman, E. and Swayne, D.E. (2013). Vaccination of gallinaceous poultry for H5N1 highly pathogenic avian influenza: current questions and new technology. *Virus Res.* 178: 121–132.

Spackman, E., Swayne, D.E., Pantin-Jackwood, M.J. et al. (2014). Variation in protection of four divergent avian influenza virus vaccine seed strains against eight clade 2.2.1 and 2.2.1.1. Egyptian H5N1 high pathogenicity variants in poultry. *Influenza Other Respir. Viruses* 8: 654–662.

Steensels, M., Bublot, M., van Borm, S. et al. (2009). Prime-boost vaccination with a fowlpox vector and an inactivated avian influenza vaccine is highly immunogenic in Pekin ducks challenged with Asian H5N1 HPAI. *Vaccine* 27: 646–654.

Suarez, D.L. and Schultz-Cherry, S. (2000). The effect of eukaryotic expression vectors and adjuvants on DNA vaccines in chickens using an avian influenza model. *Avian Dis.* 44: 861–868.

Swayne, D.E. (2006). Principles for vaccine protection in chickens and domestic waterfowl against avian influenza: emphasis on Asian H5N1 high pathogenicity avian influenza. *Ann. N.Y. Acad. Sci.* 1081: 174–181.

Swayne, D.E. (2012a). Impact of vaccines and vaccination on global control of avian influenza. *Avian Dis.* 56: 818–828.

Swayne, D.E. (2012b). The role of vaccines and vaccination in high pathogenicity avian influenza control and eradication. *Expert. Rev. Vaccines* 11: 877–880.

Swayne, D.E. (2016). The global nature of avian influenza. In: *Animal Influenza* (ed. D.E. Swayne), 177–201. Ames: Wiley.

Swayne, D.E. and Akey, B. (2005). Avian influenza control strategies in the United States of America. In: *Avian Influenza. Prevention and Control* (eds. R.S. Schrijver and G. Koch), 113–130. Dordrecht: Springer.

Swayne, D.E. and Kapczynski, D.R. (2008). Vaccines, vaccination and immunology for avian influenza viruses in poultry. In: *Avian Influenza* (ed. D.E. Swayne), 407–451. Ames: Blackwell Publishing.

Swayne, D.E. and Spackman, E. (2013). Current status and future needs in diagnostics and vaccines for high pathogenicity avian influenza. *Dev. Biol. (Basel)* 135: 79–94.

Swayne, D.E., Beck, J.R., Garcia, M., and Stone, H.D. (1999). Influence of virus strain and antigen mass on efficacy of H5 avian influenza inactivated vaccines. *Avian Pathol.* 28: 245–255.

Swayne, D.E., Beck, J.R., and Kinney, N. (2000a). Failure of a recombinant fowl poxvirus vaccine containing an avian influenza hemagglutinin gene to provide consistent protection against influenza in chickens preimmunized with a fowl pox vaccine. *Avian Dis.* 44: 132–137.

Swayne, D.E., Garcia, M., Beck, J.R. et al. (2000b). Protection against diverse highly pathogenic H5 avian influenza viruses in chickens immunized with a recombinant fowlpox vaccine containing an H5 avian influenza hemagglutinin gene insert. *Vaccine* 18: 1088–1095.

Swayne, D.E., Pavade, G., Hamilton, K. et al. (2011). Assessment of national strategies for control of high-pathogenicity avian influenza and low-pathogenicity notifiable avian influenza in poultry, with emphasis on vaccines and vaccination. *Rev. Sci. Tech. Off. Int. Epiz.* 30: 839–870.

Swayne, D.E., Spackman, E., and Pantin-Jackwood, M. (2013). Success factors for avian influenza vaccine use in poultry and potential impact at the wild bird-agricultural interface. *EcoHealth* 11: 94–108.

Swayne, D.E., Suarez, D.L., and Sims, L.D. (2020). Influenza. In: *Diseases of Poultry* (eds. D.E. Swayne, M. Boulianne, C. Logue, et al.), 210–256. Ames: Wiley.

Swayne, D.E., Suarez, D.L., Spackman, E. et al. (2015). Antibody titer has positive predictive value for vaccine protection against challenge with natural antigenic-drift variants of H5N1 high-pathogenicity avian influenza viruses from Indonesia. *J. Virol.* 89: 3746–3762.

Sylte, M.J., Hubby, B., and Suarez, D.L. (2007). Influenza neuraminidase antibodies provide partial protection for chickens against high pathogenic avian influenza infection. *Vaccine* 25: 3763–3772.

Taylor, J., Weinberg, R., Kawaoka, Y. et al. (1988). Protective immunity against avian influenza induced by a fowlpox virus recombinant. *Vaccine* 6: 504–508.

Utterback, W.W. and Schwartz, J.H. (1973). Epizootiology of velogenic viscerotropic Newcastle disease in Southern California, 1971-1973. *J. Am.Vet. Med. Assoc.* 163: 1080–1088.

van den Berg, T., Lambrecht, B., Marche, S. et al. (2008). Influenza vaccines and vaccination strategies in birds. *Comp. Immunol. Microbiol. Infect. Dis.* 31: 121–165.

Vander Veen, R.L., Mogler, M.A., Russell, B.J. et al. (2013). Haemagglutinin and nucleoprotein replicon particle vaccination of swine protects against the pandemic H1N1 2009 virus. *Vet. Rec.* 173: 344.

Veits, J., Luschow, D., Kindermann, K. et al. (2003). Deletion of the non-essential UL0 gene of infectious laryngotracheitis (ILT) virus leads to attenuation in chickens, and UL0 mutants expressing influenza virus haemagglutinin (H7) protect against ILT and fowl plague. *J. Gen. Virol.* 84: 3343–3352.

Wang, L., Suarez, D.L., Pantin-Jackwood, M. et al. (2008). Characterization of influenza virus variants with different sizes of the non-structural (NS) genes and their potential as a live influenza vaccine in poultry. *Vaccine* 26: 3580–3586.

Webster, R.G., Kawaoka, Y., Taylor, J. et al. (1991). Efficacy of nucleoprotein and haemagglutinin antigens expressed in fowlpox virus as vaccine for influenza in chickens. *Vaccine* 9: 303–308.

WHO. (2011). Cumulative number of confirmed human cases for avian influenza A (H5N1) reported to WHO, 2003–2011. www.who.int/influenza/human_animal_interface/EN_GIP_20110819CumulativeNumberH5N1casesN.pdf?ua=1

Zhang, X., Liu, M. Liu, C. et al. (2011). Vaccination with different M2e epitope densities confers partial protection against H5N1 influenza A virus challenge in chickens. *Intervirology* 54: 290–299.

Zhang, W., Tu, J., Zhao, Z. et al. (2012a). The new temperature-sensitive mutation PA-F35S for developing recombinant avian live attenuated H5N1 influenza vaccine. *Virol. J* 9: e97.

Zhang, Y., Yin, Y., Bi, Y. et al. (2012b). Molecular and antigenic characterization of H9N2 avian influenza virus isolates from chicken flocks between 1998 and 2007 in China. *Vet. Microbiol.* 156: 285–293.

Zhang, X., Chen, S., Jiang, Y. et al. (2014). Hemagglutinin glycosylation modulates the pathogenicity and antigenicity of the H5N1 avian influenza virus. *Vet. Microbiol.* 175: 244–256.

19

Rift Valley Fever

Baptiste Dungu[1] *and Michèle Bouloy*[2]

[1] *Onderstepoort Biologicazl Products SOC Ltd., Onderstepoort, South Africa*
[2] *Department of Virology, Institut Pasteur, Paris, France*

19.1 Introduction

A disease resembling Rift Valley fever (RVF) and affecting sheep was first described by Montgommery in Kenya in 1912–1913 but it was in 1930 that RVF was formally identified, during a major outbreak in a farm near Lake Naivasha in Kenya (Daubney and Hudson 1931). The virus responsible for this outbreak was isolated from blood and liver of infected sheep and called Rift Valley fever virus (RVFV). It was characterized as an arbovirus of the genus *Phlebovirus* of the family *Bunyaviridae* (Elliott and Schmaljohn 2013). In the new taxonomy, RVFV is now classified as a phlebovirus of the *Phenuiviridae* family in the Bunyavirales order (Adams et al. 2017). Until 1977, RVF appeared to affect principally ruminants, sheep being the most sensitive.

The first human fatalities directly attributable to RVFV infection were reported in South Africa in 1975 (van Velden et al. 1977). It was in 1977 that a major epidemic occurred in Egypt where 20000–200000 humans were infected, causing approximately 600 human deaths (Meegan 1979). Since then, RVF has been considered a major zoonosis (Pepin et al. 2010; Ikegami 2012; Lihoradova and Ikegami 2012; Kortekaas 2014).

Sheep, cattle, and goats are very susceptible to RVF, very young animals being the most susceptible, with almost 100% mortality rates (Swanepoel and Coetzer 2004). While adult ruminants can show subclinical or transient febrile illness, infected newborn animals die of acute hepatitis. A high rate of abortion and fetal malformation of sheep is observed almost systematically during RVF outbreaks. In humans, RVF is generally asymptomatic or develops into a mild febrile illness but in 1–2% of the cases, it can progress into a more severe disease, such as acute hepatitis, encephalitis or neurological disorders, retinitis or uveitis, which may lead to blindness and a hemorrhagic syndrome (Meegan 1979; Bird and Nichol 2012).

The virus is endemic to sub-Saharan Africa and more recently it extended its territory to the Middle East and some islands in the Indian Ocean. Beside the countries linked to the Great Rift Valley formation, which stretch from the Red Sea through East Africa to Madagascar, serious outbreaks of RVF have occurred in Egypt, Mauritania, and Senegal. Some of the major outbreaks are listed in Table 19.1. Importantly, the virus extended its territory in 2000, causing a major outbreak in Saudi Arabia and Yemen. Countries at risk include those neighboring the affected regions such as the Middle East, Europe, and North Africa. The disease is also considered to be a threat worldwide because RVFV now features on most lists of potential biological warfare agents due to its severe zoonotic nature.

The virus is transmitted by mosquitoes. More than 30 species of mosquitoes are potentially involved in RVFV transmission, the main vectors belonging to the *Aedes* and *Culex* genera (Swanepoel and Coetzer 2004; Turell et al. 2008). Ideal conditions for emergence of RVFV-infected mosquitoes occur after flooding caused by unusually heavy rains. Infected mosquitoes transmit the virus to the vertebrate hosts through their saliva when they bite. The female can also transmit the virus transovarially. During epidemics, RVFV-infected ruminants can transmit the virus to healthy animals. Transmission to humans through contact with infected animal tissues and blood appears to be a common means of infection (Gerdes 2004). This is attested by the number of human cases among butchers, veterinarians, and shepherds who contaminate themselves via

This chapter is dedicated to the memory of our friend Richard Elliott, a great scientist who was a pioneer in the field of bunyaviruses.

Veterinary Vaccines: Principles and Applications, First Edition. Edited by Samia Metwally, Gerrit Viljoen, and Ahmed El Idrissi.

Table 19.1 List of the principal RVF epizootics.

Date	Place	Reported deaths in
1930	Kenya	Sheep
1950–1951	Kenya	Sheep
1975	South Africa	Sheep, cattle, humans
1977	Egypt	Humans
1987	Mauritania, Senegal	Humans, sheep
1991, 1996–1997	Egypt	Humans, sheep
1997–1998	Kenya, Somalia, Tanzania	Humans, sheep
1998–1999	Mauritania, Senegal	Humans, sheep
2000–2001	Saudi Arabia, Yemen	Humans, sheep
2007–2008	Sudan	Humans, sheep
2008–2010	South Africa	Humans, sheep, cattle
2010	Mauritania	Humans, sheep, cattle
2010	South Africa	Humans, sheep
2010	Madagascar	Humans, sheep

abrasions of the skin, or through mucosal membranes of the respiratory tract. For this reason, it is highly recommended to veterinarians to wear gloves, gowns, and facemasks. In some cases, it has been suggested that humans become infected after consumption of raw milk; this needs to be confirmed (Mohamed et al. 2010; LaBeaud et al. 2011).

19.2 Properties of RVFV Proteins and Rationale for the Design of Safe Vaccines

The RVFV is enveloped and spherical with a diameter of 80–120 nm. Like all members of the family, it possesses a single-stranded tripartite RNA genome composed of three segments: large (L), medium (M), and small (S) (Figure 19.1) (Elliott and Schmaljohn 2013). The L segment codes for the RNA-dependent RNA polymerase L protein; the M segment codes for a single polypeptide, which is the precursor to the Gn and Gc envelope glycoproteins, after being cleaved co-translationally. The alternative use of several in-frame initiation codons gives rise to precursors generating Gn and Gc and at least two nonstructural proteins called NSm and P78, respectively 14 and 78 kDa proteins. The glycoproteins Gn and Gc form heterodimers arranged in an icosahedral lattice with T = 12 symmetry. The S segment utilizes an

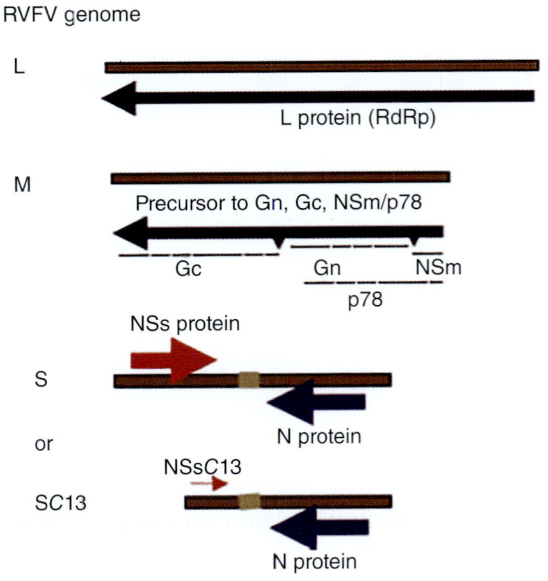

Figure 19.1 Schematic representation of the L, M, and S segments of the RVFV genome. The S segment of the attenuated Clone 13 is also represented.

ambisense strategy and codes for the N nucleoprotein in the antigenomic orientation and the nonstructural NSs protein in the genomic orientation.

Among the RVFV proteins, the glycoproteins play an essential role in protection. This was determined based on early studies of passive transfer of serum or antibodies which indicated that the viral glycoproteins induce specific antibodies neutralizing the virus and protecting from RVFV challenge. Hence, provision of these proteins is required in the design of RVFV vaccines (inactivated, live attenuated, live attenuated nonspreading particle or subunit vaccine).

The NSs protein has been studied extensively and was shown to have multiple functions, which together lead to suppression of the host immune responses and act as a potent virulence factor. Because of this critical role, it became obvious that the new live attenuated RVF vaccines should lack the NSs protein, as in the natural isolate Clone 13, which carries a large deletion of 70% in the NSs gene (Figure 19.1), and viruses obtained by reverse genetics. More recently, progress has been made in understanding the role of the NSm protein which was also shown to be implicated in virulence. The properties of the two proteins will be briefly described in the following paragraphs.

19.2.1 The NSs Protein

Most wild strains of RVFV express a nonstructural NSs protein, which is considered to be one of the main factors responsible for RVFV pathogenesis. The main functions of NSs identified so far are summarized in Figure 19.2.

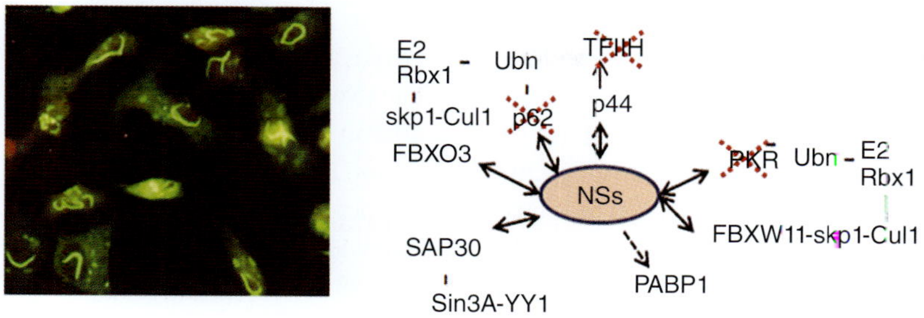

Figure 19.2 (a) Vero cells infected with a virulent strain of RVFV (ZH5). Staining with antibodies against NSs allows visualization of the protein in the cytoplasm, as well as in the nucleus, where it forms filamentous structures. (b) Representation of the NSs protein interacting with different partners and leading to proteasomal degradation of PKR and p62 or interference with the assembly of TFIIH. PABP1 was not found to interact with NSs.

Although this virus replicates in the cytoplasm, NSs is the only viral protein present in the nucleus of the host cell where it forms filamentous structures (Yadani et al. 1999) interacting with several cellular proteins and causing various effects responsible for RVFV pathogenicity. The interaction of NSs with the TFIIH (transcription factor IIH), and the general transcription factor subunits p44 and p62 leads to the sequestration of p44 within the nuclear NSs filaments and the degradation of p62 (Le May et al. 2004; Kalveram et al. 2011). These interactions are responsible for the general inhibition of cell transcription that is associated with viral infection. To destroy p62, NSs recruits the E3 ubiquitin ligase FBXO3, which results in suppression of the transcriptional upregulation of innate immunity (Kainulainen et al. 2014). RVFV NSs leads also to the sequestration of PABP1 in the nuclear speckles, creating a state within the cell that favors viral protein production (Copeland et al. 2013). NSs also downregulates protein kinase PKR posttranscriptionally, inducing its specific degradation through the proteasome pathway (Habjan et al. 2009; Ikegami et al. 2009; Kalveram et al. 2013). This is carried out by assembling NSs and PKR to the E3 ligase complex (Madhasani et al. 2016).

NSs also interacts with the cellular co-repressor SAP30 (Sin3A-associated protein, 30 kDa) via a region mapped within amino acids 210–230. A mutant RVFV with a deletion of the SAP30 interacting domain was created and was not able to interact with the interferon-β promoter, which led to the conclusion that SAP30–NSs interaction is responsible for the inhibition of interferon-β gene expression (Le May et al. 2008). However, other possible mechanisms for interferon-β suppression should be considered (Head et al. 2012; Kainulainen et al. 2014).

Through SAP30, NSs interacts with pericentromeric chromosomal sequences causing chromosomal segregation defects (Mansuroglu et al. 2009). In addition to these interactions, it was shown, using a genome-wide chromatin immunoprecipitation combined with promoter sequence microarray (ChIP-on-chip) approach, that NSs targets a wide range of host DNA regions which belong to cellular pathways that are closely related to RVFV-induced disorders, such as cell adhesion, axonal guidance, development, and coagulation (Benferhat et al. 2012).

19.2.2 The NSm Proteins

Five AUG codons are present in the NSm coding sequence of the RVFV M segment (Elliott and Schmaljohn 2013). These AUG codons are alternatively used to produce the two major structural glycoproteins Gn and Gc and at least two accessory proteins, NSm and P78, the latter consisting of a fusion between the NSm and Gn proteins. A third nonstructural NSm', a 13 kDa protein initiated at AUG 3, was also detected; it corresponds to a slightly truncated, functionally active form of NSm (Won et al. 2006; Kreher et al. 2014).

Mutant viruses with deletion of the entire NSm region and lacking expression of both NSm and P78 have been shown to be highly attenuated in rats and to be defective for virus spread in mosquitoes (Bird et al. 2011; Crabtree et al. 2012; Kading et al. 2014). Other mutant viruses, in which one or several of the AUG codons in the NSm region were knocked out, were used to show that NSm is a virulence factor in the mouse model, while P78 does not seem to have any detectable effect (Kreher et al. 2014). Strikingly, NSm has only a limited effect in the mosquito vector, whereas P78, in which NSm remains fused to Gn and associates with virus particles, critically influences RVFV dissemination in the invertebrate host.

The NSm nonstructural protein as well as its substitute NSm' is specifically transported to the surface of mitochondria (Won et al. 2007; Terasaki et al. 2013). The antiapoptotic activity of NSm requires its proper mitochondrial localization to be effective, and this activity lies within the

45 C-terminal amino acids of the protein. The association of NSm with mitochondria may also be important in regulating the cellular p38 MAPK response whose activation is triggered by increased levels of ROS (Narayanan et al. 2011).

19.3 Licensed Veterinary Vaccines

It is worth recalling that there is only one serotype of RVFV and that genome sequence analysis has revealed a high level of conservation among strains, which is a good indication that only one vaccine is needed to protect against the circulating strains of RVFV.

To date, there are three commercially available vaccines: the inactivated RVF vaccine, produced in South Africa and Egypt, the live attenuated vaccine, based on the Smithburn virus strain, produced in South Africa and Kenya, and the more recently registered RVF Clone 13, produced by Onderstepoort Biological Products (OBP) in South Africa and by MCI Santé Animale in Morocco (summarized in Table 19.2). This vaccine is more likely to become the vaccine of choice until such time that a vaccine with additional attributes such as compatibility with sero-DIVA is available.

19.3.1 Live Attenuated RVF Smithburn Vaccine

The live RVF vaccines most commonly produced and used are based on the Smithburn virus derived from the Entebbe strain isolated from mosquitoes in western Uganda in 1944 and passaged 79–85 times by intracerebral inoculation of mice. This resulted in the loss of hepatotropism, the acquisition of neurotropism, and the capacity to immunize sheep safely when administered parenterally (Smithburn 1949). The South African RVF Smithburn vaccine is based on the 103rd mouse brain passage level of the virus, while Kenya uses the 106th passage level to produce a vaccine. In both cases, the vaccines are grown in anchored baby hamster kidney cell culture systems. The two major producers of the live RVF Smithburn vaccine, OBP in South Africa and the Kenya Veterinary Vaccines Production Institute (KEVEVAPI), have produced millions of doses since 1952 and 1960 respectively, with the vaccine having been widely used throughout Africa and the Middle East (Swanepoel and Coetzer 2004).

However, the live attenuated RVF Smithburn vaccines have several disadvantages: they may induce abortions, malformations in the fetuses of vaccinated animals, hydrops amnii, and prolonged gestation in a significant proportion of vaccinated dams. Their use during an outbreak is not advised as they are based on a live virus (see section 19.4). Another reported problem with this vaccine is the poor antibody response in vaccinated cattle (Barnard 1979).

19.3.2 Inactivated RVF Vaccine

To address the problems associated with the residual virulence of the Smithburn vaccine, as well as the poor antibody response in vaccinated cattle, an inactivated vaccine has been used since the 1970s in South Africa. The vaccine is a formalin-inactivated virulent strain of RVFV formulated in aluminum hydroxide gel as adjuvant for the prophylactic immunization of cattle, sheep, and goats. It can be used in all livestock species, at different physiological stages, including pregnancy, and during outbreaks. This inactivated RVF vaccine makes it possible to vaccinate cows that can then confer colostral immunity to their offspring. However, due to the poor immunogenicity of this vaccine in cattle, it requires a booster 3–6 months after initial vaccination, followed by annual inoculations (Barnard 1979). The need for booster doses, and therefore two

Table 19.2 RVF vaccines manufactured in Africa.

Manufacturer	Country	Name and strain	Vaccine type	Country of registration and distribution
Onderstepoort Biological Products	South Africa	Smithburn	Live	South Africa, Namibia
		RVF inactivated vaccine	Killed	South Africa
		RVF Clone 13	Live	South Africa
Veterinary Serum and Vaccine Research Institute	Egypt	Smithburn	Live	Egypt
		RVF inactivated vaccine Zagazig H501	Killed	Egypt
KEVEVAPI	Kenya	Riftvax Smithburn	Live	Kenya
MCI Santé Animale	Morocco	RVF Clone 13	Live	Morocco

Disclaimer: It was the authors' intention to list all vaccine producers and are not responsible for the safety, quality, and effectiveness of the vaccines listed in the table.

vaccination campaigns within 6 months, discourages several African countries from using this vaccine, due to high overall associated costs and logistical challenges.

Inactivated RVF vaccines are currently produced in Egypt and in South Africa. Other inactivated vaccines for human use have been developed but will not be discussed in this chapter.

19.3.3 RVF Clone 13

Since 2010, a new vaccine called RVF Clone 13 has been registered by OBP in South Africa and used in South Africa, Botswana, Namibia, Zambia, and Mozambique (Kortekaas et al. 2014). It is based on an avirulent RVF virus isolated from a nonfatal case of RVF in the Central African Republic that had been passaged in mice and Vero cells, and then plaque purified in order to study the homogeneity of virus subpopulations. The clone designated Clone 13 did not react with NSs-specific monoclonal antibodies as it carries a deletion of 70% in the NSs gene. The resulting protein NSs_{C13} is truncated and unstable, being degraded rapidly by the proteasomal pathway (Muller et al. 1995) (Figure 19.1). When further investigated, it was found to be avirulent in mice, yet immunogenic (Muller et al. 1995; Vialat et al. 2000). This vaccine has been evaluated for safety and efficacy in sheep (Dungu et al. 2010) and cattle (von Teichman et al. 2011). More than 10 million RVF Clone 13 vaccine doses were used during the 2009–2010 RVF outbreak in South Africa and vaccination played a key role in the control of the disease (OBP, personal communication).

Two field trials were recently conducted with Clone 13, one in Kenya, with various commercial livestock farms (404 animals: 168 sheep, 151 goats, and 85 cattle) (Njenga et al. 2015), and the other in Senegal (Lo et al. 2015). In these studies, Clone 13 was administered according to the manufacturer's instructions and was found to be well tolerated in African breeds and safe to use in pregnant livestock. It was also highly immunogenic in sheep and goats and antibody levels persisted up to 1 year after vaccination. A moderate immunogenicity was observed in cattle in Kenya.

To anticipate a possible future incursion of RVFV in Europe, the safety of Clone 13 was assessed according to the guidelines from the World Animal Health Organization (OIE) and the regulations of the European Pharmacopoeia (EP) (Makoschey et al. 2016). To conform to these regulations, all the tests were performed with a 10–100-fold overdose of vaccine and European breeds of sheep. This study confirmed that Clone 13 can be applied safely in young lambs: it did not spread to the environment or contact lambs even after multiple administrations of an overdose via different inoculation routes and it did not revert to virulence upon animal-to-animal passage. However, overdose vaccination to gestating ewes resulted in virus transmission to the fetus, malformations, and stillbirths (Makoschey et al. 2016). These data indicate that vaccination with Clone 13 is safe and efficacious in lambs and sheep and that the recommended dose should be carefully controlled for pregnant ewes.

Altogether, the RVF Clone 13 vaccine is certainly a very relevant option for use in Africa. There are currently two manufacturers of the RVF Clone 13 vaccine: OBP in South Africa and MCI Santé Animale in Morocco, which has a thermo-tolerant version of the vaccine (Daouam et al. 2014, 2015).

The absence of the nonstructural protein NSs in new RVF vaccines potentially enables differentiation between infected and vaccinated animals (DIVA). Tests have been developed to detect antibodies against NSs in infected animals (McElroy et al. 2009; Fernandez et al. 2012). Other serological or molecular assays will be needed.

19.4 Vaccination Strategies and Guidelines

The rapid development of countermeasures against RVFV is important to minimize the impact of the disease. Besides vaccines (and eventually antivirals, of which none has yet been demonstrated to be efficient), early detection of the virus and diagnosis of the disease represent important capabilities for a government to implement to prevent further spread of RVFV. Therefore, existing detection methods (serology and genome detection) should be rapidly available and eventually, new ones developed. Nowadays, RVFV serology is based on the detection of immunoglobulin M (IgM) and immunoglobulin G (IgG) for which assays have been developed (Paweska et al. 2005). The nucleoprotein N is the major antigen inducing an immune response. The presence of RVFV-specific IgM antibodies is important to reveal a recent infection (i.e. within 1 month) in animals or humans (Paweska et al. 2005). Rapid detection of viral RNA from viremic samples can be done by conventional or real-time polymerase chain reaction (RT-PCR) (Escadafal et al. 2013), loop-mediated isothermal amplification (LAMP) (Peyrefitte et al. 2008; Le Roux et al. 2009) or recombinase polymerase amplification (RPA) assay (Euler et al. 2012). Alternatively, if viral RNA cannot be well preserved, RVFV antigens can be detected by antigen-capture (or sandwich) enzyme-linked immunosorbent assay (ELISA) (Jansen van Vuren and Paweska 2009) or by immunohistochemistry for postmortem examination.

Because RVF outbreaks occur in irregular cycles, a number of countries do not implement vaccination between outbreaks. Nonetheless, vaccination of livestock during interepidemics or ahead of outbreaks is highly recommended in preventing RVFV infection and virus spread. Yearly vaccination, practiced in a limited number of countries, such as South Africa, would contribute to increased herd immunity.

When a live attenuated vaccine is used during outbreaks, an animal infected with a wild strain and vaccinated can generate reassortants between the vaccine and the circulating wild strains. Therefore, vaccination with live attenuated virus presents a risk to generate virulent reassortants. However, the problem can be minimized if the attenuated vaccine does not induce viremia in the vaccinated livestock, which has been demonstrated for Clone 13 (Makoschey et al. 2016). Theoretically, inactivated nonreplicating vaccines have been recommended as a good alternative during outbreaks. However, inactivated RVF vaccines were produced from virulent strains, which poses a permanent risk to the manufacturer and a failure to completely inactivate some batches would lead to the reintroduction of RVFV in livestock.

Two strategies have been considered for addressing the issue of vaccine availability and improved herd immunity: (i) a RVF vaccine bank (or strategic stock), and (ii) use of combination vaccines including RVF which would then rely on the regular vaccination of animals for the second, more commonly used vaccine, such as lumpy skin disease in cattle and sheep and goat pox in sheep and goats, in order to build immunity in vaccinated animals to RVF.

19.5 Next-Generation Vaccines

To date, in addition to the three RVF vaccines described above, currently registered and in use, several strategies have been employed to develop new vaccine candidates which are now at different stages of development. Most of these technologies were reviewed during the 2011 RVF meeting organized by the Food and Agriculture Organization (FAO) (FAO 2011; Kortekaas et al. 2014). Key challenges in developing new RVF vaccines include the following needs:

- Biosecurity level (BSL) 3–4 stables for virus and animal work, and associated laboratory capacity (for serology, virus isolation, virus titration). This challenge could be overcome if the new vaccines are proven safe enough to be handled at BSL2.
- Vaccinated personnel if animal challenge studies with a virulent virus have to be conducted, unless it is in a very high-containment facility that would allow working on animals without direct contact.
- An adequate and proven challenge model. Most efficacy studies in recent years have relied on demonstrating the ability of the vaccine to prevent abortion in vaccinated pregnant ewes challenged with a virulent RVF virus (Dungu et al. 2010). The use of the above challenge model requires the involvement of well-trained veterinarians and adequate equipment and facilities to conduct estrus synchronization and subsequent artificial insemination of the dams. Kortekaas et al. (2012) established other challenge models based on the ability of the vaccine to reduce or prevent viremia in vaccinated animals postchallenge.

One reality to date is that there is little interest or commercial incentive for vaccine manufacturers to develop, register, and produce a new RVF vaccine. Hence, very few of the very promising candidate vaccines have gone beyond the experimental proof of concept stage.

19.5.1 Attenuated Viruses

A live attenuated MP-12 thermosensitive vaccine was obtained from the wild-type ZH548 strain by serial mutagenesis (Caplen et al. 1985). MP-12 is considered as a conditional vaccine for veterinary use in the USA, as well as a potential vaccine candidate for human use (FAO 2011; Wilson et al. 2014). However, the NSs of MP-12 is fully functional to inhibit host cellular responses (Billecocq et al. 2008). For this reason, a reassortant in which NSs was defective was selected after co-infection of MP12 and Clone 13. This gave rise to R566, possessing the L and M segments of MP12 and the S segment of Clone 13, which was used to vaccinate mice and lambs. R566 provided partial protection against a virulent challenge, suggesting that the thermosensitive mutations attenuate the virus too extensively (Kortekaas et al. 2014). A similar virus rMP12-C13 type also lacking functional NSs was generated by a reverse genetics system (Ikegami et al. 2006).

Using the reverse genetics technology, several groups have produced nonpathogenic RVFV lacking NSs and NSm (Bird et al. 2011; Crabtree et al. 2012) as well as RVFV nonspreading particles whose genomes lack the NSs gene and the complete M genome segment, rendering the particles unable to spread autonomously (Kortekaas et al. 2011; Dodd et al. 2012). RVFV replicon particles induced high levels of neutralizing antibodies and cytokine and chemokine responses in mice (Kortekaas et al. 2011; Dodd et al. 2012). In other RVF viruses produced by reverse genetics, the genome consists of two segments, L and S, in which the NSs gene was replaced by the glycoprotein gene (Brennan et al. 2011). As a vaccine, this provided sterilizing immunity in lambs.

19.5.2 Subunit Vaccines

Based on data showing the importance of neutralizing antibodies against the glycoproteins for RVF protection, these proteins were expressed from vaccinia virus or baculovirus and their immunogenicity tested in animal models (Schmaljohn et al. 1989). More recently, a subunit vaccine based on the Gn ectodomain (Gn-e), which is the major target for neutralizing antibodies, was developed and found to induce neutralizing antibodies after a single vaccination in mice and lambs and to protect lambs from viremia, pyrexia, and clinical signs (de Boer et al. 2010; Kortekaas et al. 2012). Adenovirus and Newcastle disease virus vectors were also used to express RVFV glycoproteins (Holman et al. 2009; Kortekaas et al. 2010). Virus-like particle-based vaccines whose efficacies were demonstrated in rodent models were also developed in various laboratories (de Boer et al. 2010; Koukuntla et al. 2012).

Experimental DNA vaccines for the control of RVFV have been developed and tested in rodent models in several laboratories but the immunogenicity in sheep is relatively low (Lorenzo et al. 2010).

19.6 Desired Specifications and Requirements of RVF Vaccines

While there are safety and efficacy attributes expected in any RVF vaccine, certain requirements may vary depending upon whether the vaccine is destined for an endemic region or a previously free country or region with an RVF incursion. Box 19.1 summarizes some of the key preferred attributes of RVF vaccines in general, but also specific attributes for an endemic or a free region.

Irrespective of the intended use, it will be critical that the RVF vaccine complies with minimum quality standards described in the RVF chapter of the OIE Manual (OIE 2019). Preferably, the vaccine should have been registered with national regulatory authorities in the vaccinating country. However, in an emergency, veterinary authorities may issue special dispensation for importing a nonregistered RVF vaccine, which should comply with quality standards as described earlier. In Africa, there is the opportunity of requesting that the vaccine batches to be used undergo quality control testing at the Pan African Vaccine Center (PANVAC) (see Chapter 3).

During planning and while implementing a RVF vaccination campaign or program, it is critical to include a monitoring program which includes sero-monitoring, clinical assessment, and data management.

Box 19.1 Key preferred attributes of RVF vaccines

- **Generic characteristics**
  - **Safety**
    - Safe to produce
    - Safe for all physiological stages of animals
    - No residual virulence
    - No risk of introduction into the environment (shedding, persistence in animals, etc.)
    - No risk of spread to human or other species
  - **Efficacy**
    - Protection of all susceptible species
    - Quick onset of protective immunity, including in young animals
    - Long-lasting immunity
    - Stop transmission: prevent amplification of RVFV in ruminants
  - **Vaccination**
    - Cost-effective for producers and users
    - Single vaccination
    - Ease of application
    - Suitable for stockpiling (vaccine or antigen bank) and quick availability
- **Endemic regions**
  - Continuous vaccination: yearly vaccination of susceptible livestock
    - Need to know how many vaccinations may be required to build life-long immunity
    - Solid protective immunity after one vaccination
- **Free regions**
    - Quick onset of protective immunity
    - Protective in young animals and possibly newborn naïve animals
    - Sterilizing immunity
    - DIVA

19.7 Summary

Control of RVF through the use of vaccines and the design of suitable vaccination strategies remains very challenging in many affected countries due to the cyclical nature of the disease and the long interepidemic periods that have been noted in all endemic countries. In many cases, countries consider the use of vaccination only at first indication of an outbreak. Control strategies that promote the establishment of good herd immunity in the livestock population in endemic regions are more likely to reduce the devastating impact of severe outbreaks.

Novel vaccines should therefore help establish long-lasting herd immunity. Given the need to use such vaccines at large scale, they should be inexpensive and should provide efficient and long duration of immunity after a single vaccination. Vaccination should be safe regardless of the physiological state of the animal, especially during pregnancy. The possibility of needle-free delivery would be advantageous, especially when the absence of virus circulation cannot be definitely established and reuse of needles represents a risk for further dissemination. Novel vaccines that enable DIVA by use of an appropriate discriminatory assay would be beneficial. Finally, the development of safe veterinary vaccines should encourage and stimulate the development of human vaccines.

References

Adams, M.J., Lefkowitz, E.J., King, A.M.Q. et al. (2017). Changes to taxonomy and the international code of virus classification and nomenclature ratified by the international committee on taxonomy of viruses (2017). *Arch. Virol.* 162 (8): 2505–2538.

Barnard, B.J.H. (1979). Rift Valley fever vaccine – antibody and immune response in cattle to a live and an inactivated vaccine. *J. S. Afr. Vet. Assoc.* 50: 155–157.

Benferhat, R., Josse, T., Albaud, B. et al. (2012). Large-scale chromatin immunoprecipitation with promoter sequence microarray analysis of the interaction of the NSs protein of Rift Valley fever virus with regulatory DNA regions of the host genome. *J. Virol.* 86 (20): 11333–11344.

Billecocq, A., Gauliard, N., Le May, N. et al. (2008). RNA polymerase I-mediated expression of viral RNA for the rescue of infectious virulent and avirulent Rift Valley fever viruses. *Virology* 378 (2): 377–384.

Bird, B.H. and Nichol, S.T. (2012). Breaking the chain: Rift Valley fever virus control via livestock vaccination. *Curr. Opin. Virol.* 2: 315–323.

Bird, B.H., Maartens, L.H., Campbell, S. et al. (2011). Rift Valley fever virus vaccine lacking the NSs and NSm genes is safe, nonteratogenic, and confers protection from viremia, pyrexia, and abortion following challenge in adult and pregnant sheep. *J. Virol.* 85 (24): 12901–12909.

Brennan, B., Welch, S.R., McLees, A., and Elliott, R.M. (2011). Creation of a recombinant Rift Valley fever virus with a two-segmented genome. *J. Virol.* 85: 10310–10318.

Caplen, H., Peters, C.J., and Bishop, D.H.L. (1985). Mutagen-directed attenuation of Rift Valley fever virus as a method for vaccine development. *J. Gen. Virol.* 66 (Pt 10): 2271–2277.

Copeland, A.M., Altamura, L.A., van Deusen, N.M., and Schmaljohn, C.S. (2013). Nuclear relocalization of polyadenylate binding protein during Rift Valley fever virus infection involves expression of the NSs gene. *J. Virol.* 87 (21): 11659.

Crabtree, M.B., Kent Crockett, R.J., Bird, B.H. et al. (2012). Infection and transmission of Rift Valley fever viruses lacking the NSs and/or NSm genes in mosquitoes: potential role for NSm in mosquito infection. *PLoS Negl. Trop. Dis.* 6: e1639.

Daouam, S., Fakri, F.Z., Ennaji, M.M. et al. (2014). Heat stability of the Rift Valley fever virus clone 13 live vaccines. *Trials Vaccinol.* 3: 61–64.

Daouam, S.G.F., Arkam, A.E., Naouli, Y. et al. (2015). Evaluation of the safety and efficacy of a live attenuated thermostable Rift Valley fever vaccine in sheep, goats and cattle. *J. Vaccines Vaccin.* 6: 295.

Daubney, R. and Hudson, J.R. (1931). Enzootic hepatitis or Rift Valley fever. An undescribed disease of sheep, cattle and man from East Africa. *J. Path. Bact.* 34: 545–579.

de Boer, S.M., Kortekaas, J., Antonis, A.F. et al. (2010). Rift Valley fever virus subunit vaccines confer complete protection against a lethal virus challenge. *Vaccine* 28: 2330–2339.

Dodd, K.A., Bird, B.H., Metcalfe, M.G. et al. (2012). Single-dose immunization with virus replicon particles confers rapid robust protection against Rift Valley fever virus challenge. *J. Virol.* 86: 4204–4212.

Dungu, B., Louw, I., Lubisi, A. et al. (2010). Evaluation of the efficacy and safety of the Rift Valley fever clone 13 vaccine in sheep. *Vaccine* 28: 4581–4587.

Elliott, R.M. and Schmaljohn, C.S. (2013). Bunyaviridae. In: *Fields Virology* (eds. D.M. Knipe and P.M. Howley), 1244–1278. Philadelphia: Lippincott, Williams and Wilkins.

Escadafal, C., Paweska, J.T., Grobbelaar, A. et al. (2013). International external quality assessment of molecular detection of Rift Valley fever virus. *PLoS Negl.Trop. Dis.* 7 (5): e2244.

Euler, M., Wang, Y., Nentwich, O. et al. (2012). Recombinase polymerase amplification assay for rapid detection of Rift Valley fever virus. *J. Clin. Virol.* 54 (4): 308–312.

FAO (2011). Rift Valley fever vaccine development, progress and constraints. Proceedings of the GF-TADs meeting, January 2011, Rome, Italy. FAO Animal Production and Health Proceedings, No. 12. www.fao.org/3/i2310e/i2310e00.htm

Fernandez, J.C., Billecocq, A., Durand, J.P. et al. (2012). The nonstructural protein NSs induces a variable antibody response in domestic ruminants naturally infected with Rift Valley fever virus. *Clin. Vaccine Immunol.* 19 (1): 5–10.

Gerdes, G.H. (2004). Rift Valley fever. *Rev. Sci. Tech.* 23: 613–623.

Habjan, M., Pichlmair, A., Elliott, R.M. et al. (2009). NSs protein of rift valley fever virus induces the specific degradation of the double-stranded RNA-dependent protein kinase. *J. Virol.* 83 (9): 4365–4375.

Head, J.A., Kalveram, B., and Ikegami, T. (2012). Functional analysis of Rift Valley fever virus NSs encoding a partial truncation. *PLoS One* 7: e45730.

Holman, D.H., Penn-Nicholson, A., Wang, D. et al. (2009). A complex adenovirus-vectored vaccine against Rift Valley fever virus protects mice against lethal infection in the presence of preexisting vector immunity. *Clin. Vaccine Immunol.* 16 (11): 1624–1632.

Ikegami, T. (2012). Molecular biology and genetic diversity of Rift Valley fever virus. *Antiviral Res.* 95 (3): 293–310.

Ikegami, T., Won, S., Peters, C.J., and Makino, S. (2006). Rescue of infectious Rift Valley fever virus entirely from cDNA, analysis of virus lacking the NSs gene, and expression of a foreign gene. *J. Virol.* 80 (6): 2933–2940.

Ikegami, T., Narayanan, K., Won, S. et al. (2009). Rift Valley fever virus NSs protein promotes post-transcriptional downregulation of protein kinase PKR and inhibits eIF2alpha phosphorylation. *PLoS Pathog.* 5 (2): e1000287.

Jansen van Vuren, P. and Paweska, J.T. (2009). Laboratory safe detection of nucleocapsid protein of Rift Valley fever virus in human and animal specimens by a sandwich ELISA. *J. Virol. Methods.* 157 (1): 15–24.

Kading, R.C., Crabtree, M.B., Bird, B.H. et al. (2014). Deletion of the NSm virulence gene of Rift Valley fever virus inhibits virus replication in and dissemination from the midgut of Aedes aegypti mosquitoes. *PLoS Negl.Trop. Dis.* 8: e2670.

Kainulainen, M., Habjan, M., Hubel, P. et al. (2014). Virulence factor NSs of Rift Valley fever virus recruits the F-box protein FBXO3 to degrade subunit p62 of general transcription factor TFIIH. *J. Virol.* 88 (6): 3464.

Kalveram, B., Lihoradova, O., and Ikegami, T. (2011). NSs protein of Rift Valley fever virus promotes posttranslational downregulation of the TFIIH subunit p62. *J. Virol.* 85: 6234–6243.

Kalveram, B., Lihoradova, O., Indran, S.V. et al. (2013). Rift Valley fever virus NSs inhibits host transcription independently of the degradation of dsRNA-dependent protein kinase PKR. *Virology.* 435: 415–424.

Kortekaas, J. (2014). One Health approach to Rift Valley fever vaccine development. *Antiviral Res.* 106 (2014): 24–32.

Kortekaas, J., de Boer, S.M., Kant, J. et al. (2010). Rift Valley fever virus immunity provided by a paramyxovirus vaccine vector. *Vaccine* 28 (27): 4394–4401.

Kortekaas, J., Oreshkova, N., Cobos-Jimenez, V. et al. (2011). Creation of a nonspreading Rift Valley fever virus. *J. Virol.* 85: 12622–12630.

Kortekaas, J., Antonis, A.F., Kant, J. et al. (2012). Efficacy of three candidate Rift Valley fever vaccines in sheep. *Vaccine* 30 (23): 3423–3429.

Kortekaas, J., Zingese, J., Ksiasek, T., and Lubroth J. (2014). Report of the *ad hoc* workshop on the current state of Rift Valley fever vaccine and diagnostics development, 5–7 March 2014, Rome, Italy. www.fao.org/3/a-i4466e.pdf

Koukuntla, R., Mandell, R.B., and Flick, R. (2012). Virus-like particle-based countermeasures against Rift Valley fever virus. *Zoonoses Public Health* 59 (Suppl. 2): 142–150.

Kreher, F., Tamietti, C., Gommet, C. et al. (2014). The Rift Valley fever accessory proteins NSm and P78/NSm-GN are distinct determinants of virus propagation in vertebrate and invertebrate hosts. *Emerging Microbes Infect.* 3 (10): e71.

LaBeaud, A.D., Muiruri, S., Sutherland, L.J. et al. (2011). Postepidemic analysis of Rift Valley fever virus transmission in Northeastern Kenya: a village cohort study. *PLoS Negl.Trop. Dis.* 5: e1265.

Le May, N., Dubaele, S., Proietti de Santis, L. et al. (2004). TFIIH transcription factor, a target for the Rift Valley hemorrhagic fever virus. *Cell* 116 (4): 541–550.

Le May, N., Mansuroglu, Z., Léger, P. et al. (2008). A SAP30 complex inhibits IFN-beta expression in Rift Valley fever virus infected cells. *PLoS Pathog.* 4 (1): e13.

Le Roux, C.A., Kubo, T., Grobbelaar, A.A. et al. (2009). Development and evaluation of a real-time reverse transcription-loop-mediated isothermal amplification assay for rapid detection of Rift Valley fever virus in clinical specimens. *J. Clin. Microbiol.* 47 (3): 645–651.

Lihoradova, O. and Ikegami, T. (2012). Modifying the NSs gene to improve live-attenuated vaccine for Rift Valley fever. *Expert Rev. Vaccines* 11 (11): 1283–1285.

Lo, M.M., Mbao, V., Sierra, P. et al. (2015). Safety and immunogenicity of Onderstepoort Biological Products' Rift Valley fever clone 13 vaccine in sheep and goats under field conditions in Senegal. *Onderstepoort J. Vet. Res.* 82 (1): 857.

Lorenzo, G., Martin-Folgar, R., Hevia, E. et al. (2010). Protection against lethal Rift Valley fever virus (RVFV) infection in transgenic IFNAR(−/−) mice induced by different DNA vaccination regimens. *Vaccine* 28 (17): 2937–2944.

Madhasani, R., Tran, J.P., Retterer, C. et al. (2016). Protein kinase R degradation is essential for Rift Valley fever virus infection and is regulated by SKP1-CUL1-F-box (SCF) FBXW11-NSs E3 ligase. *PLoS Pathog.* 12 (2): e1005437.

Makoschey, B., van Kilsdonk, E., Hubers, W. et al. (2016). Rift Valley fever vaccine virus clone 13 is able to cross the ovine placental barrier associated with foetal infections, malformations, and stillbirths. *PloS Negl. Trop. Dis* 10 (3): e0004550.

Mansuroglu, Z., Josse, T., Gilleron, J. et al. (2009). Nonstructural NSs protein of rift valley fever virus interacts with pericentromeric DNA sequences of the host cell, inducing chromosome cohesion and segregation defects. *J. Virol.* 84: 928–939.

McElroy, A.K., Albarino, C.G., and Nichol, S.T. (2009). Development of a RVFV ELISA that can distinguish infected from vaccinated animals. *Virol. J.* 6: 125.

Meegan, J.M. (1979). The Rift Valley fever epizootic in Egypt 1977–78. *Trans. R. Soc. Trop. Med. Hyg.* 73 (6): 618–623.

Mohamed, M., Mosha, F., Mghamba, J. et al. (2010). Epidemiologic and clinical aspects of a Rift Valley fever outbreak in humans in Tanzania, 2007. *Am. J. Trop. Med. Hyg.* 83 (2 Suppl): 22–27.

Muller, R., Saluzzo, J.F., Lopez, N. et al. (1995). Characterization of clone 13, a naturally attenuated avirulent isolate of Rift Valley fever virus, which is altered in the small segment. *Am. J. Trop. Med. Hyg.* 53: 405–411.

Narayanan, A., Popova, T., Turell, M. et al. (2011). Alteration in superoxide dismutase 1 causes oxidative stress and p38 MAPK activation following RVFV infection. *PLoS One* 6: e20354.

Njenga, M.K., Njagi, L., Thumbi, S.M. et al. (2015). Randomized controlled field trial to assess the immunogenicity and safety of Rift Valley fever clone 13 vaccine in livestock. *PLoS Negl.Trop. Dis.* 9 (3): e0003550.

OIE. (2019). Manual of Diagnostic Tests and Vaccines for Terrestrial Animals. www.oie.int/en/international-standard-setting/terrestrial-manual/access-online

Paweska, J.T., Burt, F.J., and Swanepoel, R. (2005). Validation of IgG-sandwich and IgM-capture ELISA for the detection of antibody to Rift Valley fever virus in humans. *J. Virol. Methods* 124 (1–2): 173–181.

Pepin, M., Bouloy, M., Bird, B.H. et al. (2010). Rift Valley fever virus (Bunyaviridae: Phlebovirus): an update on pathogenesis, molecular epidemiology, vectors, diagnostics, and prevention. *Vet. Res.* 41 (6): 61.

Peyrefitte, C.N., Boubis, L., Coudrier, D. et al. (2008). Real-time reverse-transcription loop-mediated isothermal amplification for rapid detection of Rift Valley fever virus. *J. Clin. Microbiol.* 46 (11): 3653–3659.

Schmaljohn, C.S., Parker, M.D., Ennis, W.H. et al. (1989). Baculovirus expression of the M genome segment of Rift Valley fever virus and examination of antigenic and immunogenic properties of the expressed proteins. *Virology* 170: 184–192.

Smithburn, K.C. (1949). Rift Valley fever; the neurotropic adaptation of the virus and the experimental use of this modified virus as a vaccine. *Br. J. Exp. Pathol.* 30 (1): 1–16.

Swanepoel, R. and Coetzer, J.A.W. (2004). Rift Valley fever. In: *Infectious Diseases of Livestock with Special Reference to Southern Africa*, 2e (eds. J.A.W. Coetzer and R.C. Tustin), 1037–1070. South Africa: Oxford University Press.

Terasaki, K., Won, S., and Makino, S. (2013). The C-terminal region of Rift Valley fever virus NSm protein targets the protein to the mitochondrial outer membrane and exerts antiapoptotic function. *J. Virol.* 87: 676–682.

Turell, M.J., Linthicum, K.J., Patrican, L.A. et al. (2008). Vector competence of selected African mosquito (Diptera: Culicidae) species for Rift Valley fever virus. *J. Med. Entomol.* 45: 102–108.

van Velden, D.J., Meyer, J.D., Olivier, J. et al. (1977). Rift Valley fever affecting humans in South Africa: a clinicopathological study. *S. Afr. Med. J.* 51 (24): 867–871.

Vialat, P., Billecocq, A., Kohl, A., and Bouloy, M. (2000). The S segment of rift valley fever phlebovirus (Bunyaviridae) carries determinants for attenuation and virulence in mice. *J. Virol.* 74: 1538–1543.

von Teichman, B., Engelbrecht, A., Zulu, G. et al. (2011). Safety and efficacy of Rift Valley fever Smithburn and clone 13 vaccines in calves. *Vaccine* 29: 5771–5777.

Wilson, W.C., Bawa, B., Drolet, B.S. et al. (2014). Evaluation of lamb and calf responses to Rift Valley fever MP-12 vaccination. *Vet. Microbiol.* 172 (1–2): 44–50.

Won, S., Ikegami, T., Peters, C.J., and Makino, S. (2006). NSm and 78-kilodalton proteins of Rift Valley fever virus are nonessential for viral replication in cell culture. *J. Virol.* 80 (16): 8274–8278.

Won, S., Ikegami, T., Peters, C.J., and Makino, S. (2007). NSm protein of Rift Valley fever virus suppresses virus-induced apoptosis. *J. Virol.* 81: 13335–13345.

Yadani, F.Z., Kohl, A., Prehaud, C. et al. (1999). The carboxy-terminal acidic domain of Rift Valley fever virus NSs protein is essential for the formation of filamentous structures but not for the nuclear localization of the protein. *J. Virol.* 73 (6): 5018–5025.

20

Bluetongue

Giovanni Savini[1], Piet van Rijn[4], Karin Darpel[3], Alessio Lorusso[1], Carrie Batten[3], Pascal Hudelet[6], Stéphan Zientara[5], and James MacLachlan[2]

[1] *Istituto Zooprofilattico Sperimentale dell'Abruzzo e del Molise "G. Caporale", Teramo, Italy*
[2] *School of Veterinary Medicine, University of California, Davis, California, USA*
[3] *The Pirbright Institute, Woking, Surrey, UK*
[4] *Department of Virology, Central Veterinary of Wageningen University Research Center (CVI), Lelystad, The Netherlands*
[5] *ANSES Laboratoire de Santé Animale, Maisons-Alfort, France*
[6] *Veterinary Public Health Technical Services, Merial, France*

20.1 Introduction

Bluetongue virus (BTV) continues to surprise the scientific community and requires constant adaptation of previous assumed knowledge. In the last few years, new BTV serotypes and new potential vectors have been identified, an additional nonstructural viral protein has been characterized, and the capability of some field strains/serotypes of the virus to be transmitted either vertically or horizontally, to alter their pathogenicity, host specificity, and capacity for spread was revealed. In other words, the virus is able to change and adapt to new environments and episystems. Furthermore, some serotypes/strains of BTV can cause severe clinical disease, affecting different animal species and resulting in significant losses, whereas other infections are entirely asymptomatic with minimal or insignificant economic impact.

Reassortment of viral genes between field strains, vaccine strains, and between field and vaccine strains of BTV have generated and will continue to generate novel virus genotypes. The potential for these progeny strains to be transmitted more effectively and to have increased virulence poses significant additional risks for ruminant health. Although it is an aspect still poorly understood and which requires further investigation, it is clear that the threat of exotic virus topotypes should not be underestimated and that an evaluation of their ability to cause severe clinical disease in endemic episystems is increasingly necessary.

Evolutionary dynamics and selection pressure drive the emergence of new BTV strains and, possibly, serotypes; meanwhile, the advent of improved diagnostic technology and surveillance systems has facilitated their identification. Several new virus serotypes (BTV-25, -26, -27, -28, -29, and perhaps -30) have been identified since 2008, three of them just in 2015. These viruses have novel properties, emphasizing the urgent need to characterize their biology and significance. Thus, the continued evolution of BTV strains poses a substantial challenge to the research and regulatory communities, rendering this virus extremely difficult to control.

Vaccination has the strategic role of controlling and preventing BTV infection of susceptible animals. Strategies devoted to inhibit virus replication and control their spread among hosts and vectors need to cope with these extremely heterogeneous populations. Because little or no cross-protection occurs between different serotypes of the virus, a variety of different viral antigenic types are used in vaccines. Multivalent vaccines containing two or more antigenic types are used in an attempt to provide broader protection.

This chapter deals with various aspects of the biology and potential control of BTV infection with particular reference to evolving trends in vaccines and vaccination strategies that might be used to control this economically important disease.

20.2 History and Epidemiology

Bluetongue (BT) is an arthropod-transmitted viral disease of ruminants, especially sheep (MacLachlan et al. 2009, 2015). The disease was first described in South Africa and probably existed there long before sheep farming was

Veterinary Vaccines: Principles and Applications, First Edition. Edited by Samia Metwally, Gerrit Viljoen, and Ahmed El Idrissi.

initiated (Henning 1956). The first comprehensive descriptions of the disease were published around the turn of the twentieth century (Hutcheon 1902; Spreull 1905; Theiler 1906). Spreull (1905) introduced the name "bluetongue," which is the English translation of the Afrikaans name for the disease of "*Blaauwtong*." Sir Arnold Theiler, in 1906, first showed that BT was caused by a filterable virus (Henning 1956), and he also introduced the first widely used BT vaccine that incorporated a virus strain attenuated by serial passages in sheep. This monovalent vaccine was used between 1907 and 1943, when its use was discontinued after it became clear that it did not confer immunity against the many other BTV serotypes that circulated in South Africa (Henning 1956).

The identification of *Culicoides* midges as the insect vector of BTV and African horse sickness virus is attributed to du Toit (1944). Until approximately 1950, it was thought that bluetongue was confined to Africa, the Middle East (Israel), and Mediterranean islands such as Cyprus, but the disease was then described in the USA (Hardy and Price 1952; McKercher et al. 1953). An extensive epizootic also occurred on the Iberian Peninsula in 1956–1957. It was clearly demonstrated during the second half of the twentieth century that BTV is present throughout tropical and temperate regions of the world, frequently in the absence of disease (Gibbs and Greiner 1994; MacLachlan and Osburn 2006).

To date, BTV has been isolated from ruminants and vector insects from all continents except Antarctica (MacLachlan and Mayo 2013; MacLachlan et al. 2015). Hematophagous *Culicoides* insects are biological vectors that transmit BTV from infected to susceptible ruminants and, because BTV infection of ruminants is not contagious (with the notable exception of recently identified small ruminant-associated BTVs, such as Toggenburg orbivirus [serotype 25], and serotypes 26 and 27), the global distribution of BTV coincides with the distribution of competent *Culicoides* insect vectors and warm or hot climatic conditions. With the exception of transient incursions of single virus serotypes into the Iberian peninsula and Mediterranean islands, Europe was historically free of BTV until 1998 when multiple serotypes invaded and became established in portions of the continent. Similarly, serotypes of BTV once confined to the Caribbean Islands have recently invaded North America and in 2015, for the first time, evidence of BTV infection of livestock was detected in Ontario, Canada.

It is increasingly evident that BTV exists in distinct ecosystems in different regions of the world and specific virus strains have likely co-evolved with different species of the insect vector. It is also increasingly clear that BTV infection of domestic and wild ruminants occurs throughout much of the world with minimal development of disease, but aspects of the epidemiology of BTV infection remain poorly defined (MacLachlan et al. 2015). Whereas BTV may be transmitted year-round in tropical and subtropical areas of the world, infection is seasonal in temperate areas. Recent studies clearly show that BTV can overwinter in temperate areas in adult midges that survive during the colder months (Mayo et al. 2014, 2016; Steyn et al. 2016). Viremia is transient in BTV-infected livestock and persistent infection does not occur with most BTV serotypes (MacLachlan et al. 2009, 2015), the notable exception being BTV serotype 25 (Toggenburg orbivirus; Vögtlin et al. 2013).

Although over 1000 species of *Culicoides* are known worldwide, relatively few of these species have been incriminated as vectors of BTV (Meiswinkel et al. 2007). Species of vector insects that transmit BTV differ among regions, and are especially poorly characterized in the portions of Asia that are devoid of *Culicoides imicola* (*C. imicola*), the traditional African-Asian vector of BTV (Tabachnick 2004; Jafari-Shoorijeh et al. 2010; MacLachlan 2010). BTV has also spread rapidly throughout extensive portions of Europe where *C. imicola* does not occur, utilizing apparently new vector species, including Palaearctic species such as *Culicoides obsoletus* sensu *strictu*, *C. pulicaris*, *C. dewulfi*, *C. scoticus*, and *C. chiopterus* (Caracappa et al. 2003; Savini et al. 2005; Meiswinkel et al. 2007; Dijkstra et al. 2008; Wilson and Mellor 2009; Conraths et al. 2009; Kampen and Werner 2010). These insects were all resident in Europe long before the recent emergence of multiple BTV serotypes, suggesting that environmental changes may have been responsible for their recent ability to serve as efficient vectors of the virus (Purse et al. 2005, 2008).

20.3 Costs and Trade Implications

Because of the severe economic consequences that it can cause in epidemic situations, BT is included in the list of notifiable diseases by the World Organization for Animal Health (OIE 2016). A notifiable disease is any disease that has to be reported by law to government authorities. A global estimate of the impact of bluetongue was US$ 3 billion (Bath 1989). Analyses on recent BTV-8 incursions in Europe in 2007 revealed economic costs, at national level, ranging from US$ 85 million to 1.4 billion (Tabachnick et al. 2008; Velthuis et al. 2010). Although in endemic settings the incursion of a virulent strain may still cause significant disease, as frequently seen in South India (Chand et al. 2015), the impact of BT in endemic situations generally appears to be relatively small, with infertility and vaccination being significant costs.

Restrictive, nontariff trade barriers have been instituted by some BTV-free countries, justified in part by uncertainties regarding the epidemiology of BTV infection and the putative role of persistently infected (carrier) cattle in the perceived global dissemination of BTV. Thus, although the direct economic impact of bluetongue is often minimal in endemic settings or following the incursion of low-virulent virus strains, and the concept of persistent infection of livestock is now rejected, nontariff trade barriers pertaining to bluetongue have caused substantial economic loss because of their adverse impact on animal movement and trade, particularly that of cattle and germplasm (MacLachlan and Osburn 2006). In other words, in certain scenarios the reaction to the disease may be more damaging than the direct production losses caused by the disease (Rushton and Lyons 2015).

20.4 Vaccines

Bluetongue vaccines are divided into nonreplicating and replicating vaccines. Nonreplicating BT vaccines can be subdivided based on inactivation of infectious BTV, and subunit vaccines consisting of one or more BTV proteins produced by a variety of expression systems. Replicating BT vaccines can be subdivided into vector vaccines expressing one or more BTV proteins and virus vaccines based on live attenuated or genetically modified BTV.

Inactivated, whole-virus and live attenuated virus vaccines (LAVs) are the only nonreplicating and replicating BT vaccines available in the market.

20.4.1 Live Attenuated BT Vaccines

The first generation of commercial bluetongue vaccines were LAVs. They were developed more than a century ago at Onderstepoort Veterinary Institute, South Africa. A field strain of BTV serotype 4 was passaged a limited number of times in sheep and used as a LAV for more than 40 years. Currently used LAVs have been generated by over 50 serial passages in embryonated chicken eggs and subsequently in tissue cultures of BHK_{21} cells (Dungu et al. 2004a). For most of the twentieth century, use of these vaccines was restricted mainly to southern and northern Africa, India, the Middle and Far East, and North America, and intended to limit clinical disease. South African vaccines contain, in total, 15 serotypes divided in three pentavalent vaccines serially injected with intervals of 3–4 weeks, resulting in broad cross-protection against the multiplicity of BTV serotypes endemic to the region (Dungu et al. 2004b).

In North America, similar, live attenuated vaccines for prevailing serotypes were developed and used in sheep and captive cervids since the 1950s.

In the late 1990s, the BTV incursion in southern Europe led briefly to the use of South African LAV in Italy, Corsica, and Spain (Zientara and Sanchez-Vizcaino 2013; Pérez de Diego et al. 2014). These vaccines typically elicit a strong antibody response, which is directly correlated with their ability to replicate in the vaccinated host. LAVs are inexpensive and capable of stimulating protective immunity after a single inoculation. They have proven to be effective in preventing clinical BT disease in the areas where they are used (Caporale et al. 2004; Patta et al. 2004; Savini et al. 2008). Although these LAVs have not been registered for use in cattle, vaccine formulations containing LAVs for serotypes 2, 4, 9, and 16 have been used in cattle in southern Europe and the Middle East, showing few adverse reactions (Savini et al. 2008). LAVs were used in India until 2015, followed by the introduction of inactivated vaccines (Ranjan et al. 2015).

A variety of documented or potential drawbacks are, however, attributed to BT LAVs. These include underattenuation, which may result in disease expression that varies among sheep of different breeds (BTV-16) (Breard et al. 2004; Savini et al. 2008). Adverse responses to LAV vaccination can include depressed milk production in lactating sheep, temporary infertility in rams and ewes, and abortion/embryonic death and teratogenesis in offspring when these vaccines are used in pregnant females (Savini et al. 2008). Besides, LAVs often induce viremia with a virus titer sufficient for LAV spread by midges (Monaco et al. 2004; Savini et al. 2004a; Veronesi et al. 2005; Monaco et al. 2006). Indeed, local transmission of LAVs for serotype 2 and 16 has been demonstrated (Ferrari et al. 2005; Savini et al. 2005). Furthermore, spread and uncontrolled replication of LAVs have led to virulent BTV variants through reversion to virulence or reassortment with field virus (Ferrari et al. 2005; Veronesi et al. 2005; Batten et al. 2008; Savini et al. 2012). Although instances of vaccine virus reassortment have been documented in Europe, the frequency and significance of these events remain uncertain. Natural dissemination of LAV strains is also probably responsible for the sporadic incidence of teratogenic defects in unvaccinated cattle in South Africa and North America (Savini et al. 2008).

Despite the risk and shortcomings of LAVs, these types of vaccines are used in many BT-endemic parts of the world since they are effective and cheap, whereas the adverse reactions are limited in local breeds (Bhanuprakash et al. 2009; McVey and MacLachlan 2015). On the other hand, LAV is not the preferred vaccine when eradication is the ultimate goal, due to uncontrolled spread of vaccine virus and incompatibility with differential detection of infected animals in the vaccinated population (Savini et al. 2008).

Live attenuated vaccines for serotypes other than BTV-1, -2, -4, -9, and -16 have never been approved in Europe. In 2008, evidence of circulation in Belgium, the Netherlands, and Germany of BTV serotypes 6 and 11, and most recently the circulation of BTV serotype 14 in Lithuania, Latvia, Poland, and Spain, being strains most likely derived from LAVs (de Clercq et al. 2009; Eschbaumer et al. 2009b; van Rijn et al. 2012; Nomikou et al. 2013), showed that illegal use of LAVs can lead to virus spread by midges in moderate climates.

20.4.2 Inactivated Vaccines

Inactivated BT vaccines were developed in the 1970s and 1980s, but remained experimental at that time (Parker et al. 1975; Stott et al. 1985; Stevens et al. 1985; Campbell et al. 1985). The emergence of several BTV serotypes in Europe reactivated this approach and inactivated BT vaccines were licensed and became the preferred type of vaccine in Europe. Inactivated vaccines were produced at industrial scale for several but limited serotypes. For most of these, details of production, formulation, and adjuvant have not been published but field data show convincing records of rarely seen adverse reactions and high levels of protection against clinical signs and viremia.

The first inactivated vaccine used in the field after the emergence of BT in Europe was the vaccine against BTV-2. Subsequently, inactivated monovalent BTV-4 and bivalent BTV-2 and -4 vaccines were developed and used in Corsica, Spain, Portugal, and Italy (Zientara et al. 2010). Inactivated products were then developed and commercialized for BTV-9, -1, and -8. All of the most recent European BT vaccination campaigns have exclusively used inactivated vaccines, in part owing to fears that some field viruses may be related to LAVs (Zientara et al. 2010).

Inactivated whole-virus vaccines are very safe although mild, transitory, and painless local reaction at the site of injection as well as slight fever have sometimes been reported after vaccination. If produced properly, these vaccines can be highly efficacious. Their inherent potential disadvantages include high costs of production, as vaccination requires large amounts of antigen, and the need for booster immunizations as inactivated vaccines generally induce a relatively transient immunity. Most companies producing BTV inactivated whole-virus vaccines follow the guidelines of the European Pharmacopoeia and Committee for Veterinary Medicines Products. Clinical, immunological, and virological data documenting the efficacy of these vaccines are required by the European Medicine Agency (Zientara et al. 2010).

20.4.3 Registered BT Vaccines

Live attenuated vaccines were the first generation of commercial BT vaccines. Safety considerations led to the development of safer, inactivated vaccines against the serotypes relevant to the European outbreak situation. The first commercial BT vaccine of the second generation (i.e. inactivated vaccines) was introduced by Merial in Italy in 2003, under temporary Authorization of Use (Savini et al. 2008). Several European manufacturers introduced other inactivated vaccines in Europe under the same regulatory framework: temporary authorizations of use, conditional licences, or registrations under exceptional circumstances. These temporary authorizations were later converted into full marketing authorizations (Saegerman et al. 2007; Savini et al. 2008).

Registration in Europe follows the strict regulatory guidelines set by the European Pharmacopoeia and the Committee for Medicinal Products for Veterinary Use (CVMP). Production must follow European Good Manufacturing Practices (EU-GMP).

Vaccines of the next generation (see section 20.5) have proven to be safe and effective under experimental conditions, and have the potential to address some of the weaknesses of inactivated vaccines, like compatibility with postvaccination serosurveillance for infection, rapid onset of immunity, and cross-serotype protection. However, development and registration of a new vaccine represents a major R&D investment, and would be justified financially for a manufacturer only by a significant advantage over existing inactivated vaccines. As of 2020, none has been registered and made available commercially (Table 20.1).

20.4.4 Costs and Sustainability

The cost of a vaccination campaign with inactivated vaccines is a major issue. For example, Pinior et al. (2015) have evaluated the costs of the national BTV surveillance and vaccination programs between 2005 and 2013, before, during, and after the BTV-8 outbreak in Austria commencing in 2008. The total net cost of the BTV-8 surveillance and vaccination programs arising from the outbreak amounted to €22.8 million (0.86% of the national agricultural Gross Value Added), of which 32% was allocated to surveillance and 68% to the vaccination program. Of the total program costs, the EC supplied €4.9 million, while the remaining costs (€18 million) were directly financed from national resources. Of the latter, €14.5 million was classed as public costs, including €2 million contributions in kind, and €3.4 million as private costs. The assessment of the costs revealed heterogeneous temporal and spatial distributions.

Table 20.1 Vaccines by country of registration (at time of publication).

Company	Product name	Serotype	Vaccine type[a]	Adjuvant	Countries where licensed	Indications
Vaccines licensed for use in Europe						
Bioveta	BioBos BTV8	8	I	Aluminum hydroxide, saponin	Czech Republic	Cattle, sheep
CZ Veterinaria	BLUEVAC BTV8	8	I	Aluminum hydroxide, saponin	EU	Cattle, sheep
CZ Veterinaria	BLUEVAC-1	1	I	Aluminum hydroxide, saponin	Spain, France	Cattle, sheep
CZ Veterinaria	BLUEVAC-4	4	I	Aluminum hydroxide, saponin	Spain	Cattle, sheep
Merial	BTVPUR AlSap	1, 8, 2, 4 + any combination of 2 of these strains[b]	I	Aluminum hydroxide, saponin	EU	Cattle, sheep
Merial	BTVPUR AlSap 9	9	I	Aluminum hydroxide, saponin	Italy	Cattle, sheep
MSD Animal Health	Bovilis BTV 8	8	I	Aluminum hydroxide, saponin	EU	Cattle, sheep
Syva	Syvazul-1	1	I	Aluminum hydroxide, saponin	EU	Cattle, sheep
Syva	Syvazul-1 + 8	1, 8	I	Aluminum hydroxide, saponin	Spain	Cattle, sheep
Syva	Syvazul-4	4	I	Aluminum hydroxide, saponin	Spain	Sheep
Syva	Syvazul-8	8	I	Aluminum hydroxide, saponin	Spain	Cattle, sheep
Zoetis	ZULVAC 1 + 8 Ovis	1 + 8	I	Aluminum hydroxide, saponin	EU	Sheep
Zoetis	ZULVAC 8 Ovis	8	I	Aluminum hydroxide, saponin	EU	Sheep
Zoetis	ZULVAC 8 Ovis	8	I	Aluminum hydroxide, saponin	EU	Cattle
Zoetis	ZULVAC 1 Ovis	1	I	Aluminum hydroxide, saponin	EU	Sheep
Zoetis	ZULVAC 1 Bovis	1	I	Aluminum hydroxide, saponin	EU	Cattle
Zoetis	ZULVAC 1 + 8 Bovis	1 + 8	I	Aluminum hydroxide, saponin	EU	Cattle
Zoetis	ZULVAC 4 Ovis	4	I	Aluminum hydroxide, saponin	Spain	Sheep
Vaccines licensed for use in India						
Biovet Private Limited	BioBT-Oil	1 + 2 + 10 + 16+ 23	I	Oil	India	Sheep and goats
Biovet Private Limited	BioBT-Gel	1 + 2 + 10 + 16+ 23	I	Aluminum hydroxide, saponin	India	Sheep and goats
Indian Imunologicals	Raksha Blu	1 + 2 + 10 + 16+ 23	I	Aluminum hydroxide, saponin	India	Sheep and goats
Vaccines licensed for use in China						
Yunnan Tropical and Subtropical Animal Virus Disease Laboratory	Bluetongue vaccine	1 + 16	LAV I	Unknown	China	Sheep and goats

(Continued)

Table 20.1 (Continued)

Company	Product name	Serotype	Vaccine type[a]	Adjuvant	Countries where licensed	Indications
Vaccines licensed for use in Morocco						
Biopharma	BTVAC	1 + 4	LAV		Morocco	Sheep and goats
MCI Santé Animale	OVIVAX BT1 + 4	1 + 4	LAV		Morocco	Sheep and goats
Vaccines licensed for use in Russia						
National Research Institute for Veterinary Virology and Microbiology of Russia	Bluetongue vaccine	1,6,8,4,9,16	I	Aluminum hydroxide, saponin	Russia	Sheep and goats
Vaccines licensed for use in South Africa						
Onderstepoort Biological Products	Bluetongue vaccine for sheep	A: 1 + 4 + 6 + 12 + 14 B: 3 + 8 + 9 + 10 + 11 C: 2 + 5 + 7 + 13 + 19	LAV		South Africa	Sheep
Vaccines licensed for use in Turkey						
Etlik Veterinary Control Central Research Institute	Blue-T4 ETVAC Mavi Dil Asisi	4	LAV		Turkey	Sheep
Vaccines licensed for use in the USA						
Colorado Serum Company	Bluetongue vaccine	10	LAV		USA	Sheep and goats
Newport Laboratories	Custom-made EHD + BTV vaccine	Autogenous EHD + BTV, serotypes on demand (EHD1 + 2 + 6 BTV17 + 3)	I, CM	Oil	USA	Cervids only
Poultry Health Laboratories (PHL)	BlueVac	10, 11, 17	LAV		California	Sheep

[a] CM, custom made; I, inactivated; LAV, modified live virus.
[b] BTVPUR was registered under the multistrain guideline that allows combinations of strains suited to the epidemiology.

Disclaimer: It was the authors' intention to list all vaccine producers and are not responsible for the safety, quality, and effectiveness of the vaccines listed in the table.

The assessment of contributions in kind is of importance to public authorities as it increases visibility of the available resources and shows how they have been employed. Similarly, the economic impact due to the cost and the management of animal vaccination for control and prevention of the disease using LAVs has been measured. In South Africa, approximately 7–8 million doses of the vaccine were sold per year (Grewar 2016) for an amount equal to approximately $2 million per year for farmers. Assuming a relatively stable sheep population in South Africa, this coverage amounts to approximately 25% of the population.

20.4.5 Quality Control Testing for BT Vaccines

Local requirements for product registration and quality control (QC) may vary from country to country depending on local needs, but the overall approach remains identical: to reach the required level of quality, manufacturers must implement an integrated system of quality assurance incorporating Good Manufacturing Practices (GMP), QC (tests carried out on raw materials, during production, and on final product) and quality risk management. These systems should be fully documented and their effectiveness monitored (OIE 2016; European Pharmacopoeia 2017).

Both vaccine producers and national regulatory authorities play a role in assuring the quality of licensed veterinary products. Vaccine manufacturers have the primary legal responsibility for the safety, quality, and efficacy of the products they produce and commercialize. National regulatory authorities are responsible for the approval of licence applications.

20.4.5.1 Quality Control of the Seed Lot System

Live attenuated vaccine master seed virus (MSV) is prepared from a single plaque of serially passaged, live attenuated BTV. Each MSV should be tested for transmissibility and reversion to virulence prior to vaccine manufacture. Samples of vaccine prepared from virus culture at the maximum permitted passage level should be tested in sheep for lack of residual virulence (including reversion to virulence), safety, and immunogenicity. There is no requirement to verify reversion to virulence with inactivated vaccine MSVs. Identity of the master seed lots should be adequately characterized. The serotype is usually confirmed through sequencing. MSV purity needs to be proven. MSV must be demonstrated free of contaminating bacteria, viruses, prions, fungi, and mycoplasmas. Whatever the virus propagating system, the method must be aseptic, controlled, and proven to be free from contaminating microorganisms.

20.4.5.2 Quality Control of Raw Materials

Each batch of raw materials entering the production process must be tested and quarantined until shown to meet specifications. Substances of animal origin, including serum and cells, must be checked for the presence of viable bacteria, viruses, fungi, or mycoplasma. Ingredients of animal origin should be sourced from a country with negligible risk for transmissible spongiform encephalopathies (TSEs).

20.4.5.3 In-Process Quality Controls

Infectious virus titration is used to monitor virus culture. The test is also used to quantify potency of LAVs. For BT inactivated vaccines, when the suspension reaches its maximum virus titer, the cells are disrupted and virus is harvested. Subsequently, inactivation is performed according to processes adopted by the manufacturer. The process must comply with legislation and be validated to ensure complete inactivation. Inactivation kinetics are controlled for every batch produced through regular sampling to measure for live virus by titration of infectivity. The inactivation process should not significantly alter the immunogenic properties of the antigens. For high-quality vaccines, the inactivated antigen may then undergo various downstream processes such as purification and/or concentration.

20.4.5.4 Finished Product Batch/Serial Control Tests for Release

Whatever the type of vaccine, a number of tests and controls are required on each vaccine batch before its release, to verify that the controls in place during production have been efficient and that the finished product meets the specifications agreed upon with the regulatory authority. Manufacturing practices should be such that every starting material and production step is appropriately documented to allow verification that the batch was indeed produced according to the outline of production declared by the manufacturer (OIE 2016). In addition, specific QC tests should be performed on each final product. These QC tests are performed on randomly selected vaccine vials of each batch and can be subdivided in three types:

1) QC testing on the vial itself: sterility, appearance (including volume per vial, color, etc.), pH and other measures.
2) Safety test: assessment of the safety of the batch, preferably in the target species.
3) Potency test: assessment of the strength of the batch:

   - for live attenuated vaccines, this usually consists of a virus titration on the finished product, which may be difficult with multivalent BT vaccines.

- for inactivated vaccines, this usually consists of a vaccination followed by a serotype-specific serological titration or by a challenge.

Once all quality documentation has been reviewed and all QC tests have been performed, and found to be within the product specifications, the vaccine batch can be released. The vaccine is then granted its shelf-life, as demonstrated in stability studies conducted during the development of the vaccine.

20.4.6 Possible Combination with Other Vaccines

Multivalent BTV inactivated or live attenuated vaccines are marketed by several companies. However, when LAVs are not given at the same visit, it is recommended to wait at least 3–4 weeks before giving other LAVs. For inactivated vaccines, there are no restrictions to simultaneously vaccinate animals with other vaccines. In North America, autogenous, inactivated vaccines are available. These are custom-made vaccines that contain herd-specific (homologous) antigens. They usually contain combinations of BTV and epizootic hemorrhagic disease virus antigens. Few published data are available for the evaluation of these products (McVey and MacLachlan 2015) and, in general, few studies have been published about combining the use of BTV vaccines with other vaccines.

20.4.7 Desired Specifications when Ordering Vaccines

The choice of vaccines to use depends on the strategy (and the budget dedicated to BTV control) put in place in the country or region where the vaccination has to be used. If the objective is to eradicate the virus, inactivated vaccines could be recommended. If the objective is to reduce the incidence of clinical signs, live vaccines can be used. However, when ordering vaccines, particular care should be taken to ensure that the product: (i) is registered and licensed in the country in accordance with national legislation (e.g. Regulation [EO] No. 726/2004 in the European Union (EU); https://ec.europa.eu/health/sites/health/files/files/eudralex/vol-1/reg_2004_726/reg_2004_726_en.pdf), (ii) is targeted against the serotype(s) circulating in the region, (iii) is able to prevent clinical signs and viremia due to bluetongue virus, (iv) is capable of providing immunity one year after its application, (v) has a shelf-life of at least 12 months, (vi) is applicable to cattle and sheep, (vii) is safe for use in all animal categories including young, pregnant, and lactating animals. In addition, the product leaflet for use should have text in the language of the country where vaccination is to be applied, and the age of first vaccination and revaccination should be clearly indicated, according to species and physiological status of the animals to be vaccinated.

20.4.8 Postvaccination Monitoring

Postvaccination monitoring should be put in place to check the quality of the vaccine-induced population immunity and the overall efficiency of the vaccination program. Showing the impact of a vaccination campaign on the disease is critical to justify the cost of vaccination and identify potential weaknesses in the program. It is assumed that vaccination will reduce the rate of spread of BTV if a sufficiently high coverage (>80%) is achieved (Patta et al. 2004; Szmaragd et al. 2010).

Although both humoral and cell-mediated immunities are involved, the most relevant indicator of protection is considered to be the antibody response and, particularly, the neutralizing antibody response. However, as no differentiation of infected from vaccinated animals (DIVA) products are commercially available, distinguishing immunity due to vaccination from that due to infection requires complementary polymerase chain reaction (PCR) testing for viremia to monitor the prevalence of BTV-infected animals in a population vaccinated with inactivated vaccines. In a dataset collected by the European Food Safety Authority (EFSA) containing 149 virological observations in cattle and sheep populations vaccinated with BTV inactivated vaccines, 43 were without any positive test result, and in the other 106, prevalences ranged from 0.00073 to 0.19, with a median value of 0.0065 (EFSA 2011). On the other hand, numerous BTV vaccination campaigns implemented in the last decades using either LAVs or inactivated products have been successful in controlling and, in some circumstances, eradicating the infection.

20.5 BT Vaccines in the Pipeline

Marketed vaccines are used successfully to reduce economic losses, but have particular or general shortcomings depending on the field situation (Feenstra and van Rijn 2017). Novel vaccine candidates with improved profiles are in the pipeline.

20.5.1 Nonreplicating Experimental BT Vaccines

To reduce the time necessary to initiate production of *inactivated whole-BTV vaccines* against emerging serotypes, serotype determining outer capsid proteins VP2 and VP5 can be exchanged in one virus backbone used for antigen production (Boyce et al. 2008; van Gennip et al. 2012a;

Nunes et al. 2014). This approach has been demonstrated for 16 serotypes including chimeric VP2 proteins, but has failed for other BTV serotypes (Nunes et al. 2014; Feenstra et al. 2015a). BTVs with exchanged serotype-specific proteins as well as those without dispensable NS3/NS3a protein can be processed similarly to previously produced inactivated whole-BTV vaccines (van Gennip et al. 2014). The latter will be DIVA compliant with NS3-based enzyme-linked immunosorbent assays (ELISAs) (Barros et al. 2009; Tacken et al. 2015).

All experimental *subunit vaccines* include the serotype-specific immunodominant VP2 protein. Several VP2 production systems have been studied to reduce costs per protective dose (Huismans 1985; Inumaru and Roy 1987, Urakawa et al. 1994, Athmaram et al. 2007), including those with immunostimulating complex-based adjuvant (Anderson et al. 2013, 2014), soluble fusion proteins (Mohd Jaafar et al. 2014; Legisa et al. 2015), and VP2 incorporation in MuNS microspheres (Brandariz-Nuñez et al. 2010; Marin-Lopez et al. 2014). VP2-based subunit vaccines lacking VP7 protein are DIVA vaccines compatible with the extensively validated and used ELISAs targeting serogroup-specific VP7 to detect BTV-infected animals.

Virus-like particles (VLPs) of BTV consisting of VP3, VP7, VP2, and VP5 have been generated in insect cells using baculovirus expression (French et al. 1990; Belyaev and Roy 1993; Stewart et al. 2010), and using the *Nicotiana benthamiana* plant and the cowpea mosaic virus based HyperTrans plant transient expression vector system (Rybicki 2010). VLP cocktails of several serotypes showed results varying from partial protection against some heterologous serotypes to interference in protective response against an included serotype (Roy et al. 1994; Roy 2004; Pérez de Diego et al. 2011). Despite all these efforts and promising results in huge sheep trials for more than 25 years, VLP-based vaccines have not been manufactured. Most likely, VLPs cannot compete with the currently marketed inactivated BT vaccines with regard to affordability.

VP2 subunit and VLP vaccines provide opportunities to improve the vaccine profile compared with licensed inactivated BT vaccines such as safer production and DIVA potential, because of the absence of one or more immunogenic virus proteins. The main drawback of these nonreplicating vaccine candidates is the high cost of production.

20.5.2 Replicating Experimental BT Vaccines

Vector-based vaccines only express desired BTV proteins. Consequently, vector vaccine candidates will not induce BT and have DIVA potential. Several viruses have been used for vector-based BT vaccines in experimental trials, such as canarypox virus (Boone et al. 2007), capripox viruses (Perrin et al. 2007), myxomavirus (Top et al. 2012), bovine herpes virus (Franceschi et al. 2011), and equine herpes virus (Ma et al. 2012). All these vector-based vaccines require booster vaccination, and complete protection was not achieved for most vaccine candidates. An obstacle for vector-based vaccines is preexisting immunity directed to vector-associated antigens, which could reduce their efficacy if the vector is used to successively vaccinate against different diseases or when annual revaccination is required (Ura et al. 2014).

Priming by *DNA vaccination followed by vaccination with vector-based vaccine* can partially overcome the disadvantage of preexisting immunity against the vector. However, delivery of DNA vaccines is not efficient and use on a global scale is therefore still limited (Grunwald and Ulbert 2015). This prime-boost strategy has been examined but most vaccine combinations have not been tested in the ruminant host yet (Calvo-Pinilla et al. 2009, 2012; Jabbar et al. 2013; Li et al. 2015). Although vector-based vaccines with or without DNA priming can support DIVA and safety, cost-effectiveness to control BT is questionable.

Bluetongue virus-based vaccine candidates have been developed by use of reverse genetics, enabling rescue of "synthetic" BTV indistinguishable from ancestor BTV (Boyce et al. 2008; van Gennip et al. 2012b). *Reassortants based on the vaccine platform of LAV* (BTV-6/net08; [Maan et al. 2010; van Rijn et al. 2012]) by exchange of serotype determining genome segments of serotype 8 completely protected against virulent BTV-8 (Maan et al. 2008), and a cocktail of three such "serotyped" BT vaccines induced neutralizing antibodies against all three serotypes (van Gennip et al. 2012a). Spontaneous reversion to virulence is still a potential risk, since fundamental knowledge of the attenuation of LAVs is largely missing, and therefore complete safety cannot be guaranteed.

In order to further increase safety of BTV-based vaccines, novel vaccine platforms have been developed and applied for several serotypes (van Gennip et al. 2012a; Nunes et al. 2014). Vaccination with *disabled infectious single cycle* (DISC) vaccine leads to an aborted virus replication cycle (Matsuo et al. 2011). Crude cell lysates of 10^8 PFU/animal DISC vaccine or cocktails of 10^8 PFU DISC vaccine/serotype/animal for up to seven serotypes completely protected sheep and cattle against clinical signs and viremia (Matsuo et al. 2011; Celma et al. 2013, 2017). This amount of virus is similar to that of inactivated whole-BTV vaccine. Necessarily, DISC vaccines must be manufactured in special cell lines expressing VP6 protein by *in trans* complementation. Because crude cell lysates of DISC vaccines induce antibodies against all immunogenic proteins, these have no DIVA potential.

The *disabled infectious single animal* (DISA) vaccine platform is based on LAV (BTV6/net08; [Maan et al. 2010; van Rijn et al. 2012]) with a deletion in segment 10 that lacks nonessential NS3/NS3a protein (Feenstra et al. 2014a; van Gennip et al. 2014). DISA vaccine has DIVA potential, since it is distinguishable from field BTV (van Rijn et al. 2013; Feenstra et al. 2014c). Experimental NS3-based ELISAs need further improvement and validation (Barros et al. 2009; Tacken et al. 2015). DISA vaccines are completely safe as they are not virulent, do not cause viremia (so no uptake by midges), and do not propagate in midges (Feenstra et al. 2014b,c, 2015a,b). Vaccination with 2×10^5 $TCID_{50}$ DISA vaccine resulted in rapid and complete serotype-specific protection (Feenstra et al. 2014b,c). The DISA vaccine platform has been applied for several serotypes, including for chimeric VP2 protein (Feenstra et al. 2015a). The protective dose in sheep is similar to that of LAVs but could be further reduced (van Rijn et al. 2017) by enhancing the interferon-mediated immune responses (Chauveau et al. 2013). DISA vaccine can be manufactured in established BT vaccine production systems.

As genetically modified organisms (GMOs) with segmented genomes, the safety of replicating DISC and DISA vaccine platforms needs special attention with regard to reassortment. Virulent variants cannot arise by reassortment within one vaccine platform, since all are attenuated by deficiency for VP6 or NS3/NS3a, respectively. Virulent variants are unlikely to arise by reassortment with field BTV, especially for the LAV-based DISA vaccine platform, since virulence is determined by many genome segments (Coetzee et al. 2014; Janowicz et al. 2015). Above all, a cell concomitantly infected by field BTV and vaccine virus is a prerequisite for reassortment events. The chance of this is negligible if there is no viremia and will be limited to animals infected by field BTV, shortly after vaccination with DISC or DISA vaccines.

20.6 Immune Response and Duration of Immunity

20.6.1 Immune Responses to BTV and BT Vaccines

Following infection with BTV, antibodies against all structural and nonstructural viral proteins can be detected in the serum of ruminants (Huismans and Erasmus 1981; Richards et al. 1988). The potential of BTV serum antibodies to confer serotype-restricted protection against BT was initially demonstrated in passive serum transfer and challenge experiments in sheep (Jeggo et al. 1984a). Neutralizing antibodies are the immune correlate believed to protect previously infected animals against reinfection with a BTV strain of the homologous serotype (Letchworth and Appleton 1983). Epitopes of neutralizing antibodies and serotype determination are localized in limited interactive domains of the outer coat protein VP2 (White and Eaton 1990; DeMaula et al. 2000) and sheep inoculated with purified VP2 were resistant to challenge with the same BTV serotype (Huismans et al. 1987).

Various epitopes eliciting neutralizing antibodies are highly conformation dependent and, at least for some BTV strains, it has been shown that VP5 can indirectly influence neutralization due to its conformational influence on VP2 (Cowley and Gorman 1989; DeMaula et al. 2000). The role of antibodies raised against the other BTV proteins in BTV immunity is still unknown, as further antibody-dependent mechanisms, such as any involvement in direct or complement-facilitated cell-mediated cytotoxicity, has so far not been clearly demonstrated (Jeggo et al. 1983a). Most vaccines against BTV are therefore designed and validated for their potential to induce neutralizing antibodies. Nonetheless, although the detection of neutralizing antibody at the time of challenge generally correlates well with protection against that serotype, it has also been reported that animals can still be protected in the absence of detectable neutralizing antibodies (Savini et al. 2004b; Oura et al. 2009).

Immunity in the absence of detectable neutralizing antibodies might depend on other immune mechanisms, such as cell-mediated immune (CMI) responses and immune priming to more quickly and effectively respond to challenge infection. BTV-specific cytotoxic T cells (CTLs) have been demonstrated in infected and/or vaccinated mice and sheep, but CMI responses in ruminants to BTV remain poorly characterized (Jeggo and Wardley 1982; Janardhana et al. 1999). Although $CD8^+$ cytotoxic T lymphocytes were proposed as the most likely protective candidate (Jeggo et al. 1984b, 1985), T cell dependency of the antibody response to BTV infection and/or vaccination in ruminants is largely undefined and it is currently unknown if T cell-independent antibody responses exist for BTV as shown for other viral infections of ruminants (Juleff et al. 2009).

Vaccine preparations based on replicating viruses (such as LAVs) can induce protective immunity comparable to natural infection (MacLachlan et al. 2014) and cytosolic expression of viral proteins will result in efficient major histocompatibility complex (MHC) class I as well as MHC class II presentation, thereby potentially eliciting both $CD4^+$ and $CD8^+$ T cell as well as humoral immune response. Inactivated vaccines induce a relatively slow onset of immunity. Extracellular delivery of antigens is likely to favor MHC class II presentation, although the extent of CMI responses, especially CTL generation, to these preparations is mostly unknown and can be further influenced by adjuvants (Anderson et al. 2013, 2014).

20.6.2 Confirmation of Immunity

In the absence of protective immune correlates, detection of serogroup-specific anti-VP7 antibodies as well as neutralizing antibodies is used as a conservative assessment to identify if ruminants are responding immunologically to vaccine preparations (Monaco et al. 2004; Calistri et al. 2010; Vitale et al. 2016; van Rijn et al. 2017). The large-scale use of inactivated BT vaccine, especially against BTV-8 in northern Europe, highlighted that the reliable detection of serogroup-specific anti-BTV vaccine-induced antibodies required a booster vaccination, especially in cattle, although sensitivity of antibody detection might be influenced by the specific ELISA test used (Eschbaumer et al. 2009a; Oura et al. 2009). Vaccination with LAV seemed to result in the induction of serogroup- and serotype-specific antibodies in the majority of animals following a single inoculation (Savini et al. 2004c,d). However, the limited correlation of seroconversion to protective immunity currently requires *in vivo* challenge experiments to fully assess the efficiency of vaccines (Moulin et al. 2012). Clearly, identification of immune protection correlates to screen vaccine responses *ex vivo* and therefore limiting the necessity for animal challenge studies would be highly beneficial.

20.6.3 Cross-Serotype Immunity

A major future challenge for BTV vaccinology is the urgent need for cross-serotype protective BT vaccines, as to date, 30 serotypes of BTV have been discovered and advanced molecular technologies frequently identify new serotypes. The mostly serotype-specific immunity to BTV infection would otherwise require vaccine development for each specific serotype (Alpar et al. 2009; MacLachlan et al. 2014). The co-circulation of strains from numerous serotypes in the same geographical area renders such a vaccination approach highly undesirable.

Conserved, individual neutralizing epitopes have been identified between strains from different serotypes in either a neutralizing or nonneutralizing conformation and a degree of serological cross-reactivity of certain serotypes to virus strains from other serotypes is frequently observed in neutralization assays (Ristow et al. 1988; Rossitto and MacLachlan 1992; DeMaula et al. 1993, 2000). Challenge experiments in ruminants have also occasionally reported partial protection to heterologous virus strains, but such cross-serotype protection seems to be random and unpredictable (Umeshappa et al. 2010; Breard et al. 2015).

Interestingly, sequential infection or immunization with two or more BTV serotypes can lead to the development of neutralizing antibodies against serotypes to which the animal has never been exposed (Jeggo et al. 1983b, 1986), further suggesting the existence of some common neutralization epitopes on VP2. Bivalent and multivalent vaccine preparations containing either VP2s or BTV strains from multiple serotypes have been reported to protect against challenge with those BTV strains present in the preparation, while potentially eliciting broader neutralizing capability to other heterologous strains (Savini et al. 2009; Celma et al. 2013). Occasionally, however, some animals did not develop detectable neutralizing antibodies against all serotypes in the preparation (Savini et al. 2004e). Additionally, co-infection of sheep or cattle with several BTV strains may result in the failure of some strains to induce neutralizing antibodies or even to replicate (Jeggo et al. 1984c; dal Pozzo et al. 2013). This raised concerns for polyvalent vaccine designs based on the concurrent presence of multiple VP2s.

20.6.4 Duration of Protection Following Vaccination

The economic feasibility of any vaccination campaign heavily depends on the duration of immunity induced by selected vaccines, but the exact timeframes of immune protection are rarely assessed. Currently used LAV or inactivated BTV vaccines have reported protective immunity upon challenge between 7 and 12 months and yearly revaccination is often adopted in the field (Savini et al. 2004b; Hamers et al. 2009; Oura et al. 2009; Waeckerlin et al. 2010). Booster vaccination increased the antibody responses compared with single vaccinations, and especially in cattle, repeated vaccination and a high dose are considered necessary for long-lasting protection (Hund et al. 2012). Surprisingly, however, anti-BTV antibodies including neutralizing antibodies have been reported for up to 4 years in ruminants following the BTV-8 vaccination campaign using different inactivated preparations (Eschbaumer et al. 2012; Oura et al. 2012; Batten et al. 2013). Although protection was not confirmed in challenge experiments, vaccination with inactivated vaccines may potentially protect ruminants for longer periods than initially assumed.

20.7 Vaccination Strategies

It is now commonly accepted that stamping out is not a suitable strategy to deal with a vector-borne disease such as BT, and the slaughter of all susceptible animals in the entire infected and at-risk areas cannot be considered as an alternative. The basic control strategy is based on strict movement controls of susceptible animals from zones considered affected to BTV-free zones, intensive clinical, serological, and entomological surveillance, and mass vaccination of susceptible animals. Vaccination against BTV is considered to be the main means of control.

For BT, the type of vaccine used depends on the circumstances and the aim of vaccination, since a vaccine with the ideal profile has not been developed yet (Feenstra and van Rijn 2017). Emerging outbreaks in BT-free areas need rapid onset of serotype-specific protection, whereas endemic areas with multiple serotypes require long-lasting and broad protection. Both BTV inactivated and LAVs are available in some parts of the world, and these logically should be based on the local virus strains and serotypes. There is little cross-protection between BTV serotypes, so to achieve comprehensive protection, animals should be vaccinated against all BTV serotypes that circulate in a given region. LAVs should be administered prior to breeding to avoid fetal infections (and subsequent fetal losses and teratogenic defects). LAVs also should be given prior to the seasonal period of virus transmission (late summer and fall in temperate zones) to avoid infection of vectors with the virus strains contained in the vaccine and so minimize the likelihood of recombination/reassortment of vaccine and field viruses (MacLachlan et al. 2015).

Bluetongue vaccines may be used for different purposes or vaccination strategies, depending on the epidemiological situation of the affected area and desired objectives (i.e. disease control or disease eradication). The main objectives of BT vaccination strategies are to: (i) prevent clinical disease, (ii) reduce the spread of BTV, (iii) eradicate BT from the country or region, and (iv) permit the safe movement of susceptible animals between BT-affected and BT-free zones (Savini et al. 2008). These goals have guided BT vaccination campaigns since the incursion of BTV into Europe, enabling the eradication of serotypes 1, 2, and 8 in some regions. It is therefore commonly accepted that vaccines can help limit the spread of BTV and eradicate the infection in some instances. A vaccination campaign aiming at eradication should target susceptible ruminant species, achieve a high degree of herd immunity (80%), and include extensive areas surrounding any active BT outbreak. Such campaigns should also take into account climate, geography, and the abundance of competent insect vectors and susceptible wildlife animals.

All these factors are important for vaccination outcomes and for the interseasonal reemergence (persistence) of BTV infection in an area. In the same way, it should be kept in mind that a strategy only based on either direct control measures (movement restrictions) or vaccination of sheep would not be capable of limiting the spread of infection effectively. A successful control in fact requires the contemporaneous appliance of both vaccination of susceptible animals and restricting movement of viremic animals between BT-affected and BT-free zones (Savini et al. 2008).

Recently, the European Commission requested the EFSA to assess the most suitable duration of a BT vaccination campaign intended to achieve disease freedom in a country or region. A mathematical model was developed to analyze the virus spread according to different durations of vaccination campaigns in different areas in Europe, selected for their specific patterns of disease and vector ecology (the UK, France, southern Spain, and Sardinia). It was concluded that even when the vaccination of 95% of susceptible cattle and sheep is constantly applied for 3 consecutive years, BTV is not eradicated and may reemerge after a couple of years. Only after 5 years of vaccination of 95% of susceptible cattle and sheep will the prevalence of infection become close to eradication levels, although reaching zero values for sheep only occurred in the UK, France, and Sardinia, but not Spain (EFSA 2017).

20.8 Summary

In summary, BT is a globally emerging arboviral disease of domestic and wild ruminants. Although a number of vaccine strategies have been investigated with promising results, currently LAVs and inactivated vaccines are the only vaccines commercially produced and used to prevent BT. LAVs are highly effective in providing a cost-effective strategy for serotype-specific immunization of livestock, but it is increasingly apparent that the use of these vaccines has adverse potential consequences including: (i) underattenuation and/or reversion to virulence of the LAV virus, (ii) acquisition and dissemination of LAVs by vectors with reassortment of genes of vaccine viruses with those of "field" viruses to create genetically novel progeny, (iii) altered biological properties of LAVs including the potential for transplacental transmission (particularly those LAVs propagated in embryonated chickens' eggs) and the capacity for acquisition and dissemination by species of vector midges that were not previously known to be efficient vectors of BTV. Inactivated whole virus vaccines provide a safer alternative than LAVs, but typically are more expensive to produce and induce relatively transient immunity. The latest experiences have indicated that the widespread use of an appropriate inactivated vaccine can be a highly effective method for controlling an outbreak of BTV. However, as their efficacy is limited to specific serotypes and currently it is not possible to differentiate infected from vaccinated animals, there is room for improvement.

Delays in development and production and problems with the speed of delivery and the extent of uptake also indicate considerable room for improvement. The commercial nature of vaccine production and the high costs of developing and producing a new vaccine mean that the process is unlikely to begin while any uncertainty remains over the purchase and use of the product.

New BTV vaccines can, however, be developed relatively rapidly where close links between laboratories, international organizations, governments, and industry exist. One clear area for improvement may also be in government action as placing preorders for vaccines is likely to result in more rapid delivery and earlier vaccine deployment. Meanwhile, problems with vaccine uptake can be reduced by improving the provision of information to livestock keepers about the effectiveness and safety of a given vaccine and the economic risk of not vaccinating.

Most introductions of BTV in the last decade have occurred through repetitive "gateways." It would be sensible to make the most efficient use of limited surveillance resources by targeting known routes of viral introduction. BT is an infectious disease for which, especially in Europe, vaccine or antigen banks should be available in the near future. Of course, establishing a vaccine bank for every serotype would be impractical but it would be extremely valuable for those serotypes circulating in nearby countries. Continuous monitoring of the epidemiological situation of these countries is then recommended to identify serotypes posing the greatest risk for livestock. This would advance development of vaccines against those serotypes.

The basis of protective immunity of livestock to BTV infection is increasingly defined, including the protective immunogens of BTV. Thus, a variety of new-generation vaccine candidates and platforms have also been developed, as described in detail in this review. These next-generation strategies, many with DIVA capability, include nonreplicating subunit vaccines and virus-like particles, heterologous microbial expression vectors (e.g. using poxviruses as expression vectors for immunogenic BTV proteins), and genetically engineered LAVs, including replicating but nontransmittable virus-based vaccines (DISC and DISA). Although experimental studies have confirmed the potential efficacy of several of these strategies for safe and effective immunization of livestock against BT, to date, none of these vaccine candidates have been developed commercially for use in the field.

Thanks to advanced molecular virology and the availability of genomic information on BTV, there are new opportunities to create novel concept vaccines. Focus should be on new vaccine development and improvement of existing vaccines for broader and longer term protection. Improved diagnostic and vaccination strategies are certainly crucial to tackle the growing threat of BTV infection in order to effectively prevent and control the disease in the future. It is critical to monitor BTV populations with continued nationwide surveillance to map BTV genetic diversity, and to identify and prevent spreading of relevant strains.

References

Alpar, H.O., Bramwell, V.W., Veronesi, E. et al. (2009). Bluetongue virus vaccines past and present. In: *Bluetongue* (eds. P. Mellor, M. Baylis and P. Mertens), 397–428. London: Academic Press.

Anderson, J., Hagglund, S., Breard, E. et al. (2013). Evaluation of the immunogenicity of an experimental subunit vaccine that allows differentiation between infected and vaccinated animals against bluetongue virus serotype 8 in cattle. *Clin. Vaccine Immunol.* 20 (8): 1115–1122.

Anderson, J., Breard, E., Bengtsson, K.L. et al. (2014). Purification, stability, and immunogenicity analyses of five bluetongue virus proteins for use in development of a subunit vaccine that allows differentiation of infected from vaccinated animals. *Clin. Vaccine Immunol.* 21 (3): 443–452.

Athmaram, T.N., Bali, G., Kahng, G.G., and Dwarakanath, S. (2007). Heterologous expression of bluetongue VP2 viral protein fragment in *Pichia pastoris*. *Virus Genes* 35: 265–271.

Barros, S.C., Cruz, B., Luis, T.M. et al. (2009). A DIVA system based on the detection of antibodies to non-structural protein 3 (NS3) of bluetongue virus. *Vet. Microbiol.* 137: 252–259.

Bath, G.O. (1989) Bluetongue. In: *2nd International Congress for Sheep. Veterinarians*. Massey University, Wellington, New Zealand, 349–357.

Batten, C.A., Maan, S., Shaw, A.E. et al. (2008). A European field strain of bluetongue virus derived from two parental vaccine strains by genome segment reassortment. *Virus Res.* 137: 56–63.

Batten, C.A., Edwards, L., and Oura, C.A.L. (2013). Evaluation of the humoral immune responses in adult cattle and sheep, 4 and 2.5 years post-vaccination with a bluetongue serotype 8 inactivated vaccine. *Vaccine* 31 (37): 3783–3785.

Belyaev, A.S. and Roy, P. (1993). Development of baculovirus triple and quadruple expression vectors: co-expression of three or four bluetongue virus proteins and the synthesis of bluetongue virus-like particles in insect cells. *Nucleic Acids Res.* 21: 1219–1223.

Bhanuprakash, V., Indrani, B.K., Hosamani, M. et al. (2009). Bluetongue vaccines: the past, present and future. *Expert Rev. Vaccines* 8: 191–204.

Boone, J.D., Balasuriya, U.B., Karaca, K. et al. (2007). Recombinant canarypox virus vaccine co-expressing genes encoding the VP2 and VP5 outer capsid proteins of bluetongue virus induces high level protection in sheep. *Vaccine* 25: 672–678.

Boyce, M., Celma, C.C., and Roy, P. (2008). Development of reverse genetics systems for bluetongue virus: recovery of infectious virus from synthetic RNA transcripts. *J. Virol.* 82: 8339–8348.

Brandariz-Nuñez, A., Menaya-Vargas, R., Benavente, J., and Martinez-Costas, J. (2010). A versatile molecular tagging method for targeting proteins to avian reovirus muns inclusions. Use in protein immobilization and purification. *PLoS One* 5: e13961.

Breard, E., Hamblin, C., Hammoumi, S. et al. (2004). The epidemiology and diagnosis of bluetongue with particular reference to Corsica. *Res. Vet. Sci.* 77: 1–8.

Breard, E., Belbis, G., Viarouge, C. et al. (2015). Evaluation of adaptive immune responses and heterologous protection induced by inactivated bluetongue virus vaccines. *Vaccine* 33 (4): 512–518.

Calistri, P., Giovannini, A., Savini, G. et al. (2010). Antibody response in cattle vaccinated against bluetongue serotype 8 in Italy. *Transbound. Emerg. Dis.* 57 (3): 180–184.

Calvo-Pinilla, E., Rodriguez-Calvo, T., Sevilla, N., and Ortego, J. (2009). Heterologous prime boost vaccination with DNA and recombinant modified vaccinia virus Ankara protects IFNAR(-/-) mice against lethal bluetongue infection. *Vaccine* 28: 437–445.

Calvo-Pinilla, E., Navasa, N., Anguita, J., and Ortego, J. (2012). Multiserotype protection elicited by a combinatorial prime-boost vaccination strategy against bluetongue virus. *PLoS One* 7: e34735.

Campbell, C.H., Barber, T.L., Knudsen, R.C., and Swaney, L.M. (1985). Immune response of mice and sheep to bluetongue virus inactivated by gamma irradiation. *Prog. Clin. Biol. Res.* 178: 639–647.

Caporale, V., Giovannini, A., Patta, C. et al. (2004). Vaccination in the control strategy of bluetongue in Italy. *Dev. Biol. (Basel)* 119: 113–127.

Caracappa, S., Torina, A., Guercio, A. et al. (2003). Identification of a novel bluetongue virus vector species of *Culicoides* in Sicily. *Vet. Rec.* 153 (3): 71–74.

Celma, C.C., Boyce, M., van Rijn, P.A. et al. (2013). Rapid generation of replication-deficient monovalent and multivalent vaccines for bluetongue virus: protection against virulent virus challenge in cattle and sheep. *J. Virol.* 87: 9856–9864.

Celma, C.C., Stewart, M., Wernike, K. et al. (2017). Replication-deficient particles: new insights into the next generation of bluetongue virus vaccines. *J. Virol.* 91 (1): e01892–e01816.

Chand, K., Biswas, S.K., Pandey, A.B. et al. (2015). Bluetongue in India: a review. *Adv. Anim. Vet. Sci.* 3 (11): 605–612.

Chauveau, E., Doceul, V., Lara, E. et al. (2013). NS3 of bluetongue virus interferes with the induction of type I interferon. *J. Virol.* 87: 8241–8246.

Coetzee, P., van Vuuren, M., Stokstad, M. et al. (2014). Viral replication kinetics and *in vitro* cytopathogenicity of parental and reassortant strains of bluetongue virus serotype 1, 6, and 8. *Vet. Microbiol.* 171: 53–65.

Conraths, F.J., Gethmann, J.M., Staubach, C. et al. (2009). Epidemiology of bluetongue virus serotype 8, Germany. *Emerg. Infect. Dis.* 15 (3): 433–435. https://doi.org/10.3201/eid1503.081210

Cowley, J.A. and Gorman, B.M. (1989). Cross-neutralization of genetic reassortants of bluetongue virus serotypes 20 and 21. *Vet. Microbiol.* 19 (1): 37–51.

Dal Pozzo, F., Martinelle, L., Thys, C. et al. (2013). Experimental co-infections of calves with bluetongue virus serotypes 1 and 8. *Vet. Microbiol.* 165 (1–2): 167–172.

De Clercq, K., Mertens, P., de Leeuw, I. et al. (2009). Emergence of bluetongue serotypes in Europe, part 2: the occurrence of a BTV-11 strain in Belgium. *Transbound. Emerg. Dis.* 56: 355–361.

Demaula, C.D., Heidner, H.W., Rossitto, P.V. et al. (1993). Neutralization determinants of United States bluetongue virus serotype 10. *Virology* 195 (1): 292–296.

Demaula, C.D., Bonneau, K.R., and MacLachlan, N.J. (2000). Changes in the outer capsid proteins of bluetongue virus serotype ten that abrogate neutralization by monoclonal antibodies. *Virus Res.* 67: 59–66.

Dijkstra, E., van der Ven, I.J., Meiswinkel, R. et al. (2008). *Culicoides chiopterus* as a potential vector of bluetongue virus in Europe. *Vet. Rec.* 162 (13): 422.

Du Toit, R.M. (1944). The transmission of blue-tongue and horse sickness by *Culicoides*. *Onderstepoort J. Vet. Res.* 19: 7–16.

Dungu, B., Gerdes, T., and Smit, T. (2004a). The use of vaccination in the control of bluetongue in southern Africa. *Vet. Ital.* 40: 616–622.

Dungu, B., Potgieter, C., von Teichman, B., and Smit, T. (2004b). Vaccination in the control of bluetongue in endemic regions: the south African experience. *Dev. Biol. (Basel)* 119: 463–472.

EFSA Opinion (2011). Scientific opinion on bluetongue monitoring and surveillance. *EFSA J.* 9 (6): 2192.

EFSA Opinion (2017). Bluetongue: control, surveillance and safe movement of animals. *EFSA J.* 15 (3): 4698.

Eschbaumer, M., Hoffmann, B., Koenig, P. et al. (2009a). Efficacy of three inactivated vaccines against bluetongue virus serotype 8 in sheep. *Vaccine* 27 (31): 4169–4175.

Eschbaumer, M., Hoffmann, B., Moss, A. et al. (2009b). Emergence of bluetongue virus serotype 6 in Europe – German field data and experimental infection of cattle. *Vet. Microbiol.* 143: 189–195.

Eschbaumer, M., Eschweiler, J., and Hoffmann, B. (2012). Long-term persistence of neutralising antibodies against bluetongue virus serotype 8 in naturally infected cattle. *Vaccine* 30 (50): 7142–7143.

European Pharmacopoeia. 9 (2017). Council of Europe, Strasbourg, France.

Feenstra, F. and van Rijn, P. (2017). Current and next-generation bluetongue vaccines: requirements, strategies, and prospects for different field situations. *Crit. Rev. Microbiol.* 43: 142–155.

Feenstra, F., van Gennip, R.G.P., van de Water, S.G.P., and van Rijn, P.A. (2014a). RNA elements in open reading frames of the bluetongue virus genome are essential for virus replication. *PLoS One* 9: e92377.

Feenstra, F., van Gennip, R.G., Maris-Veldhuis, M. et al. (2014b). Bluetongue virus without NS3/NS3a expression is not virulent and protects against virulent bluetongue virus challenge. *J. Gen. Virol.* 95: 2019–2029.

Feenstra, F., Maris-Veldhuis, M., Daus, F.J. et al. (2014c). VP2-serotyped live-attenuated bluetongue virus without NS3/NS3a expression provides serotype-specific protection and enables DIVA. *Vaccine* 32: 7108–7114.

Feenstra, F., Pap, J.S., and van Rijn, P.A. (2015a). Application of bluetongue disabled infectious single animal (DISA) vaccine for different serotypes by VP2 exchange or incorporation of chimeric VP2. *Vaccine* 33: 812–818.

Feenstra, F., Drolet, B.S., Boonstra, J., and van Rijn, P.A. (2015b). Non-structural protein NS3/NS3a is required for propagation of bluetongue virus in *Culicoides sonorensis*. *Parasites Vectors* 8: 476.

Ferrari, G., de Liberato, C., Scavia, G. et al. (2005). Active circulation of bluetongue vaccine virus serotype-2 among unvaccinated cattle in Central Italy. *Prev. Vet. Med.* 68: 103–113.

Franceschi, V., Capocefalo, A., Calvo-Pinilla, E. et al. (2011). Immunization of knock-out alpha/beta interferon receptor mice against lethal bluetongue infection with a BoHV-4-based vector expressing BTV-8 VP2 antigen. *Vaccine* 29: 3074–3082.

French, T.J., Marshall, J.J., and Roy, P. (1990). Assembly of double-shelled, virus-like particles of bluetongue virus by the simultaneous expression of four structural proteins. *J. Virol.* 64: 5695–5700.

Gibbs, E.P. and Greiner, E.C. (1994). The epidemiology of bluetongue. *Comp. Immunol. Microbiol. Infect. Dis.* 17: 207–220.

Grewar, J.D. (2016) The economic impact of bluetongue and other orbiviruses in sub-Saharan Africa, with special reference to southern Africa. *Vet. Ital.* 52 (3–4): 375–381.

Grunwald, T. and Ulbert, S. (2015). Improvement of DNA vaccination by adjuvants and sophisticated delivery devices: vaccine-platforms for the battle against infectious diseases. *Clin. Exp. Vaccine Res.* 4: 1–10.

Hamers, C., Rehbein, S., Hudelet, P. et al. (2009). Protective duration of immunity of an inactivated bluetongue (BTV) serotype 2 vaccine against a virulent BTV serotype 2 challenge in sheep. *Vaccine* 27 (21): 2789–2793.

Hardy, W.T. and Price, D.A (1952). Soremuzzle of sheep. *J. Am. Vet. Med. Assoc.* 120: 23–25.

Henning, M.W. (1956). *Animal Diseases in South Africa*, 3e. Johannesburg: Central News Agency Ltd.

Huismans, H. (1985). The use of recombinant DNA technology for the development of a bluetongue virus subunit vaccine. *Onderstepoort J. Vet. Res.* 52: 149–151.

Huismans, H. and Erasmus, B.J. (1981). Identification of the serotype-specific and group-specific antigens of bluetongue virus. *Onderstepoort J. Vet. Res.* 48 (2): 51–58.

Huismans, H., Vanderwalt, N.T., Cloete, M., and Erasmus, B.J. (1987). Isolation of a capsid protein of bluetongue virus that induces a protective immune-response in sheep. *Virology* 157 (1): 172–179.

Hund, A., Gollnick, N., Sauter-Louis, C. et al. (2012). A two year BTV-8 vaccination follow up: molecular diagnostics and assessment of humoral and cellular immune reactions. *Vet. Microbiol.* 154: 247–256.

Hutcheon, D. (1902). Malarial catarrhal fever of sheep. *Vet. Rec.* 14: 629–633.

Inumaru, S. and Roy, P. (1987). Production and characterization of the neutralization antigen VP2 of bluetongue virus serotype 10 using a baculovirus expression vector. *Virology* 157: 472–479.

Jabbar, T.K., Calvo-Pinilla, E., Mateos, F. et al. (2013). Protection of IFNAR (−/−) mice against bluetongue virus serotype 8, by heterologous (DNA/rMVA) and homologous (rMVA/rMVA) vaccination, expressing outer-capsid protein VP2. *PLoS One* 8: e60574.

Jafari-Shoorijeh, S., Ramin, A.G., MacLachlan, N.J. et al. (2010). High seroprevalence of bluetongue virus infection in sheep flocks in West Azerbaijan, Iran. *Comp. Immunol. Microbiol. Infect. Dis.* 33 (3): 243–247.

Janardhana, V., Andrew, M.E., Lobato, Z.I.P., and Coupar, B.E.H. (1999). The ovine cytotoxic T lymphocyte responses to bluetongue virus. *Res. Vet. Sci.* 67 (3): 213–221.

Janowicz, A., Caporale, M., Shaw, A. et al. (2015). Multiple genome segments determine virulence of bluetongue virus serotype 8. *J. Virol.* 89: 5238–5249.

Jeggo, M.H. and Wardley, R.C. (1982). The induction of murine cytotoxic T lymphocytes by bluetongue virus. *Arch. Virol* 71 (3): 197–206.

Jeggo, M.H., Wardley, R.C., and Taylor, W.P. (1983a). Host response to bluetongue virus. In: *Double-Stranded RNA Viruses* (eds. R.W. Compans and D.H.L. Bishop), 353–359. Amsterdam: Elsevier Science.

Jeggo, M.H., Gumm, I.D., and Taylor, W.P. (1983b). Clinical and serological response of sheep to serial challenge with different bluetongue virus types. *Res. Vet. Sci.* 34 (2): 205–211.

Jeggo, M.H., Wardley, R.C., and Taylor, W.P. (1984a). Role of neutralizing antibody in passive immunity to bluetongue infection. *Res. Vet. Sci.* 36 (1): 81–86.

Jeggo, M.H., Wardley, R.C., and Brownlie, J. (1984b). A study of the role of cell-mediated-immunity in bluetongue virus-infection in sheep, using cellular adoptive transfer techniques. *Immunology* 52 (3): 403–410.

Jeggo, M.H., Wardley, R.C., and Taylor, W.P. (1984c). Clinical and serological outcome following the simultaneous inoculation of three bluetongue virus types into sheep. *Res. Vet. Sci.* 37 (3): 368–370.

Jeggo, M.H., Wardley, R.C., and Brownlie, J. (1985). Importance of ovine cytotoxic T cells in protection against bluetongue virus infection. *Prog. Clin. Biol. Res.* 178: 477–487.

Jeggo, M.H., Wardley, R.C., Brownlie, J., and Corteyn, A.H. (1986). Serial inoculation of sheep with two bluetongue virus types. *Res. Vet. Sci.* 40 (3): 386–392.

Juleff, N., Windsor, M., Lefevre, E.A. et al. (2009). Foot-and-mouth disease virus can induce a specific and rapid CD4(+) T-cell-independent neutralizing and Isotype class-switched antibody response in naive cattle. *J. Virol.* 83 (8): 3626–3636.

Kampen, H. and Werner, D. (2010). Three years of bluetongue disease in Central Europe with special reference to Germany: what lessons can be learned? *Wien. Klin. Wochenschr.* 122 (Suppl. 3): 31–39.

Legisa, D.M., Perez Aguirreburualde, M.S., Gonzalez, F.N. et al. (2015). An experimental subunit vaccine based on bluetongue virus 4 VP2 protein fused to an antigen-presenting cells single chain antibody elicits cellular and humoral immune responses in cattle, Guinea pigs and IFNAR(−/−) mice. *Vaccine* 33 (22): 2614–2619.

Letchworth, G.J. and Appleton, J.A. (1983). Passive protection of mice and sheep against bluetongue virus by a neutralizing monoclonocal antibody. *Infect. Immun.* 39 (1): 208–212.

Li, J., Yang, T., Xu, Q. et al. (2015). DNA vaccine prime and recombinant FPV vaccine boost: an important candidate immunization strategy to control bluetongue virus type 1. *Appl. Microbiol. Biotechnol.* 99 (20): 8643–8652.

Ma, G., Eschbaumer, M., Said, A. et al. (2012). An equine herpesvirus type 1 (EHV-1) expressing VP2 and VP5 of serotype 8 bluetongue virus (BTV-8) induces protection in a murine infection model. *PLoS One* 7: e34425.

Maan, S., Maan, N.S., Ross-Smith, N. et al. (2008). Sequence analysis of bluetongue virus serotype 8 from the Netherlands 2006 and comparison to other European strains. *Virology* 377: 308–318.

Maan, S., Maan, N.S., van Rijn, P.A. et al. (2010). Full genome characterisation of bluetongue virus serotype 6 from the Netherlands 2008 and comparison to other field and vaccine strains. *PLoS One* 5: e10323.

MacLachlan, N.J. (2010). Global implications of the recent emergence of bluetongue virus in Europe. *Vet. Clin. North Am. Food Anim. Pract.* 26 (1): 163–171. https://doi.org/10.1016/j.cvfa.2009.10.012

MacLachlan, N.J. and Mayo, C.E. (2013). Potential strategies for control of bluetongue, a globally-emerging *Culicoides*-transmitted viral disease of ruminant livestock and wildlife. *Antiviral Res.* 99: 79–90.

MacLachlan, N.J. and Osburn, B.I. (2006). Impact of bluetongue virus infection on the international movement and trade of ruminants. *J. Am. Vet. Med. Assoc.* 228: 1346–1349.

MacLachlan, N.J., Drew, C.P., Darpel, K.E., and Worwa, G. (2009). The pathology and pathogenesis of bluetongue. *J. Comp. Pathol.* 141: 1–16.

MacLachlan, N.J., Henderson, C., Schwartz-Cornil, I., and Zientara, S. (2014). The immune response of ruminant livestock to bluetongue virus: from type I interferon to antibody. *Virus Res.* 182: 71–77.

MacLachlan, N.J., Mayo, C.E., Daniels, P.W., and Gibbs, E.P. (2015). Bluetongue: recent developments. *OIE Sci. Tech.* 34: 329–340.

Marin-Lopez, A., Otero-Romero, I., de La Poza, F. et al. (2014). VP2, VP7, and NS1 proteins of bluetongue virus targeted in avian reovirus muNS-mi microspheres elicit a protective immune response in IFNAR(−/−) mice. *Antiviral Res.* 110: 42–51.

Matsuo, E., Celma, C.C., Boyce, M. et al. (2011). Generation of replication-defective virus-based vaccines that confer full protection in sheep against virulent bluetongue virus challenge. *J. Virol.* 85: 10213–10221.

Mayo, C.E., Mullens, B.A., Reisen, W.K. et al. (2014). Seasonal and interseasonal dynamics of bluetongue virus infection of dairy cattle and *Culicoides sonorensis* midges in northern California--implications for virus overwintering in temperate zones. *PLoS One* 9 (9): e106975.

Mayo, C.E., Mullens, B.A., Gibbs, E.P., and MacLachlan, N.J. (2016). Overwintering of bluetongue virus in temperate zones. *Vet. Ital.* 52: 243–246.

McKercher, D.G., McGowan, B., Howarth, J.A., and Saito, J.K. (1953). A preliminary report on the isolation and identification of bluetongue virus from sheep in California. *J. Am. Vet. Med. Assoc.* 122: 300–301.

McVey, D.S. and MacLachlan, N.J. (2015). Vaccines for prevention of bluetongue and epizootic hemorrhagic disease in livestock: a North American perspective. *Vector Borne Zoonotic Dis.* 15: 385–396.

Meiswinkel, R., van Rijn, P., Leijs, P., and Goffredo, M. (2007). Potential new *Culicoides* vector of bluetongue virus in northern Europe. *Vet. Rec.* 161 (16): 564–565.

Mohd Jaafar, F., Belhouchet, M., Vitour, D. et al. (2014). Immunisation with bacterial expressed VP2 and VP5 of bluetongue virus (BTV) protect alpha/beta interferon-receptor knock-out (IFNAR(−/−)) mice from homologous lethal challenge. *Vaccine* 32: 4059–4067.

Monaco, F., de Luca, N., Spina, P. et al. (2004). Virological and serological response of cattle following field vaccination with bivalent modified-live vaccine against bluetongue virus serotypes 2 and 9. *Vet. Ital.* 40 (4): 657–660.

Monaco, F., Camma, C., Serini, S., and Savini, G. (2006). Differentiation between field and vaccine strain of bluetongue virus serotype 16. *Vet. Microbiol.* 116: 45–52.

Moulin, V., Noordegraaf, C.V., Makoschey, B. et al. (2012). Clinical disease in sheep caused by bluetongue virus serotype 8, and prevention by an inactivated vaccine. *Vaccine* 30 (12): 2228–2235.

Nomikou, K., Maan, S., Batten, C., and Mertens, P. (2013). Bluetongue molecular epidemiology report 30 November 2012: Poland (2012). VBD molecular epidemiology report form (2012-11-30). http://ec.europa.eu/food/animals/docs/ad_control-measures_bt_molec-epidemiology_report_20121130_poland.pdf

Nunes, S.F., Hamers, C., Ratinier, M. et al. (2014). A synthetic biology approach for a vaccine platform against known and newly emerging serotypes of bluetongue virus. *J. Virol.* 88 (21): 12222–12232.

OIE. (2016). Manual of Diagnostic Tests and Vaccines for Terrestrial Animals. www.oie.int/standard-setting/terrestrial-manual/access-online/

Oura, C.A.L., Wood, J.L.N., Sanders, A.J. et al. (2009). Seroconversion, neutralising antibodies and protection in bluetongue serotype 8 vaccinated sheep. *Vaccine* 27 (52): 7326–7330.

Oura, C.A.L., Edwards, L., and Batten, C.A. (2012). Evaluation of the humoral immune response in adult dairy cattle three years after vaccination with a bluetongue serotype 8 inactivated vaccine. *Vaccine* 30 (2): 112–115.

Parker, J., Herniman, K.A., Gibbs, E.P., and Sellers, R.F. (1975). An experimental inactivated vaccine against bluetongue. *Vet. Rec.* 96: 284–287.

Patta, C., Giovannini, A., Rolesu, S. et al. (2004). Bluetongue vaccination in Europe: the Italian experience. *Vet. Ital.* 40 (4): 601–610.

Pérez de Diego, A.C., Athmaram, T.N., Stewart, M. et al. (2011). Characterization of protection afforded by a bivalent virus-like particle vaccine against bluetongue virus serotypes 1 and 4 in sheep. *PLoS One* 6: e26666.

Pérez De Diego, A.C., Sánchez-Cordón, P.J., and Sánchez-Vizcaíno, J.M. (2014). Bluetongue in Spain: from the first outbreak to 2012. *Transbound. Emerg. Dis.* 61 (6): e1–e11.

Perrin, A., Albina, E., Breard, E. et al. (2007). Recombinant capripoxviruses expressing proteins of bluetongue virus: evaluation of immune responses and protection in small ruminants. *Vaccine* 25: 6774–6783.

Pinior, B., Lebl, K., Firth, C. et al. (2015). Cost analysis of bluetongue virus serotype 8 surveillance and vaccination programmes in Austria from 2005 to 2013. *Vet. J.* 206: 154–160.

Purse, B.V., Mellor, P.S., Rogers, D.J. et al. (2005). Climate change and the recent emergence of bluetongue in Europe. *Nat. Rev. Microbiol.* 3: 171–181.

Purse, B.V., Brown, H.E., Harrup, L. et al. (2008). Invasion of bluetongue and other Orbivirus infections into Europe: the role of biological and climatic processes. *Rev. Sci. Tech. Off. Int. Epiz.* 27: 427–442.

Ranjan, K., Minakshi, P., and Prasad, G. (2015). Bluetongue: Indian perspective. *Acta Virol.* 59 (4): 317–337.

Richards, R.G., MacLachlan, N.J., Heidner, H.W., and Fuller, F.J. (1988). Comparison of virologic and serologic responses of lambs and calves infected with bluetongue virus serotype 10. *Vet. Microbiol.* 18: 233–242.

Ristow, S., Leendersten, L., Gorham, J., and Yilma, T. (1988). Identification of a neutralizing epitope shared by bluetongue virus serotypes 2 and 13. *J. Virol.* 62 (7): 2503–2504.

Rossitto, P.V. and MacLachlan, N.J. (1992). Neutralising epitopes of the serotypes of bluetongue virus present in the United States. *J Gen. Virol.* 73: 1947–1952.

Roy, P. (2004). Genetically engineered structure-based vaccine for bluetongue disease. *Vet. Ital.* 40: 594–600.

Roy, P., Bishop, D.H., Leblois, H., and Erasmus, B.J. (1994). Long-lasting protection of sheep against bluetongue challenge after vaccination with virus-like particles: evidence for homologous and partial heterologous protection. *Vaccine* 12: 805–811.

Rushton, J. and Lyons, N. (2015). Economic impact of bluetongue: a review of the effects on production. *Vet. Ital.* 51: 401–406.

Rybicki, E.P. (2010). Plant-made vaccines for humans and animals. *Plant Biotechnol. J.* 8: 620–637.

Saegerman, C., Hubaux, M., Urbain, B. et al. (2007). Regulatory aspects concerning temporary authorisation of animal vaccination in case of an emergency situation: example of bluetongue in Europe. *Rev. Sc. Tech. Off. int. Epiz.* 26 (2): 395–414.

Savini, G., Monaco, F., Facchinei, A. et al. (2004a). Field vaccination of sheep with bivalent modified-live vaccine against bluetongue virus serotypes 2 and 9: effect on milk production. *Vet. Ital.* 40: 627–630.

Savini, G., Monaco, F., Citarella, R. et al. (2004b). Monovalent modified-live vaccine against bluetongue virus serotype 2: immunity studies in cows. *Vet. Ital.* 40 (4): 664–667.

Savini, G., Monaco, F., Calistri, P. et al. (2004c). Neutralising antibody response in cattle after vaccination with monovalent modified-live vaccine against bluetongue virus serotype 2. *Vet. Ital.* 40 (4): 668–670.

Savini, G., Tittarelli, M., Bonfini, B. et al. (2004d). Serological response in cattle and sheep following infection or vaccination with bluetongue virus. *Vet. Ital.* 40 (4): 645–647.

Savini, G., Monaco, F., Conte, A. et al. (2004e). Virological and serological response of sheep following field vaccination with bivalent modified-live vaccine against bluetongue virus serotypes 2 and 9. *Vet. Ital.* 40 (4): 631–634.

Savini, G., Goffredo, M., Monaco, F. et al. (2005). Bluetongue virus isolations from midges belonging to the Obsoletus complex (Culicoides, Diptera: Ceratopogonidae) in Italy. *Vet. Rec.* 157: 133–139.

Savini, G., MacLachlan, N.J., Sanchez-Vizcaino, J.M., and Zientara, S. (2008). Vaccines against bluetongue in Europe. *Comp. Immunol. Microbiol. Infect. Dis.* 31 (2–3): 101–120.

Savini, G., Hamers, C., Conte, A. et al. (2009). Assessment of efficacy of a bivalent BTV-2 and BTV-4 inactivated vaccine by vaccination and challenge in cattle. *Vet. Microbiol.* 133 (1–2): 1–8.

Savini, G., Lorusso, A., Paladini, C. et al. (2012). Bluetongue serotype 2 and 9 modified live vaccine viruses as causative agents of abortion in livestock: a retrospective analysis in Italy. *Transbound. Emerg. Dis.* 61 (1): 69–74.

Spreull, J. (1905). Malarial catarrhal fever (bluetongue) of sheep in South Africa. *J. Comp. Pathol. Therap.* 18: 321–337.

Stevens, D.R., Stott, J., Osburn, B.I. et al. (1985). Potency and efficacy of inactivated bluetongue virus vaccines. *Prog. Clin. Biol. Res.* 178: 649–652.

Stewart, M., Bhatia, Y., Athmaran, T.N. et al. (2010). Validation of a novel approach for the rapid production of immunogenic virus-like particles for bluetongue virus. *Vaccine* 28: 3047–3054.

Steyn, J., Venter, G.J., Labuschagne, K. et al. (2016). Possible over-wintering of bluetongue virus in *Culicoides* populations in the Onderstepoort area, Gauteng, South Africa. *J. S. Afr. Vet. Assoc.* 87 (1): e1–e5.

Stott, J.L., Barber, T.L., and Osburn, B.I. (1985). Immunologic response of sheep to inactivated and virulent bluetongue virus. *Am. J. Vet. Res.* 46: 1043–1049.

Szmaragd, C., Wilson, A.J., Carpenter, S. et al. (2010). The spread of bluetongue virus serotype 8 in Great Britain and its control by vaccination. *PLoS One* 5: e9353. https://doi.org/10.1371/journal.pone.0009353

Tabachnick, W.J. (2004). Culicoides and the global distribution of bluetongue virus infections. *Vet. Ital.* 40: 145–150.

Tabachnick, W.J., Smartt, C.T., and Connelly, C.R. (2008). *Bluetongue*. Gainesville: University of Florida http://edis.ifas.ufl.edu/pdffiles/IN/IN76800.pdf

Tacken, M.G., Daus, F.J., Feenstra, F. et al. (2015). Development of a competitive ELISA for NS3 antibodies as DIVA test accompanying the novel disabled infectious single animal (DISA) vaccine for bluetongue. *Vaccine* 33 (42): 5539–5545.

Theiler, A. (1906). Bluetongue in sheep. In: *Annual Report of the Director of Agriuclture, Transvaal for 1906*, 110–121.

Top, S., Foucras, G., Deplanche, M. et al. (2012). Myxomavirus as a vector for the immunisation of sheep: protection study against challenge with bluetongue virus. *Vaccine* 30: 1609–1616.

Umeshappa, C.S., Singh, K.P., Pandey, A.B. et al. (2010). Cell-mediated immune response and cross-protective efficacy of binary ethylenimine-inactivated bluetongue virus serotype-1 vaccine in sheep. *Vaccine* 28 (13): 2522–2531.

Ura, T., Okuda, K., and Shimada, M. (2014). Developments in viral vector-based vaccines. *Vaccines* 2: 624.

Urakawa, T., French, T.J., Adachi, Y. et al. (1994). Synthesis of recombinant baculoviruses expressing the outer capsid protein VP2 of five BTV serotypes and the induction of neutralizing antibodies to homologous and heterologous BTV serotypes. *Virus Res.* 3: 149–161.

van Gennip, R.G.P., van de Water, S.G.P., Maris-Veldhuis, M., and van Rijn, P.A. (2012a). Bluetongue viruses based on modified-live vaccine serotype 6 with exchanged outer Shell proteins confer full protection in sheep against virulent BTV8. *PLoS One* 7 (9): e44619.

van Gennip, R.G.P., van de Water, S.G.P., Potgieter, C.A. et al. (2012b). Rescue of recent virulent and avirulent field strains of bluetongue virus by reverse genetics. *PLoS One* 7 (2): e30540.

van Gennip, R.G.P., van de Water, S.G.P., and van Rijn, P.A. (2014). Bluetongue virus nonstructural protein NS3/NS3a is not essential for virus replication. *PLoS One* 9 (1): e85788.

van Rijn, P.A., Geurts, Y., van der Spek, A.N. et al. (2012). Bluetongue virus serotype 6 in Europe in

2008 – emergence and disappearance of an unexpected non-virulent BTV. *Vet. Microbiol.* 158: 23–32.

van Rijn, P.A., van de Water, S.G., and van Gennip, H.G. (2013). Bluetongue virus with mutated genome segment 10 to differentiate infected from vaccinated animals: a genetic DIVA approach. *Vaccine* 31: 5005–5008.

van Rijn, P.A., Daus, F.J., Maris-Veldhuis, M.A. et al. (2017). Bluetongue disabled infectious single animal (DISA) vaccine: studies on the optimal route and dose in sheep. *Vaccine* 35 (2): 231–237.

Velthuis, A.G.J., Saatkamp, H.W., Mourits, M.C.M. et al. (2010). Financial consequences of the Dutch bluetongue serotype 8 epidemics of 2006 and 2007. *Prev. Vet. Med.* 93: 294–304.

Veronesi, E., Hamblin, C., and Mellor, P.S. (2005). Live attenuated bluetongue vaccine viruses in Dorset Poll sheep, before and after passage in vector midges (Diptera: Ceratopogonidae). *Vaccine* 23: 5509–5516.

Vitale, N., Radaelli, M.C., Chiavacci, L. et al. (2016). Factors affecting seroconversion rates in cattle vaccinated with two commercial inactivated BTV-8 vaccines under field conditions. *Transbound. Emerg. Dis.* 63 (2): 175–183.

Vögtlin, A., Hofmann, M.A., Nenniger, C. et al. (2013). Long-term infection of goats with bluetongue virus serotype 25. *Vet. Microbiol.* 166 (1–2): 165–173.

Waeckerlin, R., Eschbaumer, M., Koenig, P. et al. (2010). Evaluation of humoral response and protective efficacy of three inactivated vaccines against bluetongue virus serotype 8 one year after vaccination of sheep and cattle. *Vaccine* 28: 4348–4355.

White, J.R. and Eaton, B.T. (1990). Conformation of the VP2 protein of bluetongue virus (BTV) determines the involvement in virus neutralization of highly conserved epitoped within the BTV serogroup. *J. Gen. Virol.* 71: 1325–1332.

Wilson, A.J. and Mellor, P.S. (2009). Bluetongue in Europe: past, present and future. *Philos. Trans. R. Soc. London, Ser. B* 364: 2669–2681.

Zientara, S. and Sanchez-Vizcaino, J.M. (2013). Control of bluetongue in Europe. *Vet. Microbiol.* 165: 33–37.

Zientara, S., MacLachlan, N.J., Calistri, P. et al. (2010). Bluetongue vaccination in Europe. *Expert Rev. Vaccines* 9 (9): 989–991.

21

Peste des Petits Ruminants

Adama Diallo[1,2] and Rabindra Prasad Singh[3]

[1] UMR CIRAD-INRA ASTRE, Montpellier, France
[2] ISRA/LNERV, Dakar Hann, Dakar, Senegal
[3] Division of Biological Products, ICAR – Indian Veterinary Research Institute, Bareilly, Uttar Pradesh, India

21.1 Introduction

Peste des petits ruminants (PPR) is a highly contagious viral disease of small ruminants. In its acute forms, it is characterized by high fever, nasal and ocular discharges, diarrhea, and death in 50–60% of cases, even more if it occurs in naïve populations (Diallo and Libeau 2014). The symptoms are like those of rinderpest, the related cattle disease that was declared officially eradicated from the world in 2011 (www.fao.org/docrep/018/i3366e/i3366e.pdf).

Rinderpest was known in the fourth century (Lefèvre 2010) but the first report on PPR dates back to only 1942 (Gargadennec and Lalanne 1942). For a long time, PPR reports were confined to West Africa. It was only after the 1970s that its geographical distribution steadily expanded across Africa (apart from southern countries), the Middle and Near East and Asia, extending from western Asia to China (Banyard et al. 2010; Libeau et al. 2014; Baron et al. 2016). Today, about 80% of the world's sheep and goat populations are threatened by PPR (Figure 21.1).

Currently, PPR is the fastest growing and potentially the most economically important disease of sheep and goats in many regions of the developing world where these domestic animals play an integral and important role in sustainable agriculture. PPR has spread so alarmingly during the last two decades that it has become a concern for the Food and Agriculture Organization of the United Nations (FAO) and the World Organization for Animal Health (OIE), which convened an international conference on the situation in April 2015 in Abidjan, Côte d'Ivoire (www.fao.org/news/story/en/item/282397/icode). At that conference, a strategy was adopted for the global control and eradication of PPR (PPR-GCES) by the year 2030 (Anonymous 2015).

21.2 Types of Vaccines Commercially Available

Peste des petits ruminants is caused by a virus, the peste des petits ruminants virus (PPRV) that belongs to the genus *Morbillivirus* within the family *Paramyxoviridae*. The other members of the *Morbillivirus* group include rinderpest virus (RPV), measles virus (MV), canine distemper virus (CDV), phocine distemper virus (PDV), dolphin morbillivirus (DMV), porpoise morbillivirus (PMV), and feline morbillivirus (FeMV) (Diallo and Libeau 2014; Parida et al. 2015). The virus particle is composed of an envelope, a genomic RNA, and six structural proteins, namely the nucleocapsid protein (N), the phosphoprotein (P), the matrix protein (M), the fusion protein (F), the hemagglutinin (H), and the large RNA-dependent polymerase RNA protein (L). While the N protein of morbilliviruses is the major viral protein, it does not induce a protective immune response, unlike the hemagglutinin (H) and fusion (F) proteins that mediate virus entry into the cell and its propagation in the host. Those two viral proteins induce immune protection against the virus infection and the disease (Barrett et al. 2006; Diallo and Libeau 2014). F and N protein gene sequences have been used for typing the different PPRV strains so far identified. They are classified into four genotypes: I, II, III, and IV (Figure 21.2).

All the four PPRV genotypes are endemic in Africa, while so far, only viruses of genotype IV have been identified in Asia (Libeau et al. 2014; Adombi et al. 2016; Baron et al. 2016). Despite this subdivision, there is only one PPRV serotype and an animal which has recovered from an infection by a PPRV strain or which has been vaccinated is protected against infection by any other PPRV strain. All PPR vaccines in use currently are live attenuated PPRV that

Veterinary Vaccines: Principles and Applications, First Edition. Edited by Samia Metwally, Gerrit Viljoen, and Ahmed El Idrissi.

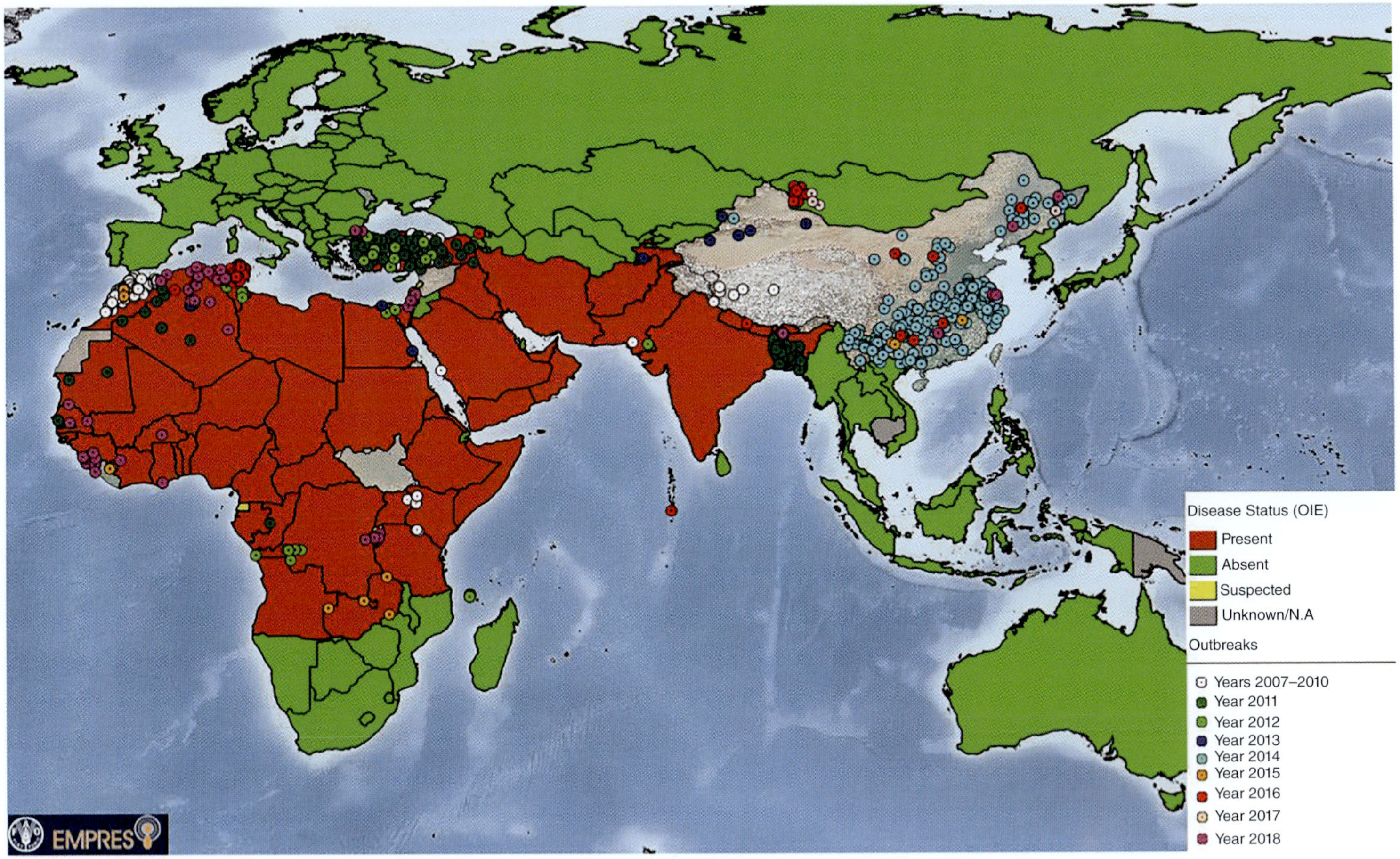

Figure 21.1 Peste des petits ruminants events from January 2007 to 31 December 2018 (by onset date). The map was produced by FAO AGAH/GLEWS using information from FAO EMPRES-i and OIE WAHIS.

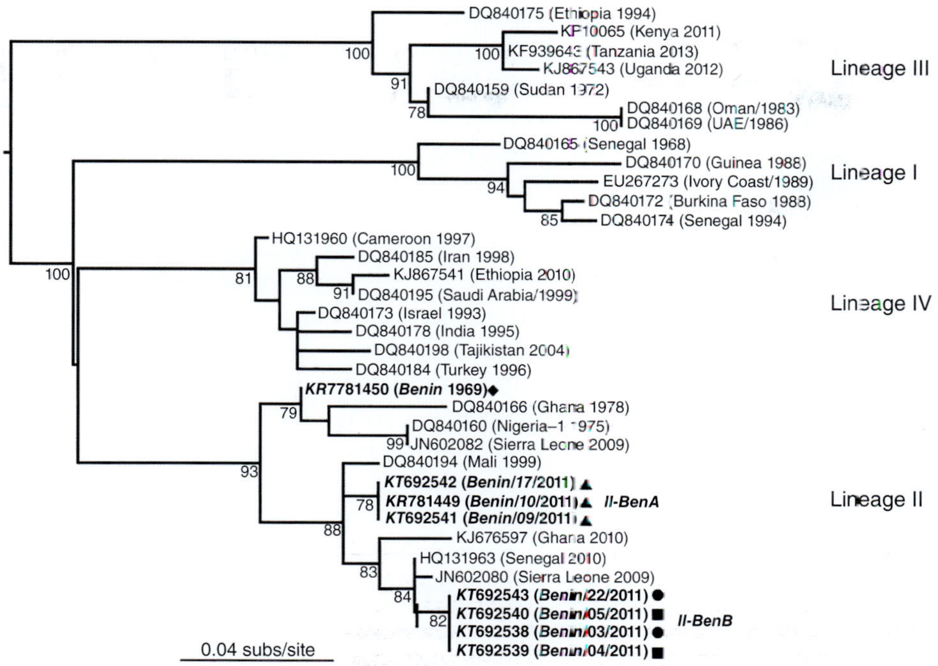

Figure 21.2 Phylogenetic tree of partial N gene sequences from different PPRV samples. Bootstrap support values (>70%) are shown. The tree is midpoint rooted for clarity only and horizontal branch lengths are scaled to the number of nucleotide substitutions per site. Source: Adombi et al. (2016).

have lost their pathogenicity through successive *in vitro* passages in cell culture (Diallo et al. 1989; Diallo 2004; Singh et al. 2009; Singh and Bandyopadhyay 2015). They all belong to genotypes II or IV (Table 21.1).

Among these attenuated PPRV vaccines, the PPRV Nigeria 75/1, lineage II and the PPRV Sungri 96, lineage IV are currently the most widely used. They are the strains for which most of the information on PPR vaccines is available (Diallo et al. 1989; Singh et al. 2009; Singh and Bandyopadhyay 2015; Hodgson et al. 2018). Both the Nigeria 75/1 and Sungri-96 vaccines have been extensively tested and validated. So far, no adverse reaction has been noted with those two vaccine strains after many years of extensive use. Their genomes have been fully sequenced (Table 21.1). The recommended vaccination dose for sheep and goats is $10^{2.5}$ $TCID_{50}$/animal (OIE 2018).

21.3 Immune Response and Duration of Immunity

The main characteristic of the pathogenesis of PPRV infection, as for all other morbilliviruses, is the profound but transient immunosuppression induced by the virus in its host with the consequence of increased susceptibility to opportunistic infections and increased mortality (Rajak

Table 21.1 Live attenuated PPRV vaccine strains commercially available (2018).

Vaccine strain	Country of origin	Animal species of origin	Lineage	Full genome sequence availability
Nigeria 75/1	Nigeria	Goat	II	Yes GenBank no. X74443
Sungri-96	India	Goat	IV	Yes GenBank no. KF727981 GenBank no. KJ867542
Arasur 87	India	Sheep	IV	Not available
Coimbatore	India	Goat	IV	Not available
Titu	Bangladesh	Goat	IV	Not available

et al. 2005). This immunosuppression is a consequence not only of the direct effect of the virus multiplying in and killing lymphoid cells but also specific morbillivirus mechanisms that overcome the host immune response, such as interference with the action of innate or induced immune responses or the blocking of interferon synthesis (Servet et al. 2003). However, although profound, the immunosuppression induced by morbilliviruses is transient and recovery from the disease is usually followed by the establishment of a strong, specific, and long-term protective immune response of the host (Servet-Delprat et al. 2003; Cosby et al. 2006).

Attenuated morbillivirus vaccines seem to have less immunosuppressive capacity compared with wild-type viruses but to have conserved their strong immune-stimulating characteristic (Cosby et al. 2006). Antibodies to PPRV are detected in animals as soon as 1 week after PPRV infection/vaccination. The vaccinated animals are protected against PPR for at least 3 years, and probably for their lifetime (Diallo et al. 2007; Sen et al. 2010; Zahur et al. 2014). Young animals born from dams that have been previously PPRV vaccinated or that have recovered from PPRV infection retain maternal anti-PPRV antibodies for up to 3–4 months (Ata et al. 1989; Bidjeh et al. 1999; Awa et al. 2002; Bodjo et al. 2006; Diallo et al. 2007; Balamurugan et al. 2012).

21.4 Desired Specifications When Ordering Vaccine

All PPR vaccines currently in use are:

- live attenuated PPR virus and are produced in Vero cells
- thermolabile so the vaccine must be supplied in conditions that minimize the loss of activity: freeze-dried or dehydrated and kept cold
- not compatible with tests that allow differentiating infected from vaccinated animals (DIVA) (Diallo et al. 2007).

All the above characteristics should be taken into consideration when ordering PPR vaccine and desired specifications are as follows:

- *Type of vaccine*: freeze-dried or dehydrated PPR attenuated cell culture vaccine, produced in Vero cells in accordance with the OIE standards (OIE 2018).
- *Quality control certificate*: vaccine quality controlled by an independent institution recognized by the OIE and/or FAO for vaccine control. The vaccine quality control certificate issued by the independent institution should be made available to the buyer.
- *Cold chain*: vaccine should be stored and supplied in a cold chain (maintained at 4–10 °C with ice packs during the transport). Each individual package should contain vaccine vial monitors (VVMs) (www.who.int/immunization/documents/IIP2015_Module2.pdf).
- *Dose of vaccine*: one dose of the attenuated virus vaccine for a sheep or goat must contain at least $10^{2.5}$ $TCID_{50}$ of live virus, the OIE recommended dose (desired dose: 10^3 $TCID_{50}$).
- *Packaging*: the vaccine is to be supplied in vials of (number of doses/vial to be specified by the buyer) with the equivalent appropriate diluent to be used for reconstituting the freeze-dried vaccine just before use. Each vial should be labeled with the number of content doses, the identification number (production lot number), and an expiry date. An instruction manual must be provided with the vaccine.

21.5 Quality Assurance and Control Testing

Each batch of vaccine, before delivery, should be tested and certified as free of extraneous agents (bacteria, fungi, mycoplasma, and other viruses). Bovine viral diarrhea virus (BVDV) is a frequent contaminant of sera used for cell culture so care has to be taken to avoid using such contaminated sera at any step of vaccine preparation.

The safety of the vaccine master seed must be tested in laboratory animals to document its freedom from nonspecific toxicity. The PPR virus identity of the vaccine must be tested and its potency must be proved in animals (test to be done only with a sample of the master seed).

As the residual moisture can affect the half-life of the vaccine during storage, its content must not exceed 2% in the final freeze-dried (or dehydrated) vaccine.

A test should prove that no virucidal activity has been detected in the diluent to be used with the vaccine.

21.6 Vaccine Application for Disease Control

21.6.1 PPR Control: The Vaccination Strategy

As PPRV transmission from excreting animals to naïve animals is mainly brought about by close contact, PPR can be controlled efficiently by application of strict sanitary preventive measures which consist of: (i) restriction of importations of susceptible animals from infected areas to disease-free areas, (ii) in case of outbreaks, implementation of a stamping-out policy, followed by disinfection of premises and compensation of affected farmers.

As most PPR-endemic areas are developing countries, these drastic measures are difficult to implement. Therefore, the main means available for the efficient prevention and control of PPR in these countries is by vaccination. In the PPR-GCES (Anonymous 2015), PPR vaccination should be carried out according to the epidemiological situation of each area/country. It is suggested that vaccination of animals older than 4 months be implemented in two successive years followed by another one or two more years of vaccination targeted to only new animals in the flock or those which were less than 4 months old during the previous vaccination rounds. This strategy takes into consideration the fact that kids and lambs born from dams previously vaccinated or having recovered from natural infection have passive immunity that lasts for about 3 months (Bidjeh et al. 1999; Awa et al. 2002; Bodjo et al. 2006). As that immunity might interfere with vaccination, it is advised not to vaccinate animals less than 4 months old in PPR-endemic areas.

The actual vaccination program and number of vaccination rounds (one or two per year) may differ from this general scheme according to the specific epidemiological situation and the animal production system in the target area. In the PPR-GCES, three major production systems have been identified: rangeland pastoralism, mixed farming, and commercial periurban and urban systems. The flock population turnover (births and other introductions of unvaccinated animals on the one hand versus deaths and off-take due to sales, for example, on the other hand) will differ from one production system to another. Animal turnover tends to be higher in the humid farming and commercial production systems compared with the pastoralist ones. Preliminary epidemiological investigations may also identify critical areas where vaccinations may be needed to stop spread of disease to currently free areas. Depending on the assessment and surveillance data, the vaccination should be time-bound, with high coverage, to achieve a population immunity rate (PIR) of at least 70%, a rate that is estimated in the PPR-GCES to be needed for PPR elimination (Anonymous 2015; Hammami et al. 2016, 2018). This threshold has been suggested according to the experience in Morocco after its first PPR outbreak in 2008 (Ettair 2012; Hammami et al. 2018). The strategy of high-coverage vaccination is more efficient for PPR control and eradication and less costly than continuous, low-coverage annual vaccination campaigns. Hammami et al. (2018) indicated that vaccination coverage must be higher than 60% in order to reach the 70% threshold of postvaccination immunity rate recommended in the PPR-GCES. It is noteworthy that with the current live attenuated PPR vaccine, emergency vaccination of animals in the face of a PPR outbreak can prevent its extension.

21.6.2 Possible Combination of PPR Vaccination With That for Other Small Ruminant Diseases

Combining PPR vaccination with vaccination for other priority diseases is highly cost-effective, as the major cost of a vaccination program is related to the delivery system (storage, transport, technical staff, etc.), the cost of which does not change much whether one or more diseases are targeted for control at the same time. The disease(s) to be controlled along with PPR must be identified as priority disease(s) for the country/region by veterinary services. Good examples of such diseases are sheep pox and goat pox, which not only have a similar distribution to PPR but also are alike in being controlled by live attenuated viral vaccines produced in cell cultures. Some preliminary studies have demonstrated the feasibility of combined PPR and sheep pox/goat pox vaccination (Martrenchar et al. 1997; Hosamani et al. 2006; Chaudhary et al. 2009).

21.7 Monitoring and Evaluation of Vaccination Campaigns and Their Effectiveness

To assess the results of a vaccination campaign, the PPR-GCES includes a postvaccination evaluation (PVE) tool (Anonymous 2015). This is a guide, based on performance indicators, describing methods to assess the immunity of small ruminant populations and to measure changes in the level of PPR outbreaks and/or small ruminant productivity. When a failure of vaccination is noted, its cause has to be investigated and corrective measures implemented. The success of a vaccination program depends upon many factors such as: (i) the vaccine quality, (ii) the effectiveness of the vaccine delivery system, and (iii) the targeted population coverage. All these factors must be monitored regularly, along with the host immune response during the vaccination campaign.

21.7.1 Vaccine Quality

It is recommended that vaccination campaigns should use vaccines that have been quality controlled independently of the manufacturer.

21.7.2 Vaccine Delivery Chain

The vaccine delivery chain that starts from the vaccine producer up to the moment of vaccination in the field is critical for the success of a vaccination campaign. As all current commercial PPR vaccines are live attenuated PPRV that are thermolabile, they must be maintained in a cold chain from production up to the moment of vaccination, in order to avoid inactivation of the virus and to ensure that the host has received the correct vaccine dose. The freeze-dried PPR vaccine is stable at +4–8 °C for at least 2–3 years. As the half-life of PPRV in suspension is about 3 hours at 37 °C (Diallo 2010), it is recommended to use the vaccine within 30–60 minutes after reconstitution of the freeze-dried product, depending on the diluent. Water, even of good quality, must never be used as a diluent to reconstitute the freeze-dried vaccine as this will result in a dramatic reduction of the vaccine titer (A. Diallo, personal observation).

The vaccination campaign must be planned and organized in a way that provides field users with sufficient vaccine at the right time. This is a challenging task in many developing countries, where veterinary services may not be well equipped and where access to remote and pastoral husbandry areas may be difficult. Such difficulties may have an important impact on the vaccine coverage. As already indicated above, it is estimated in the PPR-GCES that a coverage rate of at least 70%, based on the serology response, is needed for a successful eradication program (Anonymous 2015). Therefore, postvaccination serology surveys are important in evaluating vaccination effectiveness and success of the campaign.

21.7.3 Vaccination Campaign Coverage and Seromonitoring

Ideally, before the campaign, or on the day of vaccination, particularly in an enzootic zone, a sero-survey should be conducted to establish the baseline prevalence of PPR antibodies within the target population. Serological surveys that are conducted after vaccination will have the following objectives:

- to evaluate vaccination effectiveness by estimating the number of epidemiological units that show seroconversion after each round of vaccination
- to evaluate population immunity at a given time and over time after several vaccination campaigns by comparison with the results prior to vaccination of the target population.

Information on the age of animals from which sera are collected will allow the results to be stratified by age for more informed analysis.

In the PPR-GCES PVE tool, guidelines are provided for serum sampling protocols and for interpretation of the results. Although the prescribed test for PPR serology is the virus neutralization test (VNT), the assay that is most used currently for testing sera for PPR antibodies is the enzyme-linked immunosorbent assay (ELISA) and commercial kits that are based on this technology (Saliki et al. 1993; Anderson and McKay 1994; Libeau et al. 1995; Singh et al. 2004a; OIE 2018).

In addition to serological monitoring, the effectiveness of the vaccination campaign can be evaluated by recording PPR incidence/prevalence following passive and active surveillance. The success of the vaccination should result in a dramatic reduction of the disease incidence, even its absence, and an increase of animal productivity in the vaccinated area. Any detected vaccination failure must be investigated to identify its possible cause and required corrective actions. The possible sources of failure and that need regular checks/evaluations are as follows:

- *Vaccine quality*: vaccine samples must be collected randomly and submitted to laboratory quality control, even if a quality certificate was provided by the vaccine producer.
- *Vaccine storage*: the quality of the cold chain from the central vaccine storage up to its delivery in the field. The vaccine should always be kept cool until the moment of vaccination.
- *Quality of veterinary services*: vaccination teams, public and private, have to be trained for the task.
- *Vaccine coverage*: as indicated earlier, a coverage rate of at least 70% of the target population should be obtained. This needs careful planning, including sensitization of sheep and goat owners, to encourage them to participate in the vaccination campaign.

21.8 Availability and List of Manufacturers

More than 30 institutions in Africa, the Middle East, the Near East, and Asia produce PPR vaccines. The list in Table 21.2 may not be complete.

The Pan African Veterinary Vaccine Centre of the African Union (AU/PANVAC) provides independent testing of the quality of PPRV vaccine to be used in Africa, whether produced there or elsewhere. Its activity is recognized by both the FAO and OIE and it is now the OIE collaborating center for veterinary vaccine quality control.

21.9 Summary and Conclusions

Peste des petits ruminants is an important livestock disease, present, in 2016, in about 70 countries in Africa, the Middle East, Near East, and Asia. It threatens the production of more than 1.7 billion sheep and goats, representing

Table 21.2 List of PPR vaccine manufacturers (2018).

Name	Address	Country	Tel	Fax	Email address/website
Botswana Vaccine Institute	Broadhurst Industrial Site, Lejara Road, Private Bag 0031, Gaborone	Botswana	+267 391 27 11	+267 3956798	bvigm@mega.bw
LANAVET	BP 503 Garoua	Cameroon	+237 227 13 05/999 98 18	+237 999 9875	lanavet@iccnet.cm
National Veterinary Institute	P.O. Box 19, Debre-Zeit	Ethiopia	251-1-33 84 11	251-1-33 93 00	nvi-rt@telecom.net.et
Kenya Veterinary Vaccines Production Institute (KEVEVAPI)	P.O. Box 53260, Nairobi 00200	Kenya	+254 20 2611143; +254 20 3540071	+254 20 2472881	vaccines@wananchi.com; vaccines@kevevapi.org
Laboratoire Central Vétérinaire	BP 2295, Bamako	Mali	+223 224 33 44 /224 66 53	+223 2249809	labovetmali@labovetmali.org
Société De Productions Biologiques et Pharmaceutiques Vétérinaires BIOPHARMA	Avenue Hassan II km 2-BP 4569-10000 Rabat	Morocco	+212 537-69-16-92	+ 212 537-69-16-89	www.biopharma.ma/index.php/fr/ info@biopharma.ma
MCI Santé Animale	Lot 157, ZI Sud-Ouest P.O. Box 278, C.P. 28810, Mohammadia	Morocco	+212 5233-03132	+212 (0)5 23 30 21 30	www.mci-santeanimale.com
National Veterinary Research Institute	P.M.B. 1 Vom-Jos Plateau State, Nigeria	Nigeria	234.073.281452	+44 20 8181 7080	nvri1924@yahoo.com
Institut Sénégalais de Recherches Agricoles (ISRA) ISRA-Production	Route du Front de Terre, BP 2057, Dakar-Hann	Senegal	+221 832 27 62	+221 83221 18	productionvaccins@isra.sn www.isra.sn
Central Veterinary Research Laboratory	P.O. Box 8067, El Amarat-Khartoum	Sudan	+249 912 657 624		munaelhaj@hotmail.com
Veterinary Serum and Vaccine Research Institute	P.O. Box 131, 11381, Cairo, Abbasia, El-Sekka El-Beida St	Egypt	+202 38224406 +20223421009 +202.23421866	+202 2342821	svri@idsc.gov.eg http://vsvri-eg.com
Jordan Bio Industries Center (JOVAC)	P.O. Box 43, Amman 11941	Jordan	+96265232162/5232745	+962 6 5232210	sales@jovaccenter.com
	P.O. Box 15831, Riyadh 11454	Kingdom of Saudi Arabia	+966 1 459 09 63		m_a_alhamad@yahoo.com mzaljulaifi@yahoo.com
Central Veterinary Control and Research Institute	06020 Etlik, Ankara	Turkey	+90 3123260090 +90.4.321.1200	+90 3123211755	ehh.o@tr.net and/or etlik@vet.gov.tr www.etlikvet.gov.tr
VETAL Animal Health Products	Gölbasi Yolu Uzeri 7km, Adiyaman	Turkey	+90.416.223.20.30 or +90.416.223.24.88	90.416.223.14.56	vetal@vetal.com.tr www.vetal.com.tr

(Continued)

Table 21.2 (Continued)

Name	Address	Country	Tel	Fax	Email address/website
Dollvet	Organize Sanayi Bölgesi 8. no: 3, Cadde Merkez Sanliurfa	Turkey	+90.414.3691133	+90.414.3691662	dollvet@dollvet.com.tr www.dollvet.com.tr
Razi Vaccine and Serum Research Institute	P.O. Box 31975/148, Hessarak, Karaj	Iran	+98 26 34554658	+98 26 34552194	www.rvsri.ac.ir
Veterinary Research Institute	Al-Faisal Town, Zarar Shaheed Road 45800, Lahore Cantt	Pakistan	+92 42-99220338 +92 42-99220140		dvri@livestockpunjab.com.pk
Center for Advance Studies in Vaccinology and Biotechnology (CASVAB), University of Balochistan	Brewery Road, Quetta, 87300, Balochistan	Pakistan	+92 81-2854551	+92 81-9213134	tariqkianiraja@hotmail.com
Intervac Pvt Ltd Pakistan	113/3 Allama Iqbal Road, Ghari Shahu, Lahore 54141	Pakistan	+92-(0)42-6306957 & 6364411	+92-(0)42-6374378	info@intervacpvtltd.com intervac@brain.net.pk
PPR Section, Livestock Research Institute (LRI)	Mohakhali, Dhaka-1212	Bangladesh	+880.2.8821991	+880.2.9898896	director@lri.gov.bd
Hester Biosciences Nepal Pvt Ltd.	Arun Plaza, (HIM Service) 2nd Floor, Sundhara, Kathmandu	Nepal	Tel:+977-1-4218322		sulochana.shrestha@hester.com.np
Directorate of Animal Health Biological Products Division	Veterinary Complex, Tripuresway, GPO Box 20295, Kathmandu	Nepal	+977-01252348 +977-01-261569, 4261165	+977-01261521	bpdtri@wlink.com.np ahdt@wlink.com.np ahd@healthnet.org.np
Hester Biosciences Limited	Pushpak 1st floor, Motilal Hirabhai Road, Panchvati, Ahmedabad, Gujarat 380006	India	+91 79 2644 5106/+91 79 2644 5107	+91-79 2644 5105	mail@hester.in
Intervet India Pvt Ltd, MSD Animal Health	33, Intervet House, Behind Eden Garden, Pune Nagar Road, Maharashtra 411014	India	+91-20-66207876, +91-9890623301, +91-20 2705 1800, +91-20 6605 0400	+91-20 6605 0410	info.india@intervet.com, sreenivasulu.kilari@sp.intervet.com sreenivasulu.kilari@merck.com
Indian Immunologicals Ltd.	Rakshapuram, Gachibowli Post, Hyderabad 500032, Telangana	India	+91-9948298622, +91-9948298522, +91-40 23000211, +91-40 23000212, +91-40 23000512	+91-40 23000213	info@indimmune.com
Bio-Med Pvt. Ltd.	C-96, Site No. 1, Bulandshahar Road, Industrial Area, Ghaziabad-201 009 (U.P)	India	+91-120-2700881, +91-120-2753255, +91-120-4157534	+91-120-4340219	saryugarg@yahoo.com

Brilliant Bio Pharma Pvt. Ltd.	6-2-1012, TGV Mansions, 3rd floor, Khairatabad Rd, Indira Nagar, Khairatabad, Hyderabad, Telangana 500004	India	+91-40-66667464, +91-40-66772726	+91-40-66104915, +91-40-66772725	brilliantvetvac@rediffmail.com exports@bbpl.co.in domestic@bbpl.co.in
Telangana State Veterinary Biologicals & Research Institute (TSVBRI)	Shanthinagar, Hyderabad-28, Telangana	India	+91-40-23316366	+91-40-23307982	spgp.vbri@gmail.com vbri_ahd@ yahoo.com
Institute of Animal Health and Veterinary Biologicals (IAH&VB), Bengaluru	KVAFSU, Hebbal, Bengaluru 560024	India	+91-802341 1502	+91-8482-245107/245241	info@iahvb.com
Institute of Animal Health and Veterinary Biologicals (IAH&VB), Kerala	Palode, Pacha, Thiruvananthapuram, Kerala- 695 562	India	+91-472-2840262		dirvbi@kerala.nic.in
Xinjiang Tecon Biology Co., Ltd	Tecon Building, Changchun South Road No. 528, Urumqi, Xinjiang Uygur Autonomous Region	China	+86 09916679236	+86 09916679234	xjtcsw@tcsw.com.cn www.tcsw.com.cn
Veterinary Biologicals Factory of Tibet Autonomous Region	Tzu Chi Tong East Road No. 74, Lhasa, Tibet Autonomous Region	China	+86 08916382082	+86 08916322268	Not available
National Research Institute for Veterinary Virology & Microbiology of Russia (NRIVVaMR)	601120, Pokrov, Petushki Area, Vladimir Region	Russia	+7.49243.61407	+7 49243 62125	lunitsin@mail.ru www.vniivvim.ru
Russian Academy of Agricultural Science (RAAS)					

Disclaimer: It was the authors' intention to list all vaccine producers and are not responsible for the safety, quality, and effectiveness of the vaccines listed in the table.

nearly 80% of the global population, with a yearly loss estimated at about US$ 2.1 billion (Anonymous 2015). Indeed, Perry et al. (2002) identified PPR as one of the priority animal diseases whose control was considered important for poverty alleviation in western Africa and southern Asia.

With the success of the global rinderpest eradication that was officially achieved in 2011, a consensus is building that eradication of PPR is the next most viable candidate for livestock infectious disease eradication (Anderson et al. 2011; Baron et al. 2011; Albina et al. 2013). Indeed, a number of factors that have made possible the success of rinderpest global eradication would also apply to PPR: (i) a virus inducing life-long immunity in animals that have recovered from infection, (ii) this induced immunity is a sterile immunity as no carrier state follows the recovery from an infection (at least not known yet), (iii) existence of live attenuated vaccines that have preserved this strong immune capacity of the wild type, (iv) existence of only one virus serotype, i.e. a single vaccine strain will protect animals against all other strains (v) affordable vaccine that can be produced and delivered at low cost (Silva et al. 2008), and finally (vi) specific and highly sensitive diagnostic tests are available for the surveillance and detection of the disease (Anderson and McKay 1994; Libeau et al. 1994, 1995; Couacy-Hymann et al. 2002; Kwiatek et al. 2010; Ashraf et al. 2017).

Given the availability of modern tools, the global PPR control and eradication program being initiated by the FAO and the OIE can be started now, provided that the funds required are made available. PPR vaccines that are in use currently are thermolabile but research has been conducted to improve their thermostability (Worrall et al. 2001; Sarkar et al. 2003; Silva et al. 2011, 2014). It is expected that new products derived from this research will be commercially available in the near future.

References

Adombi, C.M., Waqas, A., Dundon, W.G. et al. (2016). Peste des petits ruminants in Benin: persistence of a single virus genotype in the country for over 42 years. *Transbound. Emerg. Dis.* 64: 1037–1044.

Albina, E., Kwiatek, O., Minet, C. et al. (2013). Peste des petits ruminants, the next eradicated animal disease? *Vet. Microbiol.* 165: 38–44.

Anderson, J. and McKay, J.A. (1994). The detection of antibodies against peste des petits ruminants virus in cattle, sheep and goats and the possible implications to rinderpest control programmes. *Epidemiol. Infect.* 112: 225–231.

Anderson, J., Baron, M., Cameron, A. et al. (2011). Rinderpest eradicated; what next? *Vet. Rec.* 169: 10–11.

Anonymous. (2015). PPR Global Control and Eradication Strategy (PPR-GCES). www.fao.org/3/a-i4460e.pdf

Ashraf, W., Unger, H., Haris, S. et al. (2017). Genetic detection of peste des petits ruminants virus under field conditions: a step forward toward disease eradication. *BMC Vet. Res.* 13 (1): 34.

Ata, F.A., Al Sumry, H.S., King, G.J. et al. (1989). Duration of maternal immunity to peste des petits ruminants. *Vet. Rec.* 124 (22): 590–591.

Awa, D.N., Ngagnou, A., Tefiang, E. et al. (2002). Post vaccination and colostral peste des petits ruminants antibody dynamics in research flocks of Kirdi goats and Foulbe sheep of north Cameroon. *Prev. Vet. Med.* 55 (4): 265–271.

Balamurugan, V., Sen, A., Venkatesan, G. et al. (2012). Study on passive immunity: time of vaccination in kids born to goats vaccinated against peste des petits ruminants. *Virol. Sin.* 27 (4): 228–233.

Banyard, A.C., Parida, S., Batten, C. et al. (2010). Global distribution of peste des petits ruminants virus and prospects for improved diagnosis and control. *J. Gen. Virol.* 91: 2885–2897.

Baron, M.D., Parida, S., and Oura, C.A. (2011). Peste des petits ruminants: a suitable candidate for eradication? *Vet. Rec.* 169: 16–21.

Baron, M.D., Diallo, A., Lancelot, R., and Libeau, G. (2016). Peste des petits ruminants virus. *Adv. Virus Res.* 95: 1–42.

Barrett, T., Banyard, A.C., and Diallo, A. (2006). Molecular biology of the Morbilliviruses. In: *Rinderpest and Peste des Petits Ruminants Virus: Plague of Large and Small Ruminants; Biology of Animal Infections* (eds. T. Barrett, P.P. Pastoret and W. Taylor), 31–67. London: Academic Press.

Bidjeh, K., Diguimbaye, C., Hendrikx, P. et al. (1999). Immunité passive colostrale chez les jeunes issus des chèvres et brebis vaccinées avec le vaccin anti-peste des petits ruminants. *Cah. Agric.* 8 (3): 219–222.

Bodjo, S.C., Couacy-Hymann, E., Koffi, M.Y., and Danho, T. (2006). Assessment of the duration of maternal antibodies specific to the homologous peste des petits ruminant vaccine "Nigeria 75/1" in Djallonké lambs. *Biokemistri* 18 (2): 99–103.

Chaudhary, S.S., Pandey, K.D., Singh, R.P. et al. (2009). A vero cell derived combined vaccine against sheep pox and peste des petits ruminants for sheep. *Vaccine* 27: 2548–2553.

Cosby, S.L., Chieko, K., and Yamanouchi, K. (2006). Immunology of rinderpest – an immunosuppression but a lifelong vaccine protection. In: *Rinderpest and Peste Des*

Petits Ruminants Virus: Plague of Large and Small Ruminants; Biology of Animal Infections (eds. T. Barrett, P.P. Pastoret and W.P. Taylor), 197–221. London: Academic Press.

Couacy-Hymann, E., Roger, F., Hurard, C. et al. (2002). Rapid and sensitive detection of peste des petits ruminants virus by a polymerase chain reaction assay. *J. Virol. Methods* 100: 17–25.

Diallo, A. (2004). Vaccination for the control of peste des petits ruminants. In: *Control of Infectious Animal Diseases by Vaccination* (eds. A. Schudel and M. Lombard). Basel: Karger.

Diallo, A. (2010). Peste des petits ruminants. In: *Infectious and Parasitic Diseases of Livestock*, vol. 1 (eds. P.C. Lefèvre, J. Blancou, R. Chermette and G. Uilenberg), 245–262. Paris: Editions TEC&DOC, Lavoisier.

Diallo, A. and Libeau, G. (2014). Peste des petits ruminants. In: *Manual of Security Sensitive Microbes and Toxins* (ed. D. Liu), 703–714. Boca Raton: CRC Press.

Diallo, A., Taylor, W.P., Lefevre, P.C., and Provost, A. (1989). Attenuation d'une souche de la virus de peste des petits ruminants: candidat pour un vaccin homologue vivant. *Rev. Elev. Med. Vet. Pays Trop.* 42: 311–319.

Diallo, A., Minet, C., Le Goff, C. et al. (2007). The threat of peste des petits ruminants: progress in vaccine development for disease control. *Vaccine* 25: 5591–5597.

Ettair, M. (2012). Stratégie de surveillance et de lutte contre la PPR au Maroc. In: *REMESA: atelier conjoint REPIVET-RESEPSA des 12 et 13 Juillet 2012*, 1–15. Tunis.

Gargadennec, L. and Lalanne, A. (1942). La peste des petits ruminants. *Bull. Serv. Zoo. A.O.F.* 5: 16–21.

Hammami, P., Lancelot, R., and Lesnoff, M. (2016). Modeling the dynamics of post-vaccination immunity rate in a population of Sahelian sheep after a vaccination campaign against peste des petits ruminants virus. *PLoS One* 11 (9): e0161769.

Hammami, P., Lancelot, R., Domenech, J., and Lesnoff, M. (2018). Ex-ante assessment of different vaccination-based control schedules against the peste des petits ruminants virus in sub-Saharan Africa. *PLoS One* 13 (1): e0190296.

Hodgson, S., Moffat, K., Hill, H. et al. (2018). Comparison of the immunogenicity and cross-lineage efficacy of live attenuated peste des petits ruminants virus vaccines PPRV/Nigeria/75/1 and PPRV/Sungri/96. *J. Virol.* 92 (24): e01471–e01418.

Hosamani, M., Singh, S.K., Mondal, B. et al. (2006). A bivalent vaccine against goat pox and peste des petits ruminants induces protective immune response in goats. *Vaccine* 24: 6058–6064.

Kwiatek, O., Keita, D., Gil, P. et al. (2010). Quantitative one-step real-time RT-PCR for the fast detection of the four genotypes of PPRV. *J. Virol. Methods* 165: 168–177.

Lefèvre, P.C. (2010). Rinderpest. In: *Infectious and Parasitic Diseases of Livestock*, vol. 1 (eds. P.C. Lefèvre, J. Blancou, R. Chermette and G. Uilenberg), 225–244. Paris: Editions TEC&DOC, Lavoisier.

Libeau, G., Diallo, A., and Parida, S. (2014). Evolutionary genetics underlying the spread of peste des petits ruminants virus. *Animal Front.* 4: 14–20.

Libeau, G., Diallo, A., Colas, F., and Guerre, L. (1994). Rapid differential diagnosis of rinderpest and peste des petits ruminants using an immunocapture ELISA. *Vet. Rec.* 134: 300–304.

Libeau, G., Préhaud, C., Lancelot, R. et al. (1995). Development of a competitive ELISA for detecting antibodies to the peste des petits ruminants virus using a recombinant nucleoprotein. *Res. Vet. Sci.* 58: 50–55.

Martrenchar, A., Zoyem, N., and Diallo, A. (1997). Study of a mixed vaccine against peste des petits ruminants and capripox infection in Northern Cameroon. *Small Rumin. Res.* 26: 39–44.

OIE. (2018). Manual of Diagnostic Tests and Vaccines for Terrestrial Animals. www.oie.int/en/international-standard-setting/terrestrial-manual/access-online

Parida, S., Muniraju, M., Mahapatra, M. et al. (2015). Peste des petits ruminants. *Vet. Microbiol.* 181: 90–106.

Perry, B.D., Randolph, T.F., McDermott, J.J. et al. (2002). *Investing in Animal Health Research to Alleviate Poverty*, 148. Nairobi: International Livestock Research Institute.

Rajak, K.K., Sreenivasa, B.P., Hosamani, M. et al. (2005). Experimental studies on immunosuppressive effects of peste des petits ruminants (PPR) virus in goats. *Comp. Immunol. Microbiol. Infect. Dis.* 28: 287–296.

Saliki, J.T., Libeau, G., House, J.A. et al. (1993). Monoclonal antibody-based blocking enzyme-linked immunosorbent assay for specific detection and titration of peste-des-petits-ruminants virus antibody in caprine and ovine sera. *J. Clin. Microbiol.* 31: 1075–1082.

Sarkar, J., Sreenivasa, B.P., Singh, R.P. et al. (2003). Comparative efficacy of various chemical stabilizers on the thermostability of a live-attenuated peste des petits ruminants (PPR) vaccine. *Vaccine* 21: 4728–4735.

Sen, A., Saravanan, P., Balamurugan, V. et al. (2010). Vaccines against peste des petits ruminants virus. *Expert Rev. Vaccines* 9: 785–796.

Servet-Delprat, C., Vidalain, P.O., Valentin, H., and Rabourdin-Combe, C. (2003). Measles virus and dendritic cell functions: how specific response cohabits with immunosuppression. *Curr. Top. Microbiol. Immunol.* 276: 103–123.

Silva, A.C., Delgado, I., Sousa, M.F. et al. (2008). Scalable culture systems using different cell lines for the production of peste des petits ruminants vaccine. *Vaccine* 9 (26): 3305–3311.

Silva, A.C., Carrondo, M.J., and Alves, P.M. (2011). Strategies for improved stability of peste des petits ruminants vaccine. *Vaccine* 29: 4983–4991.

Silva, A.C., Yami, M., Libeau, G. et al. (2014). Testing a new formulation for peste des petits ruminants vaccine in Ethiopia. *Vaccine* 32: 2878–2881.

Singh, R.P. and Bandyopadhyay, S.K. (2015). Peste des petits ruminants vaccine and vaccination in India: sharing experience with disease endemic countries. *VirusDisease* 26: 215–224.

Singh, R.P., Sreenivasa, B.P., Dhar, P. et al. (2004a). Development of monoclonal antibody based competitive-ELISA for detection and titration of antibodies to peste des petits ruminants virus. *Vet. Microbiol.* 98: 3–15.

Singh, R.P., Sreenivasa, B.P., Dhar, P., and Bandyopadhyay, S.K. (2004b). A sandwich ELISA for the diagnosis of peste des petits ruminants (PPR) infection in small ruminants using anti-nucleocapsid protein monoclonal antibody. *Arch. Virol.* 149 (11): 2155–2170.

Singh, R.K., Balamurugan, V., Bhanuprakash, V. et al. (2009). Possible control and eradication of peste des petits ruminants from India: technical aspects. *Vet. Ital.* 45: 449–462.

Worrall, E.E., Litamoi, J.K., Seck, B.M., and Ayelet, G. (2001). An ultra rapid method for the dehydration and preservation of live attenuated rinderpest and peste des petits ruminants vaccines. *Vaccine* 19: 834–839.

Zahur, A.B., Irshad, H., Ullah, A. et al. (2014). Peste des petits ruminants caccine (Nigerian Strain 75/1) confers protection for at least 3 years in sheep and goats. *J. Biosci. Med.* 2 (06): 27.

22

Brucellosis

José Maria Blasco[1], *Edgardo Moreno*[2,3], *and Ignacio Moriyón*[4]

[1] Animal Health Department IA2 CITA, Universidad de Zaragoza, Zaragoza, Spain
[2] Programa de Investigación en Enfermedades Tropicales, Escuela de Medicina Veterinaria, Universidad Nacional, Heredia, Costa Rica
[3] Instituto Clodomiro Picado, Universidad de Costa Rica, San José, Costa Rica
[4] Instituto de Saludad Tropical y Departamento de Microbiología y Parasitología, Universidad de Navarra, Pamplona, Spain

22.1 Introduction

Brucellosis is a zoonotic disease of worldwide distribution that affects a broad range of domestic and wild mammals. Members of the genus *Brucella*, a group of intracellular gram-negative bacteria, cause this disease. Presently, nine *Brucella* species have been recognized: *Brucella abortus* (infecting mainly cattle), *B. melitensis* (infecting mainly sheep and goats), *B. suis* (infecting swine and wildlife), *B. neotomae* (infecting the desert rat), *B. ovis* (infecting sheep), *B. canis* (infecting dogs), *B. ceti* (infecting cetaceans), *B. pinnipedialis* (infecting seals), and *B. microti* (infecting common voles). Proposals for new species (e.g. *B. inopinata* and *papionis*) correspond to sporadic isolates from rodents, humans, or baboons (Whatmore 2009; Whatmore et al. 2014). The *Brucella* genus and species can be identified by classic microbiological methods but DNA studies performed on isolates is currently the method of choice. Using conventional microbiological and serological tests, *B. melitensis*, *B. abortus*, and *B. suis* were divided into biovars (3, 7, and 5, respectively) several decades ago (Alton et al. 1988). Biovar typing by classic methods is difficult and not always consistent with that obtained with DNA analysis tools (Le Fleche et al. 2006).

The main clinical signs of animal brucellosis are abortion and infertility, and are not disease specific. Indeed, infected animals do not necessarily abort: this occurs frequently in the first pregnancy but becomes less likely thereafter because of sustained immunity. However, in all cases the condition is highly contagious because it is spread through contact with aborted fetuses, placentae, vaginal fluids, and milk, as well as congenitally and venereally. Humans acquire brucellosis through direct contact with infected animals (e.g. veterinarians, abattoir workers, and livestock keepers) and consumption of contaminated dairy products, but they are not a source of contagion. Thus, control of the infection in livestock, and proper food hygiene, especially pasteurization of dairy products, are the only means to reduce or avoid the disease in humans.

Human brucellosis is a debilitating chronic disease that requires prolonged and combined antibiotic therapy and, if untreated, is fatal in 1–5% of cases and may lead to permanent damage (Dalrymple-Champneys 1960; Zinsstag et al. 2011). Although some brucellae are practically not (*B. suis* biovar 2) or not at all (*B. ovis*) pathogenic for humans, most species and biovars are highly infectious. In humans, the disease lacks pathognomonic symptoms and presents a clinical picture that varies, usually according to the *Brucella* species: *B. melitensis* causes the gravest form, followed by *B. suis*, *B. abortus*, and *B. canis* (Spink 1956; Lucero et al. 2010). Two severe human brucellosis cases due to *B. neotomae* have been reported recently (Villalobos-Vindas et al. 2017). *B ceti*, *B. pinnipedialis*, and *B. microti* are confined to wildlife and have not been reported to infect humans. *B. ovis* is not infectious for humans, and *B. suis* biovar 2, present in wildlife and a cause of brucellosis outbreaks in domestic pigs throughout Europe, only infects immunocompromised people.

There are few well-documented studies on the economic impact of brucellosis that take into account all aspects of the disease. Losses depend on the prevalence, the animal species affected, and also on management, sociopolitical decisions, and marketing. An additional factor is the impact of the human disease but underreporting is common and hard data are scarce (Dean et al. 2012; Ducrotoy et al. 2014). A review of the studies available concludes that brucellosis is, in all likelihood, a major problem in low-

Veterinary Vaccines: Principles and Applications, First Edition. Edited by Samia Metwally, Gerrit Viljoen, and Ahmed El Idrissi.

income countries of Africa and Asia (McDermott et al. 2013). Nevertheless, there is general consensus that global losses can be substantially high, and the evidence indicates that the disease has a negative impact in Africa, the Middle East, Latin America, Eastern Europe, and large parts of Asia. Only Canada, USA, Japan, Australia, New Zealand, and Western and Central European countries are practically free from both *B. abortus* and *B. melitensis* in domestic animals. In these countries, eradication of *B. abortus* in cattle was achieved only after many years of costly investments in vaccination and culling. Because small ruminant breeding is often a less profitable activity practiced by farmers of marginal areas and under transhumance, eradicating *B. melitensis* has received less attention and been more difficult, and has only been achieved by some European Mediterranean countries, prompted mostly by the high impact of the human disease.

Nevertheless, globalization, environmental changes, and intensification of breeding have introduced new dimensions to zoonotic diseases (Jones et al. 2013), and from a practical standpoint, brucellosis is a disease of worldwide distribution. Indeed, there is increasing evidence that at least some countries – mostly the fast-growing economies – are currently suffering an emergence of brucellosis, often perceived as an increase in the awareness of the disease. For example, the number of human cases reported in China has increased steadily in recent decades, reaching an annual incidence as high as 1395 per 100 000 in some parts of Inner Mongolia, and analysis of over 2000 cases showed that almost 60% were initially misdiagnosed (Wang et al. 2012). The reasons for the high prevalence and incidence in many countries are diverse and, as mentioned above, include political, socioeconomic, and cultural causes. However, deficiencies in the management and application of control measures in domestic livestock are the common motif and in all likelihood the most important factor preventing progress toward control and eradication (Blasco and Molina-Flores 2011; McDermott et al. 2013).

Because of all the above circumstances, the disease poses severe economic, diagnostic, therapeutic, and prophylactic challenges to breeders, veterinarians, medical doctors, and public health authorities alike. Its socioeconomic impact, the need for One Health approaches, and the variety of hosts involved, including wildlife, make brucellosis a complex disease. This complexity is increased by the fact that, although some brucellae have a preferential host, the barriers are not strict and cross-infections can be significant in mixed husbandry systems, or in the domestic–wildlife interface, two conditions often imposed by environmental circumstances or related to cultural traditions. Thus, control and eradication are extremely difficult.

22.2 The Requirements of Brucellosis Vaccines

The conditions to be met by an ideal brucellosis vaccine have not changed since they were listed many years ago (World Health Organization 1999). In animals of both sexes and at any age, such a vaccine should: (i) be harmless and prevent infection with a single dose, (ii) not stimulate antibodies interfering with serodiagnosis, (iii) not be transmitted to humans or other animals (which includes no contamination of meat, edible organs, milk and dairy products), (iv) be stable, both *in vitro* and *in vivo*, (v) be readily cultivable under large-scale fermentation conditions, and (vi) be endowed with markers for easy differentiation from field isolates.

No current vaccine fulfills requirements (i)–(iv), so that these aspects will be discussed for each vaccine or vaccine candidate in the next sections. Suitable vaccines are available only against small ruminant and cattle brucellosis and, therefore, these discussions are limited to *B. abortus* and *B. melitensis* vaccines. Moreover, the concepts included in (i) are worth commenting on in the context of ruminant vaccines.

22.2.1 Protection

As abortion is the main clinical sign, a common misconception is to consider the rate of "protection against abortion" as a suitable index of protection against the disease and/or a useful characteristic by itself. However, infected animals that have not aborted are highly contagious and therefore of epidemiological relevance since they contribute to the perpetuation of the disease. Thus, brucellosis vaccines that reduce abortions and yet do not offer a good level of protection are counterproductive. In brucellosis, perhaps more than in other infectious diseases, the rule applies that "a bad vaccine is worse than no vaccine" because of the false security that a bad vaccine conveys (Moreno 2014).

Similarly important is to consider the challenge faced by vaccines and how this can vary according to the circumstances. For *B. abortus*, it has been estimated that up to 10^{14} bacteria are released during an abortion (Corner 1983), which means a challenge about 10^8 times higher than the estimated dose for inducing infection with 90% probability – about 10^6 bacteria – (Manthei 1959). When large numbers of stock are stabled together, the risk of exposure to such a high number of brucellae and infection is greater than when population density is low, as when the animals are bred extensively. Therefore, while intensification may provide conditions for better control, it increases the risks of transmission (Jones et al. 2013) and severely tests the efficacy of any vaccine. Indeed, herd size and animal density are well-known causes of brucellosis perpetuation in dairy farms even if vaccination is implemented (Nicoletti 1976).

It is thus critically important to understand that control and eventual eradication of brucellosis depend not only on vaccination but also on creating those conditions that minimize exposure (i.e. sound animal management, culling, restriction of animal movements, control of scavengers, hygiene, etc.). This is a relevant point when considering claims for the efficacy of vaccines that are based on observational studies carried out under favorable conditions. In brucellosis, these studies seldom include the appropriate control groups that would make the vaccine the only variable to be evaluated. Because controlled experiments allow for such groups, their interpretation looks straightforward. However, this is true only if: (i) the *Brucella* challenge infects a significant number of unvaccinated controls, (ii) the methodology (necropsy, use of the proper selective media and other bacteriological procedures, etc.) for isolating the challenge strain is sensitive enough to detect all infected animals, and (iii) the vaccines to be compared are included in the same experimental and challenge design. Regrettably, not all experiments meet these otherwise obvious conditions (Moriyón et al. 2004).

22.2.2 Vaccine Safety

It is important to consider the circumstances under which protection from abortion by a brucellosis vaccine are reported because ruminants are not uniformly susceptible throughout gestation. Moreover, safety issues are largely dependent also on the vaccine dose and vaccination route. Thus, while vaccination during the first third of pregnancy may result in no vaccine-induced abortions, the same vaccine can have a severe effect if applied during the second half, and particularly when the animals are vaccinated at mid-pregnancy. Consequently, claims about vaccine safety are only valid in this last context. Indeed, vaccination of pregnant animals is exceedingly difficult to avoid when mass vaccination strategies need to be implemented (Blasco and Molina-Flores 2011).

22.3 Brucellosis Live Vaccines

This chapter excludes vaccines claimed to be useful but on which the original experimental evidence either is not accessible – strains *B. abortus* 104-M, 82, 75/79-AB, A19, M5, and KB 17/100, and *B. melitensis* M5/90- (Deqiu et al. 2002; Denisov et al. 2013) – or has been disproved by experiments under controlled conditions – *B. suis* S2- (Xin 1986; Bosseray and Plommet 1990; Blasco et al. 1993a,b; Verger et al. 1995). For those that are well known, live vaccines have been vastly superior to inactivated (killed) products for the prevention of animal brucellosis caused by *B. abortus* or *B. melitensis* (Alton et al. 1988; Nicoletti 1990) (see also section 22.3.3). On the other hand, the brucellae are notorious for their tendency to undergo genetic drift *in vitro* and therefore, all live brucellosis vaccines should be prepared from a carefully maintained master seed and derived seed lots (see criterion (iv), section 22.2), and should pass controls for biological quality (i.e. residual virulence and immunogenicity) (Grilló et al. 2000, 2012; OIE 2017). Regrettably, this is not always the case and marketed live vaccines differ in quality. The importance of the biological controls cannot be overemphasized and it is a critical point that all potential users should keep in mind when choosing a vaccine or a vaccine manufacturer.

Brucella live vaccines are commonly classified as smooth or rough, the latter being used as differentiate between infected and vaccinated animals (DIVA) vaccines. A summary of their main characteristics is presented in Table 22.1 and they are discussed in more detail in the next sections.

22.3.1 The Classic Smooth Vaccines: *B. abortus* S19 and *B. melitensis* Rev1

22.3.1.1 Overall Characteristics

Developed more than 60 years ago, *B. abortus* S19 for cattle and *B. melitensis* Rev1 for sheep and goats remain the most effective vaccines, and their use has a great impact on the incidence of the disease in domestic ruminants and humans (Blasco 1997; Garin-Bastuji et al. 1998; Nicoletti 1990) They have been used worldwide for over 60 years and when combined with test and slaughter, they have been instrumental in almost all successful cases of eradication. The few cases where eradication has been achieved without the use of these two vaccines have been in countries or areas with exceptionally favorable epidemiological management and environmental conditions (small herds/flocks, tight control of animal movements, islands, etc.), proficient veterinary services, and the socioeconomic stability necessary for a sustained effort.

Both vaccines possess an intact smooth-type lipopolysaccharide (S-LPS) surface whose O-polysaccharide (O-PS) moiety carries the epitopes relevant in all the serodiagnostic tests of proven efficacy. Although the genomic sequence and proteome of *B. abortus* S19 and *B. melitensis* Rev1 have been described, the mechanisms for their attenuation remain elusive. Vaccine S19 was attenuated by suboptimal laboratory storage plus *in vitro* passages, and shows multiple genetic differences from virulent *B. abortus* biovar 1 counterparts (Crasta et al. 2008; Jones et al. 2013). *B. melitensis* Rev1 is a streptomycin-resistant revertant of a

Table 22.1 General characteristics of currently available brucellosis vaccines.

Vaccines	Advantages	Disadvantages	Comments
Smooth			
B. melitensis Rev 1	• Proven efficacy in control/eradication programs (France, Italy, Spain) • Effective against both *B. melitensis* and *B. ovis* • Safe in males and young replacements • Single dose affords useful protection for life • Biological quality control feasible (OIE protocol)	• Highly abortifacient • Serological interference in classic serological tests (RBT, CFT), indirect and competitive ELISAs, fluorescence polarization assay, and other S-LPS tests • Low virulence for humans; streptomycin resistant	• Safety issues minimized by avoiding vaccinating pregnant animals by the conjunctival route • Serological interference is minimized when applied to young animals by the conjunctival route • Human infections can be diagnosed using standard serological tests; treatment requires regimes that do not include streptomycin
B. abortus S19	• Proven efficacy in control/eradication programs (EU countries, USA, and Australia) • Protects cattle against both *B. abortus* and *B. melitensis* • Single dose affords useful protection for life • Biological quality control feasible (OIE protocol)	• Depending on the dose and vaccination route, can be abortifacient when used in pregnant cattle • Used subcutaneously, it is not safe in bulls (unknown safety when applied by the conjunctival route) • Serological interference in classic serological tests (RBT, CFT), indirect and competitive ELISAs, fluorescence polarization assay, and other S-LPS tests • Low virulence for humans	• Serological interference is minimized when reduced doses are applied to young animals (particularly by the conjunctival route) • Human infections can be diagnosed using standard serological tests; standard antibiotic treatment
Rough			
B. abortus RB51	• No interference in classic serological tests (RBT, CFT)	• Not recommended in pregnant cattle (abortifacient) or bulls • Less effective than S19 in inducing protective immunity (efficacy or revaccination unknown) • Unknown protection span • Protection of cattle against *B. melitensis* unknown • Serological interference in indirect and competitive ELISAs and fluorescence polarization assay • Low virulence for humans; rifampicin resistant	• No proven efficacy for eradication • No appropriate serological diagnostic tests to diagnose human infections; treatment requires regimes that do not include rifampicin

CFT, complement fixation test; ELISA, enzyme-linked immunosorbent assay; RBT, rose Bengal test; S-LPS, smooth-type lipopolysaccharide.

streptomycin-dependent mutant that carries a defect in ribosomal protein S12, in addition to other genetic differences from virulent *B. melitensis* biovar 1 counterparts. In other bacteria, S12 mutants show decreased rates of protein synthesis and, indeed, reduced fitness could account for the attenuation and S-LPS instability of Rev1 (Mancilla et al. 2013), and for the existence of inappropriate seed lots (Grilló et al. 2000; Blasco and Molina-Flores 2011).

Because both S19 and Rev1 are not protected by patents, they are marketed at relatively low cost (US$ 0.05–0.20 per dose). In controlled experiments, a single dose of these vaccines confers 50–100% protection against bacterial challenges infecting 80–100% of unvaccinated controls (Manthei 1959; Nicoletti 1990; Jacques et al. 2007; Barrio et al. 2009). In the case of S19, revaccination does not increase resistance (Beach et al. 1947; Berman et al. 1952). Moreover, some authors have concluded that the potential benefits of revaccination are outweighed by the increased interference in serological tests (reviewed in Nicoletti 1990; see also below). Indeed, it is essential to use good-quality vaccines, and there are internationally accepted biological and bacteriological quality control protocols for both vaccines (Grilló et al. 2012; OIE 2017). Nevertheless, in the experience of the authors of this chapter, vaccines of poor quality and low protective efficacy have reached the market with undue frequency in many countries.

22.3.1.2 Potential Drawbacks

Despite their efficacy, these two vaccines do not fulfill all the requisites of an optimal vaccine since: (i) vaccination of pregnant animals may induce abortions, a problem far greater in Rev1 than in S19, (ii) S19 (but not Rev1) can cause permanent genital infections when applied subcutaneously in males, (iii) both can interfere in serodiagnostic tests, an aspect that has been considered their main disadvantage, and (iv) although of low virulence, both strains can infrequently infect humans, and Rev1 is resistant to streptomycin, an antibiotic used to treat human brucellosis. The risks of accidental exposure can be greatly reduced by standard protection measures (goggles and gloves) and established protocols for handling live vaccines (OIE 2017). Similarly, the protocols of vaccination can be optimized to reduce problems (i) and (iii).

22.3.1.3 Optimizing S19 Use

The standard S19 vaccination procedure (a single subcutaneous dose of $5–10 \times 10^{10}$ colony forming units [CFU]/animal) induces long-lasting protective immunity, but may generate antibodies in a proportion of vaccinated individuals that interfere in serological tests, a problem particularly important when adult animals are immunized. Also, a significant proportion of pregnant cows can abort and/or develop S19 udder infections, with shedding of the vaccine strain in milk (Nicoletti 1990). However, under restricted management conditions, these problems can be greatly circumvented by choosing an optimal age and vaccine route and dose. Subcutaneous vaccination of young calves (between 3 and 5 months old) with a reduced dose (1/20th of the standard dose) substantially reduces the postvaccinal anti-S-LPS antibody responses, and other side effects (Alton and Corner 1981). Moreover, when applied subcutaneously, in adult cows, this reduced dose minimizes the serological response but does not abrogate the vaccine-induced abortions and udder infections (Corner and Alton 1981). This protocol still provides good immunity even under difficult conditions (Nicoletti 1990; Nicoletti et al. 1978a).

The antibody response is decreased further when the S19 vaccine is administered through conjunctival instillation rather than subcutaneously (Plommet and Fensterbank 1976, 1984; Plommet 1977, 1984; Fensterbank and Plommet 1979). The original conjunctival vaccination protocol consisted of two doses (each of 5×10^{9} CFU/animal, in a volume of 30–35 μL) administered 2–6 months apart (Plommet and Fensterbank 1976, 1984; Nicoletti et al. 1978b). Under field conditions, this method resulted in the same level of protection as the subcutaneous vaccination procedure with standard doses (Nicoletti 1984; Plommet 1984) and, in controlled experiments, it provided even better protection (Plommet 1984; Plommet and Fensterbank 1984).[1] The conjunctival method is fully safe when applied to calves of 3–5 months of age, and reduces the problem of serological interference to a minimum. Accordingly, it is the method of choice when vaccination has to be implemented simultaneously with a test and slaughter eradication program (OIE 2017). The conjunctival vaccination can be implemented under most breeding conditions, and since it minimizes abortions and milk shedding when applied to pregnant cows (Nicoletti 1990), it is the method of choice for whole-herd mass vaccination. The double conjunctival vaccination may be cumbersome under some circumstances, and experience has proved that a single conjunctival dose also provides protection useful for eradication, when combined with adequate test and slaughter, as illustrated in Figure 22.1.

It is known that subcutaneous vaccination of bulls with standard doses of S19 can cause vaccine-induced genital lesions (Lambert et al. 1964). However, a gap in knowledge that would be worth investigating is whether the reduced-dose conjunctival S19 vaccination is safe in bulls.

A general belief of inexperienced veterinarians is that conjunctival vaccination is more difficult and dangerous than the subcutaneous procedure. However, with adequate training and using simple protection measures, the conjunctival instillation of S19 or Rev1 vaccines is easily applicable at field level, regardless of the animal species and management systems (Figure 22.2).

S19 has been the cause of accidental infections in humans (Wallach et al. 2008). However, this is a very rare event and simple biosafety measures (Figure 22.2) practically abrogate the risks. Moreover, exposure or infection can be readily detected with the standard serological tests. This vaccine carries no resistance to any of the antibiotics used to treat human brucellosis.

22.3.1.4 S19 Use Against *B. melitensis* in Cattle

Cattle can become frequently infected with *B. melitensis* when herds are in contact with *B. melitensis*-infected goats or sheep (Verger 1985). One study directly demonstrated that S19 is efficient in the control of *B. melitensis* infections in cattle (Jiménez de Bagüé et al. 1991), and the evidence shown in Figure 22.1 confirms this. On the other hand, neither the protective efficacy nor the safety of Rev1 has been determined in this livestock species. Thus, Rev1 is not recommended for immunizing cattle (OIE 2017).

---

[1] Several lines of evidence show that, under natural conditions, the port of entry is the naso-oropharyngeal area (see Plommet 1977), which accounts for the effectiveness of this vaccination route. Accordingly, the accepted route for experimental infection in ruminants is the conjunctival route.

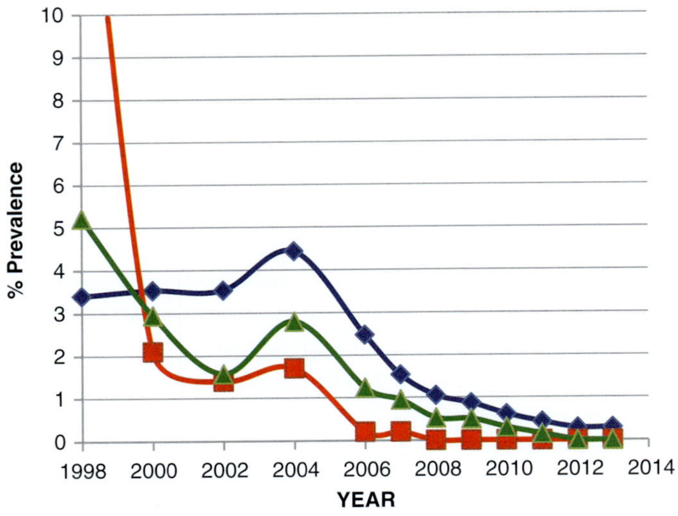

Figure 22.1 Impact of three different eradication strategies on mean herd prevalence of bovine brucellosis in Spain in the 1998–2013 period. Until 1998, *B. abortus* S19 vaccination (5–10 × 10^{10} CFU subcutaneously) was applied regularly in 3–6-month-old calves throughout Spain, with variable intensity depending upon the region. In this year, S19 vaccination was banned in all regions except Aragón (red line; see below) where herd prevalence was over 16%, mostly due to poor vaccine coverage. Events after 1998 were as follows. *Blue line* (Test and slaughter plus RB51 vaccination). Cantabria, Castilla-León, and Extremadura applied exclusively the same test and slaughter program with no vaccination, following European Union rules (Directives 77/391/CEE and 78/52/CEE). Due to the lack of progress, one of the regions (Cantabria), started a *B. abortus* RB51 mass vaccination strategy including adult cows. This RB51-based program became official also in Castilla-León and Extremadura in 2004. A total of 721 683 cows were vaccinated with RB51, simultaneously with test and slaughter, in the three regions from 2002 to 2011 (last data available). As can be seen, prevalence decreased but the disease was never eradicated from any of these three regions. *Green line* (Test and slaughter and no vaccination). Apart from Aragón (red line; see below), the remaining regions completely stopped any vaccination and applied only the European Union test and slaughter program. The disease was eradicated in 2012, and remained absent in 2013 (last data available). *Red line* (Test and slaughter and S19 conjunctival vaccination). Aragón (over 16% prevalence in 1998) implemented a compulsory *B. abortus* S19 conjunctival vaccination program (5 × 10^{9} CFU, either as one dose or two doses, administered 2–3 months apart) of 3–6-month-old calves, combined with the same test and slaughter program that was being applied in the rest of Spain. The double S19 dose was discontinued in 2000, and only one conjunctival dose was applied thereafter. The prevalence in Aragón dropped quickly and, in 2002, fell below that of the regions applying only test and slaughter (green line), remaining lower thereafter until eradication in 2008 (which has been maintained since). The sporadic outbreaks observed after 2002 in Aragón were all caused by *B. melitensis*, biovars 1 or 3, transmitted from sheep. A total of 38 754 replacement calves were vaccinated in Aragón from 2002 (no previous data are available) to 2010, when vaccination was also banned. Eradication in this region was achieved earlier than in the regions applying test and slaughter exclusively. Source: Personal compilation from RASVE data: www.mapa.gob.es/es/ganaderia/temas/sanidad-animal-higiene-ganadera/sanidad-animal/enfermedades/brucelosis/brucelosis.aspx.

22.3.1.5 Optimizing Rev1 Use

Rev1 has been essential in the eradication of *B. melitensis* infection in sheep and goats in some European Mediterranean countries heavily stricken by the disease (Figure 22.3), and is also the only available vaccine against *B. ovis* (which infects only ovines). The classic vaccination method (0.5–2 × 10^{9} CFU/animal subcutaneously) triggers a long-lasting antibody response that makes it very difficult to combine vaccination with test and slaughter policies, even if vaccination is limited to lambs and kids. However, when the same dose is administered by conjunctival instillation to lambs and kids, protection is not lessened but the antibody response is markedly reduced. Thus, Rev1 conjunctival vaccination of young replacements is compatible with test and slaughter strategies (Blasco 1997; Blasco and Molina-Flores 2011). Both S19 and Rev 1 conjunctival formulations are commercially available.

In contrast to S19, Rev1 is safe in males (Muñoz et al. 2008) but highly abortifacient and is excreted in milk by a large number of animals when applied to pregnant sheep and goats (Blasco and Molina-Flores 2011). To solve this problem, subcutaneous administration of a reduced dose (10^{3}–10^{6} CFU/animal) has been proposed in the past, but this method does not avoid abortions and confers low or no protection (Blasco 1997). Because "mass vaccination" becomes necessary under circumstances not uncommon in endemic areas, this implies that a proportion of pregnant sheep and goats would be vaccinated. Strategies for minimizing the Rev1 side effects are discussed below (see section 22.4.3). Under these circumstances, it is important that decision makers consider the balance between the side effects of vaccination and the high risk of human infections if no intervention is made.

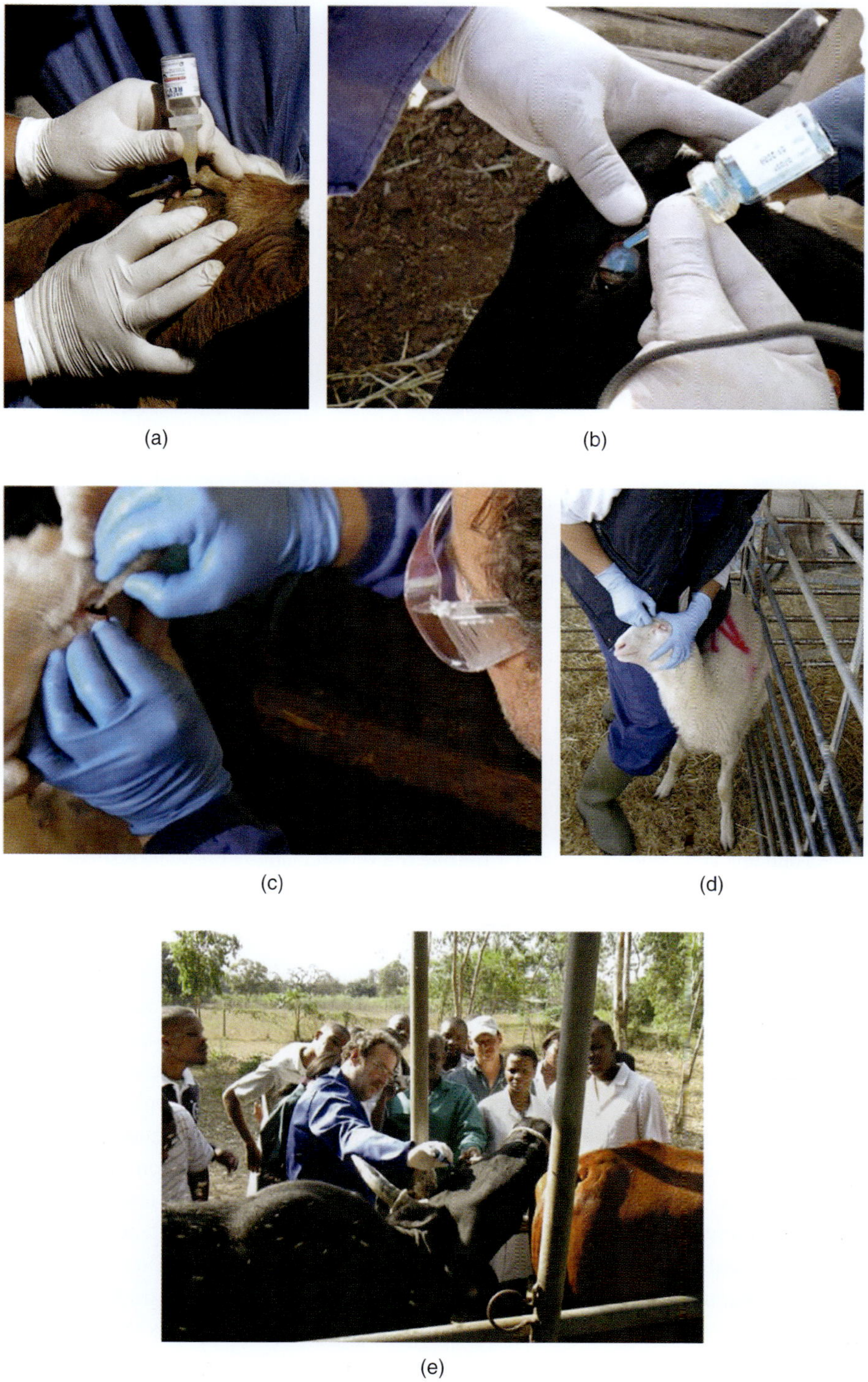

Figure 22.2 Conjunctival vaccination. (a) For animals that are not handled frequently, the easiest procedure is to place a single vaccine drop on the corneal surface. (b) The use of vaccines containing innocuous dye (Patent Blue) in the vaccine solvent helps to observe vaccine spillage. (c) Whenever possible, a better procedure is to deliver the vaccine drop in the small pouch that can be made by pinching off the lower conjunctival sac, because this facilitates vaccine adsorption by the conjunctival mucosa (persons involved in vaccination should wear adequate personal protection equipment including suitable goggles, ventilated to avoid sweating condensation, and good-quality gloves). (d) When vaccinating young lambs and kids, a trained technician can perform vaccination alone without any help. (e) However, when vaccinating cows that are not handled frequently or of aggressive breeds, an assistant should restrain the animal with appropriate equipment. In this picture, taken for teaching purposes only, the procedure was conducted with a placebo and no suitable protection goggles were used.

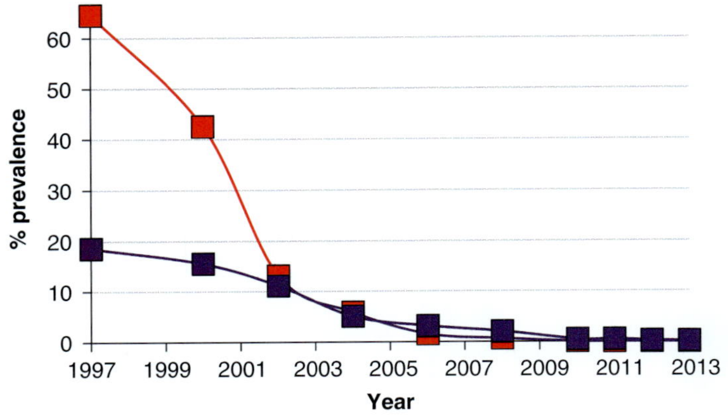

Figure 22.3 Evolution of ovine and caprine brucellosis in Spain. The plots represent the evolution of mean flock prevalence of ovine and caprine brucellosis caused by *B. melitensis* in Aragón (*red line*) and the remaining Spanish regions (*blue line*). Before 1997, Rev1 vaccination was conducted in most Spanish regions using the standard procedure (i.e. a single subcutaneous dose of $1-2 \times 10^9$ CFU applied only to 3–5-month-old sheep and goats) and, since 1990, this vaccination was combined with the official European Union test and slaughter eradication program in all Spanish regions. This eradication strategy was applied with differing intensity depending on the regions (low in Aragón), which explains why Aragón – in red – had the highest (64.2%) flock prevalence at the beginning of 1997. In this year, a mass conjunctival Rev1 vaccination (one dose of 1×10^9 CFU) program including adult sheep and goats (both males and females) was started in Aragón, covering about 50% (c. 1.2 million animals) of the regional small ruminant census. In parallel, the same conjunctival vaccination procedure was applied to the young replacements of remaining Aragón census (c. 1 million animals) combined with test and slaughter of adult animals. Mass vaccinated flocks were not tested during 1998 (to allow a reduction of prevalence by natural replacement) and only the young replacements were vaccinated (as above) in this and successive years. During 1999 and 2000, the mass vaccinated flocks in Aragón were tested annually using the native hapten gel precipitation test (Marín et al. 1999) and all positive animals culled. Since 2001, all flocks in Aragón were submitted to the same official eradication program, based on the vaccination of young replacements (with the Rev1 conjunctival vaccine) and adults tested using the European Union official rose Bengal and complement fixation tests, with seropositive animals culled. By 2002, the prevalence was significantly reduced, and the conjunctival vaccination extended officially to most Spanish regions. Since 2002 all small ruminant flocks in Spain (except for those in a few brucellosis-free regions) were submitted to the same official European Union eradication program (based on conjunctival vaccination of young replacements and test and slaughter of adults). Despite the very high initial prevalence, small ruminant brucellosis in Aragón was markedly reduced in only a few years, reaching practical eradication in 2010. Vaccination was banned in Aragón in this year and the disease remains eradicated. Source: Personal compilation from RASVE data: www.mapa.gob.es/es/ganaderia/temas/sanidad-animal-higiene-ganadera/sanidad-animal/enfermedades/brucelosis/brucelosis.aspx

As indicated above, Rev1 infrequently infects humans and is resistant to streptomycin, an antibiotic of choice in the treatment of brucellosis (Ariza et al. 2007). Although more than 50 years of experience demonstrates that risks can be minimized if simple biosafety measures (Figure 22.2) are used, these measures should never be relaxed. Standard serological tests detect human Rev1 infections readily but, as isolation would be necessary to confirm the identity of the infecting strain and cultures are not always performed, it is always advisable to use alternative regimes (such as rifampicin-doxycycline) (Ariza et al. 2007) when treating persons with a suspected Rev1 infection.

22.3.2 Brucellosis DIVA Vaccines

DIVA vaccines are those that allow the differentiation of infected from vaccinated animals. When optimized and combined with the appropriate diagnostic tests, S19 and Rev1 come close to solving the DIVA problem. Nonetheless, DIVA brucellosis vaccines have been investigated and implemented to various degrees. Two main strategies have been pursued in their development: (i) the removal in the existing vaccines (or vaccine candidate strains) of antigens present in field strains that are of diagnostic value, and (ii) the inclusion of foreign (xenogenic) antigens in the existing vaccines. Whereas the former strategy may or may not rely on new diagnostic tests, depending on the antigen removed, the latter requires a new DIVA test. The latter approach can identify animals as vaccinated, but not infection in vaccinated animals. It is important to understand that suitable DIVA vaccines replacing S19 and Rev1 would be useful only if the protection they confer is at least equivalent to that of these classic vaccines.

22.3.2.1 Rough Vaccines

These are vaccines that follow strategy (i), but do not require new *ad hoc* tests. The S-LPS of smooth (S) brucellae is made of three linked sections: O-PS, core oligosaccharide, and lipid A. Rough (R) mutants are those that lack the O-PS moiety, and in some cases the deficiency extends to sugars of the core oligosaccharide. Because the O-PS plays a prominent role in serological tests and these R mutants are attenuated, it was proposed over 60 years ago that they could serve as vaccines that would not interfere in brucellosis diagnostic tests. To this end, R mutants have been obtained by two different procedures. It has been known for a long time that S brucellae are prone to mutational losses of the O-PS, and two R vaccines, *B. abortus* 45/20 and *B. abortus* RB51 (see sections 22.3.2.1.1 and 22.3.2.1.2), are spontaneous R mutants obtained by serial passages either in animals or *in vitro*. Indeed, neither method implies that they are single and well-defined mutants (i.e. they may carry mutations in genes not related to the R phenotype), so that further attempts have been made using transposon and site-directed mutagenesis to develop new R vaccine candidates (see section 22.3.2.1.3).

Experience gathered with the existing vaccines shows that R vaccines have both disadvantages and advantages when compared with the classic smooth vaccines (Table 22.1). On the one hand, the R mutant approach has not resulted in vaccines providing the protection afforded by the classic vaccines and lacking abortifacient effects (Moriyón et al. 2004). On the other, it has been proved that some (but not all; see below) R vaccines do not interfere in serological assays that, like the rose Bengal and complement fixation tests, use whole smooth brucellae as antigens (Ducrotoy et al. 2016) and are in this diagnostic context DIVA vaccines.

However, it is important to understand that these R vaccines are not DIVA in assays that use S-LPS extracts or their hydrolytic products rather than whole cells. It is well known that the polymerization and assembly of O-PS on the core-lipid A result in heterogeneous molecules including both molecules with O-PS of variable lengths linked to the core-lipid A (i.e. a heterogeneous S-LPS) and core-lipid A molecules (i.e. R-LPS) (Freer et al. 1995). Therefore, all molecules in S-LPS extracts contain all the R-LPS epitopes and, as they become accessible in immunosorbent assays or upon S-LPS hydrolysis (Ducrotoy et al. 2016), all R vaccines induce antibodies that are detected in indirect and competitive enzyme-linked immunosorbent assay (ELISA), lateral flow immunochromatography and the fluorescence polarization assay, as shown not only for RB51 but also for several R *B. melitensis* vaccine candidates tested (Rojas et al. 2001; Nielsen et al. 2005; Barrio et al. 2009; Pérez-Sancho et al. 2014). Also worth noting is that there is a group of R mutants that are still able to synthesize internal O-PS precursors and some of these have been shown to elicit antibodies to the O-PS (Brinley Morgan et al. 1966; González et al. 2008; Barrio et al. 2009; Pérez-Sancho et al. 2014).

It is also important to understand the limitations of the R vaccine DIVA strategy in the context of prevalence. It has been proved that animals vaccinated with R vaccines develop anti-S-LPS antibodies when exposed to virulent strains (Brinley Morgan et al. 1966; Moriyón et al. 2004; Barrio et al. 2009), as expected in infected environments. Accordingly, in areas where brucellosis is present, animals immunized with R vaccines are also at risk to become positive in all S-LPS tests, particularly when prevalence is significant and exposure is repeated. Therefore, unless prevalence is very low or negligible, the validity of this DIVA strategy is uncertain. This, together with the lower protection afforded, makes the use of R vaccines uncertain where vaccination is essential for control (see section 22.4). It is also worth noting that the use of vaccines lacking antigens relevant in inducing protecting antibodies (such as S-LPS) could favor the selection of field strains harboring full antigenic and virulence factor repertoires (Moreno 2014).

***22.3.2.1.1 B. abortus* 45/20** Strain 45/20 was obtained by 20 serial passages through guinea pigs of the *B. abortus* 45/0 virulent strain, but several studies showed that it could revert to S virulent forms (Moriyón et al. 2004). Thus, 45/20 was used as a killed vaccine in oil-based adjuvants that required at least two injections. In this form, 45/20 induced antibodies detectable in some S-LPS serological tests and the protection achieved by the most common commercially available product (Duphavac) was not satisfactory (Nicoletti 1990). Results were often contradictory and unpredictable, which could be attributed to the instability of the vaccine but also to the lack of standardization of the methods. The Netherlands is the only country where 45/20 was occasionally used in a successful eradication program (Nicoletti 1990). However, since this program benefited from exceptionally favorable epidemiological conditions, highly proficient veterinary services and suitable animal management (mostly dairy farms), plus complementary measures, the contribution of 45/20 to eradication is unclear (see section 22.2.1). Indeed, other authors reported very unfavorable results when 45/20 was compared with S19 (Ray 1976) and, as the only reason to use 45/20 was to avoid vaccinating adult cattle with S19, this R vaccine was abandoned once the protocols for S19 vaccination of adult cows were optimized (see section 22.3.1.2) (Nicoletti 1990).

The experience with 45/20 illustrates that vaccination with low protective vaccines under very favorable epidemiological conditions may result in the wrong conclusion that eradication is achieved due mainly to the vaccine effect and not to other sanitary measures implemented simultaneously.

***22.3.2.1.2 B. abortus* RB51** RB51 is the only R vaccine against cattle brucellosis[2] that is currently marketed, and most of the considerations above regarding R vaccines (summarized in Table 22.1) come from evidence obtained

[2] RB51 is ineffective against brucellosis of sheep (El Idrissi et al. 2001), water buffaloes (Fosgate et al. 2003), pigs (Stoffregen et al. 2006), bison (Davis and Elzer 2002), and cervids (Kreeger et al. 2002).

with RB51. The characteristics of RB51 were selected during serial passages of virulent *B. abortus* 2308 on media containing rifampicin and penicillin, and include rifampin resistance and unpaired O-PS assembly on the bacterial surface (RB51 still expresses small amounts of intracellular O-PS) (Cloeckaert et al. 2002). The R phenotype of RB51 is stable and is caused by both an IS711 insertion in *wboA* and undefined mutations also affecting LPS genes (Moriyón et al. 2004). When compared with genetically defined R mutants in animal models, RB51 is notoriously more attenuated (Monreal et al. 2003; Moriyón et al. 2004). Very likely, this is the result of additional mutations that RB51 carries in non-LPS genes (Ma et al. 2014).

This vaccine was developed in the USA, where it was established as a conditional vaccine (1×10^{10} bacteria per dose) in 1996, once brucellosis had been practically eradicated from domestic herds through S19 vaccination plus test and slaughter strategies (Ragan 2002). Since then, RB51 has been introduced in several countries where, however, brucellosis still remains endemic or is emerging or reemerging. Although RB51 protects against mild challenges under controlled conditions (Moriyón et al. 2004), field infections in RB51-vaccinated animals have been repeatedly observed (Moriyón et al. 2004; Herrera-Lopez et al. 2010; Arellano-Reynoso et al. 2012) even in revaccinated (the duration of protection for this vaccine is unknown) animals (Olsen 2000; Luna-Martínez and Mejía-Terán 2002; Moriyón et al. 2004; Blasco and Moriyón 2005; Leal-Hernández et al. 2005; Herrera et al. 2008; Herrera-Lopez et al. 2010).

Whether RB51 protection is useful under field conditions has been a matter of debate (Blasco and Moriyón 2010; Martins et al. 2010). RB51 vaccination together with compulsory culling of animals and other complementary measures was implemented in three Azores islands, and eradication reported for Terceira but not for San Jorge or San Miguel islands. The failure in these two islands was attributed to deficiencies in the campaigns, and the usefulness of RB51 was assumed, based on the results in Terceira island (Martins et al. 2009). However, others have argued that it is not possible to discriminate the contribution of RB51 from that of the compulsory culling, plus the complementary measures implemented (Blasco and Moriyón 2010), and the fact that eradication in four other Azores islands (Corvo, Flores, Graciosa, and Pico) had been achieved by 1999 using a deficient S19 strain and vaccine 45/20 (Martins et al. 2009) seems to add weight to this argument (see section 22.2.1).

Because S19 remains as the reference vaccine for *B. abortus*, some studies have compared the protection afforded by S19 and RB51. Under controlled conditions, the few valid comparisons strongly suggest that RB51 is inferior to S19 (Moriyón et al. 2004), which is in keeping with recent comparative studies of the immunological response (Dorneles et al. 2015). The literature does not contain scientifically valid reports comparing S19 and RB51 in the same herd under field conditions (Moriyón et al. 2004). A field report on focused interventions that combined RB51 mass vaccination, complementary measures (including test and slaughter and stamping out of heavily infected herds), and S19-RB51 vaccination of heifers does not allow clear-cut conclusions on the contribution of RB51 to be obtained (Sáez et al. 2014) (see section 22.2.1). On the other hand, data comparisons between S19 and RB51 in areas where these vaccines have been implemented are in line with the controlled experiments and provide straightforward interpretation regarding the respective value of these two cattle vaccines (Figure 22.1). Contrary to S19 (see section 22.3.1.4), there is no evidence of the efficacy of RB51 against *B. melitensis* infections of cattle, a necessary condition in many endemic areas.

Concerning safety, two studies reported low rates of RB51 isolation after abortion of vaccinated animals (Martins et al. 2010; Sanz et al. 2010). However, the bacteriological diagnosis conducted in both studies used Farrell's selective media, which is highly inhibitory for RB51 (Hornsby et al. 2000). Others have found that a high proportion of animals vaccinated with RB51 abort (Mainar-Jaime et al. 2008, 2011; Dougherty et al. 2013; Fluegel et al. 2013). Presently, manufacturers explicitly warn against its use in pregnant cattle and this is not recommended by the OIE (OIE 2017).

Although rarely reported, RB51 is infectious for humans and precautions similar to those used in S19 or Rev 1 vaccination should not be relaxed (Villarroel et al. 2000; Ashford 2004; Anonymous 2013). Because rifampicin can be used in the treatment of human brucellosis (Ariza et al. 2007), the resistance of RB51 to this antibiotic should be kept in mind in all cases where RB51 infections in farmers or veterinarians handling the vaccine are suspected. This suspicion is hard to confirm because human brucellosis tests detect antibodies to the O-PS and, therefore, a negative test result is expected when RB51 infections occur. Because of this, and even though the risk may be low, it is difficult to know to what extent exposure to RB51 has resulted in infections in humans (Blasco and Moriyón 2010). However, recent reports prove that RB51 can be excreted in an important proportion of vaccinated cows, and several human infections due to RB51 have been caused after consumption of raw milk (Negrón et al. 2019).

22.3.2.1.3 Other R Vaccine Candidates No R vaccines other than 45/20 and RB51 have reached the market. Here we describe briefly those that have been tested in ruminants under controlled conditions.

Brucella abortus Δ*pgm* is a R mutant with a deletion in the gene for the phosphoglucomutase enzyme necessary for the synthesis of the LPS outer core (Ugalde et al. 2003). It has been tested experimentally, in comparison with S19, in a limited number of cattle, either as a single dose administered at 6 months of age or as double dose administered at 6 and 12 months of age (Comerci et al. 2013). Even though the results of this experiment can only be considered as preliminary, both because of the limited number of animals used and the inconsistent results, they are briefly commented upon here. A double dose of Δ*pgm* was necessary to approach the protection values obtained in the cows vaccinated with S19. However, when milk excretion of the challenge bacteria was considered, only S19 conferred significant protection. This observation was not consistent with a postmortem examination of the supramammary lymph nodes carried out 5 months after milk bacteriology. Although *B. abortus* Δ*pgm* reduced the number of abortions (Comerci et al. 2013), this criterion is not appropriate to assess true protection and may be counterproductive (see section 22.2.1). Consistent with the fact that O-PS and core synthesis follow two independent pathways (González et al. 2008), almost the totality of the Δ*pgm* revaccinated animals developed antibodies to S-LPS, which represents a response similar to or even more pronounced than that induced by conjunctival vaccination with S19 (see section 22.3.2.3). Although further research would be necessary to reach a conclusion on the protection afforded by *B. abortus* Δ*pgm*, the need for revaccination and the significant postvaccinal response to S-LPS are discouraging for a future use of this vaccine candidate in the field.

The O-PS gen *wboA*, partially responsible for the R phenotype of RB51, was deleted in *B. melitensis* to obtain strain VTMR1, which did not produce satisfactory protection in goats (reviewed in Moriyón et al. 2004). In order to investigate, in detail, the possibilities of *B. melitensis* R vaccines, an extensive random mutagenesis and screening in laboratory models led to the selection of the most promising R vaccine candidates (González et al. 2008). *B. melitensis* R mutants with changes in genes *per*, *wadA* (provisionally named *wa***), and *wbkF*, respectively involved in the synthesis of N-formylperosamine (the only O-PS sugar), the assembly of the outer core, and initial steps of O-PS polymerization, were markedly less protective than Rev1 against *B. melitensis* in sheep (Barrio et al. 2009). These same studies also showed that mutations in the *wzm*/*wzt* O-PS ABC export system synthesize internal O-PS able to induce antibodies detectable in S-LPS tests (González et al. 2008; Barrio et al. 2009). Despite this evidence, *B. melitensis* B115 (a spontaneous R mutant that carries a mutation in *wzm* and builds up internal O-PS) and a *B. melitensis* mutant deleted in *wzt* have been investigated as R vaccine candidates with inconsistent results (Adone et al. 2005, 2008; Pérez-Sancho et al. 2014). Nevertheless, in comparative experiments with Rev1 conducted almost 50 years ago, *B. melitensis* B115 did not confer protection in goats (Brinley Morgan et al. 1966).

22.3.2.2 Vaccine Candidates with Specific Protein Antigen Deletions

This DIVA approach follows strategy (i) (see section 22.3.2) and relies on the hypothesis that tests that detect antibodies to a given protein or proteins can have a diagnostic sensitivity as high as that of the S-LPS tests. Thus, a vaccine strain in which one or several of such proteins were deleted would lack a diagnostically relevant antigen(s) and a test based on the protein(s) deleted would serve as the *ad hoc* DIVA test. An intrinsic weakness of this approach is that several lines of evidence show that the antibody response to protein antigens is delayed with respect to that to the S-LPS (Trap and Gaumont 1982; Salih-Alj Debbarh et al. 1996), which means that antiprotein tests show low sensitivity in recently infected animals and, thus, at the beginning of any brucellosis outbreak (Ducrotoy et al. 2016).

Following appropriate screening, *Brucella* protein 26 (BP26) was identified as the optimal candidate for DIVA in both *B. abortus* and *B. melitensis*. Because deletion of BP26 does not generate significant attenuation, the protein was deleted in both S19 and Rev1 strains (Table 22.2). Although these BP26 deleted derivatives seemed to maintain the good vaccine properties of the parental strains, the complementary DIVA tests (indirect ELISA) did not reach optimal diagnostic performance (Table 22.2). When the BP26 deletion in Rev1 was combined with a deletion in outer membrane protein 31, the double mutant was inferior as a vaccine to the parental Rev1, and a DIVA test was not investigated. Other *Brucella* proteins have also been deleted (Table 22.2), but none of the resulting mutants fulfill the requisites of a suitable brucellosis vaccine.

22.3.2.3 Vaccines Tagged with Xenogenic Antigens

Because approach (i) (see section 22.3.2) has not been successful (Table 22.2), the introduction of foreign genes coding for suitable antigens has also been investigated to identify the vaccinated animals. Thus, although not a true DIVA approach, the underlying assumption is that vaccinated animals would produce a sustained immune response against the xenogenic antigen that would last longer than or at least as long as that to the S-LPS, the advantage being that the *ad hoc* test would complement simple assays such as the rose Bengal test or some indirect ELISA used currently for routine diagnosis. Although candidates have been proposed in the past, a S19 construct tagged with the green fluorescent protein (GFP) and its *ad*

Table 22.2 Protein-deleted *Brucella* mutants that have been tested in natural hosts.

Proteins deleted	Comments
26 kDa periplasmic protein (BP26)	Two vaccines (*B. abortus* INTA2 and *B. melitensis* CGV26) developed respectively on S19 and Rev1 that show attenuation similar to that of the corresponding parental vaccine. INTA2 was less effective than S19 (Fiorentino et al. 2008) but CGV26 induced similar protection to Rev1 against both *B. melitensis* and *B. ovis* (Jacques et al. 2007; Grilló et al. 2009). However, the DIVA test developed was less effective than S-LPS tests (Muñoz et al. 2005; Jacques et al. 2007; Grilló et al. 2009)
Outer membrane protein 31 (Omp31)	Investigated as a double BP26-Omp31 Rev1 mutant (CGV2631); the double mutant was somewhat inferior to Rev1 in protecting against either *B. melitensis* or *B. ovis* (Jacques et al. 2007; Grilló et al. 2009). No suitable DIVA test was developed
Outer membrane protein 25 (Omp25)	Compared with Rev1, preliminary experiments in goats showed less protection against infection and a more protracted serological response (Edmonds et al. 2002). DIVA test not developed and, potentially, of low sensitivity (Dubray 1997)
Heat-shock protease A (HtrA)	*B. abortus* (Elzer et al. 1996) or *B. melitensis* (Roop et al. 2001) mutants showed little attenuation in goats; limited utility of *B. melitensis* mutants as goat vaccines (Phillips et al. 1997). DIVA test not developed and, potentially, of low sensitivity (Dubray 1997)
24 kDa acid-shock protein (Asp24)	More efficacious but possibly less safe than virB2; less effective than Rev1 (Kahl-McDonagh et al. 2006); no DIVA test developed
Cytochrome bd (CydA-CydB)	*B. melitensis* mutant not attenuated in goats (Kahl-McDonagh et al. 2006); no DIVA test
Type IV secretion protein 2 (VirB2)	*B. melitensis* mutant showed reduced virulence but seemed less effective than Rev1 (Kahl-McDonagh et al. 2006); no DIVA test
Periplasmic catalase (KatE)	*B. melitensis* mutant did not result in significant attenuation in goats (Gee et al. 2004); no DIVA test developed
5′-Phosphoribosyl-5-aminoimidazole carboxylase catalytic subunit (PurE)	*B. melitensis purE* mutant showed little attenuation in goats and induced antibody responses similar to those of Rev1 (Cheville et al. 1996); no DIVA test

DIVA, differentiating infected from vaccinated animals; S-LPS, smooth-type lipopolysaccharide.

hoc ELISA-GFP is the only system that has been properly tested, thus far only in the mouse model (Chacón-Díaz et al. 2011). The S19-GFP strain maintains the biological properties (residual virulence and protection) of the parental S19, and the GFP-based test discriminates mice immunized with S19-GFP after experimental infection with virulent *B. abortus* (Chacón-Díaz et al. 2011). These works provide a "proof or concept" that should be confirmed in experiments in target species.

22.3.3 Attempts to Develop Other Vaccine Candidates

As indicated in section 22.2.1, even the good immunity triggered by S19 and Rev1 can be overcome under those circumstances where high animal and bacterial densities increase the level and frequency of the challenge inoculum. Thus, in addition to DIVA vaccines, research has also focused on the development of vaccines that could improve protection and/or eliminate some of the disadvantages of S19 and Rev1 (i.e. safety in pregnant animals and virulence for humans). Few candidates have been investigated in natural hosts (Table 22.2) because most did not match the good properties of the two classic vaccines when tested in laboratory models. A detailed discussion of the status of this research is beyond the scope of this review and only some of the strategies will be summarized here.

As can be seen in Table 22.2, these vaccine candidates include mutants with changes in outer membrane proteins, stress proteins, proteins necessary to build the type IV secretion system *virB* (critical for *Brucella* virulence), components of the electron transport chain required to adapt *Brucella* respiration to low oxygen tension, the periplasmic catalase and enzymes of purine synthesis. These attenuated strains were less protective than the corresponding classic S19 and Rev1 vaccines and although some of the deleted proteins elicit specific antibodies, the responses are weak or infrequent and thus not useful to develop *ad hoc* DIVA tests.

Although a number of recombinant or DNA vaccines have been proposed, only one has been tested in the target host. This vaccine candidate uses an influenza vector

(FluBA, based on recombinant influenza viruses of the subtypes H5N1 and H1N1) expressing *Brucella* proteins L7/L12 and Omp16 (Tabynov et al. 2014a,b). A formulation Flu-L7/L12-Omp16 in adjuvant administered twice to 3–4-months pregnant cattle was reported to be similar to S19 (about 80% and 90% protection in heifers and their calves, respectively) and superior to RB51 against a severe (5×10^8 bacteria) *B. abortus* challenge (Tabynov et al. 2014a,b). Moreover, the same Flu-L7/L12-Omp16 immunization procedure and S19 were reported not to cause abortions and to provide similar protection (90% and 100% in heifers and their calves, respectively) against a severe (10^9 bacteria) *B. melitensis* challenge (Tabynov et al. 2015). However, the authors used nonselective media and other imperfect bacteriological procedures to assess the presence of brucellae, a vaccination challenge span (2 months) that was too short, and no methodology to differentiate the challenge and vaccine strains. These critical experimental flaws preclude drawing conclusions on this recent candidate.

Vaccine Rev 1 is effective against both *B. melitensis* and *B. ovis* (Blasco 1990) and it has been shown to be innocuous in rams (Muñoz et al. 2008). Because vaccination with Rev 1 is discontinued after eradication of *B. melitensis*, alternative vaccines have been investigated to immunize sheep against *B. ovis*. These include extracts rich in outer membrane components in adjuvants as well as encapsulated attenuated mutants (Blasco et al. 1993a,b; Muñoz et al. 2006; Da Costa Martins et al. 2009; Silva et al. 2015) but none of these vaccines has been used under field conditions or marketed.

22.4 Strategies for Controlling Ruminant Brucellosis

22.4.1 Requirements and Scenarios

In addition to efficient vaccines and diagnostic tests, the control and eradication of brucellosis in ruminants are largely dependent on the following factors:

i) Identification of all flocks/herds and capacity of veterinary services to conduct the interventions on the whole population of the selected area (epidemiological unit of intervention) in a short time.
ii) Availability of funds for intervention costs.
iii) Active involvement of breeders (often through awareness campaigns and education) and other relevant stakeholders.
iv) Well-understood disease status including cross-border assessments and occurrence in humans as well as proper information on the circulating *Brucella* species in the livestock involved.
v) If eradication is the goal, all the above-listed requirements are critical. Particular emphasis has to be placed on: (a) the individual identification of the whole animal census and the full control of animal movements (at least in the epidemiological unit of intervention and ideally in the whole country), (b) the need for compensation of farmers for culling, be that directly by reimbursement at market value or by economically incentivizing the "brucellosis free" status in their farms, and (c) correct political decisions and sustained commitment of all relevant authorities and stakeholders (Blasco and Molina-Flores 2011).

When only conditions (i) to (iii) are fulfilled (a common situation in resource-limited areas), a mass vaccination program (see section 22.4.3.2) without the need to identify vaccinated animals is the simplest and most practical strategy to control brucellosis in ruminants, regardless of the initial prevalence (Blasco and Molina-Flores 2011). Only when (i)–(v) are met can eradication programs be undertaken. For this purpose, two very important additional requirements are a realistic definition of the epidemiological unit and a correct estimation of the prevalence at herd/flock level. The epidemiological unit represents the restricted area of intervention and is not necessarily demarcated by administrative or national borders or uniform for a given country. On the basis of the collective (i.e. herd/flock) prevalence in well-defined intervention areas, there are three possible strategies:

- *Very low prevalence (≤1% to 4%).* A test and slaughter eradication program and the banning of vaccination could be recommended to eradicate the disease in a short to medium timeframe.
- *Low to moderate prevalence (5–10%).* A combined eradication program based on the simultaneous application of vaccination in young replacements and test and slaughter of seropositive adult animals is recommended to eradicate the disease in a medium-long timeframe.
- *High prevalence (≥10%).* Regardless of the level of professional organization and economic resources, a mass vaccination program is the only strategy to control the disease, a step strictly necessary before undertaking any eradication program.

22.4.2 Eradication Programs

An eradication program based on testing and slaughtering in the absence of vaccination can be recommended only when the collective prevalence found in the epidemiological unit is uniformly very low (see above). However, under low to moderate prevalence conditions, a test and slaughter strategy combined with the vaccination of young (3–4 months old[3]) replacements (calves with S19 and kids and lambs with Rev1; see sections 22.3.1.3 and 22.3.1.5) is the eradication program of choice to achieve "brucellosis free" status, and has been applied successfully in many countries (see an example in Figures 22.1 and 22.3).

It has to be stressed that this effort needs to be sustained and that the premature banning of vaccination, sometimes under pressure to obtain the "brucellosis officially free" status (see below) or because of political decisions, has been a frequent error in situations close to eradication. Vaccination should never be abandoned until the collective prevalence is zero in the whole epidemiological unit, there have been no cases during at least one generation (4–8 years, depending on the breeding system), and the risk of reintroduction of the disease is negligible. The "brucellosis free" status is granted when there is no detectable disease, surveillance is ongoing and yet vaccination of replacements is maintained. Under these particular conditions, conjunctival vaccination (sections 22.3.1.3 and 22.3.1.5) is essential to minimize interference with diagnostic surveillance tests.

Combined vaccination and test and slaughter programs have not infrequently succeeded in some regions but failed in others within the same country. As exemplified by several European Mediterranean and most Latin America countries, this has generated a mosaic of prevalences with some locations free of the disease while others show low to moderate infection rates. Beyond doubt, it is recommended that the "brucellosis free" status is maintained under these circumstances because the "brucellosis officially free" status (which requires banning of vaccination) would leave the animals unprotected against accidental reintroductions from neighboring epidemiological units still infected. Thus, the risks of a premature vaccination ban, in an attempt to reach the "brucellosis officially free" status, cannot be taken lightly and should always be a matter of technical evaluations and not of political decisions. Indeed, political decisions, rather than economical or structural limitations or imperfect strategies, have often hampered control and eradication and thus promoted the persistence or spread of the disease.

22.4.3 Control Programs

When eradication is not applicable, only control is feasible and to this end the only strategies are those based exclusively on vaccination.

[3]The closer vaccination is to puberty, the more intense and protracted the antibody response. When the objective is eradication, the serological response after vaccination should be as low and short as possible. For this reason it is recommended that vaccination be ideally performed always in animals of 3–4 months of age, and never exceeding 5 months.

22.4.3.1 Vaccination of Young (3–4 Months Old) Replacements

Because the groups susceptible to brucellosis include both male and female young and adult animals, the vaccination of the whole population (see below) is a logical control option. However, a serious problem for this option is the relative lack of safety of these vaccines in pregnant animals (mainly Rev1) and males (S19 and RB51) (see sections 22.3.1.2, 22.3.1.3, 22.3.1.5). Thus, to minimize these untoward effects, a classic recommendation has been to vaccinate only the young replacements (3–4 months old) on a yearly basis, male and female small ruminants with Rev1 or calves (not males) with S19 or RB51. Because it can be estimated that, depending on the species and breeding conditions, about one-third to one-fifth of the animals correspond to young replacements each year, the entire ruminant population would be protected after 4–8 years. For follow-up, vaccinated animals should be individually identified and then, if requirements (i) to (v) (see section 22.4.1) are met, this strategy should allow the application of a test and slaughter combined eradication program. In this case, it is recommended that Rev1 and S19 vaccines be applied always by the conjunctival route to minimize the intensity and duration of the serological response. This strategy may be suitable for countries with appropriate animal health surveillance services and good management practices, such as those existing in most Latin American nations. Under these conditions, and provided the effort is not discontinued because of political decisions or other circumstances and that accompanying measures (see section 22.3.1.3) are applied simultaneously, effective control can be achieved.

Owing to practical difficulties in management and with vaccination coverage, the exclusive vaccination of young replacements is exceedingly difficult to implement in most poor-resource settings, as well as in semi-arid or arid areas. Under the typical extensive husbandry of ruminants in these areas, owners tend to keep young replacements throughout the year, depending mainly on market prices and other breeding factors. Thus, even when the vaccine is available, appointments with owners for continuous vaccination to reach 100% coverage of the epidemiological unit are very difficult. This problem is increased by the difficulties of including small farms with very few animals and with locating the animals in nomadic breeding systems. Experience shows that these circumstances result in imperfect vaccination rates of the young replacement population with the ensuing maintenance of the disease (Blasco and Molina-Flores 2011).

22.4.3.2 Mass Vaccination Strategies

As proposed already in the early 1970s, an alternative to the vaccination of only young replacements is the so-called "mass" or "whole herd" vaccination with reduced doses of S19 (female cattle) or the standard Rev1 dose (small ruminants) administered subcutaneously (see section 22.3.1) to all individuals regardless of age and physiological condition (Nicoletti 1976; Blasco 1997). The rationale for this approach is that, as test and slaughter eradication programs are not applicable under high-prevalence conditions or in resource-poor or remote areas, the serological interference caused by vaccines is irrelevant. Moreover, individual identification of vaccinated animals (necessary for serological follow-up) is not realistic in many parts of the world. Indeed, individual tagging (most commonly ear tagging) of vaccinated animals does not always allow long-term identification, is expensive, and may provoke myiasis and bacterial and fungal infections in tropical and hot climates. Therefore, a mass vaccination program without tagging is the only feasible strategy to control brucellosis in ruminants in most resource-poor or remote areas.

A problem intrinsic to this strategy is that it implies vaccination of pregnant animals whereas, as indicated above, the important side effects of subcutaneous vaccination in adult animals (Nicoletti et al. 1978b; Corner and Alton 1981; Corner 1983; Blasco 1997) should not be disregarded. In cattle, mass vaccination with S19 reduced doses given either subcutaneously or conjunctively may be recommended provided the serological interference and moderate side effects (both minimized by conjunctival vaccination) can be accepted. On the other hand, a similar strategy should never be used in small ruminants, with Rev 1, because of both the more significant safety issues and the lack of protective effect of reduced doses of this vaccine (Blasco 1997; Blasco and Molina-Flores 2011). However, beyond any doubt, the advantages of the conjunctival route (see sections 22.3.1.3 and 22.3.1.5) make mass vaccination of all small ruminants by this route with the standard dose of Rev1 or of female cattle with a reduced dosage regime of S19 the safest, cheapest, and most practical strategy to control ruminant brucellosis in the short term, in resource-poor or remote areas. Indeed, this is also the strategy of choice in high-prevalence epidemiological units of resource-abundant countries (see an example in Figure 22.1). As in other strategies, mass vaccination coverage should be close to 100%, and this high coverage needs to be maintained for several generations.

Once a first mass vaccination has been applied, the hypothetically ideal procedure to minimize vaccine side effects would be to cover only the next young replacement generations every year using individual tagging to ease the follow-up. However, as indicated above, the difficulties of vaccinating and tagging all young replacements every year make this approach unrealistic in many situations. A more practical approach after the first intervention is to consider the impact of the rates of annual replacement on the age distribution in the flocks or herds, and the different epidemiological risks according to age (Blasco and Molina-Flores 2011). For example, one year after the first mass vaccination, only 20–25% of the livestock would be composed of susceptible young replacements, if the annual replacement is 20–25%, as in many extensive management systems. Because these young replacements are sexually immature and thus excluded from the period of maximal risk of infection and spreading, it is acceptable not to vaccinate them. However, in the next year, 40–50% of the population will be unprotected and a significant proportion would be sexually mature, so that mass vaccination is again required.

Therefore, a practical and cost-effective control strategy is to repeat mass vaccination only every 2 years, and to maintain this strategy for at least one or, better, two animal generations (Blasco and Molina-Flores 2011). To minimize vaccine side effects, a "time window" should be selected to avoid vaccinating a high proportion of pregnant animals. Conjunctival vaccination with S19 (cattle) or Rev 1 (sheep and goats) during the late lambing or calving, lactation and premating periods are indeed the safest times (Blasco and Molina-Flores 2011). Under conditions of very low prevalence, mass vaccination of cattle with RB51 instead of S19 can be used if the drawbacks of the vaccine are acceptable. It may be possible to find safer "time windows" in countries where parturitions are concentrated because of the seasonal availability of pastures (for example, spring or summer in most temperate or cold climates), or where the demand for animals peaks in a given period because of cultural or religious reasons. The 2-year mass vaccination strategy with S19 or Rev 1 has been applied covering millions of ruminants in several regions, with few side effects if these adequate windows are respected. For Rev 1, it is important to stress that failure to adhere to such windows may have dramatic consequences, in terms of abortions, even if the conjunctival vaccine is used. For S19, there are experimental and field (see Figure 22.1) data proving its efficacy in the event (frequent in some countries) that bovine brucellosis is caused by *B. melitensis*. For RB51, no suitable information is available on its safety and efficacy for mass vaccination purposes in cattle, and particularly when bovine brucellosis is caused by *B. melitensis*.

After several years of successful mass vaccinations, the disease should be controlled and then it is possible to consider further interventions to move toward an eradication strategy. Provided that all (i) to (v) conditions (see section 22.4.1) are fulfilled, a combined eradication program (see section 22.4.2) can be undertaken. If such a program is not feasible, serological testing of mass vaccinated animals lacks any practical sense apart from an evaluation of the quality of the vaccine and the vaccination procedure. If these are adequate, a rose Bengal test screening of a representative sample of S19/Rev 1 vaccinated animals should result in 60–90% of positive reactors 15–21 days after vaccination (Blasco and Molina-Flores 2011). For assessing the efficacy of this control strategy, the best indicator is to follow the evolution of brucellosis at mid to long term in the exposed human population of the vaccinated area.

Moving beyond mass vaccination is not easy and requires a judicious choice of serological tests because the serological background of mass vaccinated animals living in an infected environment is not easy to interpret. Even after using the conjunctival route, the serological response induced by S19 and Rev 1 vaccines in adult animals is of higher intensity and duration than that induced in young replacements. Moreover, although protected, vaccinated animals produce anamnestic responses upon contact with field brucellae, a problem that is not resolved by the use of RB51 (see section 22.3.2.1). Under these difficult conditions, where infected and vaccinated animals co-exist, the gel precipitation test with native hapten has proved to be useful (Greiner et al. 2009; OIE 2017).

22.5 Conclusions

The strategies for using the best vaccines (S19 and Rev1) in combination with the best diagnostic tests such as rose Bengal, ELISA, and gel precipitation with native hapten (Greiner et al. 2009) were broadly defined several decades ago. R vaccines have not changed these perspectives an, if the objective is to combine maximal protection and acceptable safety, RB51 is not a clear alternative to S19. Although S19 and Rev1 vaccines are imperfect (see section 22.2), their drawbacks (see section 22.3.1) are not the main limiting factors under most epidemiological conditions (see sections 22.4.2 and 22.4.3). Indeed, there are still gaps in knowledge on some aspects of the use of these vaccines but the most important limiting factors for brucellosis control reside presently not in the vaccines/vaccination procedures but in geographical, structural, political, and sociocultural aspects (see section 22.4.1) of the areas where brucellosis is endemic or emerging (Hernández-Mora et al. 2017). Some of these aspects are aggravated by the climate, physical environment, and other problems, which are unlikely to be solved soon. Therefore, even though the standard set by S19 and Rev 1 is high, at least the latter represents a clear target for improvement because of its important safety drawbacks when used in adult animals (see section 22.3.1). Moreover, no vaccines are available for reindeer, buffaloes, yaks, camels, and pigs, all highly susceptible animals that are important for the economies of large areas of the world, and able to transmit the disease to humans.

Presently, there is an upsurge of literature of uncertain quality focused on testing questionable brucellosis vaccine candidates in laboratory models that do not truly reproduce the disease in ruminants and their immunological peculiarities. Moreover, these laboratory candidates are often based on subcellular antigens and require several immunizations, which raises additional questions on their cost-effectiveness and applicability in areas where brucellosis is endemic. Fortunately, there has also been considerable improvement in our understanding of the genetics, physiology, and structural properties of brucellae and their connection with virulence and immunity. Even though high-income countries have largely eradicated the disease, this fundamental research should not be abandoned in the present globalization epoch. Basic research on *Brucella* not only contributes to our understanding of a broad group of pathogens – the intracellular bacteria – but it is also the only path in the quest for the perfect vaccine against a group of bacteria that knows no borders and whose pathogenic potential emerges constantly.

22.6 Summary

Brucellosis is a zoonotic disease caused by intracellular α-*Proteobacteria* of the genus *Brucella*. Although these bacteria can infect a wide range of domestic and wild animals, *B. melitensis* and *B. abortus* are the most relevant species in veterinary and public health and cause brucellosis in small ruminants and cattle, respectively. Sheep, goats, cattle, and camels are the main source of human infections. In some parts of the world, swine brucellosis caused by *B. suis* is also relevant as a zoonotic infection.

Only smooth (S) *B. abortus* S19 (for cattle) and *B. melitensis* Rev1 (for sheep and goats) live vaccines have demonstrated their efficacy for eradication when combined with test and slaughter. These two live attenuated vaccines have been instrumental in successful cases of control under most epidemiological conditions and when used correctly their usefulness supersedes their disadvantages. More pronouncedly in Rev1, both vaccines are abortifacient if applied to pregnant animals and, although rarely, can infect humans. In addition, S19 can cause genital infections in bulls. As both vaccines bear a wild-type, S-LPS and the O-polysaccharide of the S-LPS is the main diagnostic antigen, S19 and Rev1 vaccination interfere with serological diagnosis. These drawbacks can be largely overcome by following standardized protocols for route, dose, and age at vaccination.

There have been many attempts to develop better vaccines. DIVA vaccines are defined as those that allow differentiation of infected from vaccinated animals. Vaccines 45/20 (inactivated and abandoned decades ago) and RB51 (live attenuated) are *B. abortus* rough (R) spontaneous mutants lacking the O-polysaccharide of the S-LPS that have been used under field conditions against cattle brucellosis, and R *B. melitensis* vaccine candidates have been systematically obtained by using genetic tools and tested in sheep. Despite lacking the O-polysaccharide, R vaccines cause significant interference in immunosorbent, lateral flow immunochromatography and fluorescence polarization diagnostic assays. Protection and immune response induced by R vaccines are lower than those obtained with S19 or Rev1. Although extensively used in some countries in the last two decades, no program relying on RB51 has achieved eradication. Moreover, RB51 does not solve the safety issues related to vaccination of pregnant cattle or human infections.

Other attempts to develop DIVA brucellosis vaccines include BP26 protein-deleted Rev1 and S19. However, ancillary serological tests based on BP26 as the antigen are not sensitive enough in field-infected ruminants. A number of attenuated mutants tested in the natural hosts have failed to provide satisfactory protection and none has allowed the development of a test to solve the DIVA problem. Approaches to develop DIVA vaccines based on the inclusion of xenogenic antigens in the classic S vaccines are presently in progress. No recombinant or subcellular brucellosis vaccine has been found suitable to control brucellosis.

A number of countries have eradicated brucellosis in domestic ruminants by sustained S19 (cattle) or Rev1 (small ruminants) vaccination of young animals in combination with test and slaughter. However, this strategy relies largely on favorable circumstances related to animal management, human behavior, and effectiveness of veterinary and public health services. Where these circumstances are not met because of economic, political, cultural, geographical, or other circumstances, this strategy has failed or is not applicable. Nevertheless, even in these situations, vaccines can still be used to reduce prevalence and thus the burden of the disease on animals and humans. Mass herd vaccination has been implemented in several countries and, although for various reasons these programs have often been discontinued, there are significant examples of areas where brucellosis prevalence has been reduced considerably. Strategies for mass vaccination with S19 and Rev1 are discussed.

There are no vaccines against brucellosis in camels, water buffalo, yaks, swine, and other domestic or semi-domestic livestock. Developments in this area and an eventual improvement of S19 and Rev1 depend on fundamental research on the bacterial and host mechanisms that make the brucellae successful intracellular parasites.

Acknowledgments

Research at the laboratories of the authors is supported by grants from FIMA, Ministerio de Ciencia y Tecnología of Spain (AGL2011-30453-C04 and AGL2014-58795-CA) and European Union's Seventh Framework Program (FP7/2007-2013) under grant agreement no 221948, ICONZ (Integrated control of Neglected Zoonoses), FS-CONARE 2012-2014, Costa Rica, and UCREA-UCR. Grants to Consolidated group A14 from Aragón Government are also acknowledged.

References

Adone, R., Ciuchini, F., Marianelli, C. et al. (2005). Protective properties of rifampin-resistant rough mutants of *Brucella melitensis*. *Infect. Immun.* 73: 4198–4204.

Adone, R., Francia, M., and Ciuchini, F. (2008). Evaluation of *Brucella melitensis* B115 as rough-phenotype vaccine against *B. melitensis* and *B. ovis* infections. *Vaccine* 26: 4913–4917.

Alton, G.G. and Corner, L.A. (1981). Vaccination of heifers with a reduced dose of *Brucella abortus* strain 19 vaccine before first mating. *Aust. Vet. J.* 57: 548–550.

Alton, G.G., Jones, L.M., Angus, R.D., and Verger, J.M. (eds.) (1988). *Techniques for the Brucellosis Laboratory*. Paris: Institute National de la Recherche Agronomique.

Arellano-Reynoso, B., Suárez-Guemes, F., Estrada, F.M. et al. (2012). Isolation of a field strain of *Brucella abortus* from RB51-vaccinated and brucellosis-seronegative bovine yearlings that calved normally. *Trop. Anim. Health Prod.* 45: 695–697.

Ariza, J., Bosilkovski, M., Cascio, A. et al. (2007). Perspectives for the treatment of brucellosis in the 21st century: the Ioannina recommendations. *PLoS Med.* 4: e317.

Ashford, D.A., di Pietra, J., Lingappa, J. et al. (2004). Adverse events in humans associated with accidental exposure to the livestock brucellosis vaccine RB51. *Vaccine* 22: 3435–3439.

Barrio, M.B., Grilló, M.J., Muñoz, P.M. et al. (2009). Rough mutants defective in core and O-polysaccharide synthesis and export induce antibodies reacting in an indirect ELISA with smooth lipopolysaccharide and are less effective than Rev1 vaccine against *Brucella melitensis* infection of sheep. *Vaccine* 27: 1741–1749.

Beach, B.A., Irwin, M.R., and Berman, D.T. (1947). Response of previously vaccinated animals to exposure in the third gestation period with a virulent strain of *Brucella abortus*. *J. Am. Vet. Med. Assoc.* 110: 355–360.

Berman, D.T., Beach, B.A., and Irwin, M.R. (1952). Studies on repeated vaccination of cattle with *Brucella abortus* strain 19. III. The response of vaccinated and revaccinated cattle to conjunctival exposure with a virulent strain of *Brucella abortus* during the third gestation period. *Am. J. Vet. Res.* 13: 351–358.

Blasco, J.M. (1990). *Brucella ovis*. In: *Animal Brucellosis* (eds. K.H. Nielsen and J.R. Duncan), 352–378. Boca Raton: CRC Press.

Blasco, J.M. (1997). A review of the use of *B. melitensis* Rev1 vaccine in adult sheep and goats. *Prev. Vet. Med.* 31: 275–283.

Blasco, J.M. and Molina-Flores, B. (2011). Control and eradication of *Brucella melitensis* infection in sheep and goats. *Vet. Clin. North Am. Food Anim. Pract.* 27: 95–104.

Blasco, J.M. and Moriyón, I. (2005). Protection of *Brucella abortus* RB51 revaccinated cows. *Comp. Immunol. Microbiol. Infect. Dis.* 28: 371–373. author reply 375–377.

Blasco, J.M. and Moriyón, I. (2010). Eradication of bovine brucellosis in the Azores, Portugal–outcome of a 5-year programme (2002–2007) based on test-and-slaughter and RB51 vaccination. *Prev. Vet. Med.* 94: 154–157.

Blasco, J.M., Gamazo, C., Winter, A.J. et al. (1993a). Evaluation of whole cell and subcellular vaccines against *Brucella ovis* in rams. *Vet. Immunol. Immunopathol.* 37: 257–270.

Blasco, J.M., Marín, C., Jiménez de Bagüés, M.P., and Barberán, M. (1993b). Efficacy of *Brucella suis* strain 2 vaccine against *Brucella ovis* in rams. *Vaccine* 11: 1291–1294.

Bosseray, N. and Plommet, M. (1990). *Brucella suis* S2, *Brucella melitensis* Rev. 1 and *Brucella abortus* S19 living vaccines: residual virulence and immunity induced against three *Brucella* species challenge strains in mice. *Vaccine* 8: 462–468.

Brinley Morgan, W.J., Littlejohn, A.I., MacKinnon, D.J., and Lawson, J.R. (1966). The degree of protection given by living vaccines against experimental infection with *Brucella melitensis* in goats. *Bull. World Health Organ.* 34: 33–40.

Chacón-Díaz, C., Muñoz-Rodríguez, M., Barquero-Calvo, E. et al. (2011). The use of green fluorescent protein as a marker for *Brucella* vaccines. *Vaccine* 29: 577–582.

Cheville, N.F., Olsen, S.C., Jensen, A.E. et al. (1996). Bacterial persistence and immunity in goats vaccinated with a PurE deletion mutant or the parental 16M strain of *Brucella melitensis*. *Infect. Immun.* 64: 2431–2439.

Cloeckaert, A., Zygmunt, M.S., and Guilloteau, L.A. (2002). *Brucella abortus* vaccine strain RB51 produces low levels of M-like O-antigen. *Vaccine* 20: 1820–1822.

Comerci, D., Serantes, D.R., Carballo, E. et al. (2013). Evaluación de la eficacia protectiva de la vacuna antibrucélica, *Brucella abortus* Delta-pgm en bovinos. *SNS* 1: 1–16.

Corner, L.A. (1983). Three aspects of bovine brucellosis: epidemiology, the role of bulls and vaccines. *New South Wales Vet. Proc.* 19: 47–48.

Corner, L.A. and Alton, G.G. (1981). Persistence of *Brucella abortus* strain 19 infection in adult cattle vaccinated with reduced doses. *Res. Vet. Sci.* 31: 342–344.

Crasta, O.R., Folkerts, O., Fei, Z. et al. (2008). Genome sequence of *Brucella abortus* vaccine strain S19 compared to virulent strains yields candidate virulence genes. *PLoS One* 3: e2193.

Da Costa Martins, R., Irache, J.M., Blasco, J.M. et al. (2009). Evaluation of particulate acellular vaccines against *Brucella ovis* infection in rams. *Vaccine* 28: 3038–3046.

Dalrymple-Champneys, W. (1960). *Brucella Infection and Undulant Fever in Man*. London: Oxford University Press.

Davis, D.S. and Elzer, P.H. (2002). *Brucella* vaccines in wildlife. *Vet. Microbiol.* 90: 533–544.

Dean, A.S., Crump, L., Greter, H. et al. (2012). Global burden of human brucellosis: a systematic review of disease frequency. *PLoS Negl.Trop. Dis.* 6: e1865.

Denisov, A.A., Sclyarov, O.D., Salmakov, K.M., and Shumilov, K.V. (2013). The Russian experience in brucellosis veterinary public health. *Rev. Sci. Tech.* 32: 229–237.

Deqiu, S., Donglou, X., and Jiming, Y. (2002). Epidemiology and control of brucellosis in China. *Vet. Microbiol.* 90: 165–182.

Dorneles, E.M.S., Lima, G.K., Teixeira-Carvalho, A.E.A. et al. (2015). Immune response of calves vaccinated with *Brucella abortus* S19 or RB51 and revaccinated with RB51. *PLoS One* 10: e0136696.

Dougherty, A.M.F., Cornish, T.E., O'Toole, D. et al. (2013). Abortion and premature birth in cattle following vaccination with *Brucella abortus* strain RB51. *J. Vet. Diagn. Invest.* 25: 630–635.

Dubray, G. (1997). New vaccination approaches to animal and human brucellosis. WHO Meeting on Development of New/Improved Brucellosis Vaccines, Geneva, Switzerland.

Ducrotoy, M.J., Bertu, W.J., Ocholi, R.A. et al. (2014). Brucellosis as an emerging threat in developing economies: lessons from Nigeria. *PLoS Negl.Trop. Dis.* 8: e3008.

Ducrotoy, M.J., Conde-Álvarez, R., Blasco, J.M., and Moriyón, I. (2016). A review of the basis of the immunological diagnosis of ruminant brucellosis. *Vet. Immunol. Immunopathol.* 17: 81–102.

Edmonds, M.D., Cloeckaert, A., Hagius, S. et al. (2002). Pathogenicity and protective activity in pregnant goats of a *Brucella melitensis* Deltaomp25 deletion mutant. *Res. Vet. Sci.* 72: 235–239.

El Idrissi, A., Benkirane, A., El Maadoudi, M. et al. (2001). Comparison of the efficacy of *Brucella abortus* strain RB51 and *Brucella melitensis* Rev. 1 live vaccines against experimental infection with *Brucella melitensis* in pregnant ewes. *Rev. Sci. Tech.* 20: 741–747.

Elzer, P.H., Hagius, S.D., Robertson, G.T. et al. (1996). Behaviour of a high-temperature-requirement (Htra) deletion mutant of *Brucella abortus* in goats. *Res. Vet. Sci.* 60: 48–50.

Fensterbank, R. and Plommet, M. (1979). Vaccination against bovine brucellosis with a low dose of strain 19 administered by the conjunctival route. IV. Comparison between two methods of vaccination. *Ann. Rech. Vet.* 10: 131–139.

Fiorentino, M.A., Campos, E., Cravero, S. et al. (2008). Protection levels in vaccinated heifers with experimental vaccines *Brucella abortus* M1-luc and INTA 2. *Vet. Microbiol.* 132: 302–311.

Fluegel, A.M., Cornish, T.E., O'Toole, D. et al. (2013). Abortion and premature birth in cattle following vaccination with *Brucella abortus* strain RB51. *J. Vet. Diagn. Invest.* 25: 630–635.

Fosgate, G.T., Adesiyun, A.A., Hird, D.W. et al. (2003). Evaluation of brucellosis RB51 vaccine for domestic water buffalo (*Bubalus bubalis*) in Trinidad. *Prev. Vet. Med.* 58: 211–225.

Freer, E., Rojas, N., Weintraub, A. et al. (1995). Heterogeneity of *Brucella abortus* lipopolysaccharides. *Res. Microbiol.* 146: 569–578.

Garin-Bastuji, B., Blasco, J.M., Grayon, M., and Verger, J.M. (1998). *Brucella melitensis* infection in sheep: present and future. *Vet. Res.* 29: 255–274.

Gee, J.M., Kovach, M.E., Grippe, V.K. et al. (2004). Role of catalase in the virulence of *Brucella melitensis* in pregnant goats. *Vet. Microbiol.* 102: 111–115.

González, D., Grilló, M.J., de Miguel, M.J. et al. (2008). Brucellosis vaccines: assessment of *Brucella melitensis* lipopolysaccharide rough mutants defective in core and O-polysaccharide synthesis and export. *PLoS One* 3: e2760.

Greiner, M., Verloo, D., and de Massis, F. (2009). Meta-analytical equivalence studies on diagnostic tests for bovine brucellosis allowing assessment of a test against a group of comparative tests. *Prev. Vet. Med.* 92: 373–381.

Grilló, M.J., Bosseray, N., and Blasco, J.M. (2000). *In vitro* markers and biological activity in mice of seed lot strains and commercial *Brucella melitensis* Rev1 and *Brucella abortus* B19 vaccines. *Biologicals* 28: 119–127.

Grilló, M.J., Marín, C., Barberán, M. et al. (2009). Efficacy of bp26 and bp26/omp31 *B. melitensis* Rev.1 deletion mutants against *Brucella ovis* in rams. *Vaccine* 27: 187–191.

Grilló, M.J., Blasco, J.M., Gorvel, J.-P. et al. (2012). What have we learned from brucellosis in the mouse model. *Vet. Res.* 43: 29.

Hernández-Mora, G., Ruiz-Villalobos, N., Bonilla-Montoya, R. et al. (2017). Epidemiology of bovine brucellosis in Costa Rica: lessons learned from failures in the control of the disease. *PLoS One* 12 (8): e0182380.

Herrera, E., Palomares, G., and Díaz-Aparicio, E. (2008). Milk production increase in a dairy farm under a six-year brucellosis control program. *Ann. N.Y. Acad. Sci.* 1149: 296–299.

Herrera-Lopez, E., Suárez-Guemes, F., Hernández-Andrade, L. et al. (2010). Epidemiological study of brucellosis in cattle, immunized with *Brucella abortus* RB51 vaccine in endemic zones. *Vaccine* 28 (Suppl): F59–F63.

Hornsby, R.L., Jensen, A.E., Olsen, S.C., and Thoen, C.O. (2000). Selective media for isolation of *Brucella abortus* strain RB51. *Vet. Microbiol.* 73: 51–60.

Jacques, I., Verger, J.M., Laroucau, K. et al. (2007). Immunological responses and protective efficacy against *Brucella melitensis* induced by bp26 and omp31 *B. melitensis* Rev.1 deletion mutants in sheep. *Vaccine* 25: 794–805.

Jiménez de Bagüés, M.P., Marín, C., and Blasco, J.M. (1991). Effect of antibiotic therapy and strain-19 vaccination on the spread of *Brucella melitensis* within an infected dairy herd. *Prev. Vet. Med.* 11: 17–24.

Jones, B.A., Grace, D., Kock, R. et al. (2013). Zoonosis emergence linked to agricultural intensification and environmental change. *Proc. Natl. Acad. Sci. U.S.A.* 110: 8399–8404.

Kahl-McDonagh, M., Elzer, P.H., Hagius, S.D. et al. (2006). Evaluation of novel *Brucella melitensis* unmarked deletion mutants for safety and efficacy in the goat model of brucellosis. *Vaccine* 24: 5169–5177.

Kreeger, T.J., Cook, W.E., Edwards, W.H. et al. (2002). *Brucella abortus* strain RB51 vaccination in elk. II. Failure of high dosage to prevent abortion. *J. Wildl. Dis.* 38: 27–31.

Lambert, G., Deyoe, B.L., and Painter, G.M. (1964). Postvaccinal persistence of *Brucella abortus* strain 19 in two bulls. *J. Am. Vet. Med. Assoc.* 145: 909–911.

Le Fleche, P., Jacques, I., Grayon, M. et al. (2006). Evaluation and selection of tandem repeat loci for a *Brucella* MLVA typing assay. *BMC Microbiol.* 6: 1–14.

Leal-Hernández, M., Díaz-Aparicio, E., Pérez, R. et al. (2005). Protection of *Brucella abortus* RB51 revaccinated cows, introduced in a herd with active brucellosis, with presence of atypical humoral response. *Comp. Immunol. Microbiol. Infect. Dis.* 28: 63–70.

Lucero, N.E., Corazza, R., Almuzara, M.N. et al. (2010). Human *Brucella canis* outbreak linked to infection in dogs. *Epidemiol. Infect.* 138 (2): 280–285.

Luna-Martínez, J.E. and Mejía-Terán, C. (2002). Brucellosis in Mexico: current status and trends. *Vet. Microbiol.* 90: 19–30.

Ma, W., Guo, F., Wang, A. et al. (2014). Complete genome sequence of *B. abortus* RB51 and genomic comparison with *B. abortus* 2308. *J. Anim. Vet. Adv.* 13: 582–588.

Mainar-Jaime, R. C., Marín, C., de Miguel, M. J., et al. (2008). Experiences on the use of RB51 vaccine in Spain. Proceedings of the Brucellosis 2008 International Conference, Royal Holloway College, University of London, UK, pp. 10–13

Mainar-Jaime, R. C., Muñoz, P. M., de Miguel, M. J., Marín, C., Dieste L. & Blasco, J. M. 2011. Abortions induced by RB51 vaccine in beef cattle in central Spain: a descriptive study. Proceedings of the Brucellosis 2011 International Research Conference, Buenos Aires, Argentina, September 21–23rd.

Mancilla, M., Grilló, M.J., de Miguel, M.J. et al. (2013). Deletion of the GI-2 integrase and the *wbkA* flanking transposase improves the stability of *Brucella melitensis* Rev1 vaccine. *Vet. Res.* 44: 105.

Manthei, C.A. (1959). Summary of controlled research with strain 19. Proceedings of the 63rd Annual Meeting of the US Livestock Sanitation Association, p. 128.

Marín, C., Moreno, E., Moriyón, I. et al. (1999). Performance of competitive and indirect enzyme-linked immunosorbent assays, gel immunoprecipitation with native hapten polysaccharide, and standard serological tests in diagnosis of sheep brucellosis. *Clin. Diagn. Lab. Immunol.* 6: 269–272.

Martins, H., Garin-Bastuji, B., Lima, F. et al. (2009). Eradication of bovine brucellosis in the Azores, Portugal-outcome of a 5-year programme (2002–2007) based on test-and-slaughter and RB51 vaccination. *Prev. Vet. Med.* 90: 80–89.

Martins, H., Garin-Bastuji, B., Lima, F. et al. (2010). Reply to letter to the editor by Blasco and Moriyon (2009) concerning the manuscript 'eradication of bovine brucellosis (BB) in the Azores, Portugal-outcome of a 5-year programme (2002–2007) based on test-and-slaughter and RB51 vaccination' by H. Martins et al. (2009). *Prev. Vet. Med.* 94: 158–162.

McDermott, J., Grace, D., and Zinsstag, J. (2013). Economics of brucellosis impact and control in low-income countries. *Rev. Sci. Tech.* 32: 249–261.

Monreal, D., Grilló, M.J., González, D. et al. (2003). Characterization of *Brucella abortus* O-polysaccharide and core lipopolysaccharide mutants and demonstration that a complete core is required for rough vaccines to be efficient against *Brucella abortus* and *Brucella ovis* in the mouse model. *Infect. Immun.* 71: 3261–3271.

Moreno, E. (2014). Retrospective and prospective perspectives on zoonotic brucellosis. *Front. Microbiol.* 5: 213.

Moriyón, I., Grilló, M.J., Monreal, D. et al. (2004). Rough vaccines in animal brucellosis: structural and genetic basis and present status. *Vet. Res.* 35: 1–38.

Muñoz, P.M., Marín, C., Monreal, D. et al. (2005). Efficacy of several serological tests and antigens for diagnosis of bovine brucellosis in the presence of false-positive serological results due to *Yersinia enterocolitica* O: 9. *Clin. Diagn. Lab. Immunol.* 12: 141–151.

Muñoz, P.M., Estevan, M., Marín, C.M. et al. (2006). *Brucella* outer membrane complex-loaded microparticles as a vaccine against *Brucella ovis* in rams. *Vaccine* 24: 1897–1905.

Muñoz, P.M., de Miguel, M.J., Grilló, M.J. et al. (2008). Immunopathological responses and kinetics of *Brucella melitensis* Rev1 infection after subcutaneous or conjunctival vaccination in rams. *Vaccine* 26: 2562–2569.

Negrón, M.E., Kharod, G.A., Bower, W.A., and Walke, H. (2019). *Notes from the Field:* human *Brucella abortus* RB51 infections caused by consumption of unpasteurized domestic dairy products – United States, 2017–2019. *MMWR Morb. Mortal Wkly Rep.* 68: 185.

Nicoletti, P. (1976). A preliminary report on the efficacy of adult cattle vaccination using strain 19 in selected dairy herds in Florida. Proceedings of the Annual Meeting of the US Animal Health Association, pp. 91–106.

Nicoletti, P. (1984). Vaccination of cattle with *Brucella abortus* strain 19 administered by differing routes and doses. *Vaccine* 2: 133–135.

Nicoletti, P. (1990). Vaccination. In: *Animal Brucellosis* (eds. K.H. Nielsen and J.R. Duncan), 283–299. Boca Raton: CRC Press.

Nicoletti, P., Jones, L.M., and Berman, D.T. (1978a). Adult vaccination with standard and reduced doses of *Brucella abortus* strain 19. Vaccine in a dairy herd infected with brucellosis. *J. Am. Vet. Med. Assoc.* 173: 1445–1449.

Nicoletti, P., Jones, L.M., and Berman, D.T. (1978b). Comparison of the subcutaneous and conjunctival route of vaccination with *Brucella abortus* strain 19 vaccine in adult cattle. *J. Am. Vet. Med. Assoc.* 173: 1450–1456.

Nielsen, K.H., Smith, P., Yu, W. et al. (2005). Towards single screening tests for brucellosis. *Rev. Sci. Tech.* 24: 1027–1037.

OIE (2017). Brucellosis (*B. abortus*, *B. melitensis* and *B. suis*) (Infection with *B. abortus*, *B. melitensis* and *B. suis*). In: *Manual of Diagnostic Tests and Vaccines for Terrestrial Animals 2017*. Paris: OIE.

Olsen, S.C. (2000). Immune responses and efficacy after administration of a commercial *Brucella abortus* strain RB51 vaccine to cattle. *Vet. Ther.* 1: 183–191.

Pérez-Sancho, M., Adone, R., García-Seco, T. et al. (2014). Evaluation of the immunogenicity and safety of *Brucella melitensis* B115 vaccination in pregnant sheep. *Vaccine* 32: 1877–1881.

Phillips, R.W., Elzer, P.H., Robertson, G.T. et al. (1997). A *Brucella melitensis* high-temperature-requirement A (HtrA) deletion mutant is attenuated in goats and protects against abortion. *Res. Vet. Sci.* 63: 165–167.

Plommet, M. (1977). Studies on experimental brucellosis in cows in France. In: *Bovine Brucellosis an International Symposium* (eds. R.P. Crawford and R.J. Hidalgo), 116–134. College Station: Texas A&M University Press.

Plommet, M. (1984). Progres recents en immunization contre l'infection à *Brucella abortus*. *Prev. Vet. Med.* 2: 205–514.

Plommet, M. and Fensterbank, R. (1976). Vaccination against bovine brucellosis with a low dose of strain 19 administered by the conjunctival route. III. Serological response and immunity in the pregnant cow. *Ann. Rech. Vet.* 7: 9–23.

Plommet, M. and Fensterbank, R. (1984). La vaccination antibrucellique administrée par voie conjonctivale. *Dev. Biol. Stand.* 56: 681–687.

Ragan, V.E. (2002). The Animal and Plant Health Inspection Service (APHIS) brucellosis eradication program in the United States. *Vet. Microbiol.* 90: 11–18.

Ray, W.C. (1976). An assessment of investigations conducted in the USA on *Brucella abortus* strain 45/20 bacterins. *Dev. Biol. Stand.* 31: 335–342.

Rojas, N., Zamora, O., Cascante, J. et al. (2001). Comparison of the antibody response in adult cattle against different epitopes of *Brucella abortus* lipopolysaccharide. *J. Vet. Med. B* 48: 623–629.

Roop, R., Phillips, R., Hagius, S. et al. (2001). Re-examination of the role of the *Brucella melitensis* HtrA stress response protease in virulence in pregnant goats. *Vet. Microbiol.* 82: 91–95.

Sáez, J.L., Sanz, C., Durán, M. et al. (2014). Comparison of depopulation and S19-RB51 vaccination strategies for control of bovine brucellosis in high prevalence areas. *Vet. Rec.* 174 (25): 634.

Salih-Alj Debbarh, H., Cloeckaert, A., Bezard, G. et al. (1996). Enzyme-linked immunosorbent assay with partially purified cytosoluble 28-kilodalton protein for serological differentiation between *Brucella melitensis*-infected and *B. melitensis* Rev.1-vaccinated sheep. *Clin. Diagn. Lab. Immunol.* 3: 305–308.

Sanz, C., Sáez, J.L., Álvarez, J. et al. (2010). Mass vaccination as a complementary tool in the control of a severe outbreak of bovine brucellosis due to *Brucella abortus* in Extremadura, Spain. *Prev. Vet. Med.* 97: 119–125.

Silva, A.P.I.C.C., Macêdo, A.E.L.A., Costa, L.F. et al. (2015). Encapsulated *Brucella ovis* lacking a putative ATP-binding cassette transporter (Δ*abcBA*) protects against wild type *Brucella ovis* in rams. *PLoS One* 10: 1–18.

Spink, W.W. (1956). The pathogenesis of brucellosis. In: *The Nature of Brucellosis*, 113–144. Minneapolis: University of Minnesota Press.

Stoffregen, W.C., Olsen, S., and Bricker, B.J. (2006). Parenteral vaccination of domestic pigs with *Brucella abortus* strain RB51. *Am. J. Vet. Res.* 67: 1802–1808.

Tabynov, K., Kydyrbayev, Z., Ryskeldinova, S. et al. (2014a). Novel influenza virus vectors expressing *Brucella* L7/L12 or Omp16 proteins in cattle induced a strong T-cell immune response, as well as high protectiveness against *B. abortus* infection. *Vaccine* 32: 2034–2041.

Tabynov, K., Yespembetov, B., and Sansyzbay, A. (2014b). Novel vector vaccine against *Brucella abortus* based on influenza A viruses expressing *Brucella* L7/L12 or Omp16 proteins: evaluation of protection in pregnant heifers. *Vaccine* 32: 5889–5892.

Tabynov, K., Ryskeldinova, S., and Sansyzbay, A. (2015). An influenza viral vector *Brucella abortus* vaccine induces good cross-protection against *Brucella melitensis* infection in pregnant heifers. *Vaccine* 33: 3619–3623.

Trap, D. and Gaumont, R. (1982). Comparaison entre électrosynérèse et épreuves sérologiques classiques dans le diagnostic de la brucellose ovine. *Ann. Rech. Vet.* 13: 33–39.

Ugalde, J.E., Comerci, D.J., Leguizamon, M.S., and Ugalde, R.A. (2003). Evaluation of *Brucella abortus* phosphoglucomutase (*pgm*) mutant as a new live rough-phenotype vaccine. *Infect. Immun.* 71: 6264–6269.

Verger, J.M. (1985). *B. melitensis* infection of cattle. In: *Brucella melitensis* (eds. J.M. Verger and M. Plommet), 197–203. Dordrech: Martinus Nijhoff.

Verger, J.M., Grayon, M., Zundel, E. et al. (1995). Comparison of the efficacy of *Brucella suis* strain 2 and *Brucella melitensis* Rev. 1 live vaccines against a *Brucella melitensis* experimental infection in pregnant ewes. *Vaccine* 13: 191–196.

Villalobos-Vindas, J.M., Amuy, E., Barquero-Calvo, E. et al. (2017). Brucellosis caused by the wood rat pathogen *Brucella neotomae*: two case reports. *J. Med. Case Rep.* 11 (1): 352.

Villarroel, M., Grell, M., and Saenz, R. (2000). Reporte de primer caso humano de aislamiento y tipificación de *Brucella abortus* RB51. *Arch. Med. Vet.* 32: 89–91.

Wallach, J.C., Ferrero, M.C., Delpino, M.V. et al. (2008). Occupational infection due to *Brucella abortus* S19 among workers involved in vaccine production in Argentina. *Clin. Microbiol. Infect.* 14: 805–807.

Wang, Y., Zhang, W., Ke, Y. et al. (2012). Human brucellosis, a heterogeneously distributed, delayed and misdiagnosed disease in China. *Clin. Infect. Dis.* 56: 750–751.

Whatmore, A.M. (2009). Current understanding of the genetic diversity of *Brucella*, an expanding genus of zoonotic pathogens. *Infect Genet Evol* 9: 1168–1184.

Whatmore, A.M., Davison, N., Cloeckaert, A. et al. (2014). *Brucella papionis* sp. nov. isolated from baboons (*Papio* spp.). *Int. J. Syst. Evol. Microbiol.* 64: 4120–4128.

World Health Organization. (1999). The development of new/improved brucellosis vaccines. Report of a WHO meeting, Geneva, Switzerland, 11–12 December 1997. Geneva: World Health Organization.

Xin, X. (1986). Orally administrable brucellosis vaccine: *Brucella suis* strain 2 vaccine. *Vaccine* 4: 212–216.

Zinsstag, J., Schelling, E., Solera, J. et al. (2011). Brucellosis. In: *Handbook of Zoonoses*, 2e (eds. S.R. Palmer, L. Soulsby, P.R. Torgeson and D.G. Brown), 54–62. Oxford: Oxford University Press.

23

Contagious Bovine Pleuropneumonia

François Thiaucourt[1], *Nick Nwankpa*[2], *and William Amanfu*[3]

[1] *CIRAD, UMR_INRA, ASTRE, Montpellier, France*
[2] *Pan African Veterinary Vaccine Center, African Union Commission, Debre Zeit, Ethiopia*
[3] *International Veterinary Consultant, Accra, Ghana*

23.1 Introduction

Contagious bovine pleuropneumonia (CBPP) is an infectious disease affecting *Bovidae* and caused by a mycoplasma: *M. mycoides* subsp. *mycoides* (Mmm) (OIE 2015). The disease is transmitted directly, from a sick animal to a susceptible one, through droplets expelled during coughing. The incubation period may vary from 3 weeks to 6 months with an average of 4–5 weeks. Within a naïve herd, the susceptibility may vary from animal to animal, some being naturally resistant, others moderately susceptible, and others highly susceptible. The proportion of susceptible animals will depend notably on the virulence of the circulating Mmm strain. In the vast majority of cases, the lesions will be unilateral.

Highly susceptible animals develop exudative pleuropneumonia lesions affecting the whole lung (left or right) with an accumulation of high quantities of pleural effusion resulting from the inflammation of the pleura (Provost et al. 1987). Affected lungs and pleural effusion are ideal environments that allow the mycoplasmas to multiply to high titers (up to $10^{9.5}$ per mL). These animals may be responsible for the rapid transmission to in-contact susceptible animals within a radius of up to 50 m. In the absence of antibiotic treatment, a high proportion of acutely infected animals will die within 10–30 days.

Moderately susceptible animals will develop a localized lesion of pneumonia which will not spread to the whole lung. In such cases, lesions will progressively be surrounded by a fibrous tissue encapsulating the affected lung. Such lesions, called "sequestra," can persist for long periods of up to 2 years and Mmm can be shed for a long time. Although it is difficult to measure the exact risk they represent, these animals may be responsible for the long-term persistence of CBPP as they are difficult to identify (Hudson 1972).

Contagious bovine pleuropneumonia recently emerged as a disease, around 300 years ago (Dupuy et al. 2012). It gained an almost worldwide distribution in the middle of the nineteenth century through cattle trade and movement. By the end of the nineteenth century and the beginning of the twentieth century, many countries regained their CBPP-free status by applying very strict control measures based on the slaughter of affected herds and the control of animal movements.

Mycoplasmas are susceptible to a number of drugs and antibiotics but, after 1950, the control of the disease was based on the use of live vaccines, obtained after empirical attenuation that followed passages in broth medium or embryonated eggs (Thiaucourt et al. 2000). In Australia, massive campaigns using the V5 strain allowed a dramatic reduction of CBPP prevalence. A switch to a strict test and slaughter policy led to the eradication of the disease from that continent (Newton 1992). Similarly, in Africa, the joint vaccination campaigns against rinderpest and CBPP, using the T1/44 or T1sr strains enabled the eradication of rinderpest and led to the efficient control of CBPP.

Following the decrease and eventual halt in vaccination efforts due to the success of the rinderpest eradication campaign, CBPP distribution and impact progressively increased in Africa (Masiga et al. 1996) (Figure 23.1). Southern Europe suffered from sporadic outbreaks of CBPP at 10–20-year intervals and the disease was eventually eliminated by test and slaughter policies at herd level. These outbreaks were due to resurgences from European Mmm strains that escaped the eradication policies and

Veterinary Vaccines: Principles and Applications, First Edition. Edited by Samia Metwally, Gerrit Viljoen, and Ahmed El Idrissi.

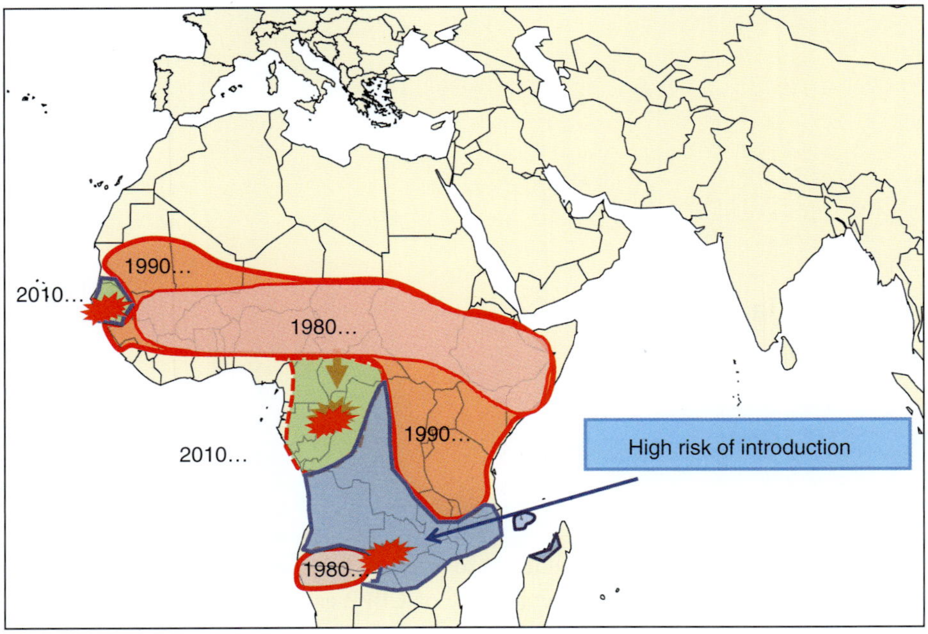

Figure 23.1 The map shows the estimated distribution of CBPP and how it has progressively extended its range in Africa. In the 1980s (salmon color) the disease was well controlled and restricted in a Sahelian zone thanks to annual vaccinations against rinderpest and CBPP. The disease distribution then progressively extended, notably at the beginning of the 1990s (orange color) until 2015, with emergence in Gabon, Congo, the Gambia, and Senegal (green color). The risk of CBPP introduction is maximal for countries bordering infected zones and CBPP could possibly spill out of Africa (dark blue color). Red flashes indicate most recent CBPP outbreaks declared in regions that were previously considered as CBPP-free.

remained undetected in between outbreaks. The last recorded CBPP outbreak occurred in 1999 and since then, Europe has been CBPP free.

Africa is currently the only continent where CBPP is highly prevalent, with areas south of the Sahara and north of the South African Development Community region affected by the disease. Insufficient funding, disorganization of centralized state veterinary services, and civil unrest are some of the reasons for inefficient vaccination campaigns and CBPP persistence (Amanfu 2009). Cattle owners are often left with the only option of treating their affected animals with antibiotics (Amanfu 2006). These treatments are also frequently suboptimal with products and regimens of nonguaranteed quality leading to higher risks of bacterial antibiotic resistance emergence.

23.2 Types of Vaccines

In the past, a number of attenuated vaccine strains were developed by successive passages in broth or embryonated eggs. Such strains included V5 (Australia), DK32 (Senegal), KH3J (Sudan), and Ben-181 (China). These vaccines were successfully used in the field but were progressively superseded by the T1/44 and T1sr strains, notably in Africa. In the early twentieth century, the search for inactivated vaccines was rapidly abandoned as live vaccines seemed both efficient and more cost-effective.

Currently, T1/44 and T1sr are the only Mmm vaccine strains that are available commercially. T1/44 was developed by passaging a naturally low-virulence Mmm strain 44 times in embryonated eggs (Sheriff and Piercy 1952). The resulting strain was sufficiently attenuated to induce a small local reaction, or no reaction at all, when injected subcutaneously while still inducing sufficient levels of protection. However, this strain may sometimes induce a local invading inflammatory reaction called "Willems reaction" (Figure 23.2). The frequency of postvaccine local reaction is quite unpredictable and may vary from 0% to 0.5%, rarely more. These reactions may occur when animals are vaccinated for the first time and not after revaccination. In such cases, appropriate antibiotic treatment must be implemented otherwise the animal may die.

T1sr is a derivative of T1/44 that has been subjected to a limited number of passages in a medium containing streptomycin to make it streptomycin resistant (Doutre et al. 1972). T1sr could then be mixed with the rinderpest vaccine that contained residues of penicillin and streptomycin; two antibiotics that were inactive against T1sr. T1sr can be used alone and has no residual virulence. The advantages and drawbacks of the T1/44 and T1sr strains are summarized in Table 23.1.

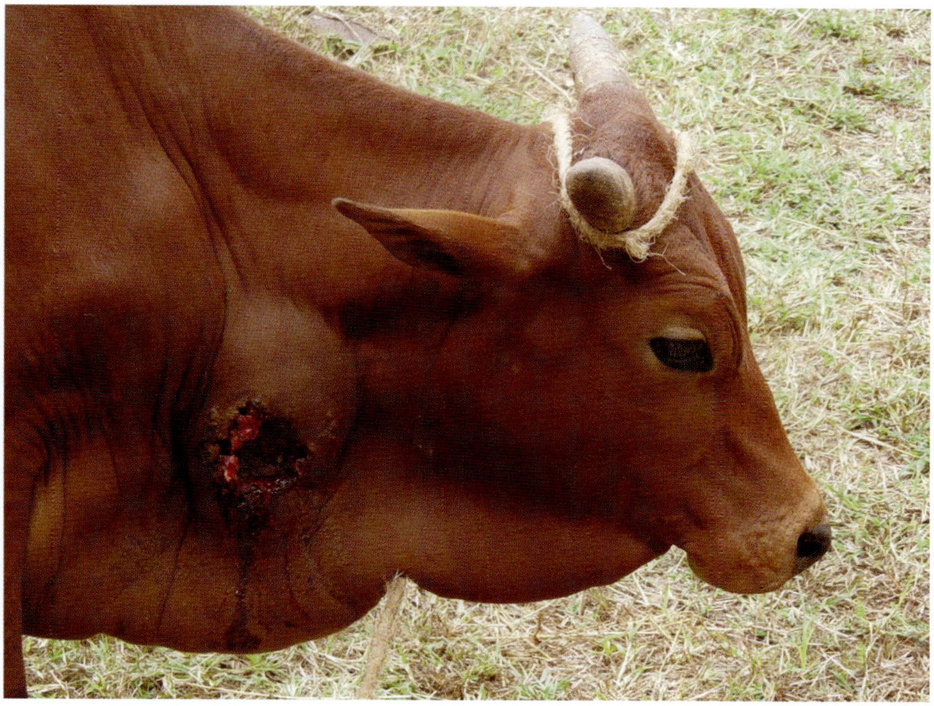

Figure 23.2 "Willems reaction" following inoculation of T1/44 vaccine. T1/44 sometimes induces an invading edema in animals vaccinated for the first time. The local subcutaneous inflammation develops slowly but steadily and can be clearly seen 15 days after vaccination. Antibiotic treatment should begin no later than 15 days to prevent further extension to dewlap or lungs that could put the animal's life at risk. When the reaction recedes, a piece of skin may slough after necrosis of the local tissue and then leave a visible scar.

These vaccines are usually provided in a freeze-dried form and must be accompanied by a proper diluent. A commercial batch of vaccine is a derivative of the grandparental stock generated by a limited number of passages, usually four, as recommended by the OIE *Manual of Diagnostic Tests and Vaccines for Terrestrial Animals* (OIE 2015). A grandparental stock of T1/44 and T1sr is kept at the African Union Pan African Veterinary Vaccine Centre (AU-PANVAC) to be distributed to vaccine producers. The absence of a cloning procedure and the limited number of passages during the vaccine production process are intended to limit the genetic drift that may otherwise occur, leading to products with unknown qualities. Mycoplasmas are bacteria with a very small genome, about 1 M base long, but with a relatively high mutation frequency. In addition, Mmm genomes are characterized by the presence of a high number of mobile genetic elements called "insertion sequences" which may undergo transposition and/or duplication events. The genome of the T1/44 strain has been published recently (Gourgues et al. 2016) and it presents a large 173 kb inversion when compared with other Mmm strains such as PG1 or Gladysdale. It is not known if this inversion was present in the original T1 strain genome or if it was acquired during the egg passages.

Recent advances in mycoplasma and molecular biology have opened promising new fields for the development of more effective CBPP vaccines that could be based on various options such as targeted attenuation of live strains, inactivated preparations, adjuvants, subunit vaccines or vectored antigens, modified and targeted delivery systems (Karst 1972; Tulasne et al. 1996; Thiaucourt et al. 2003; Dedieu-Engelmann 2008; Jores et al. 2013), or modified production processes to improve stability (March 2004; Litamoi et al. 2005). A recent FAO coordinated meeting on CBPP called for renewed efforts to be put into the development and validation of alternative CBPP vaccines (www.fao.org/ag/againfo/programmes/en/empres/news_291015b.html). However, no new vaccines are at a "near licensing" stage, to our knowledge.

23.3 Immune Response and Duration of Immunity

The mechanisms leading to protection in cattle are still poorly understood as well as the mycoplasma antigens that trigger that protection. It has been observed that animals recovering from natural CBPP were solidly immune to new infections (Rurangirwa et al. 1976). Traditional vaccination

Table 23.1 CBPP vaccines: advantages and drawbacks.

	T1/44	T1sr
Advantages		
A single "serotype" for Mmm	X	X
Low production costs	X	X
Long conservation at −20 °C when freeze dried	X	X
Easy subcutaneous administration	X	X
Transient seroconversion allowing detection of outbreaks	X	X
Relative thermostability when reconstituted (3 h at 37 °C)	X	X
Inocuity		X
Drawbacks		
Need for revaccinations to induce strong protection	X	XX
Vaccination alone not allowing eradication of CBPP	X	X
Weak seroconversion not allowing monitoring of vaccination campaigns	X	X
Need for a cold chain	X	X
No *in vitro* assay correlating with protection	X	X
No small experimental animal allowing vaccine efficacy testing	X	X
Short-lived protection (6 months)		X
Possible residual virulence	X	

procedures followed by the Peul tribes in West Africa in the nineteenth century were certainly derived from this observation. They reproduced CBPP lesions by inserting infectious material at the bridge of the nose which resulted in localized inflammation and solid immunity after recovery. In contrast, it also seems that some mycoplasma antigens and effective immune stimulation could lead to an absence of protection or, worse, an increased sensitivity to CBPP (Hübschle et al. 2003; Mulongo et al. 2015). In fact, animals that developed sequestra after an artificial infection had higher antibody titers than those that did not (Schieck et al. 2014).

In the case of T1/44 and T1sr, there is a consensus that the protective immunity is cell mediated. Vaccination with either T1/44 or T1sr triggers a short-lived and limited antibody response, irrespective of the test used for measurement (complement fixation test, indirect enzyme-linked immunosorbent assay [ELISA] or cELISA). Furthermore, revaccination does not induce a classic anamnestic antibody response. This limited antibody response can be seen as a practical advantage for the surveillance of CBPP. Serological tests can be used to detect CBPP cases in regions where vaccination has been implemented, provided the sera are gathered at least 3 months after the last vaccination. On the other hand, cell-mediated immunity can be monitored by proliferation assays performed on peripheral blood mononuclear cells (PBMCs) or $CD4^+$ T cells. While limited cell-mediated responses are observed after one or two vaccinations, these responses are notable after three vaccinations (Totte et al. 2013). Such tests are used experimentally but not on a routine basis to assess the immune status of vaccinated animals.

These observations corroborated what has been observed experimentally or in the field. Controlled experiments have shown that T1/44 and T1sr induced similar levels of protection when they were used to vaccinate naïve cattle (Yaya et al. 1999); vaccination achieved a 60% protection level in both cases. What differentiated T1/44 and T1sr was the duration of immunity which was estimated at 1 year for T1/44 (Gilbert et al. 1970) and only 6 months for T1sr. Experimental and field experiences have shown that repeated annual vaccinations in a herd, region, or compartment led to very satisfactory protection levels (Masiga and Windsor 1974; Provost 1975; Wesonga and Thiaucourt 2000). This explains the control of CBPP in Africa after repeated vaccination campaigns organized to eradicate rinderpest. It also explains the very limited CBPP prevalence in northern Namibia where annual vaccinations have been performed for many years. Residual foci of CBPP are likely to be caused by the influx of infected cattle from neighboring countries.

23.4 Desired Specifications When Ordering Vaccine

- The name of the vaccine strain: T1/44 or T1sr.
- The dose and number of doses per vial: vaccine producers often produce 100 doses per vial. However, these vials usually contain numbers of live mycoplasmas that are only marginally above the threshold indicated by the OIE (10^7 per dose). It is probable that loss will occur along the vaccination chain and that some vaccinated animals will not receive the recommended minimum dose. Provost (1987) has suggested that it would be preferable to use vials containing 10^8 mycoplasmas per dose. This idea has been reinforced during a FAO/OIE/AU-IBAR CBPP consultative group meeting with the suggestion that each vial should be meant for 40–50 doses which would increase the number of viable

mycoplasmas per dose and also reduce the titer drop once the vial is reconstituted.

- Vaccines should be supplied with an appropriate diluent (usually sterile saline or phosphate-buffered saline) (Karst 1972).
- The supplied vaccine comes from a batch which has been subjected to an independent quality control.

23.5 Quality Assurance and Control Testing

Two types of certificates should accompany the vaccine order: one from the vaccine producer (compulsory) and one from an independent laboratory such as the AU-PANVAC (highly recommended).

The producer certificate should include: (i) the name of the vaccine strain, (ii) the unique batch number, (iii) the date of production, (iv) the expiry dates when the vials are kept at −20 °C or +4 °C, (v) a statement on the purity of the product (absence of any bacterial or fungal contaminants), (vi) a statement on the uniformity of the batch, (vii) an estimation of the number of viable mycoplasmas per vial after reconstitution in the appropriate diluent (expressed in colony forming unit or color change unit) with an estimate of the uncertainty of this estimate, (viii) instructions for reconstitution of the vial in the diluent, (ix) recommendations on the permissible delay to administer the vaccine after it has been reconstituted, (x) warning on the possible postvaccine reactions when using T1/44 and ways to cope with these reactions.

The AU-PANVAC provides international independent quality control of veterinary vaccines in Africa and was designated as an OIE collaborating centre for quality control of veterinary vaccines in May 2015 by the OIE General Assembly (see Chapter 3). It is desirable that a formal preshipment request be made to the AU-PANVAC before the submission of vaccines for quality control. The AU-PANVAC sends templates of all documents required for the submission of samples which should be filled and sent at least 1 week before the vaccines are dispatched. These forms are necessary to secure import permits for the vaccines before they arrive and will ensure prompt clearance from the custom authorities.

23.5.1 Tests Indicated for Quality Control of CBPP Vaccines at AU-PANVAC

23.5.1.1 Identity

Polymerase chain reaction (PCR) technique for the *in vitro* identification of mycoplasmas is used as a CBPP vaccine identity test. Two types of PCR tests are used at the AU-PANVAC for CBPP vaccine identity. A specific PCR test for the identification of the vaccine strains T1, T1/44, and T1sr using specific primer pair MmmSCP1-T1M2 (Lorenzon et al. 2000) is used to amplify the 700 bp long DNA fragment in the T1 vaccine strains. This PCR enables the T1 strain to be distinguished from all other vaccine or pathogenic strains. A group-specific PCR is used for the detection of members of the Mycoplasma group (van Kuppeveld et al. 1994). A positive result for both tests confirms the identity of the T1/44 strain in the vaccine. A single positive result with the group-specific PCR may indicate a mycoplasma contamination.

23.5.1.2 Sterility and Freedom from Contamination

Sterility is defined as the absence of living organisms apart from the Mmm used for vaccination. The Standard Procedures for determination of freedom from contamination of CBPP vaccines used by the AU-PANVAC include test procedures for the detection of viable bacteria and fungi in biological materials described in the OIE Terrestrial Manual and ELISA test for the detection of mycoplasmas.

23.5.1.3 Potency

This is determined indirectly by estimating the number of mycoplasmas per dose. The titration method is based on a series of primary 10-fold dilutions, followed by inoculation in liquid or on solid mycoplasma medium. The titers are then expressed in colony forming units (CFUs), in the agar plate method or in viable mycoplasmas (broth method), according to standard calculations.

A minimum of 10^7 per dose is required but higher titers are recommended to take into account the decrease in titer likely to occur at each critical phase (transport to central storage, storage in the field, reconstitution, and delay before administration).

23.5.1.4 Safety

Safety studies for CBPP vaccines during registration include the safety of a single dose, of an overdose, and of repeated single doses. However, for batch control testing of CBPP vaccines, larger dose studies are required at 10 times the normal dose. Due to the cost and space required for using large animals, safety studies for batch control of CBPP vaccines are usually implemented in laboratory animals such as guinea pigs and mice.

23.5.1.5 Stability

Freeze-drying of vaccines is done mainly for preservation, i.e. to ensure that the viability and potency of the vaccine remain stable during its shelf-life when stored at −20 °C or +4 °C. It is important to determine the level of residual moisture in the vaccine as this ensures that the manufacturers' freeze-dry cycle was properly done. The residual moisture is determined at the AU-PANVAC by the gravimetric method and the recommended limit is set at 3%. NB: at −20 °C, freeze-dried CBPP vaccines are theoretically very stable (>5 years). Stability at +4 °C may be more variable and it is the responsibility of the vaccine producer to ensure that its products contain a minimum of 10^7 live mycoplasmas per dose at the end of the expiry date.

23.5.1.6 AU-PANVAC Certificate

Usually, the AU-PANVAC issues a Certificate of Quality together with a report to the manufacturer if the vaccine passes all the prescribed tests. However, if the vaccine fails, only a test report is issued. If a vaccine quality control test request is made by persons other than the manufacturer, only a test report is issued at the end. The Certificate of Quality is issued with respect to the batch of vaccine tested and the sampled vials received by the AU-PANVAC.

23.6 Vaccine Application for Disease Control

Only T1/44 and T1sr vaccines will be discussed here, as they are the only ones currently available on the market.

23.6.1 Epidemiological Settings and Objectives

The design of a cost-effective CBPP control strategy, with a vaccination program, must be based on a reliable evaluation of CBPP prevalence in the various relevant epidemiological compartments. It should also take into account the risks for CBPP spread, especially animal movements (legal or illegal), which are the basis for CBPP spread, maintenance or reintroduction. The surveillance programs have to be tailored for each case (not the subject of this paper) and may include tools such as participatory epidemiological approaches, detection of CBPP lesions at slaughter slabs or slaughterhouses, serological surveys using OIE prescribed tests and performed within a quality management system, detection of outbreaks, and confirmation by detecting Mmm by isolation or molecular techniques.

23.6.2 Vaccination Strategy

In the case of CBPP, the epidemiological unit is the herd. All animals above 6 months should be vaccinated. After primary vaccination, the expected protection rate is about 60% (Nkando et al. 2012). This rate will increase after repeated vaccinations that could take place after 6 months or 1 year. In that case, full protection of the herd is expected after three vaccinations.

It is quite difficult to describe a single vaccination strategy for CBPP, as this will depend on the losses which are due to the disease, the means allocated by the state or requested from cattle owners, and the objectives of the strategy which could span from limited control to reduce CBPP prevalence to an "acceptable level," a near complete control or even an elimination or eradication (Provost 1996; Geering and Amanfu 2002). Once the final objectives have been decided, the strategy should then consider space and time considerations. It should define the scale and locations where the strategy will be applied (one herd, one compartment, a region, a country or a continent) and how it will be sequentially applied. CBPP is one of the few diseases for which the OIE can endorse official control programs. These programs must be clearly described in their objectives, progression, and means of application. This information can be summarized by a questionnaire (OIE Terrestrial Animal Health Code, Chapter 1.10: www.oie.int/index.php?id=169&L=0&htmfile=chapitre_selfdeclaration_CBPP.htm).

The full cooperation of the cattle owners is of paramount importance for the success of the strategy. This means that initial communication is needed to convince owners that CBPP vaccination is the most cost-effective way to cope with the disease and to eventually eliminate it. Great care should be taken to design a uniform strategy for cost recovery and price settings (Kairu-Wanyoike et al. 2014). Warnings about possible postvaccinal reactions when using T1/44 for the first time will have to be clearly mentioned, as otherwise these could jeopardize all future efforts. Alternatively, vaccination campaigns may start using T1sr, before a switch to T1/44.

As vaccine vials usually contain titers which are only marginally above the minimum threshold, it will be of paramount importance to organize the vaccination campaign to limit losses in viability all along the vaccination chain. This includes keeping the vials at −20 °C, limiting the time of storage at +4 °C, using proper diluents, and limiting the time between reconstitution and administration.

It should be noted that historical experience has shown that a strategy based on vaccination alone (with the same live vaccines used today) has never allowed the eradication of the disease. This has to be taken into consideration when designing the final steps of the strategy. The approach should include the implementation of efficient surveillance systems allowing swift detection and confirmation of suspected cases, policies concerning control of animal movement, and slaughter of confirmed CBPP cases. In this last case, great attention should be given to the compensations awarded to owners, as failure to do so will likely lead to smuggling of positive cases and rampant dissemination of CBPP.

23.6.3 Possible Combination with Vaccines for Other Diseases

Past experience during the combined rinderpest and CBPP vaccination campaigns has shown that these two vaccines could be used in combination without any loss of activity to either component (Provost 1969; Jeggo et al. 1987; Rossiter and Kariuki 1987). However, there is a lack of information about possible interference between CBPP vaccine and other types of vaccines. As some vaccines may orientate the immune response toward Th1 or Th2 responses, it is expected that they may have an impact on CBPP vaccination efficiency. This is a field where further research is urgently needed.

23.6.4 Use of Vaccine in the Face of an Outbreak

Here again, no single recommendation can be made, as requirements will depend upon the epidemiological context and the strategy that has been adopted, in the zone where the outbreak occurred.

In the past, Australian veterinary services designed a very precise strategy to reduce CBPP prevalence and eventually to eliminate CBPP from affected herds. All animals were subjected to a serological test (field complement fixation test) and positive animals were sent to slaughter (Mmm is not a zoonotic agent) and the remaining cattle vaccinated. This procedure was implemented at 3-month intervals, until two consecutive tests showed that there were no more positive animals in the herd, or any animal showing clinical symptoms.

Such a strategy may be difficult to implement in many African countries at present. Vaccinating animals that do not show any clinical symptoms is always recommended. The fate of affected animals is more debatable. Slaughtering them would be the ultimate way to reduce the contamination risk but it will not completely eliminate the risk as some animals in the incubation or recovery phase will still shed mycoplasmas. Treating these affected animals with antibiotics could be another option, as it will also reduce the contamination risk. In fact, a strategy based on combining well-applied antibiotic treatments to affected animals with vaccination of the remaining cattle could lead to gradual elimination of the disease in the herd. This is what is suggested by computer models but such a strategy has never been tested experimentally or in the field.

23.6.5 When Vaccination Is Not Recommended

Vaccines are not recommended for countries that wish to regain their CBPP-free status rapidly, which should instead base their eradication strategy on sanitary measures including slaughter and movement control in combination with efficient surveillance systems. Past experiences include the slaughter of affected herds (Europe) or slaughter of the whole cattle population located in an infected zone (Botswana).

Such recommendations may be modified once inactivated DIVA vaccines are available, allowing the differentiation of infected from vaccinated animals and postvaccination seroprevalence studies.

23.7 Monitoring and Vaccine Effectiveness (with the T1/44 Vaccines)

23.7.1 Postvaccination Monitoring

This is an important point to clarify for CBPP vaccines. In contrast to viral vaccines such as rinderpest or peste des petits ruminants (PPR), CBPP vaccines *do not* induce constant and long-lasting seroconversions irrespective of the serological test used (Hudson 1968; Gilbert and Windsor 1971). Hence, serology is not a good tool to monitor the immunity induced by vaccination campaigns.

On the other hand, as antibody titers wane rapidly (after 3 months), serology can be used to detect outbreaks and evaluate CBPP prevalence which should be declining sharply when the vaccination campaigns are successful. The impact of vaccination campaigns on disease can naturally be evaluated with all the surveillance tools applied to CBPP (participatory epidemiology, slaughter slab surveillance, detection of outbreaks). The epidemiological unit that makes sense for CBPP is the herd. Sampling frames should take that fact in consideration and organize a random selection of herds in which selected animals will be targeted, notably those having shown suspicious symptoms previously or older animals. When using a serological test with very high specificity, this sampling strategy should be more cost-effective while enhancing the sensitivity of positive herd detection.

23.7.2 Outbreaks in Vaccinated Animals

The protection afforded by the vaccine should be obtained between 2 and 4 weeks after vaccination. Hence, vaccinated animals can still develop CBPP if the vaccine was not correctly applied or if the animal was already in the incubation period of the disease when vaccinated.

23.8 Vaccine Adverse Reactions

Contagious bovine pleuropneumonia vaccine strain T1/44 sometimes induces a localized invading inflammatory reaction called a "Willems reaction" (Figure 23.2). This reaction develops progressively and can be clearly visible 2 weeks after vaccination. At this time, such reacting animals must receive antibiotic treatment if the reaction becomes large and invading (>20 cm diameter) and does not seem to regress naturally. The percentage of reactors may vary from one place to another (Lindley 1971; Revell 1973) and therefore, this percentage has to be evaluated at the beginning of the vaccination campaign, to adapt the strategy accordingly, possibly switching to T1sr vaccine strain where necessary. Such adverse reactions may be due to a reversion to virulence of the vaccine strain when it is propagating in its natural host (Davies and Gilbert 1969).

Vaccine manufacturers should give clear warnings about adverse reactions in the leaflets that are inserted with the vaccine vials.

23.9 Availability and List of Manufacturers

Contagious bovine pleuropneumonia vaccine is produced by at least eight laboratories in Africa. The global production of CBPP vaccines can be accessed through the OIE website (www.oie.int/wahis_2/public/wahid.php/Countryinformation/Vaccines). The global production varied from 51 to 41 million doses between 2013 and 2015. This is a small proportion of the cattle at risk within Africa. The laboratories producing CBPP vaccine in Africa include the following by country, in alphabetical order:

- Botswana Vaccine Institute (BVI), Gaborone, Botswana. www.bvi.co.bw/content/id/27/Products
- Laboratoire National Vétérinaire (LANAVET), Garoua, Cameroon. www.lanavet.com/Lanavet_WEB
- National Veterinary Institute (NVI), Debre Zeit, Ethiopia. www.nvi.com.et/CBPP.html
- Kenya Veterinary Vaccine Production Institute (KEVEVAPI), Muguga, Kenya. www.kevevapi.org/index.php
- Laboratoire Central de l'Elevage (LABOCEL), Niamey, Niger
- National Veterinary Research Institute (NVRI), Vom, Nigeria. www.nvri.gov.ng/Vaccines_Product.php
- Laboratoire National d'Elevage et de Recherches Vétérinaires (LNERV), Dakar, Senegal
- Laboratoire Central Vétérinaire (LCV), Bamako, Mali

23.10 Summary

Contagious bovine pleuropneumonia is an infectious disease affecting *Bovidae* and caused by a mycoplasma: *M. mycoides* subsp. *mycoides* (Mmm). Presently, Africa is the only continent where CBPP is highly prevalent; insufficient funding, disorganization of centralized state veterinary services, and civil unrest are some of the reasons for inefficient vaccination campaigns and CBPP persistence. In the past, a number of attenuated vaccine strains were successfully used in the field but were progressively superseded, notably in Africa, by two strains, T1/44 and T1sr, and these are now the only Mmm vaccine strains that are available commercially. T1/44 produces longer protective immunity but can induce a local invading inflammatory reaction called "Willems reaction" while T1sr does not. The mechanisms leading to protection in cattle are still poorly understood but it has been observed that animals recovered from natural CBPP infection were solidly protected.

The grandparental stock of T1/44 and T1sr is kept at the African Union Pan African Veterinary Vaccine Centre which is an OIE collaborating centre for distribution to vaccine producers. Recent advances in mycoplasmology and molecular biology have opened promising new fields in the development of more effective CBPP vaccines and a recent FAO coordinated meeting on CBPP issues called for renewed efforts to be put into the development and validation of alternative CBPP vaccines.

This paper discusses issues related to use of current CBPP vaccines, especially requirements for ensuring the production and use of good-quality CBPP vaccines and strategies for disease control. Specific consideration is given to vaccine specifications and quality assurance; quality control testing of CBPP vaccines; the application of vaccine for CBPP disease control; CBPP vaccination strategy; possible combinations of CBPP vaccine with vaccines of other diseases; and CBPP vaccination monitoring. A list of CBPP vaccine producers is also provided.

References

Amanfu, W. (2006). The use of antibiotics for CBPP control: the challenges. In: *CBPP Control: Antibiotics to the Rescue* (ed. J. Lubroth), 7–11. Rome: FAO.

Amanfu, W. (2009). Contagious bovine pleuropneumonia (lungsickness) in Africa. *Onderstepoort J. Vet. Res.* 76: 13–17.

Davies, G. and Gilbert, F.R. (1969). Contagious bovine pleuropneumonia vaccination in East Africa. *Bull. Epizoot. Dis. Afr.* 17: 21–26.

Dedieu-Engelmann, L. (2008). Contagious bovine pleuropneumonia: a rationale for the development of a mucosal sub-unit vaccine. *Comp. Immunol. Microbiol. Infect. Dis.* 31: 227–238.

Doutre, M.P., Chambron, J., and Bourdin, P. (1972). Valeur de l'immunité conférée par un vaccin mixte antibovipestique-antipéripneumonique lyophilisé préparé à l'aide de la souche T1 (S(R)). *Rev. Elev. Med. Vet. Pays Trop.* 25: 1–14.

Dupuy, V., Manso-Silvan, L., Barbe, V. et al. (2012). Evolutionary history of contagious bovine pleuropneumonia using next generation sequencing of *Mycoplasma mycoides* subsp. *mycoides* "small colony". *PLoS One* 7: e46821.

Geering, W.A. and Amanfu, W. (2002). Preparation of contagious bovine pleuropneumonia contingency plans. In: *FAO Animal Health Manual*, vol. 14. Rome: FAO. www.fao.org/3/a-y4143e.pdf.

Gilbert, F.R. and Windsor, R.S. (1971). The immunizing dose of T1 strain *Mycoplasma mycoides* against contagious bovine pleuropneumonia. *Trop. Anim. Health Prod.* 3: 71–76.

Gilbert, F.R., Davies, G., Read, W.C.S., and Turner, G.R.J. (1970). The efficacy of T1 strain broth vaccine against contagious bovine pleuropneumonia: in-contact trials carried out six and twelve months after primary vaccination. *Vet. Rec.* 86: 29–33.

Gourgues, G., Barré, A., Beaudoing, E. et al. (2016). Complete genome sequence of *Mycoplasma mycoides* subsp. *mycoides* T1/44, a vaccine strain against contagious bovine pleuropneumonia. *Genome Announc.* 4: e00263–e00216.

Hübschle, O.J., Tjipura-Zaire, G., Abusugra, I. et al. (2003). Experimental field trial with an immunostimulating complex (ISCOM) vaccine against contagious bovine pleuropneumonia. *J. Vet. Med. B Infect. Dis. Vet. Public Health* 50: 298–303.

Hudson, J.R. (1968). Contagious bovine pleuropneumonia. Experiments on the susceptibility and protection by vaccination of different types of cattle. *Aust. Vet. J.* 44: 83–89.

Hudson, J.R. (1972). *La péripneumonie contagieuse des bovidés*, vol. 86. Rome: FAO.

Jeggo, M.H., Wardley, R.C., and Corteyn, A.H. (1987). A reassessment of the dual vaccine against rinderpest and contagious bovine pleuropneumonia. *Vet. Rec.* 120: 131–135.

Jores, J., Mariner, J., and Naessens, J. (2013). Development of an improved vaccine for contagious bovine pleuropneumonia: an African perspective on challenges and proposed actions. *Vet. Res.* 44: 122.

Kairu-Wanyoike, S.W., Kaitibie, S., Heffernan, C. et al. (2014). Willingness to pay for contagious bovine pleuropneumonia vaccination in Narok South District of Kenya. *Prev. Vet. Med.* 115: 130–142.

Karst, O. (1972). Contagious bovine pleuropneumonia: lyophilised (T 1) vaccine. *Bull. Epizoot. Dis. Afr.* 20: 69–76.

Lindley, E.P. (1971). Experiences with a lyophilised contagious bovine pleuropneumonia vaccine in the Ivory Coast. *Trop. Anim. Health Prod.* 3: 32–42.

Litamoi, J.K., Ayelet, G., and Rweyemamu, M.M. (2005). Evaluation of the xerovac process for the preparation of heat tolerant contagious bovine pleuropneumonia (CBPP) vaccine. *Vaccine* 23: 2573–2579.

Lorenzon, S., David, A., Nadew, M. et al. (2000). Specific PCR identification of the T1 vaccine strains for contagious bovine pleuropneumonia. *Mol. Cell. Probes* 14: 205–210.

March, J.B. (2004). Improved formulations for existing CBPP vaccines – recommendations for change. *Vaccine* 22: 4358–4364.

Masiga, W.N. and Windsor, R.S. (1974). The efficacy of T1 strain broth culture vaccine against contagious bovine pleuropneumonia: the effect of revaccination of cattle 6 months and 1 year after primary vaccination and prolonged exposure. *Bull. Epizoot. Dis. Afr.* 22: 27–31.

Masiga, W.N., Domenech, J., and Windsor, R.S. (1996). Manifestation and epidemiology of contagious bovine pleuropneumonia in Africa. *Rev. Sci. Tech. Off. Int. Epiz.* 15: 1283–1308.

Mulongo, M., Frey, J., Smith, K. et al. (2015). Vaccination of cattle with the N terminus of LppQ of *Mycoplasma mycoides* subsp. *mycoides* results in type III immune complex disease upon experimental infection. *Inf. Immun.* 83: 1992–2000.

Newton, L.G. (1992). Contagious bovine pleuropneumonia in Australia: some historic highlights from entry to eradication. *Aust. Vet. J.* 69: 306–317.

Nkando, I., Ndinda, J., Kuria, J. et al. (2012). Efficacy of two vaccine formulations against contagious bovine pleuropneumonia (CBPP) in Kenyan indigenous cattle. *Res. Vet. Sci.* 93: 568–573.

OIE. (2015). Contagious bovine pleuropneumonia. In: *Manual of Diagnostic Tests and Vaccines for Terrestrial Animals*. Paris: OIE.

Provost, A. (1969). Principes de production d'un vaccin mixte associé antibovipestique-antipéripneumonique inoculé en un seul temps. *Bull. Epizoot. Dis. Afr.* 17: 7–10.

Provost, A. (1975). La péripneumonie en Afrique centrale. Situation épizootologique. Appréciation des mesures prophylactiques. *Bull. Off. Int. Epizoot.* 84: 403–411.

Provost, A. (1996). Strategies for prevention and eradication of contagious bovine pleuropneumonia with or without vaccination. *Rev. Sci. Tech. Off. Int. Epiz.* 15: 1355–1371.

Provost, A., Perreau, P., Breard, A. et al. (1987). Contagious bovine pleuropneumonia. *Rev. Sci. Tech. Off. Int. Epiz.* 6: 625–679.

Revell, S.G. (1973). Local reactions following C.B.P.P. vaccination in Zambia. *Trop. Anim. Health Prod.* 5: 246–252.

Rossiter, P.B. and Kariuki, D.P. (1987). Single and combined rinderpest vaccines. *Vet. Rec.* 121: 230–231.

Rurangirwa, F.R., Masiga, W.N., and Mtui, B. (1976). An anamnestic response to challenge with virulent *Mycoplasma mycoides* subsp. *mycoides* of cattle immune to contagious bovine pleuropneumonia. *J. Comp. Pathol.* 86: 381–386.

Schieck, E., Liljander, A., Hamsten, C. et al. (2014). High antibody titres against predicted mycoplasma surface proteins do not prevent sequestration in infected lung tissue in the course of experimental contagious bovine pleuropneumonia. *Vet. Microbiol.* 172: 285–293.

Sheriff, D. and Piercy, S.E. (1952). Experiments with an avianised strain of the organism of contagious bovine pleuropneumonia. *Vet. Rec.* 64: 615–621.

Thiaucourt, F., Yaya, A., Wesonga, H. et al. (2000). Contagious bovine pleuropneumonia. A reassessment of the efficacy of vaccines used in Africa. *Ann. N.Y. Acad. Sci.* 916: 71–80

Thiaucourt, F., Dedieu, L., Maillard, J.C. et al. (2003). Contagious bovine pleuropneumonia vaccines, historic highlights, present situation and hopes. *Dev. Biol.* 114: 147–160.

Totte, P., Yaya, A., Sery, A. et al. (2013). Characterization of anamnestic T-cell responses induced by conventional vaccines against contagious bovine pleuropneumonia. *PLoS One* 8: e57509.

Tulasne, J.J., Litamoi, J.K., Morein, B. et al. (1996). Contagious bovine pleuropneumonia vaccines: the current situation and the need for improvement. *Rev. Sci. Tech. Off. Int. Epiz.* 15: 1373–1396.

van Kuppeveld, F.J., Johansson, K.E., Galama, J.M. et al. (1994). Detection of mycoplasma contamination in cell cultures by a mycoplasma group-specific PCR. *Appl. Environ. Microbiol.* 60: 149–152.

Wesonga, H. and Thiaucourt, F. (2000). Experimental studies on the efficacy of T1sr and T1/44 vaccine strains of *Mycoplasma mycoides* subsp. *mycoides* SC against a field isolate causing contagious bovine pleuropneumonia in Kenya- effect of a revaccination. *Rev. Elev. Med. Vet. Pays Trop.* 53: 313–318.

Yaya, A., Golsia, R., Hamadou, B. et al. (1999). Essai comparatif d'efficacité de deux souches vaccinales T1/44 et T1sr contre la péripneumonie contagieuse bovine. *Rev. Elev. Med. Vet. Pays Trop.* 52: 171–179.

24

Classic Swine Fever

Klaus Depner[1], Marie-Frédérique Le Potier[2], and Klaas Dietze[1]

[1] *FAO Reference Centre for Classical Swine Fever, Friedrich-Loefler-Institute, Greifswald, Germany*
[2] *ANSES – Laboratoire de Ploufragan/Plouzané/Niort, National Reference Laboratory for Classical Swine Fever, Zoopole Les Croix, Ploufragan, France*

24.1 Introduction

Classic swine fever (CSF) is one of the most devastating diseases for pig production. It is widely distributed apart from some free regions, such as North America, the European Union (EU), Australia, and Africa, except Madagascar. The etiological agent is a RNA virus and a member of the genus *Pestivirus*, family *Flaviviridae*. Currently, on the basis of phylogenetic analysis, classic swine fever virus (CSFV) can be divided into three groups with three or four subgroups but only one serogroup is recognized. Wild and domestic suids are the only known reservoir of the virus.

The main routes of transmission are oronasal by direct or indirect contact with infected wild or domestic pigs, or oral by ingestion of contaminated foodstuffs (Edwards 2000). Airborne spread of CSFV seems less important under field conditions, even if it has been experimentally demonstrated (Weesendorp et al. 2009). Transmission by semen is possible as experimental studies have shown that infected boars can shed CSFV in semen (Floegel et al. 2000). CSF is characterized by cutaneous hyperemia or cyanosis and diverse rather nonspecific symptoms. In the acute form, the initial clinical signs include anorexia, lethargy, conjunctivitis, respiratory signs, and constipation followed by diarrhea. In the chronic form, the same clinical signs are observed, but the pigs survive for 2–3 months before dying. Other nonspecific signs, e.g. intermittent hyperthermia, chronic enteritis, and wasting, may also be seen.

Differential diagnosis from other diseases characterized by cutaneous hyperemia or cyanosis is only possible by laboratory analysis. The one constant sign in the acute clinical form of CSF is hyperthermia, usually greater than 40 °C, and piglets are often seen piled in a corner (Floegel-Niesmann et al. 2009). CSFV is able to cross the placenta of pregnant sows and infect fetuses at any stage of pregnancy and can cause abortion and stillbirths. However, infection at 50–70 days of gestation can lead to the birth of persistently viremic piglets. Such piglets initially appear clinically normal, but subsequently begin to waste or develop congenital tremors (Vannier et al. 1981). Depending on the virulence of the virus strain and the age and breed of the host (Depner et al. 1997), infected pigs can show clinical signs within 3–6 days of exposure to the virus and die rapidly, recover, or develop chronic disease which is invariably fatal. Animals may start to shed virus within a few days of infection and before the onset of clinical signs. With less virulent strains, the time to the onset of disease can be as long as 13–19 days (Durand et al. 2009). However, due to the nonspecific nature of clinical signs, especially with strains of moderate or low virulence, the diagnosis can be delayed in a herd for 6–8 weeks, promoting virus spread.

To control or eradicate the disease, vaccination has been carried out widely for decades. Modified live viruses (MLVs) were mostly used as they were generally safe and efficacious. However, it was not possible to differentiate infected from vaccinated animals (DIVA). Because of the impossibility of applying a DIVA strategy with MLV, subunit or marker vaccines have been developed, as recently reviewed (Blome et al. 2017). Despite the numerous publications during the last decade, only a few marker vaccine candidates have been commercialized. These vaccines and their possible use in the field are described in this chapter.

24.2 Types of Vaccines

Two types of CSFV vaccines are commercially available:

- the MLV, including the well-known, live, lapinized "Chinese" C strain, the Japanese GPE-strain, and the French cell-adapted Thiverval strain

Veterinary Vaccines: Principles and Applications, First Edition. Edited by Samia Metwally, Gerrit Viljoen, and Ahmed El Idrissi.

- the newer marker vaccines that allow differentiation of field virus-infected versus vaccinated animals (DIVA principle). These include the baculovirus-expressed E2 recombinant protein, subunit vaccine, which contains no live virus (Bouma et al. 1999), and the live chimeric pestivirus CP7_E2Alf (Reimann et al. 2004).

Both types, MLV and marker vaccines, have been licensed for intramuscular inoculation (www.ema.europa.eu). Additionally, one MLV has also a license for oral vaccination of wild boar in some EU member states.

Currently, MLVs are often used for the prophylactic vaccination of domestic pigs. They are suitable tools for reducing the disease and virus spread by decreasing virus replication (EFSA 2009). For oral vaccination, only live attenuated vaccines are suitable. The application of mass oral vaccination to wild boars through a baiting system containing the C-strain "Riems" vaccine proved to be efficacious to control and eradicate the infection in western European wild boar populations (Rossi et al. 2015). However, these MLVs do not permit differentiation of vaccine antibodies from field virus-induced antibodies and this can interfere with the evaluation of an eradication program (Saubusse et al. 2016).

Subunit vaccines based on E2 baculo-expressed proteins are efficacious and fully safe (Bouma et al. 1999), but not suitable for oral vaccination. Although some results indicated that the efficacy of these vaccines was not ideal for an emergency application (Depner et al. 2001; Uttenthal et al. 2001), their use as an additional tool in an eradication plan could be considered, if the matching DIVA diagnostic tool is available. This serological test should permit the detection of specific antibodies to CFSV proteins other than E2, even in the presence of vaccine-derived antibodies. Enzyme-linked immunosorbent assay (ELISA) kits that can detect specific antibodies to other CSFV proteins, such as Erns or NS3, are commercially available. However, because of cross-reactions between CSFV and other pestiviruses such as bovine viral diarrhea virus (BVDV), the specificity of these kits is often not sufficient to rule out a serological suspicion of CSF (Schroeder et al. 2012). Today, there is one CSFV E2 subunit vaccine commercialized, based on the purified E2 glycoprotein expressed in baculovirus, administered in a water-in-oil adjuvant (Porcilis® Pesti, MSD Animal Health).

The CSF eradication program in Romania is an example of the implementation of a DIVA vaccination scheme. In the later course of this eradication program, before vaccination was phased out, the commercial production sector switched from C-strain vaccine to a DIVA vaccine, allowing this sector to finish compulsory vaccination more quickly.

The chimeric pestivirus CP7_E2Alf is currently the most promising new live vaccine as it has been demonstrated to be safe and able to induce an effective protective immunity (Tignon et al. 2010; Blome et al. 2014), even if the efficacy of vaccination with CP7_E2Alf in the presence of maternal-derived antibodies (MDAs) seems to be slightly less than in their absence. On a population level, the results suggest that the CP7_E2Alf vaccine is an effective tool in the control and eradication of CSF. Moreover, it can be applied for both intramuscular and oral use even for young age groups, with MDAs having a limited effect on efficacy (Rangelova et al. 2012), or in pigs with antibodies to other pestiviruses (Drager et al. 2016). CP7_E2Alf has been licensed and commercialized as Suvaxyn® CSF Marker by Zoetis. New ELISAs have been developed to specifically detect antibodies to CSFV Erns and, therefore, distinguish them from antibodies derived from the pestivirus backbone of the vaccine (Aebischer et al. 2013), but fully validated kits are not currently available.

24.3 Immune Response and Duration of Immunity

From an evolutionary point of view, CSFV is relatively stable for a RNA virus and only one serogroup has so far been recognized. Convalescent or vaccinated pigs present a long and stable immunity against all the variants of CSFV, based on neutralizing antibodies against NS3, E2, and Erns viral proteins. However, among these three membrane glycoproteins, E2 is the most immunogenic. This protein can induce neutralizing antibodies 2 weeks after intramuscular inoculation of live virus, while antibodies to Erns or NS3 are often detected 1 week later and at a lower titer.

The traditional MLVs induce a high level of protection against clinical disease and neutralizing antibodies are detectable at 2 weeks postvaccination. Moreover, vaccination closer to challenge can confer some, but not complete, protection against clinical disease and virus dissemination (Graham et al. 2012), even when vaccination is by the oral route (Renson et al. 2013). The duration of immunity is at least 6–12 months, regardless of the route of administration (intramuscular or oronasal), and even the offspring are protected (Kaden et al. 2008).

The efficacy of the baculovirus-expressed E2 protein vaccines has been extensively evaluated in vaccination challenge and transmission trials, but with variable results. At least 14 days were needed to develop clinical protection in growing pigs vaccinated with a single dose (Bouma et al. 2000). If challenged earlier, no protection against clinical disease and no reduction of virus shedding were observed

(Uttenthal et al. 2001). Vaccination with a double dose protected pregnant gilts from clinical disease but did not prevent the “carrier sow syndrome” with the subsequent birth of infected piglets exhibiting the late-onset form of CSF (Depner et al. 2001). In conclusion, these subunit E2 marker vaccines need more than one parenteral application to be fully effective and are not indicated for oral vaccination.

The chimeric pestivirus CP7_E2Alf has also been widely assessed for its safety and potency (Koenig et al. 2007). Like the C-strain, it is able to induce neutralizing antibodies from 2 weeks after vaccination by either the intramuscular or oral route (Blome et al. 2014). It was also still able to protect pigs vaccinated 6 months earlier, even when challenged with a highly virulent CSF strain. Cell-mediated immunity seems to play an important role in long-term protection (Renson et al. 2014).

24.4 Desired Specifications When Ordering Vaccine

In Chapter 3.8.3. on CSF in the OIE *Manual of Diagnostic Tests and Vaccines for Terrestrial Animals* (www.oie.int/fileadmin/Home/eng/Health_standards/tahm/3.08.03_CSF.pdf), the minimum requirements for information on vaccine safety, efficacy, and protocol schedules are described (OIE 2017). Manufacturers of CSF vaccine should be able to provide these details for their products.

A lot of C-strain vaccines are locally produced but safety and potency have only been assessed for a few commercialized vaccines. Further studies using comparable approaches on the quality of available CSF vaccines would facilitate decision making on vaccine purchase. Vaccines that have been authorized for sale in markets with known demanding standards, for example the EU, can be considered safe and efficacious.

However, the detailed requirements may differ depending on the epidemiological situation (emergency outbreak/endemic), targeted animals (domestic or wild), and the purpose of the vaccination (disease prevention/virus eradication). The use of a marker vaccine only adds value if there is a validated companion diagnostic kit available for DIVA serology and the capacity to conduct postvaccination monitoring.

24.5 Quality Assurance and Control Testing

Different properties of each vaccine batch have to be assessed before it can be released with, at least, a demonstration of the absence of contaminants, the minimum dose (virus titer for MLV or protein concentration for subunit vaccine), the stability of the vaccine with the appropriate storage conditions (temperature, light, etc.). For detailed procedures, see the OIE *Manual of Diagnostic Tests and Vaccines for Terrestrial Animals* and the two sections on (i) principles of veterinary vaccine production and (ii) tests of biological materials for sterility and freedom from contamination.

24.6 Vaccine Application for Disease Control

24.6.1 Vaccination Strategy

Vaccination has to be considered as one tool in a range of measures, as part of a complex strategy. In the past, the use of vaccines in emergencies was limited by the possibility that vaccinated animals might spread the virus further. Moreover, infected animals could not be easily and rapidly identified or distinguished from vaccinated but uninfected animals.

To control CSF outbreaks, vaccination can be implemented either as a vaccination-to-live or a vaccination-to-kill strategy. Protective vaccination or vaccination-to-live means that vaccinated animals are kept to the end of a normal production cycle and their meat eventually marketed. Suppressive vaccination or vaccination-to-kill means that animals around an infected farm are vaccinated to reduce the spread of infection and to gain time. Those animals will eventually be destroyed. Vaccination-to-kill might be an option in an emergency situation to regain the free status of the region as quickly as possible. Another option is to vaccinate only the growing pigs, to protect them until the time for them to be slaughtered, but not the sows, to avoid long-lasting maternally derived antibodies interfering in future diagnostic serology.

24.6.2 Epidemiological Settings and Objectives

The overall epidemiological setting will inform the key components of the CSF control strategy and the possible use of vaccine, within the corresponding vaccination plan. In general, two epidemiological settings can be considered for the domestic pig population: (i) CSF is endemic in the country, and (ii) CSF is not present in the country but there is a risk of incursion. A separate strategy is needed for dealing with CSF in wild boar as the tools and options differ significantly.

In an endemic situation, the objectives for vaccine application can be very distinct. When aiming for overall control of the disease by pushing the pathogen out of the domestic pig population, vaccination can be helpful where other tools for control (e.g. stamping out, zoning with restrictive measures, etc.) may prove to be insufficient or too costly to eradicate CSFV from the domestic pig sector. In this case, it is recommended to work out a step-by-step, progressive control plan that will allow efficient and strategic use of vaccine. The plan should be implemented on the basis of a value chain analysis providing details on production systems with the highest risk of spreading the disease (often medium-sized breeding farms) and with the potential to act as a reservoir (often seen in the backyard sector).

In an endemic setting where no larger scale, coordinated control of CSF is implemented, farmers should consider vaccination as a means to reduce the disease incidence on-farm and therefore reduce losses attributed to CSF. For regions where swine production plays an important role for household food security of poor people, support in CSF vaccination for small-scale producers will contribute to protecting the livelihoods of these farming communities. In these settings, the live attenuated vaccines without DIVA principle are sufficient and represent the economically sensible alternative. Yearly vaccination intervals should be aimed for, covering all pigs in the target population.

In an emergency situation, such as increased outbreaks within an already affected country or the incursion of CSF into a free country or area, emergency vaccination should be considered.

These different settings will form the respective starting points of a vaccination effort that should be clearly linked to a defined objective. For CSF in domestic pigs, as for wild boar, this could be the overall eradication of the disease, the prevention of further spread, or just the reduction of losses due to clinical CSF in the affected population. All these objectives will require different efforts and have different "endpoints" for the vaccination efforts involved.

24.6.3 Possible Combination with Vaccines for Other Diseases

Vaccines against CSF are commonly monovalent. When CSF vaccination is applied as a routine vaccination for breeding animals and their offspring, it may be possible for the vaccination schedule to be harmonized with other routine vaccinations for the specific age groups; however, interference with vaccination from maternally derived antibodies has to be taken into account. Unless specifically mentioned in the manufacturer's product description, the vaccine should be administered separately (separate injection) and not mixed with other vaccines.

24.6.4 Use of Vaccine in the Face of an Outbreak

Emergency vaccination in a crisis situation is increasingly seen as complementary to other zoosanitary measures, and as a means to reduce reliance on culling alone. There have been significant advances in the development of diagnostic tests and modern vaccines, and new techniques that enable detection of an infected herd reliably within a short time so that preventive culling can be minimized. In principle, live attenuated vaccine and subunit marker vaccines can be used in preventive vaccination and emergency vaccination. Currently, MLVs are often used for prophylactic vaccination of domestic pigs since they are cheaper. However, if a DIVA strategy is envisaged, marker vaccines have to be used.

In particular, when outbreaks happen in a country where a large proportion of the pig sector is kept in smaller, so-called backyard operations, often with very particular production practices, the decision whether to vaccinate or not must be carefully judged. Table 24.1 based on Annex V of Directive 2001/89 EC provides some decision criteria to be considered (EC 2001).

The following approaches are likely to improve the effectiveness of vaccination:

Table 24.1 Vaccination decision criteria.

Criteria	Decision: For vaccination	Decision: Against vaccination
The epidemiological situation and outbreak circumstances are clear	No	Yes
Sufficient biosecurity measures are implemented on all pig holdings	No	Yes
There has been a high number of outbreaks over recent months	Yes	No
The likelihood of new outbreaks in the coming months is high	Yes	No
The use of illegal swill feeding is suspected	Yes	No

- The emergency vaccination program should be compulsory.
- Vaccination should be limited in time and unconditionally linked to management improvements within the domestic pig production sector (see below).
- Where possible, a regional approach with mutually independent areas, in which the vaccination is organized, implemented and controlled, should be preferred.

Management measures needed for a successful vaccination program include:

- identification and registering of holdings and pigs
- minimal standards for biosecurity in all pig holdings (including nonprofessional holdings)
- safe trading of pigs from nonprofessional holdings, and in the longer term, banning of such trade
- the correct implementation of all control measures as foreseen in legislation when a CSF outbreak is detected
- the establishment and execution of an education campaign for all nonprofessional pig keepers to improve their understanding of CSF
- the establishment and execution of a training program for veterinarians and staff.

Regular assessment of the situation is needed to demonstrate progress with regard to these minimal conditions.

Emergency vaccination has not been considered a first-hand option for countries trying to regain a CSF-free status as quickly as possible, yet with the availability of marker vaccines it should in general be seen in a new light. Diagnostic tools substantiating that vaccinated animals, or meat and other products obtained from vaccinated animals, are free from pathogens and can be traded safely, make the vaccinate-to-live approach viable to export-oriented production sectors.

24.6.5 When Vaccination Is Not Recommended

With the overall good availability of safe and efficacious vaccines for administration by either intramuscular inoculation or the oral route, there are very few scenarios where vaccination against CSF cannot be recommended. At the level of the individual pig, animals with maternal antibodies, or which are sick or incubating the disease should not be vaccinated.

In CSF-free areas, a nonvaccination policy is often applied for international trade purposes. Markets with a CSF-free status may not accept products from vaccinated animals, even though they are as safe for human consumption as those derived from unvaccinated animals. In the future, to accept vaccination, the livestock industry needs sufficient guarantees that products from vaccinated animals are marketable without price reductions. This is a crucial issue which must be resolved to guarantee the free movement of goods while encouraging the use of vaccination as a preventive animal health measure, avoiding unnecessary losses.

The OIE requires assurance that no vaccination has taken place in the said population for at least 12 months for the official CSF-free status to be granted, in accordance with the Terrestrial Code, unless a vaccine allowing the DIVA principle has been used. As these vaccines have only become licensed since the early 2000s, countries with a longer standing CSF freedom have not applied them in eradication programs.

The decision to vaccinate against CSF as a response to an outbreak in a country that is facing a new introduction of the disease and has previously had the official OIE status "free of CSF" must therefore be judged carefully. In such situations, where assured early detection and proper surveillance are in place, and where rigorous stamping-out practices can be implemented, the disease-free status may be regained more quickly without vaccination, with a reduced negative impact from trade restrictions on the exporting pig sector.

24.6.6 Vaccine Application in Wildlife and Feral Pigs

Control and eradication of CSF in wild boar cannot be managed as in domestic pigs, i.e. using an exhaustive culling or vaccination strategy. Alternatively, hunting and vaccination can be used in order to stop transmission by reducing the number of susceptible individuals. According to the scientific opinion of the Panel on Animal Health and Welfare of the European Food Safety Authority on Control and Eradication of CSF in Wild Boar (EFSA 2009), the disease will fade out in small populations of less than 1500 animals and will persist for several years among areas containing more than 2000 annually shot wild boars.

Oral vaccination with a live attenuated bait vaccine (C-strain) has been used in order to stop virus transmission by reducing the number of susceptible individuals (Kaden et al. 2002). Vaccination represents a potential tool to control the spread and intensity of infection under certain circumstances. In combination with immunity generated by circulation of field virus, vaccination decreases virus circulation, which finally may eliminate the virus in an area.

Areas to be vaccinated should be designated according to the landscape structure (forested areas, motorways, rivers, lakes, etc.) and the spatial distribution and connectivity of the wild boar, rather than relying on administrative boundaries. Vaccination strategies also require strictly defined epidemiological and sampling units. The vaccination process increases population immunity progressively: the maximum population immunity is only reached after three double campaigns (one year). Thereafter, the rapid turnover of animals requires a continuous vaccination effort to maintain population immunity. Therefore, one isolated vaccination campaign cannot increase population immunity sufficiently to control CSF. Moreover, a significant protective effect of preventive vaccination, especially within municipalities that had been vaccinated at least one year before disease emergence, has been described (Rossi et al. 2010).

Vaccination coverage is important. A minimum target of 40% of susceptible animals should be vaccinated, considering the level of infection and the population parameters. If 60% of animals are vaccinated, there is a high probability of eradication, whereas vaccination of 20% or less of susceptible animals is likely to be associated with endemic stability (the infection can spread in neighboring patches with low incidence). In the field, the average proportion of immune animals is often up to 60% but immunity is much lower in animals less than 1 year old, due to the failure of piglets less than 6 months to consume the vaccine baits currently on the market. The low immunity observed in 3–12-month-old wild boar might explain the persistence of wild-type virus in vaccinated populations.

Control strategies require a holistic approach which takes into consideration the biology of the disease, the biology of the wild boar population, and interfering human activities like feeding, hunting, and vaccination.

Classic swine fever does not persist in a wild boar population when, following virus introduction, most of the survivors become immune and so insufficient susceptible pigs remain available to maintain the chain of infection. Principally, CSFV can persist in a wild boar population only when there is a viremic animal which transmits the virus to at least one further susceptible wild boar ($R_0 > 1$). However, monitoring and understanding a disease in an open ecosystem is rather a complex exercise because several parameters, such as the population structure and dynamics, population size, or herd immunity status, remain unknown or can only be estimated.

24.7 Monitoring and Vaccine Effectiveness

24.7.1 Postvaccination Monitoring

Postvaccination monitoring based on serosurveillance for undisclosed infection and the analysis of outbreak data should be seen as an essential component for all vaccination programs. Experience gained in the rather complex requirements for postvaccination monitoring in wild boar is described in the following section. The same principles can be applied to postvaccination monitoring in domestic pigs, where implementation is much simpler.

After completing oral immunization, the age class of wild boar that should be examined serologically to detect a new or reemerging infection depends on the season in which vaccination was completed and the length of time since completion.

Two years after an oral immunization campaign, piglets younger than 6 months might still have maternal antibodies, and boars older than 12 (or 18) months probably still have vaccination antibodies. Hence, a wild boar population is considered as CSF free if the antibody prevalence in the age class 6–12 (or 18) months is below a certain detection level (i.e. <5%, 95% confidence interval).

In the third and subsequent years after oral vaccination, animals aged 6–24 months should be free from CSFV antibodies. Animals older than 3 years will probably be serologically positive due to vaccination, and animals <6 months might have maternal antibodies.

After the end of the vaccination campaign, the following monitoring plan is proposed:

- first year after vaccination: no serological monitoring, focus on virological testing
- second year after vaccination: serological monitoring of wild boar 12–24 months old
- third year after vaccination and following: serological monitoring of piglets and young wild boar (6–24 months).

Minimum number of samples per metapopulation each year: 59 (5% prevalence with 95% confidence interval).

In addition to serological examinations, virological tests should be conducted in all age classes. However, emphasis has to be put on piglets, on all diseased wild boar, and on animals found dead. If CSF is suspected, all shot or found dead wild boar within a radius of 3–5 km have to be examined virologically for at least 1 month.

24.7.2 Outbreaks in Vaccinated Animals

When using a good-quality vaccine according to the manufacturer's instructions, including proper handling during shipment and storage and proper implementation of the vaccination itself, CSF outbreaks should not occur in vaccinated populations. In this case, outbreaks should rather be seen as an indicator for a malfunctioning of the vaccination scheme that will require revision. In addition, the potential of vaccine failure due to evasion of vaccine-induced immunity needs to be taken into account if no evident mistakes can be identified in the implementation of the vaccination. As most vaccines used globally are based on CSFV genotype

1, it has been described that populations infected with genetically more distant genotype 2 CSFVs might not be adequately protected despite proper use of the vaccine itself (Yoo et al. 2018). Another potential reason for vaccination failure is the absence of response to vaccination in piglets persistently infected with CSFV, as has been experimentally demonstrated by Munoz-Gonzalez et al. (2015).

24.8 Adverse Reactions to Vaccination

Severe adverse reactions to CSF vaccines are uncommon with vaccines that comply with the OIE requirements. For any specific vaccine, indications on adverse reactions can be found in the manufacturer's product information. In general, adverse reactions are often dependent on the adjuvants used. It is highly recommended to inform the manufacturer if adverse reactions are observed when using the vaccine.

24.9 Availability and List of Manufacturers

Vaccines against CSF are widely available globally. Most international companies active in the field of veterinary vaccines have a CSF vaccine in their portfolio. In addition, in many countries, one or more local producers supply the domestic market. The market in China, for example, is supplied by over 50 companies offering vaccines against CSF (Luo et al. 2014). Two newer vaccines allowing the application of the DIVA principle have been officially authorized by the European Medicines Agency. The Porcilis Pesti, based on baculovirus-expressed E2 protein, has been authorized since 2000 and the Suvaxyn CSF Marker, a live recombinant E2 gene switched BVDV containing CSF E2 (CP7_E2alf), since 2015.

24.10 Summary

Classic swine fever remains one of the major burdens of global pig production. As well as massive losses in affected swine populations, the disease hampers development of the commercial pig sector due to trade restrictions. These problems continue, although the necessary tools for CSF control and eradication have been available for many decades. These tools include detailed knowledge of the key epidemiological risk factors for CSF spread, the availability of robust laboratory detection systems and, last but not least, the availability of safe and efficacious vaccines that provide lasting immunity. Even in difficult to manage populations such as wild boars and feral pigs, the available tools can lead to successful control and eradication. In summary, from the biological perspective, CSF is a disease that is relatively easy to control, yet the efforts required to do so are long lasting and should not be underestimated.

Modified live vaccines have played a dominant role in CSF control based on vaccination. From the early 2000s on, modern vaccines that would allow application of the DIVA principle have been on the market and bring with them the potential to substantially reduce the need to cull animals in large numbers, especially in epidemics, when applied within a vaccinate-to-live control strategy.

References

Aebischer, A., Müller, M., and Hofmann, M.A. (2013). Two newly developed Erns-based ELISAs allow the differentiation of classical swine fever virus-infected from marker-vaccinated animals and the discrimination of pestivirus antibodies. *Vet. Microbiol.* 161 (3–4): 274–285.

Blome, S., Gabriel, C., Schmeiser, S. et al. (2014). Efficacy of marker vaccine candidate CP7_E2alf against challenge with classical swine fever virus isolates of different genotypes. *Vet. Microbiol.* 169 (1–2): 8–17.

Blome, S., Moss, C., Reimann, I. et al. (2017). Classical swine fever vaccines – state-of-the-art. *Vaccine* 35 (46): 6297–6301.

Bouma, A., de Smit, A.J., de Kluijver, E.P. et al. (1999). Efficacy and stability of a subunit vaccine based on glycoprotein E2 of classical swine fever virus. *Vet. Microbiol.* 66 (2): 101–114.

Bouma, A., de Smit, A.J., de Jong, M.C. et al. (2000). Determination of the onset of the herd-immunity induced by the E2 sub-unit vaccine against classical swine fever virus. *Vaccine* 18 (14): 1374–1381.

Depner, K.R., Hinrichs, U., Bickhardt, K. et al. (1997). Influence of breed-related factors on the course of classical swine fever virus infection. *Vet. Rec.* 140 (19): 506–507.

Depner, K.R., Bouma, A., Koenen, F. et al. (2001). Classical swine fever (CSF) marker vaccine – trial II. Challenge study in pregnant sows. *Vet. Microbiol.* 83 (2): 107–120.

Drager, C., Schroder, C., Konig, P. et al. (2016). Efficacy of Suvaxyn CSF Marker (CP7_E2alf) in the presence of pre-existing antibodies against bovine viral diarrhea virus type 1. *Vaccine* 34 (39): 4666–4671.

Durand, B., Davila, S., Cariolet, R. et al. (2009). Comparison of viraemia- and clinical-based estimates of within- and between-pen transmission of classical swine fever virus from three transmission experiments. *Vet. Microbiol.* 135 (3–4): 196–204.

EC. (2001). Council Directive 2001/89/EC of 23 October 2001 on Community measures for the control of classical swine fever. Official Journal of the European Communities. L 316/5.

Edwards, S. (2000). Survival and inactivation of classical swine fever virus. *Vet. Microbiol.* 73 (2–3): 175–181.

EFSA (2009). Control and eradication of classic swine fever in wild boar. *EFSA J.* 7 (1): 932.

Floegel, G., Wehrend, A., Depner, K.R. et al. (2000). Detection of classical swine fever virus in semen of infected boars. *Vet. Microbiol.* 77 (1–2): 109–116.

Floegel-Niesmann, G., Blome, S., Gerß-Dülmer, H. et al. (2009). Virulence of classical swine fever virus isolates from Europe and other areas during 1996 until 2007. *Vet. Microbiol.* 139 (1–2): 165–169.

Graham, S.P., Everett, H.E., Haines, F.J. et al. (2012). Challenge of pigs with classical swine fever viruses after C-strain vaccination reveals remarkably rapid protection and insights into early immunity. *PLoS One* 7 (1): e29310.

Kaden, V., Lange, E., Fischer, U., and Strebelow, G. (2002). Oral immunisation of wild boar against classical swine fever: evaluation of the first field study in Germany. *Vet. Microbiol.* 115: 179–185.

Kaden, V., Lange, E., Steyer, H. et al. (2008). Classical swine fever virus strain "C" protects the offspring by oral immunisation of pregnant sows. *Vet. Microbiol.* 130 (1–2): 20–27.

Koenig, P., Lange, E., Reimann, I., and Beer, M. (2007). CP7_E2alf: a safe and efficient marker vaccine strain for oral immunisation of wild boar against classical swine fever virus (CSFV). *Vaccine* 25 (17): 3391–3399.

Luo, Y., Li, S., Sun, Y., and Qiu, H.J. (2014). Classical swine fever in China: a minireview. *Vet. Microbiol.* 172 (1–2): 1–6.

Munoz-Gonzalez, S., Perez-Simo, M., Munoz, M. et al. (2015). Efficacy of a live attenuated vaccine in classical swine fever virus postnatally persistently infected pigs. *Vet. Res.* 46: 78.

OIE. (2017). Manual of Diagnostic Tests and Vaccines for Terrestrial Animals. www.oie.int/en/standard-setting/terrestrial-manual/access-online

Rangelova, D., Nielsen, J., Strandbygaard, B. et al. (2012). Efficacy of marker vaccine candidate CP7_E2alf in piglets with maternally derived C-strain antibodies. *Vaccine* 30 (45): 6376–6381.

Reimann, I., Depner, K., Trapp, S., and Beer, M. (2004). An avirulent chimeric *Pestivirus* with altered cell tropism protects pigs against lethal infection with classical swine fever virus. *Virology* 322 (1): 143–157.

Renson, P., Le Dimna, M., Keranflec'h, A. et al. (2013). CP7_E2alf oral vaccination confers partial protection against early classical swine fever virus challenge and interferes with pathogeny-related cytokine responses. *Vet. Res.* 44: 9.

Renson, P., Le Dimna, M., Gabriel, C. et al. (2014). Cytokine and immunoglobulin isotype profiles during CP7_E2alf vaccination against a challenge with the highly virulent Koslov strain of classical swine fever virus. *Res. Vet. Sci.* 96 (2): 389–395.

Rossi, S., Pol, F., Forot, B. et al. (2010). Preventive vaccination contributes to control classical swine fever in wild boar (*Sus scrofa* sp.). *Vet. Microbiol.* 142 (1–2): 99–107.

Rossi, S., Staubach, C., Blome, S. et al. (2015). Controlling of CSFV in European wild boar using oral vaccination: a review. *Front. Microbiol.* 6: 1141.

Saubusse, T., Masson, J.D., Le Dimma, M. et al. (2016). How to survey classical swine fever in wild boar (*Sus scrofa*) after the completion of oral vaccination? Chasing away the ghost of infection at different spatial scales. *Vet. Res.* 47: 21.

Schroeder, S., von Rosen, T., Blome, S. et al. (2012). Evaluation of classical swine fever virus antibody detection assays with an emphasis on the differentiation of infected from vaccinated animals. *Rev. Sci. Tech.* 31 (3): 997–1010

Tignon, M., Kulcsar, G., Haegeman, A. et al. (2010). Classical swine fever: comparison of oronasal immunisation with CP7E2alf marker and C-strain vaccines in domestic pigs *Vet. Microbiol.* 142 (1–2): 59–68.

Uttenthal, A., Le Potier, M.F., Romero, L. et al. (2001). Classical swine fever (CSF) marker vaccine trial I. Challenge studies in weaner pigs. *Vet. Microbiol.* 83 (2): 85–106.

Vannier, P., Plateau, E., and Tillon, J.P. (1981). Congenital tremor in pigs farrowed from sows given hog cholera virus during pregnancy. *Am. J. Vet. Res.* 42 (1): 135–137.

Weesendorp, E., Stegeman, A., and Loeffen, W. (2009). Dynamics of virus excretion via different routes in pigs experimentally infected with classical swine fever virus strains of high, moderate or low virulence. *Vet. Microbiol.* 133 (1–2): 9–22.

Yoo, S.J., Kwon, T., Kang, K. et al. (2018, 2018). Genetic evolution of classical swine fever virus under immune environments conditioned by genotype 1-based modified live virus vaccine. *Transbound. Emerg. Dis.* 65: 735–745.

25

Newcastle Disease

Ian Brown[1], Peter Cargill[2], Ralph Woodland[3], and Thierry van den Berg[4]

[1] *Animal and Plant Health Agency, Addlestone, Surrey, UK*
[2] *Wyatt Poultry Veterinary Services, Hereford, UK*
[3] *Formerly Veterinary Medicines Directorate, UK*
[4] *Veterinary and Agrochemical Research Centre, Brussels, Belgium*

25.1 Introduction

Newcastle disease (ND) is one of the most important diseases in poultry worldwide and causes devastating losses to the poultry industry, while impacting food security in many regions of the world. The cause of the disease is Newcastle disease virus (NDV) which belongs to the avian orthoavulavirus type 1 (AOAV-1) serotype, formerly avian paramyxovirus type. An important characteristic of AOAV-1 strains is their ability to cause distinct clinical signs and different levels of disease severity even in the same species. Typically, disease produced in chickens can be classified into five pathotypes: (i) viscerotropic velogenic, causing highly virulent infection with hemorrhagic lesions in the intestinal tract; (ii) neurotropic velogenic, causing high mortality following nervous signs; (iii) mesogenic, causing respiratory and sometimes nervous signs with low to moderate mortality; (iv) lentogenic, causing mild respiratory and/or unapparent enteric infection; (v) avirulent asymptomatic.

Historically, there have been waves of panzootics affecting domestic birds. All outbreaks are caused by a single serotype, but not all strains of AOAV-1 are classified as NDV. The classification of these viruses is based on international criteria for determining virulence in chickens (OIE 2018). Although chickens appear to be the domestic species most susceptible to NDV, the virus is capable of infecting a wide range of avian species. In some species, such as ducks, there are few signs of disease, even when infected with strains virulent for chickens. Importantly, other species can act as reservoir hosts, such as Columbiformes (including pigeons and doves) which may be significant in the spread and transmission of disease. The mode of transmission from bird to bird is dependent on the tropism of the virus, with birds that show respiratory disease shedding virus in droplets and aerosolized mucus which may be inhaled by susceptible birds. Viruses restricted to replication in the gastrointestinal tract may be transferred by ingestion of contaminated feces either directly or in contaminated food or water or by the inhalation of small infective particles produced in dried feces. As a result of these modes of spread, the virus may be able to transmit rapidly, for instance within an intensively enclosed fully stocked broiler house, whereas spread in caged layers may be slower.

The agency of humans has a central role in the spread of NDV, mainly through the movement of live birds, fomites, personnel, and poultry products from infected premises to susceptible birds. For these reasons, control and eradication of the disease presents significant challenges to the poultry industry worldwide, and therefore the use of vaccination has been applied for many decades as an important control tool.

25.2 Types of Vaccines

There are a large number of vaccines against ND available worldwide. Although some new vaccines have been produced using molecular biology techniques, the vast majority of commercially available vaccines are conventionally produced. Both live and inactivated (sometimes referred to as killed) vaccines are available. Live vaccines may be further divided into "traditionally attenuated" and "vector vaccines."

Veterinary Vaccines: Principles and Applications, First Edition. Edited by Samia Metwally, Gerrit Viljoen, and Ahmed El Idrissi.

25.2.1 "Traditionally Attenuated" Live Vaccines

Vaccine strains, in common with ND field viruses, vary in their relative tropism for respiratory, enteric, and nervous systems as well as their intracerebral pathogenicity index (ICPI). The OIE recommends that the maximum ICPI be <0.7. In the European Union (EU), the permissible maximum ICPI index is defined by Commission Decision 93/152/EEC (and endorsed in the European Pharmacopoeia) (EUR-Lex 1993) which defines a maximum ICPI of 0.4 (10^7 EID_{50}) or 0.5 (10^8 EID_{50}). These standards are in place in order to prevent adverse neurological side effects of vaccines and are respected by most but not all vaccine manufacturers across the world. The ICPI index of the commonly used vaccines has been shown not to impact the level of protection conferred (Orsi et al. 2009) and therefore ICPI index should not be a consideration when choosing vaccines for use. While there is minor variation in the ICPI index of the various vaccine strains, the most important differentiating attribute is the relative differences in tissue tropism between the respiratory and enteric systems.

Due to their live nature, these vaccines require controlled storage conditions (+2 °C to +8 °C) although some vaccines possess thermostable properties that allow short-term exposure at higher temperatures, which can be advantageous for transport to remote farms in hot climates where administration techniques are limited (Oakeley 2000). In particular, thermostable ND vaccine strains, such as V4 and I-2, have been used extensively to protect village chickens against ND, due to their decreased dependence on cold chain for transport and storage while retaining their antigenicity. These viruses survive for several weeks at temperatures in excess of 20 °C when stabilized with a carrier (Echeonwu 2008).

Combination live ND vaccines, usually combined with infectious bronchitis (IB), are commercially available as are combined multivalent inactivated ND vaccines and are discussed later in the chapter.

Live ND vaccines are the most commonly used across the world, partly due to their ability to be administered via mass vaccination techniques. The strains used for these vaccines are most commonly lentogenic (e.g. Hitchner-B1, LaSota, Ulster 2C, VG/GA, and the thermostable vaccines V4 and C2) but mesogenic strains such as Komarov and Roakin, which are more pathogenic, may be used primarily in countries where ND is endemic (OIE 2018). The vaccine viruses may be propagated in specific pathogen-free (SPF) hen's eggs or cell cultures. They are frequently provided in freeze-dried form and must be reconstituted in a suitable diluent or chlorine-free water for administration. Administration is typically via eye-drop, spray, or drinking water, although a live vaccine for *in ovo* use has also been developed.

Exposure to live, traditionally attenuated vaccines results in a comprehensive immune response resulting in the generation of circulating, local (mucosal) and cell-mediated immunity (CMI). Although these vaccines are capable of reducing or eliminating clinical signs and mortality, they do not prevent infection with field virus or field virus shedding (Alexander et al. 1999). Live vaccines have also been shown to initiate a more rapid cell-mediated immune response than inactivated vaccines (Popovic et al. 2010). Live attenuated vaccines are commonly used to vaccinate 1-day-old chicks but in some cases repeated doses are recommended if prolonged immunity is required (Alexander and Senne 2008).

A recent development has been the production of vaccine incorporated into effervescent tablets provided in blister packs which, although they still need to be stored and transported refrigerated, have the advantage that packaging is more convenient and lighter for transportation.

25.2.2 Live Vectored Vaccines

There are several vectored NDV vaccines available (reviewed by Dimitrov et al. 2017). They are usually based on either turkey herpesvirus (HVT) or avian poxvirus (POX) vaccines as the vector, which due to their large genomes facilitate insertion of the necessary genetic sequences that code for key protective ND antigens without adversely affecting the viability and efficacy of the vaccine vector itself. As the vector replicates in the bird, the immune system is exposed to the key ND antigens. The pathogenesis of HVT and POX is distinct from that of NDV which, in addition to exposure only to a limited number of ND virus epitopes, results in a distinguishable immune response compared with traditionally attenuated ND vaccines, although vaccine efficacy is good. As there is no exposure to live ND virus, no consideration for ND virus tropism or the level of attenuation is required; only the vector tropism needs to be considered when choosing the product to use.

Due to the nature of the vectors employed in commercially available vaccines, mass vaccination techniques cannot be used, administration being possible only by injection of individual birds, or eggs, via specialized *in ovo* equipment. In addition, these products are only available as frozen presentations requiring storage and transport in liquid nitrogen. These features may present practical and logistical complications that may not be possible to overcome in some situations.

Only a few recombinant vector vaccines have been authorized in certain countries. A cell-associated live recombinant turkey herpes virus (rHVT/ND) expressing the fusion protein of NDV D-26 lentogenic strain (Vectormune® ND) was recently authorized in the EU with indications for efficacy against Marek's disease in addition to ND. A similar vaccine (Innovax®-ND) is authorized in the USA. Some other vaccines that contain recombinant fowlpox virus expressing ND antigens have been authorized in the USA (Trovac®-NDV, VectorVax® FP-N). Although all these innovative products have the potential for immunizing against two diseases at the same time, it is possible that existing immunity against the vector might interfere with the development of immunity against NDV. Furthermore, the need for the recombinant turkey herpes virus vaccines and Trovac-NDV to be stored and transported in liquid nitrogen may limit their applicability in some environments.

25.2.3 Inactivated Vaccines

Inactivated vaccines need to be administered by injection of individual birds and are typically used to boost the immunity of older birds such as layers and breeders that have previously been primed by a live vaccine. The vaccine virus may be propagated in fowls' eggs that can be obtained either from an SPF or healthy flock. Vaccine virus inactivation must comply with regulatory requirements, such as those of the European Pharmacopoeia (Ph. Eur), according to the type of inactivant (e.g. formaldehyde or β-propiolactone) and the concentration used and the duration of treatment. Either virulent or avirulent strains can be used as seed virus but from the point of view of safety, the use of avirulent strains may be considered more suitable. They are usually presented in liquid form incorporating an adjuvant (typically an oil emulsion) to enhance the immune response. Inactivated NDV antigens are often included in multicomponent vaccines in combination with inactivated antigens of other avian pathogens such as IBV, avian metapneumovirus (avian rhinotracheitis), avian reovirus, infectious bursal disease (IBD) virus, and egg drop syndrome virus.

Inactivated vaccines consist of ND virus formulated with an adjuvant which is usually a water and oil emulsion or may also be an aluminum hydroxide adjuvant; however, experimental work has been performed with other adjuvants such as *Sargassum pallidum* polysaccharides (Li et al. 2012).

Although inactivated, the Ph. Eur requires that the ND antigens contained in inactivated vaccines comply with the ICPI requirements previously detailed in order to minimize the risk of disease in case of inactivation failure. Some data are available suggesting that the use of viruses with higher ICPIs induces protective antibodies for a longer duration (Roy et al. 1999), but the risk of iatrogenic disease due to poor inactivation outweighs their potential benefit.

Immunological priming with live ND vaccines greatly potentiates the level of protection generated by inactivated vaccines which require individual administration via injection and those commercially available vary in dose from 0.1 to 0.5 mL per bird, although 0.3–0.5 mL dose per bird is most common.

As the ND virus is inactivated, tissue tropism is irrelevant and the adjuvanted nature of the products provides long-term immune stimulation that results in high levels of circulating antibody for a number of months, but little or no mucosal immunity. The currently available inactivated vaccines utilize the common live vaccine strains for antigen, but some vaccines utilizing local endemic NDV strains, such as genotype VII (reclassified and split into genotypes VII.1.1, VII.1.2, VII.2) (Dimitrov et al. 2019), are in development for some geographic areas and the use of homologous viruses as vaccine strains may have some benefit in terms of improved protection and reduction of virus shedding (Miller et al. 2007; Roohani et al. 2015).

25.2.4 Alternative Technology Vaccines

Several alternative technology experimental vaccines have been developed, such as an antibody/antigen complex vaccine that may be used by "*in ovo*" administration (Kapczynski et al. 2012) and a recombinant pDNA expressing ND virus fusion proteins but these are either not commercially available or in late pipeline development.

Infectious bursal disease and infectious laryngotracheitis (ILT) experimental vaccines have been produced and evaluated utilizing ND virus as a vector. In addition, ND virus as a vector for delivering avian influenza (AI) antigens has been developed and applied in the field, particularly in China and Mexico. The focus of these field applications was, however, to control AI and so utility for control of ND in the field was not reported. In China, these vaccines were withdrawn after 2012, possibly due to challenges in overcoming ND maternally derived immunity (Basavarajappa et al. 2014; Kim et al. 2014).

25.3 Immune Response and Duration of Immunity

For the efficient design of a vaccine, it is important to know the optimal type of immune response that will afford full protection – the so-called immunological correlates of protection (Plotkin 2010). For certain viruses, antibody-dependent immunity might be sufficient, while for others, cell-mediated immunity is essential. A protective immune response to vaccination will be related to the production of antibodies (humoral immunity), the action of sensitized T lymphocytes

(CMI), or a combination of both. Moreover, mucosal immunology is increasingly gaining attention as an area of great potential for the development of vaccines. Indeed, mucosal surfaces are the major site of entry of many infectious agents into the host. The mucosae contain several defined lymphoid tissues that respond specifically to invading antigens and this immune response can be either cellular and/or humoral (IgA). Mucosal immunology research has been hampered by the difficulty and labor-intensive nature of collecting samples and by the lack of information in poultry. For example, to date, there are limited data available on IgA mucosal responses or cytotoxic T cells to viruses in chickens. This information is essential to ensure that a given *in vitro* potency test is also relevant for assessing *in vivo* efficacy, and for making sure that the relevant immune response is being measured against adequate antigens.

Ideally, vaccination against NDV should result in sterilizing immunity against infection and replication of the virus with, as a result, no excretion and transmission. Realistically, ND vaccination does not fully reach this goal but usually protects the birds from the more serious consequences of disease, although virus replication and shedding may still occur, albeit at a reduced level (Alexander and Senne 2008). Although a good correlation between humoral immunity and protection has been demonstrated (Beard and Brugh 1975), cell-mediated (Russell et al. 1997) and local (or mucosal) (Takada and Kida 1996) immune responses are known to play an important role to decrease the excretion and dissemination of the virus.

Antibodies can be detected against NDV approximately 6–10 days postinfection, while specific CMI after stimulation of antigen-specific cytotoxic T cells (CTLs) generally requires about 7–10 days. As the mean time of death following infection with NDV is 2–6 days, the presence of preexisting antibodies prior to infection appears to be the most critical mechanism for protection from clinical disease (Kapczynski and King 2005). In studies using cyclosporin A and cyclophosphamide to suppress B and T cells, respectively, chickens with CMI specific for NDV were not protected from lethal challenge in the absence of ND antibodies as determined by hemagglutination inhibition (HI) tests. However, birds with NDV-specific antibodies were shown to be protected. The results indicate that antibodies are the key modulators of protection, but that CMI likely contributes to decrease viral shedding through targeted killing of NDV infected cells (Russell et al. 1997).

25.3.1 Humoral Immunity

The induction of neutralizing antibodies is one of the main goals of vaccination and either the anti-HN (anti-hemagglutinin-neuraminidase) or anti-F (anti-fusion protein) neutralizing antibodies protect against disease and infection (Reynolds and Maraqa 2000a). In the chicken, IgM, IgY (avian IgG equivalent), and IgA antibodies are produced as part of the immune response. Antibodies are detected at the site of infection and in the blood starting at 6 days after infection or live virus vaccination and levels peak 21–28 days after infection. Antibodies neutralize the ND virus particles by binding and preventing attachment of the virus to host cells (Al-Garib et al. 2003). The antibody response, measured as HI titers, is currently used in chickens as a serological marker of immunological response or measure of efficacy to the vaccine, but enzyme-linked immunosorbent assay (ELISA) tests can be more sensitive. Levels of serum antibody correlate with immune protection against clinical disease. Single vaccination with live lentogenic virus will produce a response in susceptible birds of about 2^4–2^6, but HI titers as high as 2^8 or more may be obtained following a vaccination program involving oil-emulsion vaccine. After vaccination with only an inactivated vaccine, the immune response will mainly be humoral, not cell mediated. Therefore, the antibody titers necessary to get full protection against mortality, clinical signs, and virus shedding respectively become extremely high. This has been illustrated by two studies using inactivated vaccines (Allan et al. 1978; Westbury et al. 1984) and emphasizes the complementary role of CMI in full protection against NDV. In addition, it has been shown that the efficacy of vector vaccines against NDV often does not correlate with serum IgG levels (Rauw et al. 2010).

25.3.2 Cell-Mediated Immunity

Cell-mediated immunity responses to NDV may be detected shortly after vaccination with a live NDV vaccine (Reynolds and Maraqa 2000b). It is feasible to measure CMI by proliferation tests or release of interleukins such as ChIFNγ *ex vivo*. Based on several studies in poultry, the development of a capture ELISA for the measurement of ChIFNγ released by T cells from spleen or blood after *ex vivo* stimulation has proved to be a good way to evaluate CMI in the chicken, after different ND vaccination regimens (Lambrecht et al. 2004).

Currently, most Th1-associated cytokines in chickens have been identified, and can be monitored as immunological correlates, either by cytokine-specific ELISA in supernatants of *ex vivo* antigen-restimulated cells or by enzyme-linked immunospot (ELISPOT) assays (Ariaans et al. 2008). Several studies have compared CMI responses between birds receiving live versus inactivated NDV vaccines. Results indicated increased CMI with the live NDV vaccination whereas CMI derived from inactivated NDV vaccines took longer to develop and were not as robust

(Lambrecht et al. 2004). Also, the virulence of the virus appears to play a role in CMI stimulation as Rauw et al. (2009) demonstrated an earlier and shorter CMI induced by a less virulent NDV vaccine strain, compared with a stronger and longer CMI mediated by a more virulent vaccine strain. NDV-specific CMI was detected up to 12 weeks postvaccination in the peripheral blood and spleen of commercial layer chickens vaccinated at 1 day old according to different vaccination regimens (Rauw et al. 2014). In contrast, relatively little is known about the relevance of CTL responses for the control of NDV. It seems that pulmonary cellular immunity and especially $CD8^+$ T cells expressing ChIFNγ may be very important in protecting the naïve natural host against lethal respiratory viruses (Kapczynski et al. 2013). Classic cell lysis assays have been established to measure functional CTL activity against IB (Seo and Collisson 1997) or AI (Kapczynski 2014) but have been poorly investigated for NDV. In general, however, these cell culture-based assays requiring inbred chicken lines are difficult to establish and to reproduce.

25.3.3 Local Immunity

As mucosal surfaces represent the main route of entry of NDV, it is essential that vaccination induces a good level of local (mucosal) immunity. This immune response after vaccination can be investigated by detection of local accumulation of specific immune cell populations (Jayawardane and Spradbrow 1995). Following infection or vaccination with NDV, local head-associated lymphoid tissue (HALT) immunity is principally evaluated by the detection of specific IgA in the tears corresponding to the accumulation of immune cells, mainly B cells, in the Harderian gland, a lymphoid tissue located close to the lacrimal glands of the birds (Rauw et al. 2009). In the gut-associated lymphoid tissues (GALTs), specific IgA in bile or in the supernatant of *ex vivo* cultures of intestinal tissue has also been detected till 12 weeks post live ND vaccination (Al-Garib et al. 2003). Additionally, in the bronchial-associated lymphoid tissues (BALTs) and particularly in the lung secretions, virus-neutralizing antibody against NDV in tracheal washes can also been demonstrated (Rauw et al. 2009). Finally, local NDV-specific CMI in the digestive tract and in the lung was detected till 10 weeks postvaccination in commercial layer chickens vaccinated at 1 day old with a live NDV (Rauw et al. 2014).

25.3.4 Maternal-Derived Antibody

Maternal-derived antibody (MDA) is passively transferred in the egg from the mother to the embryo from the 18th day of incubation and is crucial in early life to provide protection against pathogens previously encountered by the dam. However, beside these benefits, MDA has disadvantages by affecting the induction of specific active immune responses induced by vaccination. Indeed, MDA can interfere by reducing the replication of vaccine and consequently reducing the induction of specific active immune responses (Rauw et al. 2009). In addition, the level of maternal immunity in young chickens may vary considerably from farm to farm, batch to batch, and among individual chickens. Therefore, vaccination at day-old by spray followed by a boost after 2 weeks in drinking water or spray are usually recommended in order to prime early immune responses, especially locally, as soon as possible in the presence of MDA.

The duration of immunity depends on the vaccination program chosen. The actual titers obtained and their relationship to the degree and duration of immunity for any given flock and program are difficult to predict. For this reason, one of several strategies is employed. Either the birds are not vaccinated until 2–4 weeks of age after waning of MDA, when most of them will be susceptible, or 1-day-old birds are vaccinated by conjunctival instillation or by the application of a coarse spray at the hatchery. Alternatively, embryos can be vaccinated *in ovo* after approximately 18 days incubation. This will establish active infection in some birds that will persist until maternal immunity has waned. A boost is then carried out 2–4 weeks later. Revaccination of layers should only be done if there is a very high risk of field challenge. All EU-registered vaccines, for example, are intended for use in layers and breeders and have to be proven to provide protection at end of lay. It should be noted that the use of live vaccines in birds in lay is very risky and can cause egg drop or even mortality, particularly if birds are mycoplasma positive.

The duration of immunity following three methods of triple vaccination was followed in an 18-month-long controlled experiment (Dardiri and Yates 1962). The three methods provided equal levels of protection against an intramuscular challenge with GB Texas NDV. As the period between vaccination and challenge increased, the number of birds with low antibody titer, virus isolation from the trachea and eggs, and mortality and appearance of clinical signs increased. Interestingly, a single vaccination with a recombinant rHVT-ND vaccine at 1 day of age provided complete or almost complete (95–100%) clinical protection against NDV challenges from 4 weeks up to 72 weeks of age when the latest challenge was done (Palya et al. 2014).

25.4 Desired Specifications when Ordering Vaccine

There are many aspects to vaccine specification that should be considered in the context of the epidemiological situation where it will be used. A detailed account of all aspects of ND vaccines, including their production and use, has been published (Allan et al. 1978). The fundamental considerations should be safety, quality, and efficacy.

Various internationally recognized standards covering these points are in place such as the Ph. Eur in Europe and similar standards in the USA (US Pharmacopeia) and Australia (Australian Pharmaceutical Formulary). They are useful references for good practice when considering the use of vaccine not produced according to these systems. Although uncommon, in some geographic areas counterfeit vaccine may be present in the market. This is usually relabeled vaccine that has either expired or may not contain ND antigen. It is recommended to only purchase vaccine from reliable sources that can be validated by the relevant vaccine manufacturer.

25.4.1 Safety

Newcastle disease vaccines should be demonstrated to be both safe and efficacious for the target species. Safety should be tested in accordance with VICH guideline 44 (VICH 2008) using specially formulated batches that contain the maximum titer or amount of antigen per dose that may be contained in commercial batches. As mentioned previously, the strains of virus used in live vaccines for use in countries where the disease is not endemic should have an ICPI of less than 0.4 or 0.5, depending on the dose of vaccine given.

Neurological side effects of ND vaccines are unlikely when vaccine use is restricted to strains with a low ICPI value. However, respiratory reactions with some strains available may result in reduced feed conversion, reduced growth, and potential mortality (depending on the environmental management standards in place and concurrent disease). Inappropriate administration techniques might also lead to these effects.

25.5 Quality Assurance and Control Testing

Each batch of vaccine should be subject to a range of quality control tests sufficient to demonstrate that it complies with the specifications that have been determined to be safe and efficacious. As an example, suitable testing regimes are indicated in the Ph. Eur monographs 0450 (for live vaccines) and 0870 (for inactivated vaccines) (European Pharmacopoeia 2016).

The following range of tests are considered suitable for live vaccines:

- The identity of the vaccine virus is confirmed by neutralization with monospecific NDV antiserum. The strain of vaccine virus may be identified by a suitable method, for example using monoclonal antibodies or by genetic sequencing.
- Vaccines intended for administration by injection should be shown to be sterile. Frozen or freeze-dried vaccines produced in embryonated fowls' eggs and not intended for administration by injection may contain a maximum of one nonpathogenic microorganism per dose.
- The vaccine should be shown to be free from contamination with mycoplasmas and extraneous viruses.
- The titer of live vaccine virus should be within the range that has been determined to be safe and efficacious.

The following range of tests are suitable for inactivated vaccines:

- The identity of the vaccine antigen may be confirmed by injection into naïve birds (i.e. no antibodies against NDV) resulting in the production of antigen-specific antibodies.
- The batch of vaccine should be shown to be sterile and free from avian pathogens.
- The batch of vaccine should be tested to confirm the absence of residual live NDV, either during the manufacturing process or in the finished product.
- The vaccine batch should be tested for potency to confirm that it is equivalent to one that meets the 50 PD_{50} (protective dose) per dose specification. It is not necessary to carry out the PD_{50} test for each batch and an alternative method that gives adequate assurance of equivalence with a 50 PD_{50} vaccine can be used. The Ph. Eur describes an *in vitro* ELISA test for hemagglutinin-neuraminidase antigen content which can be used together with a test for the adjuvant if it has been adequately validated and shown to correlate with *in vivo* potency. Alternatively, a serological test in vaccinated chickens can be used when a minimum antibody titer of 4.0 $\log_2$, at 17–21 days after vaccination, is required for a satisfactory batch.

Freedom from extraneous agents is a critical requirement for ND vaccines as the nature and scale of poultry production systems facilitate rapid and efficient dissemination of extraneous agents on a global basis, as experienced with egg drop syndrome in 1976 (Smyth 2013). The level of extraneous agents testing should be considered when choosing an ND vaccine to use along with the screening of embryonated fowls' eggs or other culture systems utilized in production. In addition, the sensitivity and specificity of the techniques employed for testing should be considered.

Clear definition of the minimum protective dose of ND vaccines and assurance of the appropriate vaccine titer at the end of the defined shelf-life are also very important aspects to consider. Vaccine manufacturers should be in a position to provide data on these specifications for their vaccines. When reviewing the data provided, consideration for the challenge strain and vaccine dose employed as well as the route of vaccination and challenge if different vaccines are to be compared is advised.

25.5.1 Efficacy

While there may be differences in the relative efficacy of the various ND vaccines available, the success or failure of them is more influenced by the effectiveness of their administration and clear definition and implementation of the overall ND control strategy. It is important to be aware that there are no ND vaccines available that prevent birds from becoming infected with field strain ND viruses. However, the vaccines will ameliorate the adverse effects of the field strain, reduce viral shedding and therefore positively impact the epidemiology of field strain ND viruses. The level of ameliorative effect and rate of impact on ND epidemiology will be dependent on the virulence of the field ND strain present and the effectiveness of the control strategy.

Efficacy should be tested using batches formulated to contain the minimum titer or amount of antigen per dose that may be contained in commercial batches. The European Pharmacopoeia monograph 0450 (European Pharmacopoeia 2016) specifies that live vaccines should be capable of protecting at least 90% of vaccinated chickens that have been challenged with a dose of virulent virus sufficient to kill 100% of unvaccinated control chickens. Inactivated vaccines should contain at least 50 PD_{50} per dose (Ph. Eur. monograph 0870) (European Pharmacopoeia 2016).

Other than the technical specification, there are several other practical points that require consideration when choosing an ND vaccine:

- Availability – since ND vaccine manufacturing capacity is finite and this will potentially impact choice.
- Cost benefit – vaccine and administration costs, in relation to the benefit derived, should be considered within the context of the relevant local epidemiological situation.
- Vaccine presentation – various presentations of vaccine are available which vary from 1000 to 15 000 doses; frozen vaccine in glass vials requiring storage and transport in liquid nitrogen; freeze-dried vaccine in glass vials requiring storage and transport at +2 to +8 °C.

The presentation and storage conditions should be reviewed in relation to the practical environment where vaccine will be used. The technical attributes of the vaccines available, moderated by the above practical considerations, should be reviewed in relation to the epidemiological situation present before making a final decision (see section 25.6):

- Endemic NDV.
- Freedom from NDV/low-virulence AOAV-1 and low risk of introduction.
- Freedom from NDV/low-virulence AOAV-1 and high risk of introduction.
- Vaccination in the face of virulent or low-virulence virus outbreak.

25.6 Vaccine Application for Disease Control

25.6.1 Vaccination Strategy

In some countries, legislation affects the use and quality of vaccines. Policies generally are linked to the enzootic nature of the disease or the perceived threat for new incursion. There are extremes of policy ranging from a total ban on vaccination, to no regulation, to compulsory vaccination. This may include specifications on the characteristics of vaccine strains used, for example, with regard to the master seed of live vaccines and the number of protective doses included, as well as the permitted ICPI value (e.g. less than 0.4). Such approaches are used within the EU and elsewhere (Council Directive 92/66). Furthermore, the master seed of viruses for inactivated vaccine production must have an ICPI value of less than 0.5; the OIE sets down recommended international guidelines (OIE 2000). However, in epidemiological situations where ND is endemic, a more aggressive approach can include mesogenic strains being used for vaccines. These strains will have ICPI values >0.5 and therefore cause some mortality and increased side effects due to clinical disease.

As mentioned previously, regardless of vaccine choice and strategy defined, the efficiency and accuracy of vaccine administration are crucial to success in preventing or controlling ND, while it must be accepted that vaccination alone will not eliminate ND. Vaccines must be used in conjunction with sound biosecurity and good sanitary measures for any control program to be successful. In situations of extreme challenge, no vaccines are likely to offer complete protection. Furthermore, the concept of "national flock protection" is important to consider, such that all susceptible birds within the same geographic area or epidemiological system must be efficiently vaccinated to bring under control clinical ND.

The only stage in a bird's life where total control of vaccine administration is possible is at the hatchery and as such, depending upon the epidemiological situation, the opportunity to vaccinate in the hatchery should be taken via *in ovo*, day-old injection, spray or gel application.

The various ND vaccine types available have been reviewed earlier and although inactivated vaccines are generally only employed in laying and breeding birds, administration of inactivated ND vaccines to day-old birds in the hatchery, in addition to live ND vaccine, is practiced in some countries where ND is endemic or there is a high risk of introduction. This practice is gradually being replaced by the use of vaccination *in ovo* or at day old, with vector vaccines, even though the *in ovo* use of pox-vectored ND vaccines may reduce hatchability (Peter Cargill, personal communication; Stone et al. 1997; Ramp et al. 2012).

Some fundamental approaches to vaccination strategies in various epidemiological situations are listed in Table 25.1, but a detailed strategy must consider the practical environment and its restrictions, as well as any political or regulatory influences, or impact on the ability to export both live birds and poultry products. Importantly, any vaccination strategy can be developed based on clear principles but must be adapted according to local factors as a single approach will not be applicable to all settings, risks, and conditions.

Table 25.1 and the text below set out the principles that should be adopted in order to prevent and control ND in various situations. However, the following country situations may be used as examples of ND vaccination strategies at the time of writing:

- South Africa – large poultry population, endemic ND field challenge that fluctuates in terms of level and viral genotype responsible.
- Thailand – large poultry population, endemic ND challenge, various genotypes of virus.
- Germany – large poultry population, nonendemic, compulsory ND vaccination.
- United Kingdom – large poultry population, ND free, low risk of ND incursion.
- Denmark – small poultry population, ND free, vaccination prohibited.
- St Helena, South Atlantic – very small poultry population, isolated geographically, naïve population. However, ND incursion has occurred; emergency vaccination applied.

25.6.1.1 South Africa

- Endemic nature results in constant risk of circulation of existing virus as well as new virus incursion.
- Vaccination programs tend to vary in intensity in relation to the perceived and measured risk of ND outbreaks.

Table 25.1 Vaccination strategies for different epidemiological scenarios.

Epidemiological situation	Vaccination strategy[a]
NDV freedom – low risk of introduction	• Vaccination of breeders and layers (long lived, economically important, difficult to cull) • No vaccination of broilers, due to vaccine cost and potential negative impact on economic performance • Nonvaccinated birds act as sentinels facilitating early identification of virus incursion • Routine monitoring for ND incursion • Detailed contingency plans required in event of an outbreak • Security stocks of ND vaccine advisable
NDV freedom – high risk of introduction	• Hypervaccination of breeders and layers strongly advised • Vaccination of broilers with a low reactive strain in order to minimize negative impact on economic performance • Detailed contingency plans required in event of an outbreak • Security stocks of ND vaccine advisable
Outbreak of virulent NDV[b] or virus endemic	• Additional, live vaccination of breeders and layers in lay regardless of risk of adverse effect on egg production • Live vaccines should be used but if birds not previously ND vaccinated, drops in egg production may be encountered • Choice of route of vaccination should be based on what is considered to be most reliable in terms of vaccine delivery (i.e. spray or drinking water) and what is most practical to facilitate vaccination of all susceptible birds as quickly as possible • Repeat live vaccination at week 4 to 6 intervals to optimize protection • Implement vaccination of breeders and layers in rear if not in place (vaccination starting at day old) Broilers • Vaccinate all broilers which are more than 14 days from slaughter with live vaccine (spray or drinking water) by the most practical route to facilitate vaccination of susceptible birds at the earliest opportunity. • Vaccinate all broilers *in ovo* or at day old by spray or gel • Repeat vaccination during growing period on at least one occasion depending upon risk of disease

[a] These are examples and any plan should be adapted to take account of local specified factors.
[b] NDV by definition is virulent avian avulavirus-1 (formerly APMV-1).

- Vaccine choice depends on the prevailing risk; milder, less reactive vaccines preferred.
- Vaccination of all bird types essential; choice of vaccine depends on the current risk and incidence of ND balanced with the potential adverse effects of less attenuated vaccines.
- Application of live vaccine to day-old birds plus boost with inactivated or vector vaccines is common.
- Multiple live vaccines administered throughout the rearing/growing period.
- Multiple inactivated vaccines used in long-lived and valuable stock.
- Use of live vaccines "in lay" common although potential risk to egg production.
- Widespread vaccination compromises the ability to identify low-level circulation of ND field virus.
- Due consideration for the effects of immunosuppressive diseases such as IBD and Marek's disease is essential as these impact the efficacy and subsequent value of ND vaccination.

25.6.1.2 Thailand

All comments related to South Africa are relevant other than the following:

- The size, nature, and structure of the industry facilitate circulation of existing ND viruses, while the geographic location is such that new virus incursion is highly likely.
- Vaccination programs tend to remain at a high level due to the constant risk.
- Vaccine choice orientated toward more reactive, immunogenic vaccines.

25.6.1.3 Germany

- Geographic location results in constant, medium-level risk of ND incursion.
- Legislative measures in place; ND vaccination of all commercial poultry is compulsory and responsibility for protection is delegated to the field veterinarians responsible for the farms.
- Compulsory vaccination can compromise the ability to detect new virus incursions.
- Vaccine choice varies according to the perceived risk, with the less reactive vaccines preferred especially in growing birds.
- Day-old vaccination of all bird types is in place; field boosters are dependent on bird type and perceived risk.

25.6.1.4 United Kingdom

- Geographic location results in moderately low risk of incursion, but trade links with mainland Europe increase risk of incursion.
- Vaccination of long-lived stock with live followed by inactivated ND vaccine is routinely applied; however, ND vaccine is used intradermally at day old, but not routinely practiced.
- Nonvaccination of broilers provides a large sentinel population that facilitates early identification of virus incursion.
- Vaccination programs are revised based on new epidemiological information from neighboring countries.

25.6.1.5 Denmark

- ND vaccination prohibited in all bird types.
- Incursion of ND virus easily identified due to naïve poultry population.
- Lower size and density of poultry population allow control and eradication by use of a slaughter policy.

25.6.1.6 St Helena, South Atlantic

- An extremely isolated island geographically, but susceptible to ND virus incursion due to trade links with other countries.
- Incursion of ND likely to devastate key local food supplies.
- Reactive vaccination in the event of virus incursion, live plus inactivated vaccination of all susceptible poultry in the face of an outbreak.
- Small population size facilitates individual bird vaccine administration which results in rapid high-level protection.

25.6.2 Vaccinating Small Flocks and High-Value Birds

The most secure method of vaccinating birds against ND is by concurrent administration of live and inactivated ND vaccine. Live vaccine should be given by individual eye-drop and inactivated vaccine may be administered during the same handling process.

Eye dropping diluent and dropper tips are available for use with commercial ILT vaccine and are suitable for use with ND vaccines, but for ease of use, ND vaccine should be sourced in 1000 dose presentations as the ILT diluent accommodates 1000 doses.

25.6.3 Epidemiological Settings and Objectives

When considering the circumstances under which vaccination should be applied, it must be emphasized that vaccination should not be regarded as an alternative to good management practice and biosecurity or the adoption of adequate control policies for the prevention of introduction and spread. While vaccines can reduce disease burden, prevent death, protect and reduce susceptibility to infection, and interrupt or abrogate transmission under field conditions, they cannot realistically be expected to provide 100% protection, therefore vaccination should be used in combination with other measures for control of ND.

Vaccination should be adapted and designed according to the local epidemiological factors; this will have a fundamental influence on the effectiveness of the vaccination program once implemented. Key factors that need to be considered when designing a vaccination program include:

- the type of poultry production (for example, commercial or rural)
- the structure and organization of the industry
- poultry population density (including spectrum of species)
- the prevailing disease situation
- vaccine suitability and availability
- use of other vaccines
- incidence of other diseases in populations to be vaccinated
- availability of suitable resources (people and equipment)
- costs of program (including benefit analysis).

The objectives should have a clear purpose, taking into account all of the aforementioned factors to achieve a practical outcome. The results from vaccination can be categorized as follows:

- protection against clinical disease
- reduce susceptibility to infection with the consequence of reduced virus shedding (quantity and duration) and increasing host resistance to initial infection by requiring a higher infectious dose to initiate infection
- reduce the risk of transmission between vaccinated birds and from vaccinated to nonvaccinated birds.

Interruption of transmission at flock level will be necessary to abrogate onward spread. For vaccination to achieve success in reducing clinical disease, it must be effective at the individual level but reducing susceptibility, reducing virus shedding, and interrupting transmission will benefit all vaccinated flocks within a region. The desired outcomes at flock or country/region/compartment level should be clearly defined at the outset before applying the program. At flock level, if a single bird is not immunized, it has a chance of being infected but this is inversely proportional to the level of protection achieved at the flock level and generally the broad principle is that vaccination should be applied successfully to 80% of birds within a flock to mitigate risk of spread within the flock (Miller et al. 2013).

By geographical region, the higher the prevalence of vaccinated flocks in an area, the lower the probability of infection in unvaccinated flocks located in the same area. This is important because it will not be appropriate to necessarily vaccinate all production types (Table 25.1). Except during epizootics of ND, vaccination of birds beyond 3 weeks of age is usually only practiced in egg-laying birds, since these are longer lived and therefore by definition are more likely to encounter infection during their production lifetime. Because ND can infect all production sector types, creating challenges in both large commercial production sectors but also rural poultry, flexibility of design of the vaccination program will be important to achieve a successful outcome. Therefore, the structure and organization of the local poultry sector where the program is to be applied will be important in shaping design.

Systems for vertical integration typically lead to relatively high concentrations of production units in certain regions and areas and by definition present increased challenges for risk of major epidemics and subsequent control (Marangon and Busani 2007). It is important, therefore, that the relevant and appropriate vaccines together with their appropriate administration, using the correct antigen combinations (especially considering live vaccines in combination with other approaches) and optimal virus virulence, as appropriate, have become essential elements in managing and balancing risk at competitive cost. In rural communities, in developing countries, ND is a well-defined problem of village poultry where the virus is often endemic and such populations act as reservoirs for the virus. Increased use of thermostable lentogenic viruses, including those that can be delivered via food, has met with some success (Oakeley 2000; Wambura et al. 2000; Alexander et al. 2004). However, education of communities on concepts of basic hygiene and disease prevention approaches is needed to complement the vaccination of village poultry. Key problems in this sector are appropriate delivery and maintenance of cold chain of the product to ensure vaccine efficacy.

The use of vaccination requires adjustment in diverse conditions according to the local risk for disease occurrence, level of biosecurity practice in key poultry production systems and practical use with each type of poultry operation. Considering these factors together, it should be possible to target appropriate areas/populations where vaccination can provide effective outputs. Considering current threats for virus incursion, it is important that a surveillance program complements vaccination using reliable diagnostic tests, such that adaptations or changes to the program can be made, should the epidemiological situation change. Furthermore, such approaches will also provide assurance or not of the success of vaccination through the determination of induced antibody levels.

In principle, there are three basic strategies that can be applied. First, routine vaccination, which is commonly used in areas where NDV is endemic or the threat of repeated incursion is high. When properly applied, this approach is effective in reducing mortality and production losses and may be able to lower the prevalence of infection at population level such that other eradication measures may be applied, i.e. culling of infected flocks, if this is the desired outcome. The reality is that in many counties, routine vaccination is applied with limited monitoring and without close alignment to the disease threat. Second, preventive vaccination may be transiently applied whenever the risk for introduction of virus and further spread increases. The rationale behind this strategy is that a level of protective immunity in a target population exists which can be boosted in the case of immediate risk or evidence of introduction of field virus. The use of this type of approach in the absence of a disease outbreak but in combination with other measures including biosecurity may maximize poultry protection if a risk of exposure exists. Many countries require preventive vaccination of all poultry, even in the absence of outbreaks, due to perceived disease threat. As a result, many poultry around the globe are vaccinated in this way but it does compromise assessing the real disease threat and distribution of infection on an active basis. Ideally, a clearly defined exit strategy should be formulated before preventive vaccination is undertaken.

A vaccination program designed to ultimately result in the eradication of infection would require phasing and targeting to specific sectors at greatest risk. Continuous increase in population immunity in a defined region monitored through surveillance can provide a focus for targeted application of other control measures such as culling infected flocks in order to reduce infection pressure and ensure that correlates of between-flock transmission risk are reduced to a level whereby infection cannot be maintained in a population.

Under field conditions, vaccination alone is not sufficient to bring about effective control of ND and needs to be accompanied by good hygiene practices. In poorly managed, overcrowded, badly ventilated conditions, for example, underlying bacterial infections can be common and even the mildest live vaccine strains may then produce disease sufficiently severe to mimic ND. It is essential, therefore, that good hygiene practices complemented by good management are vital in flocks being vaccinated and not merely during disease outbreaks. In particular, where preventive or emergency vaccination is used to underpin the surveillance program, the choice of vaccine may be important, as it will influence the tools and the evidence base to track and monitor vaccinated infected flocks. Vaccines compatible with differentiating vaccinated from infected animals (DIVA) testing are now available (see section 25.2.2) but data are lacking on their use for this purpose in a field setting. However, they offer the possibility to monitor immune responses discriminating field challenge from vaccinal immunity (Peeters et al. 2001; Park et al. 2006). These approaches are particularly important if the exit strategy is eradication, since early detection of infected vaccinated flocks is important as they present a source of virus for onward transmission.

An alternative to the use of a DIVA vaccine is a monitoring program that applies the use of sentinel birds. These are unvaccinated birds that are placed in contact with the vaccinated population and regular monitoring would reveal the presence of active ND infection in the vaccinated flock. However, there are logistical and practical challenges in the use of such systems to provide total assurance for reliable detection of infected flocks.

25.6.4 Vaccination of Turkeys

Turkeys tend to be refractory to live ND vaccines. Seroconversion to live ND vaccines can be poor, although birds appear to be protected when the more reactive live vaccines are employed. Very few live vaccines are registered for use in turkeys, but one such vaccine has recently achieved registration in the EU. Inactivated ND vaccine should be administered to turkeys with care and the breast muscle avoided as a site of injection, due to potential adjuvant damage to the most valuable portion of the carcass.

25.6.5 Vaccination of Birds Other than Chickens and Turkeys

Due to the current regulatory systems in place around the world, most ND vaccines are licensed for chickens and some for turkeys An ND vaccine is available for pigeons in some countries and is aimed at use in racing pigeons.

There is a large variation in the susceptibility of "other species" such as ducks, pheasant, and partridge to the commercially available ND vaccines. However, both live and inactivated vaccines are commonly used in these species with few or no adverse effects reported. When considering any ND control program, these "minor species" should be considered in terms of their number/location and involvement in any epidemiological system and a decision made on vaccination strategy. On balance, due to the relative bird numbers usually involved and lack of evidence of adverse effects of ND vaccines, these species should be vaccinated as a routine in most epidemiological situations, other than where vaccination is prohibited or the country is considered to be ND free.

25.6.6 Possible Combination with Vaccines for Other Diseases

In general, ND vaccines should not be used in combination with vaccines for other diseases unless data are available to demonstrate their compatibility. Combined use of live ND vaccines with other viral respiratory disease vaccines should be considered carefully as the results can be variable due to potential synergistic effects with respect to adverse respiratory reaction and/or potential interference rendering one or both vaccines ineffective (e.g. combined use with live ILT vaccines), or potentially beneficial in terms of serological response (such as some NDV and avian metapneumovirus vaccines) (Ganapathy et al. 2006). If data exist to support combination use, then this should be clearly indicated in the vaccine's data sheet or summary of product characteristics. In particular, some live ND vaccines have indications for compatibility with the manufacturer's own live vaccines against other avian diseases, such as IB, ILT, IBD, and Marek's disease. Some combined live NDV and IB vaccines are commercially available and have well-considered balanced titers of each virus in order to ensure efficacy of both components.

Additionally, as noted previously, inactivated ND virus antigens are often included in multicomponent vaccines in combination with inactivated antigens of other avian pathogens such as IB, avian metapneumovirus (avian rhinotracheitis), avian reovirus, IBD, egg drop syndrome virus, and infectious coryza. The concurrent use of live and inactivated NDV vaccines carries no risk and is a useful approach when vaccinating naïve birds during an outbreak (Senne et al. 2004).

The variable properties of the commercially available live respiratory virus vaccines are such that advice should be sought from the relevant manufacturers before combining products with ND vaccines.

Combined use of live ND vaccines and live *Escherichia coli* is generally nonproblematic, but advice should also be sought from manufacturers prior to use. Combined use with traditionally attenuated *Mycoplasma synoviae* (Ms) and *Mycoplasma gallisepticum* (Mg) vaccines should be avoided, whereas combined use of some ND vaccines with temperature-sensitive Ms and Mg vaccines is a general practice in place in some countries. Nevertheless, advice from manufacturers should always be sought prior to use.

There are numerous combined inactivated NDV vaccines commercially available which may include the following antigens in addition to NDV:

- infectious bronchitis
- avian metapneumovirus
- egg drop syndrome
- reovirus
- infectious bursal disease
- infectious coryza.

25.6.7 Use of Vaccine in the Face of an Outbreak

When a new outbreak of ND occurs in a previously unaffected country, area, or compartment and the epidemiological situation indicates that there could be rapid and extensive spread of infection, emergency vaccination to mitigate the threat can be considered. In many countries where vaccination is voluntary or even prohibited, this may be a necessary tool and a cost–benefit analysis should ideally be available to inform the decision making. Such programs of vaccination should be under the official control of the competent veterinary authority in the country or region concerned and, therefore, subject to certain specifications and monitoring. A decision to apply emergency vaccination would depend on a number of factors, including availability of adequate resources for prompt deployment of appropriate vaccines. Consideration needs to be given to the period in which nonvaccinated birds remain susceptible to infection after vaccine administration. As such, the deployment of such programs requires careful planning and speed of action. These programs require systematic vaccination of all flocks in a defined area. The EU sets out specified conditions for the application of such measures (92/66/EEC).

Under such programs, poultry that are moved into disease control areas should be vaccinated and transport of animals from vaccination areas to slaughter, for example, should only be permitted following appropriate health certification of birds from affected flocks. These licensed movements need to take account of the infection risk within the vaccination zone related to the period since vaccination began, with the perceived risk being lower once the vaccination program is complete and susceptible birds have seroconverted to the vaccine (see section 25.3). A key component of any emergency vaccination program is close monitoring of infection status (in actively infected flocks) in the vaccinated population. In addition, consideration may also be given, based on local factors, to vaccination of other populations, e.g. racing pigeons, which may be a risk for potential onward spread of infection.

25.6.8 When Vaccination Is Not Recommended

There are several situations when vaccination with live NDV vaccines should be avoided:

- In situations where there is a low/medium risk of introduction of NDV to a flock, it is logical to not vaccinate

broilers due to the potential adverse impact of vaccination on bird performance. The added benefit of this approach is that the largest sector of the bird population that generally has the lowest level of biosecurity acts as a sentinel population, where NDV incursion can be identified easily and serological surveillance implemented.
- Birds already infected with NDV should not be vaccinated as the vaccination is likely to complicate the disease and exacerbate morbidity and mortality.
- Where trade in poultry or poultry products may be adversely affected, as many countries will not accept importation of vaccinated live birds or poultry products from ND-vaccinated birds.
- Vaccination of *M. synoviae* and *M. gallisepticum*-positive birds should be avoided, if possible, as these two agents act synergistically with ND vaccines and vaccination may result in chronic respiratory disease (CRD).
- Where poor administration of ND vaccines is likely to result in adverse respiratory reactions and lead to CRD. Poor administration may consist of incomplete vaccination of a flock and/or bacterial contamination of vaccination equipment.

There are a few situations where use of inactivated NDV vaccines should be avoided:

- Small birds that may suffer adverse effects from the oil adjuvant.
- Ducks and geese that do not tolerate oil adjuvant well and may suffer mortality. If vaccination is considered essential, oil-based vaccines should be administered carefully by the subcutaneous route rather than the intramuscular route.
- Use of inactivated NDV (and other inactivated) vaccines should be avoided in unhealthy birds due to the impact of the oil adjuvant.

25.7 Monitoring and Vaccine Effectiveness

25.7.1 Postvaccination Monitoring

There are several serological techniques available for efficiently detecting the humoral response to ND vaccines. However, the results of these tests do not necessarily correlate with the effectiveness of the vaccine in use, as local immunity in the respiratory tract and digestive tract is important in protecting birds and humoral antibody levels do not represent levels of local immunity (see section 25.3). Vaccine effectiveness should be evaluated in relation to the epidemiological situation in question, bearing in mind that vaccines cannot prevent infection with or some degree of morbidity and mortality due to very virulent ND strains in a vaccinated commercial poultry production environment. Ultimately, the basic poultry production parameters such as feed conversion efficiency, weight gain, mortality rates, and average weight at slaughter should be used to gauge vaccine effectiveness (Marangon and Busani 2007).

Postvaccination monitoring should include the following factors:

- Reporting of any postvaccination respiratory reactions and investigation to determine the presence/absence of field ND strains or other pathogens. This may include circulation of lentogenic or avirulent field strains that might compromise interpretation of any monitoring data. The presence of these viruses should be definitively determined in the laboratory with accurate identification and appropriate adjustments made to the correct interpretation of data.
- Serological monitoring at least 14 days subsequent to vaccination. Various techniques are available (ELISA, HI, VN). ELISA and HI are most commonly employed. If there is circulation of lentogenic or avirulent strains, these will compromise and potentially influence serological profiles. Comparators in similar flocks vaccinated under the same conditions but without incursion of these viruses would be required to determine expected flock profiles in order to deduce any possible negative impacts of such events or, perhaps more likely, increased titer magnitude. Expected ELISA titers will differ depending on the assay system and particular vaccine in use, as well as the impact of any field challenge. ELISA kit and vaccine manufacturers are usually able to provide advice on parameters associated with vaccination and vaccination plus field challenge which will boost the ND titers detected. Serological responses may also vary between bird strains and species; turkeys, for example, are slow to develop detectable humoral antibodies. HI tests are also in common use and although results may vary slightly depending on the particular vaccine and antigen in use, postvaccinal HI titers expected from use of live ND vaccines are dependent on the vaccine in use but are generally between 2^3 and 2^7. Titers in excess of 2^7 would probably imply that some field ND challenge has occurred. ND HI titers after sequential vaccination with live and killed ND vaccines may be between 2^5 and 2^8. Highly variable titers may indicate poor vaccine administration and/or ND field challenge.
- Polymerase chain reaction (PCR) detection techniques are available for use with both tracheal and cloacal swabs and can be useful in monitoring vaccine administration but more commonly are used to detect AOAV-1 strains (see above regarding lentogenic or avirulent strains). However, these techniques should be interpreted with caution, particularly if not fully validated for use on field samples.

Postvaccination monitoring techniques have many limitations and, as such, a focus on ensuring that vaccine administration is accurate and efficient is critical to the success of any ND vaccination program and should include:

- a physical audit of the vaccination equipment and process
- ensuring the cold chain for vaccine is maintained
- ensuring the correct dose is being given
- the use of dyes to evaluate vaccination efficiency on farm or in the hatchery
- the use of gel administration equipment when available and audit of tongue staining.

25.7.2 Outbreaks in Vaccinated Animals

As noted previously, no ND vaccines will prevent morbidity or mortality when there is extensive challenge with very virulent ND field virus. Vaccination will, however, reduce the mortality, morbidity, and shedding of field virus and therefore impact the dynamics of spread.

In cases where protection after vaccination is far below expectation, this is usually due to one or a combination of the following factors:

- Breach of the cold chain and reduced/absent vaccine titer.
- Poor administration, resulting in failure to deliver vaccine to birds (c.f. data on flock coverage required).
- Vaccine strain in use is inappropriate in terms of its immunogenicity for the field strain present.
- Early challenge with field virus prior to the development of a protective immune response from the vaccine.
- Poor environmental management resulting in high ammonia and dust levels.
- Co-infection with another respiratory pathogen (i.e. ILT, Ms, Mg, AI).
- Extremely high level of field challenge due to sustained breaches in biosecurity.

25.8 Vaccine Adverse Reactions

Adverse reactions to ND vaccines may occur in both birds and humans under certain circumstances. Adverse reactions in birds are usually associated with respiratory symptoms but if severe may also cause morbidity and mortality and increased factory condemnations at slaughter.

The main factors contributing to adverse reactions (including induction of mild respiratory signs) to live ND vaccines are as follows:

- Inappropriate spray equipment used to apply vaccine.
- Bacterial contamination of vaccination equipment (usually *E. coli* or *Pseudomonas* spp.).
- Vaccine applied to birds with low or no maternal antibody to ND.
- Birds suffering from immunosuppressive diseases (IBD/Marek's/chicken anemia virus).
- Vaccine overdose.
- Failure to vaccinate the complete flock.
- Co-infection with other pathogens (ILT/IB/mycoplasma/low-pathogenicity AI).
- Poor chick quality:
  - Dehydration
  - Concurrent bacterial infection.
- Poor environmental management resulting in high ammonia and dust levels.

Adverse reactions to inactivated ND vaccines are caused by the physical effects of the adjuvant or injection processes, as the ND antigen is inactivated.

- The irritant nature of the adjuvant can cause reduced mobility and appetite over a period of a few days.
- Bacterial contamination of the vaccine or vaccinating equipment can lead to local abscess formation at the site of infection or bacterial septicemia and mortality.
- Inadvertent injection of vaccine into the liver due to inappropriate needle length or site of breast injection usually results in death within a few minutes.
- Physical damage to leg bones or nerves due to needle impact leading to lameness and periosteal reaction.

Few adverse reactions are generally seen after vaccination against ND if the products are applied in accordance with the manufacturers' recommendations. In the case of live conventional vaccines, these are limited to mild respiratory signs such as coughing or sneezing. A slight transient swelling may be observed at the injection site for 2–3 weeks after administration of inactivated vaccines.

25.8.1 Adverse Reactions in Humans

Newcastle disease virus is capable of infecting humans, causing a mild transient conjunctivitis which is self-limiting with no permanent effect; however, no human-to-human transmission has been reported (Alexander 2000)

Conjunctival infection usually occurs due to physical introduction into the eye by operatives manipulating vaccines prior to vaccination of birds, usually with a finger or by splashing vaccine. Vaccine virus titers are generally high, so the number of viral particles introduced to the eye by these methods can be substantial. The conjunctivitis is often unilateral. Oral consumption of vaccine has occurred in the past with no adverse effects reported (Crosby et al. 1986). Spray administration of ND is a common practice globally, although conjunctivitis is rarely reported, indicating that direct physical introduction into the eye is the most likely means of infection. Operatives should ensure that hands are washed thoroughly after handling NDV vaccine and protective eyewear in the form of goggles is helpful in preventing introduction into the eyes.

25.9 Availability and List of Manufacturers

The list of global vaccine manufacturers is extensive and no single site contains a comprehensive list (Table 25.2). It is important, however, that the quality of vaccine should be assured and recommended criteria referred to in this chapter, with proven properties, considered when selecting an appropriate vaccine and regimen.

25.10 Summary

Newcastle disease is one of the most important diseases in poultry worldwide and is endemic in many parts of the world. It causes devastating losses to the poultry industry, while impacting food security in many countries. The cause of the disease is NDV which belongs to the avian orthoavulavirus type 1 serotype.

A key tenet for control and reduction of disease incursion and/or spread is the use of vaccines, broadly divided into live attenuated and inactivated vaccines. Live attenuated vaccines vary in their relative tropism for respiratory, enteric, and nervous systems but they are controlled to prevent adverse clinical side effects. These vaccines can be further divided into traditionally attenuated and vector vaccines. The benefit of live vaccines is that they can be applied using mass vaccination techniques, including in the hatchery. Furthermore, they have the ability to induce a broad immune response including humoral, mucosal, and CMI. Vectored vaccines normally contain a NDV gene insert (fusion or hemagglutinin-neuraminidase gene) into a virus vector delivery system which induces immunity to the protective ND antigens. Inactivated vaccines need to be administered by injection of individual birds and are typically used to boost the immunity of older birds such as layers and breeders that have previously been primed by a live vaccine. These vaccines are safe and immune responses can be elevated by the use of adjuvants. They are often delivered in combination with other inactivated antigens for avian pathogens such as infectious bronchitis virus.

Newcastle disease vaccination protects the birds from more serious consequences of the disease but virus replication and shedding may still occur, including transmission, albeit at a reduced level. Generally, there is a good correlation between humoral immunity and protection against clinical disease. Antibodies are generally induced 6–10 days postinfection/-vaccination whilst CMI responses generally require a few days longer. Humoral antibodies neutralize ND virus particles, and a commonly used method to determine levels of antibody is the hemagglutination inhibition test. The titers generated in this assay are used as a correlate for predicted protection against clinical disease. Maternally derived antibodies that are naturally transmitted passively from the mother to the offspring are crucial in early life to provide protection. However, MDA also have some disadvantages by affecting the induction of specific active immune responses by vaccination. To overcome some of these effects, birds are often not vaccinated until 2–4 weeks of age or by the vaccination of 1-day-old birds at the hatchery through aerosol spray or eye drop, thereby establishing infection of mucosal and conjunctival surfaces and circumventing humoral protective responses.

When determining vaccine specification, three fundamental considerations should be safety, quality, and efficacy. International standards are laid down that normally require a vaccine to be able to protect 90% of vaccinated birds from a lethal challenge dose of virulent virus. In considering the choice of vaccine, it is also important to do a cost–benefit analysis and consider the practicality of delivery, including any requirements for vaccine thermostability.

Vaccination strategies will vary by country and region and could be subject to legislative control, ranging from a total ban on vaccination to no regulation or even compulsory vaccination. Vaccination alone will not resolve persistent or endemic infection but will reduce the disease burden within a national flock. Each program should be tailored according to the local epidemiological scenario which will range from continuous circulation of virus within an endemically infected population to a population with low risk of introduction and historically free. Vaccination, to be successful, should be applied in conjunction with other practices such as good management, biosecurity, and adequate policies for controlling and preventing introduction and spread. Key elements to consider when designing a vaccination program would be the type of poultry production, the structure and organization of the industry, the poultry density in the defined region, the prevailing disease situation, vaccine suitability and availability, incidence of other diseases in populations to be vaccinated, availability of resources, and costs of implementation.

There are three basic outcomes from a vaccination program: first, protection against clinical disease; second, to reduce susceptibility to infection within a population with the consequence of reduced shedding and

Table 25.2 List of Newcastle disease vaccine manufacturers.

Company name	URL	Company address	Type of vaccine (killed or attenuated)	Strain
Merial Limited	http://avian.merial.com/live-inactivated-vaccines-0	Ellesfield Avenue, Bracknell, Berkshire RG12 8YS, UK	Live	VG/GA-AVINEW, LaSota
			Inactivated	Ulster 2C
Ceva Animal Health LLC	www.ceva.us	10 Avenue de la Ballastière, 33 500 Libourne, France	Live	F Protein
Elanco Lohmann	www.elanco.com www.elanco.us/poultry-vaccines	2500 Innovation Way, Greenfield, IN 46140, USA	Inactivated	B1 type, LaSota
			Live	B1 type, LaSota
Qingdao Yebio Bioengineering Co. Ltd.	https://ybcloq.en.china.cn	Quanda Road, Dayang Village E. Hongdao Town, Qingdao, Shandong, China	Live	Clone-30
			Inactivated	LaSota
Zoetis Inc.	www.zoetis.com	10 Sylvan Way, Parsippany, NJ 07054, USA	Killed	Queensland V4
			Live	B1
FATRO SpA	www.fatro.it	Via Molino Emili 2, 25 030 Maclodio, Italy	Live	Hitchner B1, LaSota, Clone 30
			Killed	LaSota
Kyoto Biken	www.kyotobiken.co.jp/en	24-16 Makishima-cho, Uji-shi, Kyoto 611-0041, Japan	Live	B1
Vaksindo (Vaksindo Satwa Nusantara Pt.)	https://vaksindo.fm.alibaba.com	Jl. Pembangunan II, Bogor Propinsi Jawa Barat, Indonesia	Live	B1, LaSota
			Killed	LaSota
Sindh Poultry Vaccine Center	www.livestocksindh.gov.pk/pdf/spvc-karachi.pdf	Sindh Poultry Vaccine Center, Animal Sciences Complex, Korangi Karachi-74 900, Pakistan	Live	Mukteswar, Komarov, LaSota
Merck Animal Health	www.msd-animal-health.co.uk	Walton Manor, Walton, Milton Keynes MK7 7AJ, UK	Live	C2, Hitchner B1, Clone 30
	www.msd-animal-health.ph/products/products.aspx?productclass=vaccines-poultry		Inactivated	Clone 30
Harbin Veterinary Research Institute (HVRI)	www.hvri.ac.cn/en	No. 678 Haping Road, Xiangfang District, Harbin 150 069, China	Live	LaSota
Zhejiang Ebvac Biotech Co. Ltd.	http://english.ebvhz.com	401 23rd Street, Lower Sha Economic and Technological Development Zone, Hangzhou, China	Live	L-Line clone/CS2, Clone 30, LaSota
			Inactivated	LaSota
Hester Biosciences Ltd.	www.hester.in	Pushpak 1st floor, Motilal Hirabhai Road, Panchvati Circle, Ahmedabad, Gujarat 380 006, India	Live	B1, LaSota, R2B- Mukteswar
			Inactivated	LaSota

Please note this is not an exhaustive list of all vaccine manufacturers. When making a decision on vaccine type and source, we would direct you to the relevant information in this chapter of factors to consider. It may be that there are local manufacturers of vaccine strains that better meet the specification and criteria. The authors cannot accept any liability or responsibility for the accuracy or relevance of this information.

transmission; third, to reduce and interrupt transmission between vaccinated and nonvaccinated birds. A key component of any vaccination program is close monitoring of the "field" infection status in the vaccinated population.

There are a number of situations where vaccination is not recommended, including where there is a low risk of introduction of ND into an area or production sector. For example, broilers, being short-lived animals, are less likely to become infected, plus there are adverse impacts of vaccination on their performance. Trade may also be a factor in considering when to vaccinate, as well as the presence of other pathogens, the impact of which may be exacerbated through the use of ND vaccines. Furthermore, some hosts do not respond effectively to vaccination, such as turkeys and domestic waterfowl, so careful balancing of the benefits by sector is required. Adverse reactions in any species can occur under certain circumstances and are often associated with respiratory symptoms which may impact upon morbidity and mortality rates.

In summary, vaccination for ND has been shown over many years to be an important tool for disease prevention and control, while in some settings it is also invaluable in protecting food security.

References

Alexander, D.J. (2000). Newcastle disease and other avian paramyxoviruses. *OIE Rev. Sci. Tech.* 19 (2): 443–462.

Alexander, D. and Senne, D. (2008). Newcastle disease, other avian paramyxoviruses and pneumoviruses infection. In: *Diseases of Poultry*, 12e (eds. Y.M. Saif, A.M. Fadly, J.R. Glisson, et al.), 75–115. Ames: Blackwell Publishing Ltd.

Alexander, D.J., Manvell, R.J., Banks, J. et al. (1999). Experimental assessment of the pathogenicity of the Newcastle disease viruses from outbreaks in Great Britain in 1997 for chickens and turkeys, and the protection afforded by vaccination. *Avian Pathol.* 28 (5): 501–511.

Alexander, D.J., Bell, J.G., and Alders, R.G. (2004). A technology review: Newcastle disease, with special emphasis on its effect on village chickens. www.fao.org/3/y5162e/y5162e00.htm

Al-Garib, S.O., Gielkens, A.L., Gruys, D.E. et al. (2003). Immunoglobulin class distribution of systemic and mucosal antibody responses to Newcastle disease in chickens. *Avian Dis.* 47 (1): 32–40.

Allan, W.H., Lancaster, J.E., and Toth, B. (1978). *Newcastle Disease Vaccines*. Rome: FAO.

Ariaans, M.P., van de Haar, P.M., Lowenthal, J.W. et al. (2008). ELISPOT and intracellular cytokine staining: novel assays for quantifying T cell responses in the chicken. *Dev. Comp. Immunol.* 32 (11): 1398–1404.

Basavarajappa, M.K., Kumar, S., Khattar, S.K. et al. (2014). A recombinant Newcastle disease virus (NDV) expressing infectious laryngotracheitis virus (ILTV) surface glycoprotein D protects against highly virulent ILTV and NDV challenges in chickens. *Vaccine* 32 (28): 3555–3563.

Beard, C.W. and Brugh, M. (1975). Immunity to Newcastle disease. *Am. J. Vet. Res.* 136: 509–512.

Council Directive 92/66/EEC. (1992). Community measures for the control of Newcastle Disease. http://eur-lex.europa.eu/legal-content/en/TXT/?uri=CELEX%3A31992L0066

Crosby, A.D., d'Andrea, G.H., and Geller, R.J. (1986). Human effects of veterinary biological products. *Vet. Hum. Toxicol.* 28 (6): 552–553.

Dardiri, A.H. and Yates, V.J. (1962). Duration of immunity in layers after the use of live- or killed-virus Newcastle disease vaccine. *Am. J. Vet. Res.* 23: 330–337.

Dimitrov, K.M., Afonso, C.L., Yu, Q., and Miller, P.J. (2017). Newcastle disease vaccines. A solved problem or a continuous challenge? *Vet. Microbiol.* 206: 126–136.

Dimitrov, K.M., Abolnik, C.,Afonso, C.L. et al. (2019). Updated unified phylogenetic classification system and revised nomenclature for Newcastle disease virus. *Infection, Genetics and Evolution*, 74, p.103917.

Echeonwu, G.O.N. (2008). Survival of Newcastle disease virus (NDV) strain V4-UPM coated on three grain offal and exposed to room temperature. *Afr. J. Biotech.* 15: 2688–2692.

EUR-Lex. (1993). Access to European Union law. 93/152/EEC: Commission Decision of 8 February 1993 laying down the criteria for vaccines to be used against Newcastle disease in the context of routine vaccination programmes. https://eur-lex.europa.eu/legal-content/EN/TXT/?qid=1557326971591&uri=CELEX:31993D0152

European Pharmacopoeia. (2016). 9th edition. Strasbourg: European Directorate for the Quality of Medicines and Healthcare (EDQM).

Ganapathy, K., Todd, V., Cargill, P. et al. (2006). Interaction between a live avian pneumovirus vaccine and two different Newcastle disease virus vaccines in broiler chickens with maternal antibodies to Newcastle disease virus. *Avian Pathol.* 35 (6): 429–434.

Jayawardane, G.W. and Spradbrow, P.B. (1995). Mucosal immunity in chickens vaccinated with the V4 strain of Newcastle disease virus. *Vet. Microbiol.* 46 (1-3): 69–77.

Kapczynski, D.R. (2014). Detection of cell-mediated immune response to avian influenza viruses. *Methods Mol. Biol.* 1161: 199–215.

Kapczynski, D.R. and King, D.J. (2005). Protection of chickens against overt clinical disease and determination of viral shedding following vaccination with commercially available Newcastle disease virus vaccines upon challenge with highly virulent virus from the California 2002 exotic Newcastle disease outbreak. *Vaccine* 23 (26): 3424–3433.

Kapczynski, D.R., Martin, A., Haddad, E.E., and King, D.J. (2012). Protection from clinical disease against three highly virulent strains of Newcastle disease virus after in ovo application of an antibody-antigen complex vaccine in maternal antibody-positive chickens. *Avian Dis.* 56 (3): 555–560.

Kapczynski, D.R., Afonso, C.L., and Miller, P.J. (2013). Immune responses of poultry to Newcastle disease virus. *Dev. Comp. Immunol.* 41 (3): 447–453.

Kim, S.H., Paldurai, A., Xiao, S. et al. (2014). Modified Newcastle disease virus vectors expressing the H5 hemagglutinin induce enhanced protection against highly pathogenic H5N1 avian influenza virus in chickens. *Vaccine* 32 (35): 4428–4435.

Lambrecht, B., Gonze, M., Meulemans, G., and van Denberg, T.P. (2004). Assessment of the cell-mediated immune response in chickens by detection of chicken interferon-gamma in response to mitogen and recall Newcastle disease viral antigen stimulation. *Avian Pathol.* 33 (3): 343–350.

Li, L.-J., Li, M.-Y., Li, Y.-T. et al. (2012). Adjuvant activity of Sargassum pallidum polysaccharides against combined Newcastle disease, Infectious Bronchitis and avian influenza inactivated vaccines. *Mar. Drugs* 10 (12): 2648–2660.

Marangon, S. and Busani, L. (2007). The use of vaccination in poultry production. *Rev. Sci. Tech. - Off. Int. Epizoot.* 26 (1): 265–274.

Miller, P.J., King, D.J., Afonso, C.L., and Suarez, D.L. (2007). Antigenic differences among Newcastle disease virus strains of different genotypes used in vaccine formulation affect viral shedding after a virulent challenge. *Vaccine* 25 (41): 7238–7246.

Miller, P.J., Afonso, C.L., El Attrache, J. et al. (2013). Effects of Newcastle disease virus vaccine antibodies on the shedding and transmission of challenge viruses. *Dev. Comp. Immunol.* 41 (4): 505–513.

Oakeley, R.D. (2000). The limitations of a feed/water based heat-stable vaccine delivery system for Newcastle disease-control strategies for backyard poultry flocks in sub-Saharan Africa. *Preventative Vet. Med.* 47 (4): 271–279.

OIE. (2000). Report of a meeting of the OIE Standards Commission, November 2000. OIE, Paris. www.oie.int/doc/ged/D1281.PDF

OIE (2018). Chapter 3.3.14). Newcastle disease (infection with Newcastle disease virus). In: *Manual of Diagnostic Tests and Vaccines for Terrestrial Animals*. Paris: OIE www.oie.int/fileadmin/Home/eng/Health_standards/tahm/3.03.14_NEWCASTLE_DIS.pdf

Orsi, M.A., Doretto Junior, L., Reischak, D. et al. (2009). Newcastle disease virus vaccine strains: immunogenicity is not influenced by ICPI. *Braz. J. Poultr. Sci.* 11 (2): 129–133.

Palya, V., Tatár-Kis, T., Mató, T. et al. (2014). Onset and long-term duration of immunity provided by a single vaccination with a Turkey herpesvirus vector ND vaccine in commercial layers. *Vet. Immunol. I.mmunopathol* 158 (1-2): 105–115.

Park, M.S., Steel, J., García-Sastre, A. et al. (2006). Engineered viral vaccine constructs with dual specificity: avian influenza and Newcastle disease. *Proc. Natl. Acad. Sci.* 103 (21): 8203–8208.

Peeters, B.P., de Leeuw, O.S., Verstegen, I. et al. (2001). Generation of a recombinant chimeric Newcastle disease virus vaccine that allows serological differentiation between vaccinated and infected animals. *Vaccine* 19 (13): 1616–1627.

Plotkin, S.A. (2010). Correlates of protection induced by vaccination. *Clin. Vaccine Immunol.* 17 (7): 1055–1065.

Popovic, M., Balenovic, M., Kabalin, A. et al. (2010). Evaluation of CD45(+) cells kinetics in the blood of fattening chickens immunized with live or inactivated Newcastle disease vaccine. *Vet. Arhiv* 80 (1): 61–69.

Ramp, K., Topfstedt, E., Wäckerlin, R. et al. (2012). Pathogenicity and immunogenicity of different recombinant Newcastle disease virus clone 30 variants after in ovo vaccination. *Avian Dis.* 56 (1): 208–217.

Rauw, F., Gardin, Y., Palya, V. et al. (2009). Humoral, cell-mediated and mucosal immunity induced by oculo-nasal vaccination of one-day-old SPF and conventional layer chicks with two different live Newcastle disease vaccines. *Vaccine* 27 (27): 3631–3642.

Rauw, F., Gardin, Y., Palya, V. et al. (2010). Improved vaccination against Newcastle disease by an in ovo recombinant HVT-ND combined with an adjuvanted live vaccine at day-old. *Vaccine* 28 (3): 823–833.

Rauw, F., Gardin, Y., Palya, V. et al. (2014). The combination of attenuated Newcastle disease (ND) vaccine with rHVT-ND vaccine at 1 day old is more protective against ND virus challenge than when combined with inactivated ND vaccine. *Avian Pathol.* 43 (1): 26–36.

Reynolds, D.L. and Maraqa, A.D. (2000a). Protective immunity against Newcastle disease: the role of antibodies specific to Newcastle disease virus polypeptides. *Avian Dis.* 44 (1): 138–144.

Reynolds, D.L. and Maraqa, A.D. (2000b). Protective immunity against Newcastle disease: the role of cell-mediated immunity. *Avian Dis.* 44 (1): 145–154.

Roohani, K., Tan, S.W., Yeap, S.K. et al. (2015). Characterisation of genotype VII Newcastle disease virus (NDV) isolated from NDV vaccinated chickens, and the efficacy of LaSota and recombinant genotype VII vaccines against challenge with velogenic NDV. *J. Vet. Sci.* 16 (4): 447–457.

Roy, P., Koteeswaran, A., and Manickam, R. (1999). Comparative efficacy of two different inactivated oil emulsion Newcastle disease vaccines in chickens. *Cheiron* 28 (3): 71–74.

Russell, P.H., Dwivedi, P.N., and Davison, T.F. (1997). The effect of cyclosporin A and cyclophosphamide on the populations of B and T cells and virus in the Harderian gland of chickens vaccinated with the Hitchner B1 strain of Newcastle disease virus. *Vet. Immunol. Immunopathol* 60: 171–185.

Senne, D.A., King, D.J., and Kapczynski, D.R. (2004). Control of Newcastle disease by vaccination. *Dev. Biol. (Basel)* 119: 165–170.

Seo, S.H. and Collisson, E.W. (1997). Specific cytotoxic T lymphocytes are involved in in vivo clearance of infectious bronchitis virus. *J. Virol.* 71 (7): 5173–5177.

Smyth, J.A. (2013). Atadenovirus (egg drop syndrome and related infections). In: *Diseases of Poultry*, 13e (eds. D.E. Swayne, J.R. Glisson, L.R. McDougald, et al.), 301–309. Ames: Wiley Blackwell.

Stone, H., Mitchell, B., and Brugh, M. (1997). In ovo vaccination of chicken embryos with experimental Newcastle disease and avian influenza oil-emulsion vaccines. *Avian Dis.* 41 (4): 856–863.

Takada, A. and Kida, H. (1996). Protective immune response of chickens against Newcastle disease, induced by the intranasal vaccination with inactivated virus. *Vet. Microbiol.* 50: 17–25.

VICH. (2008). International Cooperation on Harmonisation of Technical Requirements for Registration of Veterinary Medicinal Products (VICH) GL44: guideline on target animal safety for veterinary live and inactivated vaccines. www.vichsec.org/guidelines/biologicals/bio-safety/target-animal-safety.html

Wambura, P.N., Kapaga, A.M., and Hyera, J.M.K. (2000). Experimental trials with a thermostable Newcastle disease virus (strain I 2) in commercial and village chickens in Tanzania. *Preventive Vet. Med.* 43 (2): 75–83.

Westbury, H.A., Parsons, G., and Allan, W.H. (1984). Duration of excretion of virulent Newcastle disease virus following challenge of chickens with different titres of serum antibody to the virus. *Aust. Vet. J.* 61 (2): 44–46.

26

Porcine Reproductive and Respiratory Syndrome

Antonio Garmendia[1], Waithaka Mwangi[2], and Gourapura Renukaradhya[3]

[1] Department of Pathobiology and Veterinary Science, University of Connecticut, Storrs, Connecticut, USA
[2] Department of Diagnostic Medicine/Pathobiology (DMP), College of Veterinary Medicine, Kansas State University, Manhattan, Kansas, USA
[3] Food Animal Health Research Program, OARDC, Veterinary Preventive Medicine, The Ohio State University, Wooster, Ohio, USA

26.1 Introduction

Porcine reproductive and respiratory syndrome (PRRS) is one of the most important infectious diseases of swine worldwide (Wensvoort et al. 1991; Murakami et al. 1994; Done et al. 1996; Beltran-Alcrudo et al. 2007). Only a few countries (Argentina, Australia, Brazil, Cuba, Finland, New Zealand, Norway, Sweden, and Switzerland) have been reported to be free of PRRS (Beltran-Alcrudo et al. 2007; Zimmerman et al. 2015). Losses caused by PRRS are primarily due to reproductive failure in sows and gilts and respiratory disease in suckling and growing pigs (Done et al. 1996; Neumann et al. 2005; Holtkamp et al. 2013). There is a substantial negative economic impact, especially to nursery and finisher herds, from PRRS virus (PRRSV) infection (Neumann et al. 2005). There are also significant economic losses in breeding herds due to significant decrease in weaned pigs (Linhares et al. 2014).

The etiological agent, PRRSV, is a single-stranded, positive-sense, enveloped, RNA virus. The virion is approximately 62 nm in diameter, and is a member of the family *Arteriviridae*, in the order Nidovirales (Benfield et al. 1992; Meulenberg et al. 1993). The RNA genome, approximately 15 kb in length, is capped at the 5′ end and polyadenylated at the 3′ end, and contains nine open reading frames (ORFs) flanked by untranslated regions at each end (Meulenberg et al. 1993; Meng et al. 1994; Meng 2000). ORFs 1a and 1b code for nonstructural proteins (NSP), involved in replication and pathogenesis, ORFs 2–7 code for virion-associated structural proteins (Meulenberg et al. 1993).

Two PRRSV genotypes are recognized: (i) the European genotype (genotype 1, PRRSV-1) which contains Lelystad virus (LV) (the prototype strain) and at least four subtypes (Stadejek et al. 2008), and (ii) the American genotype (genotype 2, PRRSV-2) with VR2332 as the prototype virus, with at least nine lineages (reviewed by Shi et al. 2010). Genetic or antigenic relatedness between isolates can be demonstrated by molecular (Mardassi et al. 1994) or serological techniques (Nelson et al. 1993), respectively. Nucleotide identity in ORFs 2–5 between genotypes ranges from 61% to 66%, whereas ORFs 6 and 7 are relatively conserved among genotypes (reviewed by Meng 2000). Nucleotide sequence identities of ORF1a and ORF1b between genotypes are about 55% and 63%, respectively. The greatest divergence between genotypes is found in the ORF1a-encoded nsp2, which share about 32% amino acid identity.

A high rate of continuous genetic mutation and potential recombination events results in emergence of multiple viral strains (Forsberg et al. 2002; Wang et al. 2019), which show marked variation in clinical presentation, severity of disease, degree of cross-protection, and vaccine efficacy. PRRSV recombination events could not be reproduced experimentally in pigs (Murtaugh et al. 2002a). The variability in disease severity depends on the age of the animal, physiological status (Hirose et al. 1995; Halbur et al. 1996), and virus strain (Park et al. 1996; Thacker 2003). Severe "atypical PRRS" outbreaks with meningoencephalitis in neonatal pigs have been reported in the USA (Halbur 1997). The virulence of the "atypical" strains has been experimentally assessed (Mengeling et al. 1998). Highly pathogenic PRRSVs causing devastating disease in swine have been reported in China (Li et al. 2007; Tian et al. 2007) and recently in the USA (Wang et al. 2015).

Veterinary Vaccines: Principles and Applications, First Edition. Edited by Samia Metwally, Gerrit Viljoen, and Ahmed El Idrissi.

26.2 Types of Vaccines

There are vaccines against both genotypes that are modified live virus (MLV) or killed virus (KV) (Table 26.1) (Murtaugh and Genzow 2011; Renukaradhya et al. 2015a, 2015b). MLV vaccines are generally more efficacious than KV vaccines (Mengeling 2005). The downside of MLV vaccines is their potential to revert to virulence (Mengeling 2005) and infect susceptible animals. Recently, attenuation of wild-type strains by codon deoptimization or by molecular breeding of envelope genes from divergent viruses was reported (Ni et al. 2013, 2014). The codon deoptimized virus was shown to be stable for up to 10 serial passages in porcine alveolar macrophages and in experimentally infected pigs.

Killed virus vaccines are obtained after physical and or chemical inactivation of the virus (Vanhee et al. 2009), and generally require multiple immunizations and potent adju-

Table 26.1 List of manufacturers of vaccines for PRRS.

Manufacturer	Vaccines Vaccine type[a]/genotype[b]/strain	Country
Aptimmune Biologics Mucosal Vaccine United States	Barricade PRRS	USA
Bestar Laboratories Ltd.	MLV(2)/KV	Singapore
Bioveta	KV/G1+G2	Czech Republic
Boehringer Ingelheim Vetmedica, Inc.	MLV/G2KV/G1	International
CAVAC (ChoongAng Vaccine Laboratories Co., Ltd.)	KV	Korea
Chengdu TECBOND Biological Products Co., Ltd.	MLV/G2/CH-1R	China
Dyntec	KV/VDE1-VDE2-VDA1	Czech Republic
	KV/VDE1-VDE2-VDA1	Russia
	KV/VDE1-VDE2	Czech/Portugal
ELANCO PREVACENT PRRS	MLV/G2/lineage 1	USA
FGBI – Federal Centre for Animal Health	KV/VI94+KPR96	Belarus
	KV/VI94+KPR97	Kazakhstan, Russia
Harbin Veterinary Research Institute	MLV/G2/HuN4-F112 KV/G2/Ch-1a	China
Hipra	MLV/G1-KV/G1	Russia, Spain, Philippines, Greece, Poland
Merial España[c]	KV	Spain
Merial Norden A/S	KV	Denmark, Finland, Norway, Sweden
Merial Russia	KV/G1/P120	Russia
Merial UK	KV/G1/P120	UK
MSD Animal Health (Merck)	MLV/G1/DV	International W. Europe
Philippines Bureau of Animal Industry	MLV/G1/VP-046	Philippines
Qilu Animal Health Products Factory	KV/G1/NVDC-JXA1	China
Ringpu (Tianjin) Bio-Pharmacy Co., Ltd.	KV/G1/NVDV-JXA1(1)	China
SYVA Laboratorios	MLV/G1/All-183	Spain
Tiankang Biopharmacuetical	MLV	China
Zoetis Animal Health	US MLV/G2	USA
Zoetis Canada	MLV/G2	Canada
Zoetis China	MLV/G2/TJM-F92	China
Zoetis Spain	KV/G1/Strain 218	Spain

This list of vaccines does not represent any authentication of the quality or efficacy of the products.
[a] Vaccine type – MLV, modified live virus vaccines; KV, killed virus vaccines.
[b] Genotype G1 or G2 – genotype 1 or 2 respectively; strain indicated when available; number in parenthesis indicates number of vaccines available.
[c] Merial has merged with Boehringer Ingelheim.
Source: Adapted from Murtaugh and Genzow (2011) and Papatsiros (2012).

vants to induce immune responses. Virus inactivation by ultraviolet light, binary ethyleneimine, or γ-radiation (Delrue et al. 2009) affects the viral genome rather than proteins, and preserves macrophage entry-associated protein domains. These virus inactivation methods and some adjuvants improved the levels of protective virus-neutralizing antibody response induced by a KV vaccine (Vanhee et al. 2009). Repeated vaccination of PRRSV-free pigs with MLV or KV vaccines, or priming with MLV vaccines followed by boosting with KV vaccines, induced both virus-neutralizing antibodies and cellular immunity (Diaz et al. 2013). The use of KV vaccines in PRRS-positive herds was regarded as a "therapeutic" vaccination (Nilubol et al. 2004).

Viral strains isolated from field outbreaks have been used as seed to generate KV autogenous vaccines for application at the point of origin, and research suggests that they are effective in boosting protection (Geldhof et al. 2013; Larcher et al. 2019). The use of antigenic grouping technology (MJPRRS-Phibro) for autogenous vaccines takes into consideration physical and immunological features of the virus to provide a broader range of immune presentations for local circulating strains. However, autogenous vaccines may not be uniformly efficient (Klopfenstein et al. 2012).

Experimental vaccines include those employing live virus vectors such as adenovirus, pseudorabies virus, transmissible gastroenteritis virus, fowl pox virus, etc., to deliver defined protective PRRSV antigens (Dee et al. 1996; Kim and Yoon 2008; Diaz et al. 2009; Li et al. 2009; Cruz et al. 2010; Zhou et al. 2010; Hu and Zhang 2014; Renukaradhya et al. 2015a). Delivery of recombinant virus antigens that are expressed in baculovirus, transgenic plants, or via DNA vaccines is also under investigation (Renukaradhya et al. 2015b; Cui et al. 2019; Oh et al. 2019; Cho et al. 2020). Reverse genetics technology has opened up many possibilities for the development of new-generation vaccines, such as gene-deleted vaccines, chimeric vaccines, dendritic cell-targeting vaccines, T-regulatory cell-suppressing vaccines, etc. (reviewed by Huang and Meng 2010). There is active research into next-generation PRRS vaccines with expanded breadth and depth (Vu et al. 2015; Cao et al. 2018; Sun et al. 2018; Cui et al. 2019).

Mucosal vaccination aimed at inducing immunity at the natural site of infection is an interesting alternative (Han et al. 2011; Hu et al. 2012). However, mucosal vaccines require potent adjuvants and antigen delivery systems to stimulate strong responses (Renukaradhya et al. 2012) and achieve cross-protection. A nanotechnology-based vaccine delivery system for mucosal delivery of killed PRRSV to achieve increased breadth of cross-protection and safety was found to be promising (Binjawadagi et al. 2014a,b; Renukaradhya et al. 2015b).

The major barrier to the control of PRRS is the extensive genetic and antigenic heterogeneity among PRRSV isolates (Katz et al. 1995; Park et al. 2014; Balka et al. 2018; Cortey et al. 2018). Currently available vaccines induce protection from clinical disease, but do not prevent infection or reinfection and provide no or variable cross-protection (Cano et al. 2007b; Diaz et al. 2012; Mateu 2013; Park et al. 2014; Choi et al. 2016; Renson et al. 2017; Jeong et al. 2018a, 2018b; Yang et al. 2020), and generally induce poor or no anamnestic response (Murtaugh and Genzow 2011; Charerntantanakul 2012; Lyoo 2015). Recently, it was reported that previously infected adult animals had significant levels of cross-neutralizing antibodies in serum (Robinson et al. 2015), which has renewed interest in elucidating mechanisms of induction of such antibodies.

Vaccination provokes reduction in the magnitude and duration of viremia, reduces clinical signs, improves production, and reduces viral shedding and transmission (Cano et al. 2007a,b; Mateu 2013; Linhares et al. 2014, 2015; Chase-Topping et al. 2020; Madapong et al. 2020). Vaccines mitigate negative effects of infection but have limitations. The narrow range of protection remains a major concern. However, it is technically possible to attain a broader range of protection using bioengineering and bioinformatics tools (Dwivedi et al. 2011; Roca et al. 2012; Vu et al. 2015; Cui et al. 2020). Several approaches are under investigation for PRRSV and other similarly variable viruses, including molecular breeding through DNA shuffling, consensus sequence vaccines, mosaic virus vaccines, etc. (Tong et al. 2006; Fischer et al. 2007; Thurmond et al. 2008; Barouch et al. 2010; Zhou et al. 2013; Hu and Zhang 2014; Renukaradhya et al. 2015b; Vu et al. 2015; Cui et al. 2016; Tian et al. 2017; Cui et al. 2019, 2020). It is important to keep in mind that while vaccination against PRRSV has beneficial effects, the control of PRRS also requires sound management practices and biosecurity.

26.3 Immune Response and Duration of Immunity

Natural infection and vaccination induce specific antibody and cellular immune responses (Nelson et al. 1994; Murtaugh et al. 2002b; Batista et al. 2004; Charerntantanakul et al. 2006). However, key mechanisms for complete protection are not fully understood (Pol and Steverink 2000; Xiao et al. 2004; Murtaugh and Genzow 2011; reviewed by Loving et al. 2015). During natural infection or live virus vaccination, virus-neutralizing antibody responses are delayed, while there is a relatively strong early nonneutralizing antibody response. Cellular responses, such as virus-specific lymphocyte proliferation and interferon (IFN)-γ secretion, are detectable 2–4 weeks after vaccination and are relatively weak. Delayed adaptive responses to PRRSV are attributed to a dampened type I IFN response (Albina et al. 1998; Dwivedi et al. 2012), and enhanced production of antiinflammatory cytokine IL-10 (reviewed by Thanawongnuwech and Suradhat 2010). In *in vitro* studies, the virus was also shown to downregulate the expression of co-stimulatory molecules CD80/86 and major histocompatibility complex (MHC) class II on antigen-presenting cells and increase secretion of IL-10 by mature dendritic cells, which result in impaired adaptive responses (Flores-Mendoza et al. 2008).

The infection with PRRSV is complex, partly because the virus modulates the host response to gain replication advantage (Mateu and Diaz 2008; Kimman et al. 2009; Darwich et al. 2010; Loving et al. 2015). The weak and delayed adaptive responses (Vezina et al. 1996; Plagemann 2006; Darwich et al. 2010; reviewed by Loving et al. 2015) result in chronic, persistent infection in lymphoid tissues for up to 200 days (Albina et al. 1994; Bilodeau et al. 1994; Christopher-Hennings et al. 1995; Chung et al. 1997; Batista et al. 2004; Xiao et al. 2004; Renukaradhya et al. 2012; Zimmerman et al. 2015). Viral proteins critical to protection or virulence have been identified (Pol and Steverink 2000; Kimman et al. 2009). Epitopes that invoke virus-neutralizing and nonneutralizing antibodies have been identified in viral proteins coded by ORFs 3–7 and in NSP2 (Meulenberg et al. 1997; Plana-Duran et al. 1997; Gonin et al. 1999; Yang et al. 2000; Plagemann et al. 2002; Plagemann 2004; Kim and Yoon 2008; Costers et al. 2010; reviewed by Loving et al. 2015). GP5 is a major envelope glycoprotein which has both virus-neutralizing, and nonneutralizing decoy epitopes (Plagemann et al. 2002; Ostrowski et al. 2002; Plagemann 2004). Glycan shielding of neutralizing epitopes on GP5 and GP3 has been recognized as a potential mechanism of immune evasion by PRRSV (reviewed by Loving et al. 2015). GP5 was also shown to have apoptogenic properties (Suarez et al. 1996). T cell epitopes have been identified in ORFs 2–7 (Bautista et al. 1999; Vashisht et al. 2008; Diaz et al. 2009).

Interferon-γ expression or lymphocyte proliferation responses induced by virus recall stimulation of peripheral blood lymphocytes are markers of cellular immunity activation (Vezina et al. 1996; Bautista and Molitor 1997; Zuckermann et al. 1998, 2007; Meier et al. 2003; Royaee et al. 2004; Rompato et al. 2006; Gómez-Laguna et al. 2009; Ferrari et al. 2013). However, these *ex vivo* tests have to be interpreted cautiously as the expression of IFN-γ and other cytokines, and the participation of different T cell subsets in the response is variable (Xiao et al. 2004; Gómez-Laguna et al. 2009; Costers et al. 2009).

Passive transfer of immunoglobulins to pregnant sows protected both dam and offspring from infection and disease (Osorio et al. 2002). However, in natural infections, virus and antibodies can co-exist in infected pigs, reflecting the complexity of PRRSV immunobiology (Bilodeau et al. 1994; Kimman et al. 2009).

26.4 Desired Specifications When Ordering a Vaccine

Vaccines that are safe, cross-protective, consistent, confer long duration of immunity (DOI), and do not evade or suppress the host immune response are highly desirable to control the global menace of PRRS. Current commercial vaccines do not induce sterilizing immunity, but generally reduce the effects of infection, such as reducing preweaning mortality, improving health and daily body weight gain, and reducing virus shedding as well as vertical and horizontal transmission of PRRSV (Dee et al. 1996; Mateu 2013; Amadori and Razzuoli 2014; Pileri et al. 2015; Renukaradhya et al. 2015a; Chase-Topping et al. 2020). The specifications pig farmers need when ordering PRRSV vaccines are the following: information about the use, safety, and efficacy against the respiratory or the reproductive form of the disease, cross-protection attributes, ideal age of vaccination, route of administration, vaccination schedule, number of boosters required, and shelf-life.

The main considerations when implementing and scheduling vaccinations are the PRRS status of the herd and the intended goal. Therefore, there are different potential vaccination/control scenarios (Jeong et al. 2014). There are commercially available MLV and KV vaccines for both genotypes 1 and 2 PRRSV and one KV vaccine that contains both genotypes (Table 26.1). These generally induce protection against cognate strains, but protection needs to be assessed on a case-by-case basis. MLV vaccines are generally preferred for priming, while boosting can be done with either MLV or KV vaccines. As a general criterion, vaccines for use in PRRS-positive herds should match the virus circulating in the area as much as possible and the disease should be monitored closely.

Generally, PRRSV MLVs are given intramuscularly (IM) in the neck musculature caudal to the ear lobe in 2 mL doses that may contain approximately $10^{3.5}$ to $10^{6.3}$ tissue culture infectious doses 50 ($TCID_{50}$), and $10^{3.8}$ to $10^{6.3}$ $TCID_{50}$ of PRRSV prior to inactivation in KV vaccines (Papatsiros 2012). There are two commercially available genotype 1 vaccines licensed for use by either IM or intradermal (ID) injection. The latter can be given with needleless devices in 0.2 mL volumes, requiring less restraint and handling than the former and with apparently equally good results. Keep in mind that some vaccines are labeled as safe for use during pregnancy while others are not. Vaccines should preferably be given to gilts and sows a few weeks prior to breeding. As a precaution, epinephrine should be at hand in case of allergic reactions during vaccination.

26.5 Quality Assurance and Control Testing

26.5.1 Vaccine Safety

Basic vaccine safety checks should include testing for sterility, purity, and freedom from infectious agents, including fungi, bacteria, and viruses. Vaccine master seed virus (MSV) must be free from transmissible gastroenteritis virus, porcine respiratory coronavirus, porcine epidemic diarrhea virus, porcine adenovirus, porcine circovirus 1 and 2, porcine hemagglutinating encephalitis virus, porcine parvovirus, reovirus, and rabies (OIE 2018). The MSV and the fetal bovine serum used in culture should be free of bovine viral diarrhea virus (BVDV). The MSV should be identified and its origin and passage history should be recorded. The shelf half-life of the virus should be determined experimentally.

Three major concerns with MLV vaccines are shedding of vaccine virus, risk of infection and disease in susceptible animals, and potential for reversion to virulence (Botner et al. 1997; Madsen et al. 1998; Mengeling et al. 1999a; Nielsen et al. 2001, 2002; Martínez-Lobo et al. 2013; Xia et al. 2015).

The clinical safety of MLV vaccines can be ascertained in young pigs (Pol and Steverink 2000; Xia et al. 2015) and infection of alveolar macrophages can be used as an indicator of the potential for vaccine virus transmission (Martínez-Lobo et al. 2013). Vaccinated animals and controls are observed for clinical signs and lesion development. Vaccine safety is also tested in pregnant sows during the third trimester of gestation (Pol and Steverink 2000) in which reproductive performance, including length of gestation, occurrence of abortions, stillbirths, mummified fetuses, number of healthy piglets born, etc., is evaluated. The vaccines are regarded as clinically safe if they do not cause clinical signs, although mild lung lesions may be expected upon vaccination (Martínez-Lobo et al. 2013). Vaccination of piglets with an attenuated form of the highly pathogenic PRRSV recovered in China resulted in protection with minimal adverse effects, except for mild lung lesions observed in some animals which received the lowest dose of the vaccine (Yu et al. 2015).

To test for possible reversion to virulence, successive serial passages of the vaccine virus in naïve weaned piglets and pregnant animals is done (Xia et al. 2015; OIE 2018). In these tests, virus vaccine recovered from blood or tissues is successively passaged 5–10 times (depending on the country) in naïve animals. The final virus recovered is sequenced (ORF5) and compared with the MSV to search for any changes in sequence that could reflect reversion to virulent virus. Vaccine shedding should also be tested by co-mingling vaccinated animals with PRRSV-naïve sentinel animals, including lactating sows and piglets. The sentinel pigs can be monitored for viremia, seroconversion, and lesion development and any virus detected can be evaluated by sequencing.

Vaccine virus persistence and mutation into virulent forms have been demonstrated experimentally (Mengeling et al. 1999a) and represent a serious risk. Replication/shedding of vaccine virus may produce short-term impact on fertility, transplacental infection of the fetus, shedding in semen, and transmission to sows and gilts (Botner et al. 1997; Nielsen et al. 2002). In a recent study, experimental vaccination of seronegative pregnant gilts with a MLV vaccine during peak fetal susceptibility did not result in abortion, but did result in a higher preweaning mortality and lower average daily weight gain of the litters (Schelkopf et al. 2014). The frequency and severity of adverse reactions to vaccination, including lung lesions, inflammatory reactions at injection sites, and prolonged systemic reactions, should be recorded. There is a remote chance of anaphylactic reactions to vaccines.

26.5.2 Vaccine Efficacy/Vaccine Test Trial Results

To be effective, vaccines should have an antigenic composition that reflects the predominant circulating strains. The protective efficacy of the vaccine and DOI should be ascertained by the manufacturers by vaccine challenge trials (Pol and Steverink 2000; Yu et al. 2015). Vaccines should stimulate adaptive immunity against circulating field strains and should not cause immunosuppression. Ideally, vaccines should also prevent infection and virus transmission, including transplacental transmission (reviewed by Amadori and Razzuoli 2014). Vaccines should show evidence of measurably reducing the basic reproduction number (Rose and Andraud 2017).

Two test systems are available. First, the respiratory model, wherein 3-week-old piglets are vaccinated with the highest passage of MLV vaccine and challenged 2–16 weeks later, intranasally. Second, the reproductive model wherein sows are vaccinated with the MLV vaccine and challenged with a virus intranasally at approximately 85 days of gestation and followed by evaluation of reproductive performance. In both models, challenge is with homologous virus. Protection is ascertained by evaluating clinical disease, virus load in serum and tissues, pulmonary lesion scores, average daily body weight gain, weight at market, reproductive performance, number of successful live births, number of weaned piglets, etc., compared with age-matched, sex-matched, nonvaccinated control animals receiving the same challenge virus. Determination of the degree of protection should be based on the preceding IFN-γ and neutralizing antibody responses which are also the markers of immunity (Diaz et al. 2006; Zuckermann et al. 2007).

26.6 Vaccine Application for Disease Control

In order to adopt vaccination as a control measure for PRRS, the herd has to first be extensively tested to determine the infection status (Dee 2003; Thanawongnuwech and Suradhat 2010; Holtkamp et al. 2011; Lowe et al. 2012).

Enzyme-linked immunosorbent assay (ELISA) is recommended to test for antibodies, whereas real-time polymerase chain reaction (RT-PCR) and sequencing is recommended for virus detection and characterization. Testing should be implemented on weaned pigs, nursery piglets, finisher, and breeding herds using serum or oral fluids collected following recommended guidelines (Holtkamp et al. 2011; Lowe et al. 2012; Cano 2013; Linhares et al. 2014). In North America, the tests used to classify PRRS status are interpreted using definitions approved by the American Association of Swine Veterinarians (AASV) Board of Directors in 2010 and a team of researchers at the United States Department of Agriculture-funded PRRS-Coordinated Agricultural Project. The herd PRRS status classification that follows may serve as a general guide which can be adapted and modified as needed for use in different countries or regions. This classification (summarized in Table 26.2) is based on detection of specific antibodies (indicates exposure to virus) and/or detection of virus (indicates active shedding and transmission of virus), and "pig" refers to growing pigs (Holtkamp et al. 2011). Control guidelines are available from the AASV and similar professional associations throughout the world.

Table 26.2 Categorization of PRRSV infection status in swine herds.[a]

Category test results
I Positive unstable [(SowAb+[b]/PigAb+)/(SowVirus+[c]/PigVirus+)]
II-A Positive short-term stable [(SowAb+/PigAb+)/(SowVirus−/PigVirus+)]
II-B Positive stable eliminating [(SowAb+/PigAb+)/(SowVirus−/PigVirus−)]
II-C Long-term stable [(SowAb+/PigAb+/GiltAb+)/(SowVirus+/PigVirus−/GiltVirus−)]
III Provisionally negative [(SowAb+/−/PigAb+/−/GiltAb−)/(SowVirus−PigVirus−/GiltVirus−)]
IV Negative [(SowAb−/PigAb−/GiltAb−)/(SowVirus−/PigVirus−/GiltVirus−)]

[a] Adapted from Holtkamp et al. (2011).
[b] Test positive for antibody to PRRSV (ELISA).
[c] Test positive for PRRSV (RT-PCR).

There is no single strategy that can be applied to control PRRS in all herds. Vaccination recommendations are based on herd PRRS status, manner in which the virus is spreading, type of production systems, and goals. Once the PRRS status of a herd is defined, measures to control the disease, including herd flow management, replacement management, and vaccination, should be implemented in consultation with a veterinarian. Strict biosecurity and air filtration methods are crucial to achieve control for PRRS.

To bring an infected herd back to a stable status (i.e. reproductive and productive performance is brought to optimal levels and vertical transmission is stopped), a combination of control methods must be applied. These will depend on the distribution of infection and patterns of transmission in the herd, herd density, transmission potential (R), risk of herd reinfection, etc. One approach consists of obtaining all the animal replacements at one time point, and temporarily closing the herd for an extended period (at least 30 weeks), followed by exposing the breeding stock to the circulating virus or by vaccination and assessing herd status continuously. This approach is also known as load, close, and homogenize (LCH) or herd closure. Other management practices include whole herd depopulation and repopulation, test and removal, movement of pigs all-in all-out by room in farrowing and nursery, along with mass vaccination at multiple times in a year (Dee et al. 1996; McCaw 2000; Torremorell et al. 2002, 2003; Opriessnig et al. 2007; Rowland and Morrison 2012; Cano 2013; Linhares et al. 2014; Jeong et al. 2014; Zimmerman et al. 2015; Rose and Andraud 2017).

In herds where there is vertical transmission, as evidenced by viremic piglets soon after birth, vaccination and boosting of the breeding herd until the vertical transmission is controlled as shown by RT-PCR testing is indicated (Dee et al. 1996; Cano 2013). A good indicator of stabilization is to achieve PRRSV-negative piglets and bring the herd back to baseline production at the shortest possible time period (Linhares et al. 2014).

The decision to vaccinate young pigs has to be carefully considered, especially in unstable herds, as it may not evoke protective immune responses or may yield variable results due to immune immaturity, presence of maternal antibodies, or presence of virus. In a recent report, experimental vaccination of piglets at 2 and 3 weeks of age, in the presence of maternal immunity, protected them against challenge (Kraft et al. 2019). Growing pigs in stable herds may be vaccinated if infection with PRRSV does not usually occur until 6–7 weeks of age (Mateu 2013). Vaccination can be given to growing pigs in provisionally negative herds, depending on the risk of exposure to virus of these animals. When vaccination is adopted, wild-type virus shedding, and vertical and horizontal transmission should be eventually reduced, leading to herd stabilization. Vaccination may be discontinued depending on how the herd PRRS status evolves over time. MLV mass vaccination can eliminate naïve susceptible animals and thus homogenize the immune status of a herd (Guillespie 2003; Cano et al. 2007a), and can potentially help in eliminating PRRSV infection when administered in conjunction with controlled pig flow (Dee and Philips 1998).

Repeated vaccination of sows and young pigs with KV vaccine in herds having outbreaks resulted in improvements in overall health and production (Thacker et al. 2003). In swine herds where the prevalence is decreased to less than 10% and piglets are PRRSV negative, it is recommended to eliminate virus-positive sows, introduce only PRRSV-negative gilts and boars, and reinforce biosecurity to eventually achieve a PRRSV-negative status.

When introducing PRRSV-negative replacement animals into positive herds, acclimatization by vaccination or exposure to the PRRSV that is circulating in the farm is given while in quarantine, in order to bring the immunity of the introduced animals up before they are placed with the breeding herd (Opriessnig et al. 2007; Linhares et al. 2014; Zimmerman et al. 2015). Vaccination is preferred over direct exposure to the field virus, since the latter may introduce other pathogens to the replacement gilts. If vaccination is chosen for newly introduced gilts, boosting after 4 weeks is recommended. The frequency of introduction of new stock should be quarterly, or semiannually, with a period of acclimatization of at least 60 days before their transfer into the sow herd. These guidelines should also be followed when introducing boars to PRRSV-positive herds.

26.7 Consideration of Epidemiological Factors and Control Objectives

Porcine reproductive and respiratory syndrome virus is transmitted both vertically and horizontally. The virus is viable for only short periods in nonliving matter, and while it becomes rapidly inactivated at 25–27 °C, it may survive for a few days in well or city water. The virus is inactivated by chloroform, ether, quaternary ammonium, sodium hypochlorite, or iodine compounds. However, the ability of the virus to persist in the host together with prolonged virus shedding perpetuates transmission and disease (Christopher-Hennings et al. 1995; Chung et al. 1997; Wills et al. 1997; Rowland and Morrison 2012).

Estimation of exact prevalence is confounded by use of current vaccines, which all lack differentiating between infected and vaccinated animals (DIVA) features (Zimmerman et al. 2015). The prevalence of PRRSV infection in most swine-producing countries may be conservatively estimated at over 50%. Infected animals shed the virus from multiple sites and for prolonged periods, possibly for well over 150 days after infection. Virus or viral RNA can be recovered from tonsils of infected pigs for up to 200 days, an important source of persistent virus beyond 6 months within a herd. There are no good ways to identify animals shedding virus, especially since viremia or serum antibody may be absent in carrier animals.

It is very important to realize that the virus is shed in semen even in the absence of viremia or serum antibodies. The virus is transmitted through direct contact or by fomites (Thacker et al. 2003). Airborne transmission is possible, especially between PRRSV-positive farms less than 9 km apart (Dee et al. 2012). The use of air filtration should be considered based on the overall regional PRRS status, distances between farms, and temperature, humidity, and wind velocity patterns in the area (Dee et al. 2012, 2009). It is also important to know the PRRS status of the source farm(s) for breeding replacements and semen for artificial insemination.

While vaccination is feasible and readily accessible and can be implemented quite quickly with positive returns, it should never be used as a stand-alone method of control. For regional control of PRRS, sequence information of local circulating viruses is important. Sequencing can be used to monitor virus circulation patterns and, most importantly, to identify newly emerging strains.

26.8 Combination Vaccines for PRRSV and Other Diseases

Porcine reproductive and respiratory syndrome virus infection may predispose pigs to secondary microbial infections such as *Streptococcus suis*, *Salmonella cholerasuis*, *Actinobacillus pleuropneumoniae*, *Mycoplasma hyopneumoniae*, *Pasteurella multocida*, *Bordetella bronchiseptica*, etc. (Halbur 2003). Co-infection of PRRSV and *S. suis* may be particularly difficult to control. Generally, dual vaccination with PRRSV vaccine and *S. suis* bacterin is necessary to control such infections; control may be further enhanced by judicious use of antibiotics. However, caution should be exercised when using MLV PRRS vaccines in herds where *S. suis*-associated disease is endemic as this may exacerbate the latter (Thanawongnuwech et al. 2000).

The use of multivalent vaccines to prevent or mitigate complex diseases such as the porcine respiratory disease complex (PRDC) (Opriessnig et al. 2011) is logistically attractive. In PRDC, viruses and bacteria such as PRRSV, PCV2, *M. hyopneumoniae* and *P. multocida* play an important role. Vaccines containing live attenuated PRRSV and killed PCV2 and *M. hyopneumoniae*, or live attenuated PRRSV in combination with parvovirus and *Leptospira* are commercially available. Such combination vaccines can eliminate the need to administer multiple injections.

26.9 Use of Vaccine in the Face of an Outbreak

The goal when facing an outbreak is to bring the herd to pre-outbreak production levels, achieve a PRRS-free stable status as soon as possible, and prevent transmission between herds. Curtailing vertical transmission by vaccination of sows and flow management is key to control and will help generate PRRSV-negative piglets. During an outbreak, vaccination might bring the herd back to pre-outbreak production levels relatively quickly, and it will significantly reduce weaned pig losses and wild-type virus shedding, and control respiratory disease in grow-to-finish pigs. Booster vaccinations are given either once or twice. Additional boosters reduced the duration of virus shedding, but had no effect on virus loads in tissues or the number of persistently infected animals (Cano et al. 2007b). Animals challenged with a highly pathogenic heterologous strain 3 months after their initial infection and vaccination had reduced clinical severity but still became infected.

While matching a vaccine with the circulating field strain would be ideal in the face of an outbreak, this may not always be possible. Emergency administration of a genotype-matched MLV vaccine at the time of exposure of pigs to PRRSV has been reported as beneficial in alleviating the effects of highly pathogenic virus (reviewed by Amadori and Razzuoli 2014; Renson et al. 2017).

26.9.1 When is Vaccination Not Recommended?

Vaccination is not recommended for PRRS-free herds or positive herds that have moved into Category IV (PRRS negative) or sows in Category III (provisionally negative herds). As a general rule, animals showing clinical signs, such as cough, fever, etc., should not be vaccinated. The decision to vaccinate pregnant animals with MLV vaccines must be carefully considered because there are serious concerns regarding administration of MLV vaccines to pregnant animals, especially during late gestation (Dee et al. 1996; Dewey et al. 1999). Strict adherence to vaccine label instructions and consultation with a veterinarian are recommended. Vaccines should preferably be administered to gilts or sows before breeding (Mengeling et al. 1999b). Where vaccination is not practiced, farms must maintain strict biosecurity measures and adequate herd flow management and only PRRSV-negative animals should be used for replacement. Semen for artificial insemination should be PRRSV negative.

26.10 Monitoring and Vaccine Effectiveness

26.10.1 Postvaccination Monitoring

Monitoring vaccination efficacy involves testing the breeding and growing herds for antibody in sera or oral fluids by ELISA, and more importantly for wild-type virus infection and shedding by RT-PCR analysis (Lowe et al. 2012). Herd productivity and reproductive performance can be measured as described above to confirm vaccine efficacy. Thus, duration of gestation, return to estrus, number of viable piglets, preweaning mortality, average body weight gain, and market body weight are good indicators of general herd health and reflect successful effects of controlling viral infections. Vaccination should reduce infection and shedding and transmission of virus, improve health, reduce preweaning mortality, and increase average daily weight gain and market weight.

26.10.2 Outbreaks in Vaccinated Animals

Vaccines may protect pigs from clinical disease but not from infection. Reversion of MLV vaccines to virulence has been documented to cause disease outbreaks (Botner et al. 1997; Madsen et al. 1998; Nielsen et al. 2001). In general, vaccination against PRRSV does not cross-protect nor does it induce a robust anamnestic response, thus allowing infection by variant field viruses and reinfection resulting in virus shedding and transmission. Typically, at any given time, there is a proportion of animals that are naïve to PRRSV and therefore susceptible to infection and to clinical disease. Outbreaks are usually associated with the introduction of a new strain and inadequate acclimatization of newly introduced replacement stocks, and this needs prompt attention. Herd closure along with vaccination may be indicated until the sow herd becomes stable again (Dee et al. 1996; Dee 2003). Autogenous KV vaccines may have value under these circumstances. However, this needs to be coupled with strict biosecurity and proper animal flow management.

26.11 Vaccine Adverse Reactions

When using MLV vaccines, major concerns are that the vaccine virus can potentially cause disease in pregnant sows and piglets, due to residual pathogenicity, shedding of vaccine virus, and possible reversion to virulence through mutations and recombination. While KV vaccines are safer, they are generally less efficacious than MLV for primary vaccination. Adverse reactions include occasional transient inflammation and swelling at the injection site (this may be more pronounced with KV vaccines due to presence of irritant adjuvant/s), and very rarely anaphylactic reactions.

26.12 Summary

Porcine reproductive and respiratory syndrome virus is a complex, high-impact disease of swine worldwide. Control of PRRS has proven challenging due to several pathogenic features of the virus. The virus can evade host immune responses by escaping type I IFN and NK cell cytotoxicity, delaying the production of neutralizing antibodies and secretion of IFN-γ, and by stimulating production of Tregs and other immunosuppressive mediators which result in chronic viral persistence and intermittent virus excretion for over 200 days. The virus has high mutation rates and exists in multiple variant forms; this is perhaps the major challenge to the swine industry. Current vaccines are relatively inefficient, as they are unable to protect swine herds from reinfection or against heterologous field virus infections.

There are commercially available MLV and KV vaccines. MLV perform better than KV vaccines for primary immunization. KV vaccines are better at boosting the immune response of previously infected and/or MLV-immunized animals. Vaccines should not be used as a stand-alone PRRS control method; their use needs to be complemented with strict biosecurity measures, and flow management in growing and breeding herds and replacement animals.

There is an urgent need for next-generation vaccines that address the challenges outlined above. Numerous experimental vaccines have been reported, including live vectored, viral subunits expressed in baculovirus, DNA vaccines, and nanoparticle-based intranasal delivery of KV formulated with a potent adjuvant. The latter method, under experimental conditions, showed great promise for controlling heterologous challenge virus infection. The use of reverse genetics has provided more options for new-generation vaccines such as gene-deleted vaccines, chimeric vaccines, dendritic cell-targeted vaccines, and Treg cell-suppressing vaccines. Several approaches are being explored to induce better cross-protection, including built-in biologic adjuvants, molecular breeding through DNA shuffling, consensus sequence vaccines, mosaic virus vaccines, etc. Any new vaccine must undergo safety, immunogenicity, and efficacy testing before reaching final approval for use in animals. Clear understanding of the host response to PRRSV and the mechanisms of protection against PRRSV are fundamental to the formulation of new control measures.

Acknowledgments

The authors acknowledge Drs Montserrat Torremorell, Herbert van Kruiningen, and Joan Smyth for review of the chapter and valuable comments and suggestions.

References

Albina, E., Madec, F., Cariolet, R., and Torrison, J. (1994). Immune response and persistence of the porcine reproductive and respiratory syndrome virus in infected pigs and farm units. *Vet. Rec.* 134 (22): 567–573.

Albina, E., Carrat, C., and Charley, B. (1998). Interferon-alpha response to swine arterivirus (PoAV), the porcine reproductive and respiratory syndrome virus. *J. Interferon Cytokine Res.* 18 (7): 485–490.

Amadori, M. and Razzuoli, E. (2014). Immune control of PRRS: lessons to be learned and possible ways forward. *Front. Vet. Sci.* 1 (2): 1–13.

Balka, G., Podgórska, K., Singh Brar, M. et al. (2018). Genetic diversity of PRRSV 1 in Central Eastern Europe in 1994–2014: origin and evolution of the virus in the region. *Sci. Rep.* 8: 7811.

Barouch, D.H., O'Brien, K.L., Simmons, N.L. et al. (2010). Mosaic HIV-1 vaccines expand the breadth and depth of cellular immune responses in rhesus monkeys. *Nat. Med.* 16 (3): 319–323

Batista, L., Pijoan, C., Dee, S. et al. (2004). Virological and immunological responses to porcine reproductive and respiratory syndrome virus in a large population of gilts. *Can. J. Vet. Res.* 68 (4): 267–273.

Bautista, E.M. and Molitor, T.W. (1997). Cell mediated immunity to porcine reproductive and respiratory syndrome virus in swine. *Viral Immunol.* 10 (2): 83–94.

Bautista, E.M., Suarez, P., and Molitor, T. (1999). T cell responses to the structural polypeptides of porcine reproductive and respiratory syndrome virus. *Arch. Virol* 144 (1): 117–134.

Beltran-Alcrudo, D., Lubroth, J., Njeumi, F., et al. (2007). Porcine reproductive and respiratory syndrome (PRRS): regional awareness. www.fao.org/3/a-ai340e.pdf

Benfield, D.W., Nelson, E., Collins, J.E. et al. (1992). Characterization of swine infertility and respiratory syndrome (SIRS) virus (ATCC VR-2332). *J. Vet. Diagn. Invest.* 4: 127–133.

Bilodeau, R., Archambault, D., Vezina, S.A. et al. (1994). Persistence of porcine reproductive and respiratory syndrome virus infection in a swine operation. *Can. J. Vet. Res.* 58 (4): 291–298.

Binjawadagi, B., Dwivedi, V., Manickam, C. et al. (2014a). An innovative approach to induce cross-protective immunity against porcine reproductive and respiratory syndrome virus in the lungs of pigs through adjuvanted nanotechnology-based vaccination. *Int. J. Nanomed.* 9: 1519–1535.

Binjawadagi, B., Dwivedi, V., Manickam, C. et al. (2014b). Adjuvanted poly(lactic-co-glycolic) acid nanoparticle-entrapped inactivated porcine reproductive and respiratory syndrome virus vaccine elicits cross-protective immune response in pigs. *Int. J. Nanomed.* 9: 679–694.

Botner, A., Strandbygaard, B., Sorensen, K.J. et al. (1997). Appearance of acute PRRS -like symptom in sow herds after vaccination with modified-live PRRS-vaccine. *Vet. Rec.* 141: 497–499.

Cano, J.P. (2013). PRRS surveillance programs for farms, companies and regions. www.pig333.com/what_the_experts_say/prrs-surveillance-programs-for-farms-companies-and-regions_6789/

Cano, J.P., Dee, S.A., Murtaugh, M.P. et al. (2007a). Effect of vaccination with modified-live porcine reproductive and respiratory syndrome virus vaccine on dynamics of homologous viral infection in pigs. *Am. J. Vet. Res.* 68 (5): 565–571.

Cano, J.P., Dee, S.A., Murtaugh, M.P., and Pijoan, C. (2007b). Impact of a modified-live porcine reproductive and respiratory syndrome virus vaccine intervention on a population of pigs infected with a heterologous isolate. *Vaccine* 25 (22): 4283–4291.

Cao, Q.M., Ni, Y.Y., Cao, D. et al. (2018). The recombinant MLV virus expressing the membrane-bound IL-15 cytokine greatly enhanced NK cell and γδ T cell responses and also conferred improved protection against heterologous challenge with the PRRSV NADC20 strain. *J. Virol.* 92 (13): ii.

Charerntantanakul, W. (2012). Porcine reproductive and respiratory syndrome virus vaccines: immunogenicity, efficacy and safety aspects. *World J. Virol.* 1 (1): 23–30.

Charerntantanakul, W., Platt, R., Johnson, W. et al. (2006). Immune responses and protection by vaccine and various vaccine adjuvant candidates to virulent porcine reproductive and respiratory syndrome virus. *Vet. Immunol. Immunopathol.* 109 (1–2): 99–115.

Chase-Topping, M., Xie, J., Pooley, C. et al. (2020). New insights about vaccine effectiveness: impact of Attenuated PRRS-strain vaccination on heterologous strain transmission. *Vaccine* 38 (14): 3050–3061. doi: 10.1016/j.vaccine.2020.02.015. Epub 2020 Feb 29.

Cho, Y., Heo, Y., Choi, H. et al. (2020). Porcine endogenous retrovirus envelope coated baculoviral DNA vaccine against porcine reproductive and respiratory syndrome. *Virus Anim. Biotechnol.* 31 (1): 32–41. doi: 10.1080/10495398.2018.1531014. Epub 2018 Dec 20.

Choi, K., Park, C., Jeong, J. et al. (2016). Comparison of commercial type 1 and type 2 PRRSV vaccines against heterologous dual challenge. *Vet. Rec.* 178 (12): 291.

Christopher-Hennings, J., Nelson, E.A., Hines, R.J. et al. (1995). Persistence of porcine reproductive and respiratory virus in serum and semen of adult boars. *J. Vet. Diagn. Invest.* 7 (4): 456–464.

Chung, W.B., Lin, M.W., Chang, W.F. et al. (1997). Persistence of porcine reproductive and respiratory syndrome virus in intensive farrow-to-finish pig herds. *Can. J. Vet. Res.* 61 (4): 292–294.

Cortey, M., Arocena, G., Pileri, E. et al. (2018). Bottlenecks in the transmission of porcine reproductive and respiratory syndrome virus (PRRSV1) to naïve pigs and the quasi-species variation of the virus during infection in vaccinated pigs. *Vet. Res.* 49: 107–117.

Costers, S., Lefebvre, D.J., Goddeeris, B. et al. (2009). Functional impairment of PRRSV-specific peripheral CD3+CD8high cells. *Vet. Res.* 40: 46–60.

Costers, S., Lefebvre, D.J., van Doorsselaere, J. et al. (2010). GP4 of porcine reproductive and respiratory syndrome virus contains a neutralizing epitope that is susceptible to immunoselection in vitro. *Arch. Virol* 155: 371–378.

Cruz, J.L., Zúñiga, S., Bécares, M. et al. (2010). Vectored vaccines to protect against PRRSV. *Virus Res.* 154 (1–2): 150–160.

Cui, J., O'Connell, C.M., Smith, J.D. et al. (2016). A GP5 Mosaic T-cell vaccine for porcine reproductive and respiratory syndrome virus is immunogenic and confers partial protection to pigs. *Vaccine Rep.* 6: 77–86.

Cui, J., O'Connell, C., Costa, A. et al. (2019). A PRRSV GP5-Mosaic vaccine: protection of pigs from challenge and *ex vivo* detection of IFNγ responses against several genotype 2 strains. *PLoS One* 14 (1): e0208801.

Cui, J., O'Connell, C.M., Hagen, C. et al. (2020). Broad protection of pigsagainst heterologous PRRSV strains by a GP5-mosaic DNA vaccine prime/GP5-mosaic vaccinia (VACV) vaccine boost. *Vaccines* 8(1): 106. doi: 10.3390/vaccines8010106. PMID: 32121277

Darwich, L., Díaz, I., and Mateu, E. (2010). Certainties, doubts and hypotheses in porcine reproductive and respiratory syndrome virus immunobiology. *Virus Res.* 154 (1–2): 123–132.

Dee, S. (2003). Principles in prevention, control, and eradication. In: *The 2003 PRRS Compendium – A Reference for Pork Producers* (eds. J.Z. Zimmerman, K.-J. Yoon, E. Neumann and D.A. Benfield), 78–87. Clive: National Pork Board.

Dee, S. and Philips, R. (1998). Using vaccination and unidirectional pig flow to control PRRSV transmission. *Swine Health Prod.* 6 (1): 21–25.

Dee, S., Collins, J., Halbur, P. et al. (1996). Control of porcine reproductive and respiratory syndrome (PRRS) virus. *J. Swine Health Prod.* 4 (2): 95–98.

Dee, S., Otake, S., Oliveira, S., and Deen, J. (2009). Evidence of long distance airborne transport of porcine reproductive and respiratory syndrome virus and *Mycoplasma hyopneumoniae*. *Vet. Res.* 30: 39–51.

Dee, S., Cano, J.P., Spronk, G. et al. (2012). Evaluation of the long-term effect of air filtration on the occurrence of new PRRSV infections in large breeding herds in swine dense regions. *Viruses* 4: 654–662.

Delrue, I., Delputte, P.L., and Nauwynck, H.J. (2009). Assessing the functionality of viral entry-associated domains of porcine reproductive and respiratory syndrome virus during inactivation procedures, a potential tool to optimize inactivated vaccines. *Vet. Res.* 40 (6): 62–76.

Dewey, C.E., Wilson, S., Buck, P., and Leyenaar, J.K. (1999). The reproductive performance of sows after PRRS vaccination depends on stage of gestation. *Prev. Vet. Med.* 40 (3–4): 233–241.

Diaz, I., Darwich, L., Pappaterra, G. et al. (2006). Different European-type vaccines against porcine reproductive and respiratory syndrome virus have different immunological properties and confer different protection to pigs. *Virology* 351 (2): 249–259.

Diaz, I., Pujols, J., Ganges, L. et al. (2009). In silico prediction and ex vivo evaluation of potential T-cell epitopes in glycoproteins 4 and 5 and nucleocapsid protein of genotype-I (European) porcine reproductive and respiratory syndrome virus. *Vaccine* 27: 5603–5611.

Diaz, I., Gimeno, M., Darwich, L. et al. (2012). Characterization of homologous and heterologous adaptive immune responses in porcine reproductive and respiratory syndrome virus infection. *Vet. Res.* 43 (1): 30–44.

Diaz, I., Gimeno, M., Callén, A. et al. (2013). Comparison of different vaccination schedules for sustaining the immune response against porcine reproductive and respiratory syndrome virus. *Vet. J.* 197 (2): 438–444.

Done, S.H., Paton, D.J., and White, M.E. (1996). Porcine reproductive and respiratory syndrome (PRRS): a review, with emphasis on pathological, virological and diagnostic aspects. *Br. Vet. J.* 152: 153–174.

Dwivedi, V., Manickam, C., Patterson, R. et al. (2011). Cross-protective immunity to porcine reproductive and respiratory syndrome virus by intranasal delivery of a live virus vaccine with a potent adjuvant. *Vaccine* 29: 4058–4066.

Dwivedi, V., Manickam, C., Binjawadagi, B. et al. (2012). Evaluation of immune responses to porcine reproductive and respiratory syndrome virus in pigs during early stage of infection under farm conditions. *Virol. J.* 9: 45.

Ferrari, L., Martelli, P., Saleri, R. et al. (2013). Lymphocyte activation as cytokine gene expression and secretion is related to the porcine reproductive and respiratory syndrome virus (PRRSV) isolate after in vitro homologous and heterologous recall of peripheral blood mononuclear cells (PBMC) from pigs vaccinated and exposed to natural infection. *Vet. Immunol. Immunopathol.* 151 (3–4): 193–206.

Fischer, W., Perkins, S., Theiler, S.J. et al. (2007). Polyvalent vaccines for optimal coverage of potential T-cell epitopes in global HIV-1 variants. *Nat. Med.* 13 (1): 100–106.

Flores-Mendoza, L., Silva-Campa, E., Resendiz, M. et al. (2008). Porcine reproductive and respiratory syndrome virus infects mature porcine dendritic cells and up- regulates IL10 production. *Clin. Vaccine Immunol.* 15 (4): 720–725.

Forsberg, R., Storgaard, T., Nielsen, H.S. et al. (2002). The genetic diversity of European type PRRSV is similar to that of the North American type but is geographically skewed within Europe. *Virology* 299 (1): 38–47.

Geldhof, M.F., van Breedam, W., de Jong, E. et al. (2013). Antibody response and maternal immunity upon boosting PRRSV-immune sows with experimental farm-specific and commercial PRRSV vaccines. *Vet. Microbiol.* 167 (3–4): 260–271.

Gómez-Laguna, J. Salguero, F.J., de Marco, M.F. et al. (2009). Changes in lymphocyte subsets and cytokines during European porcine reproductive and respiratory syndrome: increased expression of IL-12 and IL-10 and proliferation of CD4(-) CD8(high). *Viral Immunol.* 22 (4): 261–271.

Gonin, P., Pirzadeh, B., Gagnon, C.A., and Dea, S. (1999). Seroneutralization of porcine reproductive and respiratory syndrome virus correlates with antibody response to the GP5major envelope glycoprotein. *J. Vet. Diagn. Invest.* 11: 20–26.

Guillespie, T.G. (2003). Control with modified-live virus (MLV) PRRS vaccine. In: *The 2003 PRRS Compendium – A Reference for Pork Producers* (eds. J.Z. Zimmerman, K.-J. Yoon, E. Neumann and D.A. Benfield), 105–108. Clive: National Pork Board.

Halbur, P.G. (1997). Understanding recent severe acute PRRS/SAMs outbreaks. www.ncsu.edu/project/swine_extension/healthyhogs/book1997/halbur1.htm

Halbur, P. (2003). "PRRS Plus" – PRRS virus infection in combination with other agents. In: *The 2003 PRRS Compendium – A Reference for Pork Producers* (eds. J.Z. Zimmerman, K.-J. Yoon, E. Neumann and D.A. Benfield), 19–24. Clive: National Pork Board.

Halbur, P.G., Paul, P.S., Meng, X. et al. (1996). Comparative pathogenicity of nine US porcine reproductive and respiratory syndrome virus (PRRSV) isolates in a five-week-old-cesarean-derived colostrum-deprived pig model. *J. Vet. Diagn. Invest.* 8: 11–20.

Han, Y.W., Kim, S.B., Rahman, M. et al. (2011). Systemic and mucosal immunity induced by attenuated *Salmonella enterica* serovar Typhimurium expressing ORF7 of porcine reproductive and respiratory syndrome virus. *Comp. Immunol. Microbiol. Infect. Dis.* 34 (4): 335–345.

Hirose, O., Shilbata, I., Kudou, H. et al. (1995). Experimental infection of SPF piglets with porcine reproductive and respiratory syndrome (PRRS) viruses isolated from two farms. *J. Vet. Med. Sci.* 57 (6): 991–995.

Holtkamp, D.J., Polson, D.D., Torremorell, M. et al. (2011). Terminology for classifying swine herds by porcine reproductive and respiratory syndrome virus status. *J. Swine Health Prod.* 19 (1): 44–56.

Holtkamp, D.J., Kliebestein, M.S., Neumann, E.J. et al. (2013). Assessment of the economic impact of porcine reproductive and respiratory syndrome virus on United States pork producers. *J. Swine Health Prod.* 21 (2): 73–84.

Hu, J. and Zhang, C. (2014). Porcine reproductive and respiratory syndrome virus vaccines: current status and strategies to a universal vaccine. *Transbound. Emerg. Dis.* 61 (2): 109–120.

Hu, J., Ni, Y., Dryman, B.A. et al. (2012). Immunogenicity study of plant-made oral subunit vaccine against porcine reproductive and respiratory syndrome virus (PRRSV). *Vaccine* 30 (12): 2068–2074.

Huang, Y.W. and Meng, X.J. (2010). Novel strategies and approaches to develop the next generation of vaccines against porcine reproductive and respiratory syndrome virus (PRRSV). *Virus Res.* 154 (1–2): 141–149.

Jeong, J., Aly, S.S., Cano, J.P. et al. (2014). Stochastic model of porcine reproductive and respiratory syndrome virus control strategies on a swine farm in the United States. *Am. J. Vet. Res.* 75 (3): 260–267.

Jeong, J., Kang, I., Kim, S. et al. (2018a). A modified-live porcine reproductive and respiratory syndrome virus (PRRSV)-1 vaccine protects late-term pregnancy gilts against heterologous PRRSV-1 but not PRRSV-2 challenge. *Transbound. Emerg. Dis.* 65 (5): 1227–1234.

Jeong, J., Park, C., Oh, T. et al. (2018b). The vaccination of gilts with PRRSV-2 MLV vaccine can provide cross-protection against PRRSV-1 challenge and improve reproductive performance. *Vet. Microbiol.* 223: 119–125.

Katz, J.B., Shafer, A.L., Eernisse, K.A. et al. (1995). Antigenic differences between European and American isolates of porcine reproductive and respiratory syndrome virus (PRRSV) are encoded by the carboxy-terminal portion of viral open reading frame 3. *Vet. Microbiol.* 44 (1): 65–76.

Kim, W.I. and Yoon, K.J. (2008). Molecular assessment of the role of envelope-associated structural proteins in cross neutralization among different PRRS viruses. *Virus Genes* 37: 380–391.

Kimman, T.J., Cornelissen, L.A., Moormann, R.J. et al. (2009). Challenges for porcine reproductive and respiratory syndrome virus (PRRSV) vaccinology. *Vaccine* 27: 3704–3718.

Klopfenstein, C., Bonneau, M., Morin, M. et al. (2012). Regional PRRS control with an autogenous vaccination strategy. *Journées Recherche Porcine* 44: 93–94. www.pig333.com/swine_abstracts/regional-prrs-control-with-an-autogenous-vaccination-strategy_6119/

Kraft, C., Hennies, R., Dreckmann, K. et al. (2019). Evaluation of PRRSv specific, maternally derived and induced immune response inIngelvac PRRSFLEX EU vaccinated piglets in the presence of maternally transferred immunity. PLoS One. 14 (10): e0223060. doi:10.1371/journal.pone.0223060. eCollection 2019. PMID: 31577832

Larcher, T., Fablet, C., Renson, P. et al. (2019). Assessment of pulmonary tissue responses in pigs challenged with PRRSV Lena strain shows better protection after immunization with field than vaccine strains. *Vet. Microbiol.* 230:249–259. doi: 10.1016/j.vetmic.2019.01.022. Epub 2019 Feb 14. PMID:30827397

Li, Y., Wang, X., Bo, K. et al. (2007). Emergence of a highly pathogenic porcine reproductive and respiratory syndrome virus in the Mid-Eastern region of China. *Vet. J.* 174 (3): 577–584.

Li, B., Xiao, S., Wang, Y. et al. (2009). Immunogenicity of the highly pathogenic porcine reproductive and respiratory syndrome virus GP5 protein encoded by a synthetic ORF5 gene. *Vaccine* 27: 1957–1963.

Linhares, D.C.L., Cano, J.P., Torremorell, M., and Morrison, R.B. (2014). Comparison of time to PRRSV-stability and production losses between two exposure programs to control PRRS in sow herds. *Prev. Vet. Med.* 116: 111–119.

Linhares, D.C., Johnson, C., and Morrison, R.B. (2015). Economic analysis of immunization strategies for PRRS control (corrected). *PLoS One* 10 (12): e0144265. Erratum in: PLoS One. 2016;11(4):e0150444.

Loving, C., Osorio, F.A., Murtaugh, M., and Zuckermann, F.A. (2015). Innate and adptive immunity agaisnt porcine reproductive and respiratory syndrome virus. *Vet. Immunol. Immunopathol.* 167: 1–14.

Lowe, J.F., DeBuse, N., Morrison, R. et al. (2012). A systematic management strategy for breeding herds based on PRRS herd status. AASV Annual Meeting: Integrating Science, Welfare and Economics in Practice, pp. 517–522. www.aasv.org/aasv/documents/Lowe2012.pdf

Lyoo, Y.S. (2015). Porcine reproductive and respiratory syndrome virus vaccine does not fit in classical vaccinology. *Clin. Exp. Vaccine Res.* 4 (2): 159–165.

Madapong, A., Saeng-Chuto, K., Chaikhumwang, P. et al. (2020). Immune response and protective efficacy of intramuscular and intradermal vaccination with porcine reproductive and respiratory syndrome virus 1 (PRRSV-1) modified live vaccine against highly pathogenic PRRSV-2 (HP-PRRSV-2) challenge, either alone or in combination with of PRRSV-1. *Vet. Microbiol.* 244:108655. doi:10.1016/j.vetmic.2020.108655. Epub 2020 Mar 27.

Madsen, K.G., Hansen, C.M., Madsen, E.S. et al. (1998). Sequence analysis of porcine reproductive and respiratory syndrome virus of the American type collected from Danish swine herds. *Arch. Virol* 143 (9): 1683–1700.

Mardassi, H., Wilson, L., Mounir, S., and Dea, S. (1994). Detection of porcine reproductive and respiratory syndrome virus and efficient differentiation between Canadian and European strains by reverse transcription and PCR amplification. *J. Clin. Microbiol.* 32 (9): 2197–2203.

Martínez-Lobo, F.J., de Lome, L.C., Díez-Fuertes, F. et al. (2013). Safety of porcine reproductive and respiratory syndrome modified live virus (MLV) vaccine strains in a young pig infection model. *Vet. Res.* 44: 115–128.

Mateu, E. (2013). Vaccination against PRRSV: a practical approach.www.pig333.com/prrs/vaccination-against-porcine-reproductive-and-respiratory-syndrome-viru_7485/

Mateu, E. and Diaz, I. (2008). The challenge of PRRS immunology. *Vet. J.* 177: 345–351.

McCaw, M. (2000). Effect of reducing cross-fostering at birth on piglet mortality and performance during an acute outbreak of porcine reproductive respiratory syndrome. *J. Swine Health Prod.* 8 (1): 15–21.

Meier, W.A., Galeota, J., Osorio, F. et al. (2003). Gradual development of the interferon-γ response of swine to porcine reproductive and respiratory syndrome virus infection or vaccination. *Virology* 309: 18–31.

Meng, X.J. (2000). Heterogeneity of porcine reproductive respiratory syndrome virus: implications for current vaccine efficacy and future vaccine development. *Vet. Microbiol.* 74: 309–329.

Meng, X.J., Paul, P.S., and Halbur, P.G. (1994). Molecular cloning and nucleotide sequencing of the 3' terminal genomic RNA of the porcine reproductive and respiratory syndrome virus. *J. Gen. Virol.* 75 (7): 1795–1801.

Mengeling, W.L. (2005). The porcine reproductive and respiratory syndrome quandary. Part II: vaccines and vaccination strategy. *J. Swine Health Prod.* 13 (3): 152–156.

Mengeling, W.L., Lager, K.M., and Vorwald, A.C. (1998). Clinical consequences of exposing pregnant gilts to strains of porcine reproductive and respiratory syndrome (PRRS) virus isolated from field cases of "atypical" PRRS. *Am. J. Vet. Res.* 59 (12): 1540–1544.

Mengeling, W.L., Vorwald, A.C., Lager, K.M. et al. (1999a). Identification and clinical assessment of suspected vaccine-related field strains of porcine reproductive and respiratory syndrome virus. *Am. J. Vet. Res.* 60 (3): 334–340.

Mengeling, W.L., Lager, K.M., and Vorwald, A.C. (1999b). Safety and efficacy of vaccination of pregnant gilts against porcine reproductive and respiratory syndrome. *Am. J. Vet. Res.* 60 (7): 796–801.

Meulenberg, J.J., Hulst, M.M., de Meijer, E.J. et al. (1993). Lelystad virus, the causative agent of porcine epidemic abortion and respiratory syndrome (PEARS), is related to LDV, and EAV. *Virology* 192: 62–72.

Meulenberg, J.J.M., van Nieuwstadt, A.P., van Essen-Zandbergen, A., and Langeveld, J.P.M. (1997). Posttranslational processing and identification of a neutralization domain of the GP4 encoded by ORF4 of Lelystad virus. *J. Virol.* 71 (8): 6061–6067.

Murakami, Y., Kato, A., Tsuda, T. et al. (1994). Isolation and serological characterization of porcine reproductive and respiratory syndrome (PRRS) viruses from pigs with reproductive and respiratory disorders in Japan. *J. Vet. Med. Sci.* 56 (5): 891–894.

Murtaugh, M.P. and Genzow, M. (2011). Immunological solutions for treatment and prevention of porcine reproductive and respiratory syndrome (PRRS). *Vaccine* 29 (46): 8192–8204.

Murtaugh, M.P., Yuan, S., Nelson, E.A., and Faaberg, K.S. (2002a). Genetic interaction between porcine reproductive and respiratory syndrome virus (PRRSV) strains in cell culture and in animals. *J. Swine Health Prod.* 10 (1): 15–21.

Murtaugh, M.P., Xiao, Z., and Zuckermann, F. (2002b). Immunological responses of swine to porcine reproductive and respiratory syndrome virus infection. *Viral Immunol.* 15 (4): 533–547.

Nelson, E.A., Christopher-Hennings, J., Drew, T. et al. (1993). Differentiation of U.S. and European isolates of porcine reproductive and respiratory syndrome virus by monoclonal antibodies. *J. Clin. Microbiol.* 31 (12): 3184–3189.

Nelson, E.A., Christopher-Hennings, J., and Benfield, D.A. (1994). Serum immune responses to the proteins of porcine reproductive and respiratory syndrome (PRRS) virus. *J. Vet. Diagn. Invest.* 6 (4): 410–415.

Neumann, E.J., Kliebestein, J.B., Johnson, C.D. et al. (2005). Assessment of the economic impact of porcine reproductive respiratory syndrome on swine production in the United States. *J. Am. Vet. Med. Assoc.* 227: 385–392.

Ni, Y.Y., Opriessnig, T., Zhou, L. et al. (2013). Attenuation of porcine reproductive and respiratory syndrome virus by molecular breeding of virus envelope genes from genetically divergent strains. *J. Virol.* 87 (1): 304–313.

Ni, Y.Y., Zhao, Z , Opriessnig, T. et al. (2014). Computer-aided codon-pairs deoptimization of the major envelope GP5 gene attenuates porcine reproductive and respiratory syndrome virus. *Virology* 450–451: 132–139.

Nielsen, H.S., Oleksiewicz, M.B., Forsberg, R. et al. (2001). Reversion of a live porcine reproductive and respiratory syndrome virus vaccine investigated by parallel mutations. *J. Gen. Virol.* 82 (6): 1263–1272.

Nielsen, J., Botner, A., Bille-Hansen, V. et al. (2002). Experimental inoculation of late term pregnant sows with a field isolate of porcine reproductive and respiratory syndrome vaccine-derived virus. *Vet. Microbiol.* 84 (1–2): 1–13.

Nilubol, D., Platt, K.B., Halbur, P.G. et al. (2004). The effect of a killed porcine reproductive and respiratory syndrome virus (PRRSV) vaccine treatment on virus shedding in previously PRRSV infected pigs. *Vet. Microbiol.* 102 (1–2): 11–18.

Oh, T., Kim, H., Park, K.H. et al. (2019). Effectiveness of a commercial porcine reproductive and respiratory syndrome virus (PRRSV) subunit vaccine against heterologous PRRSV-1 and PRRSV-2 challenge in late-term pregnant gilts. *Can. J. Vet. Res.* 83(4): 248–254.

OIE. (2018). Chapter 3.8.6. Porcine reproductive and respiratory syndrome. In: Manual of Diagnostic Tests and Vaccines for Terrestrial Animals. www.oie.int/fileadmin/Home/eng/Health_standards/tahm/3.08.06_PRRS.pdf

Opriessnig, T., Baker, R.B., and Halbur, P.G. (2007). Use of an experimental model to test the efficacy of planned exposure to live porcine reproductive and respiratory syndrome virus. *Clin. Vaccine Immunol.* 14 (12): 1572–1577.

Opriessnig, T., Giménez-Lirola, L.G., and Halbur, P.G. (2011). Polymicrobial respiratory disease in pigs. *Anim. Health Res. Rev.* 12 (2): 133–148.

Osorio, F.A., Galeota, J.A., Nelson, E. et al. (2002). Passive transfer of virus-specific antibodies confers protection against reproductive failure induced by a virulent strain of porcine reproductive respiratory syndrome virus and establishes sterilizing immunity. *Virology* 302: 9–20.

Ostrowski, M., Galeota, J.A., Jar, A.M. et al. (2002). Identification of neutralizing and nonneutralizing epitopes in the porcine reproductive and respiratory syndrome virus GP5 ectodomain. *J. Virol.* 76 (9): 4241–4250.

Papatsiros, V.G. (2012). Porcine respiratory and reproductive syndrome virus vaccinology: a review for commercial vaccines. *Am. J. Anim. Vet. Sci.* 7 (4): 149–158.

Park, B.K., Yoon, J.J., and Joo, H.S. (1996). Pathogenesis of plaque variants of porcine reproductive and respiratory syndrome virus in pregnant sows. *Am. J. Vet. Res.* 57 (3): 320–333.

Park, C., Seo, H.W., Han, K. et al. (2014). Evaluation of the efficacy of a new modified live porcine reproductive and respiratory syndrome virus (PRRSV) vaccine (Fostera PRRS) against heterologous PRRSV challenge. *Vet. Microbiol.* 172 (3–4): 432–442.

Pileri, E., Gibert, E., Soldevila, F. et al. (2015). Vaccination with a genotype 1 modified live vaccine against porcine reproductive and respiratory syndrome virus significantly reduces viremia, viral shedding and transmission of the virus in a quasi-natural experimental model. *Vet. Microbiol.* 175 (1): 7–16.

Plagemann, P.G.W. (2004). The primary GP5 neutralization epitope of North American isolates of porcine reproductive and respiratory syndrome virus. *Vet. Immun. Immunopathol.* 102: 263–275.

Plagemann, P.G.W. (2006). Neutralizing antibody formation in swine infected with seven strains of porcine reproductive and respiratory syndrome virus as measured by indirect ELISA with peptides containing the GP5 epitope. *Viral Immunol.* 19 (2): 285–293.

Plagemann, P.G.W., Rowland, R.R.R., and Faaberg, K.S. (2002). The primary neutralization epitope of porcine reproductive and respiratory syndrome virus strain VR-2332 is located in the middle of the GP5 ectodomain. *Arch. Virol* 147: 2327–2347.

Plana-Duran, J., Climent, I., Sarraseca, J. et al. (1997). Baculovirus expression of proteins of porcine reproductive and respiratory syndrome virus strain Olot/91. Involvement of ORF 3 and ORF 5 proteins in protection. *Virus Genes* 14 (1): 19–29.

Pol, J.M.A. and Steverink, P.J.G.M. (2000). Vaccinology of PRRS. *Vet. Res.* 31 (1): 92–93.

Renson, P., Fablet, C., Le Dimna, M. et al. (2017). Preparation for emergence of an Eastern European porcine reproductive and respiratory syndrome virus (PRRSV) strain in Western Europe: immunization with modified live virus vaccines or a field strain confers partial protection. *Vet. Microbiol.* 204: 133–140.

Renukaradhya, G.J., Dwivedi, V., Manickam, C. et al. (2012). Mucosal vaccines to prevent porcine reproductive and respiratory syndrome: a new perspective. *Anim. Health Res. Rev.* 13 (1): 21–37.

Renukaradhya, G.J., Meng, X.J., Calvert, J.G. et al. (2015a). Live porcine reproductive and respiratory syndrome virus vaccines: current status and future direction. *Vaccine* 33 (33): 4069–4080.

Renukaradhya, G.J., Meng, X.J., Calvert, J.G. et al. (2015b). Inactivated and subunit vaccines against porcine reproductive and respiratory syndrome: current status and future direction. *Vaccine* 33 (27): 3065–3072.

Robinson, S.R., Li, J., Nelson, E.A., and Murtaugh, M.P. (2015). Broadly neutralizing antibodies against the rapidly evolving porcine reproductive and respiratory syndrome virus. *Virus Res.* 203: 56–65.

Roca, M., Gimeno, M., Brugera, S. et al. (2012). Effects of challenge with a virulent genotype II strain of porcine reproductive respiratory syndrome virus on piglets vaccinated with an attenuated genotype I strain vaccine. *Vet. J.* 193: 92–96.

Rompato, G., Ling, E., Chen, H.X. et al. (2006). Positive inductive effects of IL2 on virus specific cellular responses elicited by a PRRSV ORF7 DNA vaccine in swine. *Vet. Immunol. Immunopathol.* 109 (1–2): 151–160.

Rose, N. and Andraud, M. (2017). The use of vaccines to control pathogen spread in pig populations. *Porcine Health Manag.* 3: 8.

Rowland, R.R. and Morrison, R.B. (2012). Challenges and opportunities for the control and elimination of porcine reproductive and respiratory syndrome virus. *Transbound. Emerg. Dis.* 59 (Suppl 1): 55–59.

Royaee, A.R., Husmann, R.J., Dawson, H.D. et al. (2004). Deciphering the involvement of innate immune factors in the development of the host response to PRRSV vaccination. *Vet. Immunol. Immunopathol.* 102: 199–216.

Schelkopf, A., Nerem, J., Cowles, B. et al. (2014). Reproductive, productivity, and mortality outcomes in late-gestation gilts and their litters following simulation of inadvertent exposure to a modified-live vaccine strain of porcine reproductive and respiratory syndrome (PRRS) virus. *Vaccine* 32 (36): 4639–4643.

Shi, M., Lam, T.T., Hon, C.C. et al. (2010). Phylogeny-based evolutionary, demographical, and geographical dissection of North American type 2 porcine reproductive and respiratory syndrome viruses. *J. Virol.* 84 (17): 8700–8711.

Stadejek, T., Oleksiewicz, M.B., Scherbakov, A.V. et al. (2008). Definition of subtypes in the European genotype of porcine reproductive and respiratory syndrome virus: nucleocapsid characteristics and geographical distribution in Europe. *Arch. Virol* 153 (8): 1479–1488.

Suarez, P., Diaz-Guerra, M., Prieto, C. et al. (1996). Open reading frame 5 of porcine reproductive and respiratory syndrome virus as a cause of virus-induced apoptosis. *J. Virol.* 70 (5): 2876–2882.

Sun, H., Workman, A., Osorio, F.A. et al. (2018). Development of a broadly protective modified-live virus vaccine candidate against porcine reproductive and respiratory syndrome virus. *Vaccine* 36 (1): 66–73.

Thacker, B. (2003). PRRS virus infection and disease. In: *The 2003 PRRS Compendium – A Reference for Pork Producers* (eds. J.Z. Zimmerman, K.-J. Yoon, E. Neumann and D.A. Benfield), 11–16. Clive: National Pork Board.

Thacker, E., Thacker, B., Wilson, W., and Ackerman, M. (2003). Control with inactivated virus PRRS vaccine. In: *The 2003 PRRS Compendium – A Reference for Pork Producers* (eds. J.Z. Zimmerman, K.-J. Yoon, E. Neumann and D.A. Benfield), 109–110. Clive: National Pork Board.

Thanawongnuwech, R. and Suradhat, S. (2010). Taming PRRSV: revisiting the control strategies and vaccine design. *Virus Res.* 154 (1–2): 133–140.

Thanawongnuwech, R., Brown, G.B., Halbur, P.G. et al. (2000). Pathogenesis of porcine reproductive and respiratory syndrome virus-induced increase in susceptibility to *Streptococcus suis* infection. *Vet. Pathol.* 37 (2): 143–152.

Thurmond, J., Yoon, H., Kuiken, C. et al. (2008). Web-based design and evaluation of T-cell vaccine candidates. *Bioinformatics* 24 (14): 1639–1640.

Tian, K., Yu, X., Zhao, T. et al. (2007). Emergence of fatal PRRSV variants: unparalleled outbreaks of atypical PRRS in China and molecular dissection of the unique hallmark. *PLoS One* 2 (6): e526.

Tian, D., Cao, D., Lynn Heffron, C. et al. (2017). Enhancing heterologous protection in pigs vaccinated with chimeric porcine reproductive and respiratory syndrome virus containing the full-length sequences of shuffled structural genes of multiple heterologous strains. *Vaccine* 35 (18): 2427–2434.

Tong, J.C., Tan, T.W.S., and Ranganathan (2006). Methods and protocols for prediction of immunogenic peptides. *Briefings Bioinf.* 8 (2): 96–108.

Torremorell, M., More, C., and Christianson, W.T. (2002). Establishment of a herd negative from porcine reproductive and respiratory syndrome virus from PRRSV-positive sources. *J. Swine Health Prod.* 10 (4): 153–160.

Torremorell, M.C., Henry, S., and Christianson, W.T. (2003). Eradication using herd closure. In: *The 2003 PRRS Compendium – A Reference for Pork Producers* (eds. J.Z. Zimmerman, K.-J. Yoon, E. Neumann and D.A. Benfield), 157–160. Clive: National Pork Board.

Van Gucht, S., Labarque, G., and van Reeth, K. (2004). The combination of PRRS virus and bacterial endotoxin as a model for multifactorial respiratory disease in pigs. *Vet. Immunol. Immunopathol.* 102: 165–178.

Van Reeth, K., Labarque, G., Nauwynck, H., and Pensaert, M. (1999). Differential production of proinflammatory cytokines in the pig lung during different respiratory virus infections: correlations with pathogenicity. *Res. Vet. Sci.* 67 (1): 47–52.

Vanhee, M., Delputte, P.L., Delrue, I. et al. (2009). Development of an experimental inactivated PRRSV vaccine that induces virus-neutralizing antibodies. *Vet. Res.* 40 (6): 63–77.

Vashisht, K., Goldberg, T.L., Husmann, R.J. et al. (2008). Identification of immunodominant T-cell epitopes present in glycoprotein 5 of the North American genotype of porcine reproductive and respiratory syndrome virus. *Vaccine* 26: 4747–4753.

Vezina, S.A., Loemba, H., Fournier, M. et al. (1996). Antibody production and blastogenic response in pigs experimentally infected with porcine reproductive and respiratory syndrome virus. *Can. J. Vet. Res.* 60 (2): 94–99.

Vu, H.L., Ma, F., Laegreid, W.W. et al. (2015). A synthetic porcine reproductive and respiratory syndrome virus strain confers unprecedented levels of heterologous protection. *J. Virol.* 89 (23): 12070–12083.

Wang, X., Marthaler, D., Rovira, A. et al. (2015). Emergence of a virulent porcine reproductive and respiratory syndrome virus in vaccinated herds in the United States. *Virus Res.* 210: 34–41.

Wang, A., Chen, Q., Wang, L. et al. (2019). Recombination between vaccine and field strains of porcine reproductive and respiratory syndrome virus. *Emerg. Infect. Dis.* 25 (12): 2335–2337. doi:10.3201/eid2512.191111.

Wensvoort, G., Terpstra, C., Pol, J.M. et al. (1991). Mystery swine disease in the Netherlands: the isolation of Lelystad virus. *Vet. Q* 13: 121–130.

Wills, R.W., Zimmerman, J.J., Yoon, K.J. et al. (1997). Porcine reproductive and respiratory syndrome virus: a persistent infection. *Vet. Microbiol.* 55 (1–4): 231–240.

Xia, M., Wang, W., and Wu, H. (2015). Evaluation of reversion to virulence on a modified live highly pathogenic porcine reproductive and respiratory syndrome vaccine strain in pigs. *Austin Virol Retrovirol.* 2 (1): 1012–1018.

Xiao, Z., Batista, L., Dee, S. et al. (2004). The level of virus-specific T-cell and macrophage recruitment is independent of virus load. *J. Virol.* 78: 5923–5933.

Yang, L., Frey, M.L., Yoon, K.J. et al. (2000). Categorization of North American porcine reproductive and respiratory syndrome viruses: epitopic profiles of the N, M, GP5 and GP3 proteins and susceptibility to neutralization. *Arch. Virol* 145: 1599–1619.

Yang, S., Oh, T., Cho, H. et al. (2020). A comparison of commercial modified-live PRRSV-1 and PRRSV-2 vaccines against a dual heterologous PRRSV-1 and PRRSV-2 challenge in late term pregnancy gilts. *Comp. Immunol. Microbiol. Infect. Dis.* 69: 101423. doi: 10.1016/j.cimid.2020.101423. Epub 2020 Jan 17.

Yu, X., Zhou, Z., Cao, Z. et al. (2015). Assessment of the safety and efficacy of an attenuated live vaccine based on highly pathogenic porcine reproductive and respiratory syndrome virus. *Clin. Vaccine Immunol.* 22 (5): 493–502.

Zhou, J.X., Xue, J.D., Yu, T. et al. (2010). Immune responses in pigs induced by recombinant canine adenovirus 2 expressing the glycoprotein 5 of porcine reproductive and respiratory syndrome virus. *Vet. Res. Commun.* 34 (4): 371–380.

Zhou, L., Ni, Y.Y., Piñeyro, P. et al. (2013). Broadening the heterologous cross-neutralizing antibody inducing ability of porcine reproductive and respiratory syndrome virus by breeding the GP4 or M genes. *PLoS One* 8 (6): e66645.

Zimmerman, J., Benfield, D., Christopher-Hennings, J. et al. (2015). Porcine reproductive and respiratory syndrome (PRRS). Pork Industry Handbook.

Zuckermann, F.A., Osorio, F., and Husmann, R.J. (1998). Analysis of the cell-mediated immune response of pigs to PRRS virus. Proceedings of the American Association of Swine Practitioners, pp. 339–400. www.pork.org/wp-content/uploads/2007/08/97-1978-Zuckerman-U-of-Ill.pdf

Zuckermann, F.A., Garcia, E.A., Luque, I.D. et al. (2007). Assessment of the efficacy of commercial porcine reproductive and respiratory syndrome virus (PRRSV) vaccines based on measurement of serologic response, frequency of gamma-IFN-producing cells and virological parameters of protection upon challenge. *Vet. Microbiol.* 123 (1-3): 69–85.

27

Anthrax

Antonio Fasanella[1], Giuliano Garofolo[2], Adelia Donatiello[1], and Emanuele Campese[1]

[1] *Anthrax Reference Institute of Italy, Istituto Zooprofilattico Sperimentale della Puglia e della Basilicata, Foggia, Italy*
[2] *National and OIE Reference Laboratory for Brucellosis, Istituto Zooprofilattico Sperimentale dell'Abruzzo e del Molise "G. Caporale", Teramo, Italy*

27.1 Introduction

Anthrax is an infectious, usually fatal, disease caused by *Bacillus anthracis,* with clinical features similar to those of hemorrhagic fevers and acute or hyperacute symptoms. It became a matter of global public interest after the bioterrorist attacks in the USA during the autumn of 2001. The concern of politicians and civil authorities everywhere toward this emergency led to a significant research effort for the prevention of new bioterrorist acts.

Anthrax is primarily a disease that affects livestock and wildlife; it is distributed worldwide and can represent a danger to humans, especially when it occurs in areas considered to be free and in atypical seasons and climatic conditions. This may lead to misdiagnosis and, consequently, inappropriate management of affected carcasses with a consequent and inevitable increase in the risk of human infection.

The causative agent of anthrax, *B. anthracis,* was demonstrated by Robert Koch in 1876. Due to its high pathogenicity, this microorganism also aroused the interest of people with less noble intentions. From 1932 to 1945, the bacteriologists of Japanese Army Unit 731 tested it as a biological weapon on Manchurian prisoners (Hudson et al. 2008). Despite the signing of a treaty banning bacteriological arms, a severe outbreak of human anthrax occurred in Sverdlovsk, USSR (now Ekaterinburg, Russia) in April 1979 (Meselson et al. 1994). Soviet officials attributed the outbreak to the consumption of contaminated meat, but western governments suspected the inhalation of spores accidentally released from a nearby military research facility to have been the cause. DNA analysis of tissue samples obtained from 11 victims, attesting to the presence of at least four different anthrax strains, confirmed this hypothesis (Jackson et al. 1998). The 2001 bioterrorist attacks in the USA, in which five letters containing small quantities of anthrax spores contaminated more than 30 000 people, killed five and infected 17 (Jernigan et al. 2002). This event represents a turning point in the history of highly pathogenic agents and their use as a means of aggression against civil populations: that which until then was considered only a remote possibility had become a terrible reality and a dangerous example that could be imitated by anyone (Fasanella et al. 2010).

The disease is characterized by outbreaks that normally involve a small number of herbivores, usually kept on pasture, but it can sometimes turn into an epidemic with potentially very serious consequences for humans, where the disease can take three forms, depending on the route of entry of *B. anthracis* spores: cutaneous, gastrointestinal, or pulmonary. Recently a fourth form, injectional anthrax, due to the intake of contaminated heroin, has been documented (Berger et al. 2014). The pathogenic action of *B. anthracis* is closely linked to the following two plasmids: (i) pXO1, 182 Kb, which contains the genes encoding the three anthrax protein factors: the edema factor (EF), the lethal factor (LF) and the protective antigen (PA) (Okinaka et al. 1999); (ii) pXO2, 96 Kb, which contains the genes encoding the biosynthesis of the capsule (Uchida et al. 1997). The capsule is a linear polymer of D-glutamic acid, which plays an important role in the ability of anthrax to resist phagocytosis by macrophages.

One of the most important ways to fight anthrax is the prophylactic administration of vaccines to individuals at risk.

27.2 Types of Vaccines

27.2.1 Conventional Anthrax Vaccines

The history of the anthrax vaccine has in Louis Pasteur one of its most important actors. Pasteur demonstrated the

Veterinary Vaccines: Principles and Applications, First Edition. Edited by Samia Metwally, Gerrit Viljoen, and Ahmed El Idrissi.

effectiveness of his vaccine during an experiment at the small French village of Poully-le-Fort in May 1881. He reported:

> In brief, we now possess a vaccine of anthrax which is capable of saving animals from this fatal disease; a virus-vaccine that is itself never lethal; a live vaccine. One that can be cultivated at will and transported without alteration. Finally, this vaccine is prepared by a procedure that we believe can be generalized since, the first time around, this was the method we used to develop a fowl cholera vaccine. Based on all the conditions that I list here, and by looking at everything only from a scientific point of view, the development of a vaccination against anthrax constitutes significant progress beyond the first vaccine developed by Jenner, since the latter had never been obtained experimentally. (Pasteur et al. 2002).

The history and theory of anthrax vaccines for veterinary use are closely linked to the first developments in the science of modern vaccinology. Louis Pasteur, a pioneer in this field, developed the first anthrax vaccine in 1881 (Pasteur et al. 2002). His method was widely used for livestock immunization until the 1930s. Pasteur's schedule consisted of a first inoculation of *B. anthracis* cells from cultures incubated at 42–43 °C for 15–20 days (Pasteur type I) followed by an inoculation, after 14 days, of less attenuated *B. anthracis* cells from cultures incubated at 42–43 °C for 10–12 days (Pasteur type II) (Shlyakhov et al. 1996). The vaccine soon showed limits related to residual virulence and efficacy. This vaccine was administered in a single dose, suspended in a 50% solution of glycerol. The use of saponin as adjuvant, at variable concentrations (1–4%), in Pasteur's type II vaccines was also introduced in this period (Turnbull 1991).

For a while, around 1935, a vaccine named Carbosap was popular. The Carbosap vaccine, initially produced at the *Istituto Sieroterapico Milanese*, was evidently quite effective and consisted of less attenuated strains suspended in a 10% saponin solution. The manufacturing procedure was never revealed, however. Carbosap, a vaccine used in Italy until 2006, belongs to this family of vaccines (Garofolo et al. 2007). Cilli's research group in the *Istituto Vaccinogeno di Asmara* selected the anthrax strain used to produce Carbosap during the Second World War when Carbosap was no longer available in Italy due to supply difficulties (Cilli 1951). Here, too, the method of attenuation is unknown, but probably followed the Carbosap procedure.

Declining potencies and troublesome variations in virulence resulting in loss of vaccinated animals related not only to the virulence of the strains but also to the toxic activity of saponin in certain particularly susceptible species. These were the problems that N. Stamatin in 1931 and M. Sterne in 1937 overcame. Stamatin's anthrax cultures were cultivated and attenuated on horse blood agar. The attenuated colonies were then used for his 1190R vaccine (Shlyakhov et al. 1996). Another vaccine is obtained from the Sterne strain (34F2) by growing the bacterial isolate on 50% horse serum nutrient agar with incubation under 30% CO_2 for 24 hours (Sterne 1937).

Thus, the live attenuated vaccines can be divided into three main categories: Pasteur vaccines, Carbosap vaccine, and Sterne vaccines. The division is not merely historical but based on different attenuation mechanisms (Mikesell et al. 1983). The Pasteur method of attenuation results in loss of the pXO1 plasmid that encodes the major virulence factors (PA, LF, EF), thus producing a nontoxigenic and capsulated (pXO1−, pXO2+) vaccine. The Sterne type is a *B. anthracis* strain lacking the pXO2 plasmid encoding the capsule. It is, therefore, a toxigenic and noncapsulated strain (pXO1+, pXO2−), resulting in a nonvirulent stable phenotype which still conserves the main antigen, anthrax toxins (Hambleton et al. 1984). The Carbosap attenuation mechanism is still unknown, but studies on Carbosap vaccine demonstrated the presence of both plasmids (pXO1+, pXO2+), placing this strain in the category of toxigenic and capsulated and suggesting different mechanisms of attenuation (Fasanella et al. 2001).

Currently, the most used vaccines are Sterne vaccines. The active ingredients of these vaccines are the spores of the 34F2 "Sterne" strain. The Sterne 34F2 strain is a toxigenic and noncapsulated strain and is used worldwide, with the exception of Russia and Romania, where other, analogous toxigenic and noncapsulated strains are used (55-VNIIVV strain and 1190 R Stamatin strain respectively). Generally, the formulation of Sterne vaccine consists of about 10^7 spores suspended either in glycerin with saponin or in physiological solution with saponin (about 1.3×10^7 living spores in 0.1% saponin solution). The Sterne vaccine is undoubtedly the animal anthrax vaccine most widespread in the world. Despite its use for many decades, its mechanism of action is still not quite clear, and although it has never been proven, it is assumed that the injected spores generate the vegetative forms. These vegetative cells proliferate in vaccinated animals but being devoid of the capsule, they are quickly neutralized by the host immune system. However, the cell proliferation cycles, while having a limited time duration, are sufficient to produce a quantity of toxins able to stimulate the production of antibodies that protect the animal. The same toxins are not able to give clinical signs of disease. The Sterne strain 34F2 livestock vaccine has been in use for well over half a century and is frequently administered in response to outbreaks.

As outbreaks generally occur in summer or hotter seasons, pregnant animals are frequently among those vaccinated. Although few cases of side effects have been reported in the recent past, and the vaccination of pregnant and lactating animals appears to be safe, difficulties in the vaccination of wildlife and antibody dynamics remain the weaknesses of the Sterne vaccine. However, live attenuated Sterne vaccine in rabbit models showed that a week after the first vaccination, only 80% of the animals were protected, while 10 days after the second vaccination (carried out 3 weeks after the first), 100% of vaccinated animals were protected (Fasanella et al. 2008). In the same study, it was shown that 6 months after the second vaccination, no animals were protected.

27.2.2 New-Generation Anthrax Vaccines

The first studies on the use of recombinant or edible anthrax vaccines for veterinary use were reported by Fasanella et al. (2008). These proved the efficacy of two experimental vaccines against *B. anthracis* for veterinary use: an rPA mutant vaccine and a trivalent vaccine (TV) composed of rPA, an inactive LF mutant (mLF-Y728A; E735A) and an inactive EF mutant (mEF-K346R), both emulsified with mineral oils. Although this was only a preliminary study in a rabbit model, the possibility of administering these vaccines with antibiotics to halt incubating infections or during an anthrax epidemic was underlined. Preliminary attempts to generate transgenic PA-producing plants successfully explored the possibility to create a safe and protective vaccine (Watson et al. 2004; Brodzik et al. 2005).

An edible vaccine would be useful for the vaccination of herbivores, both domesticated and feral. For example, searching for an alternative, less expensive method to produce PA, a transgenic tobacco chloroplast was developed that expressed the 83 kDa immunogenic *B. anthracis* PA. Crude plant extracts contained up to 2.5 mg full length PA/g of fresh leaf tissue and this showed exceptional stability for several months in stored leaves or crude extracts. The recently demonstrated efficacy of the plant-expressed domain 4 of *B. anthracis* PA opens new horizons for the mass vaccination of animals in areas where the risk of anthrax is high (Gorantala et al. 2011). In fact, follow-up studies have successfully expressed PA in mustard using *Agrobacterium*-mediated transformation and in tobacco using plastid transformation. The PA produced in these crops generates systemic and mucosal immune response upon intraperitoneal or oral immunization. This could be an ideal vaccine fulfilling both human and veterinary vaccination needs.

27.3 Immune Response and Duration of Immunity

The immune response is elicited by the toxins. Toxin formation is known to occur when PA binds to receptors on cells (Bradley et al. 2001; Little et al. 2004a), undergoes proteolysis to expose a binding site for LF or EF (Klimpel et al. 1992), and forms heptamers (Milne et al. 1994). The shared cell-binding component, PA, when combined with LF, forms a lethal toxin, which kills laboratory animals (Stanley and Smith 1961; Beall and Dalldorf 1966) and is cytotoxic to certain macrophage cell lines (Friedlander 1986). When combined with EF, on the other hand, PA forms edema toxin, which causes edema and inhibits neutrophil functions (Stanley and Smith 1961; O'Brien et al. 1985) due to the calmodulin-dependent adenylate cyclase activity of EF (Smith et al. 1955).

Clearly, then, blocking PA leads to the neutralization of the toxic activity of anthrax. The protection of certain animal models (guinea pig, rabbit, nonhuman primate) against infection with *B. anthracis* can be achieved by inoculation with a variety of vaccine preparations that contain PA as their main immunogen (Ivins et al. 1990, 1992, 1998). Moreover, a strong correlation has been found between the level of PA-specific toxin-neutralizing antibodies (TNAs) and protection. Toxin neutralization is probably not the only antibody-mediated mechanism of protection. The kinetics of PA production during *B. anthracis* growth and the role of anti-PA antibody in host immunity are not clearly defined, however. Anti-PA antibodies (Abs) have also been shown to exhibit antispore activities (Stepanov et al. 1996; Welkos et al. 2001; Cote et al. 2005). Rabbit anti-rPA polyclonal Abs (pAbs) were shown to enhance the phagocytosis and subsequent killing of spores by macrophages (Welkos et al. 2001, 2002), and to partially inhibit spore germination *in vitro* (Stepanov et al. 1996; Welkos et al. 2001). Further, PA was found to be associated with spores, and to induce anti-PA Abs that delay germination *in vitro*, and enhance the phagocytic and sporicidal activities of macrophages (Cote et al. 2005).

An important aspect of the protective ability of the immune system is the persistence of PA-specific IgG memory B cells allowing animals to remain resistant to infection even after their serum Ab response has waned (Ivins et al. 1994; Tross and Klinman 2008). In a study on mice, for example, half of the animals immunized with CpG-adjuvanted anthrax vaccine adsorbed (AVA), which developed anti-PA titers 10-fold below the protective baseline, survived a 100 LD_{50} Sterne strain spore challenge. This contrasted with only 1/35 mice with the same Ab titer that had been immunized with AVA alone. These findings suggest that an important goal of anthrax vaccine development should be attaining a vaccine able to generate a durable pool of high-affinity memory B cells (Tross and Klinman 2008).

Another important aspect of immunity concerns T cells, which may play a role beyond simply enhancing adaptive humoral response. Immunization with formaldehyde-inactivated *B. anthracis* spores resulted in the generation of CD4 T lymphocytes, which responded in an MHC-restricted manner by producing interferon (IFN)-γ (Glomski et al. 2007). This suggested that the production of IFN-γ leads to the activation of phagocytes and consequently increases sporicidal and bactericidal activity. IFN-γ was shown to protect up to 60% of mice against lethal inhalational anthrax (Walberg et al. 2008).

Finally, intranasal (IN) immunization of deeply anesthetized rabbits with rPA + IL-1α consistently induced rPA-specific serum IgG enzyme-linked immunosorbent assay (ELISA) titers that were not significantly different from those induced by intramuscular (IM) immunization with rPA + alum, although lethal toxin-neutralizing titers induced by IN immunization were lower than those induced by IM immunization (Gwinn et al. 2010). The generated immune response is also affected by species differences.

27.4 Desired Specifications when Ordering Vaccine

When ordering the vaccine, it is advisable to follow at least the following requirements: (i) the recommended vaccine type is the Sterne strain $34F_2$, (ii) the usable forms are the liquid saline solution, the liquid saponin solution, or the freeze-dried formulation, (iii) the dosage ranges from 10^6 to 10^7 spores per animal, (iv) the vaccine can be used only for cattle, sheep, goats, and horses and vaccines are not specifically produced for use in wild animals, (v) shipping conditions should maintain the cold chain from the manufacturer to the field.

In China and the Russian Federation, live spore vaccines are prepared and licensed for human use. In the USA and UK, acellular, nonliving human vaccines have been produced since the 1950s. The human anthrax vaccines are not publicly available and the four vaccines produced are essentially restricted to specific national needs.

27.5 Quality Assurance and Control

Most veterinary vaccines are manufactured broadly in accordance with the *Requirements for anthrax spore vaccine (live – for veterinary use)*, *Requirements for biological substances No.13* (WHO 1967), the *Manual for the Production of Anthrax and Blackleg Vaccines* (FAO 1991), the *Manual of Diagnostic Tests and Vaccines for Terrestrial Animals* (OIE 2017), *Anthrax in Humans and Animals* (WHO 2008), and the updated European Pharmacopoeia (European Pharmacopoeia 2017).

Accurate control tests must follow the production of Sterne vaccine according to OIE standards. The counting of spores is important to ensure the correct concentration in the vaccine. The vaccine is subjected to a further check for purity control to detect the presence of contaminants, which could be aerobic bacteria, anaerobic bacteria, or fungi. These controls are performed during the vaccine production process and on packed bottles sampled randomly. When the vaccine passes all the quality control tests, a quality certificate is issued. After production, immunological efficacy tests, like ELISA or complement fixation test (CFT), can be performed on vaccinated animals.

27.6 Vaccine Application for Disease Control

27.6.1 Vaccination Strategy

In its natural state, anthrax is primarily a disease of herbivorous animals and therefore its control in both animals and humans depends to a very great extent on its prevention in livestock (principally cattle, sheep, goats, and horses), good hygienic practices when an animal dies of anthrax, and antibiotic treatment when a case occurs.

A key element in animal disease control is the use of safe vaccine, harmless, cheap, and able to induce a complete and rapid protection against the disease. The vaccination strategy may include preventive vaccination of animals or could be part of outbreak management. All animals within a buffer zone, a few to several kilometers wide, around the infected sites should be vaccinated. The vaccine should be provided as soon as possible, with two shots over 2 weeks in order to achieve the right immunological response for combating the disease and avoiding spread of the outbreak. Animals should be quarantined for 20 days after the vaccination is completed. During vaccination, it is important to be careful with the use of antibiotics. In fact, antibiotics given with Sterne vaccine promptly kill the live vaccine and therefore livestock have to be first treated with antibiotics and then vaccinated 7–10 days later when the antibiotic titer in the blood is too low to impact the live Sterne vaccine.

Human anthrax is rare and mainly occupationally related to those people at risk from working with infected wool or skins. In the bioterrorist attack scenario involving anthrax, anthrax vaccine, where available, might be recommended after exposure.

27.6.2 Considering Epidemiological Settings and Objectives

The prevalence of anthrax is declining worldwide due to the action of control programs. However, surveillance is defective in many areas because the disease is rare and the veterinary services are not prompt in recognizing it. On the other hand, anthrax is still prevalent in many natural parks where wildlife are affected, and the disease can complete its life cycle in a natural way. The epidemiology of the disease can be determined by surveillance to identify the presence of contaminated fields. In such areas, long-lasting programs of vaccination for livestock are required. The primary objective in such zones is to achieve a good level of herd immunity to manage the disease and prevent the occurrence of an outbreak.

27.6.3 Possible Combination with Vaccines for Other Diseases

The use of anthrax vaccine in conjunction with other vaccines was proposed and reported by several authors in the past (Griazin et al. 1970; Brown et al. 1976; Pankratov et al. 1977; Odarenko et al. 1978). Anthrax is endemic in most of the countries where small ruminants are reared and where several diseases either with similar ecology or with impact on animal husbandry and animal health are prevalent. The ecology of the disease suggests the possibility of having overlaps with the spore-forming bacteria that cause blackleg and malignant edema.

Reducing the vaccination efforts for dealing with several diseases was the primary objective of public veterinary services in countries with shortage of resources. At present, no official combined vaccine is registered and future studies are needed to test the feasibility of combining antigens for protecting livestock against diseases that occur in the same area.

27.7 Management of Anthrax Outbreaks

It has been proposed to classify anthrax outbreaks based on the source of infection and the risk level for humans (Fasanella et al. 2014). Three different types of animal outbreaks were defined with the most effective procedures for their management and prevention: classic sporadic outbreaks, atypical outbreaks, and epidemic outbreaks.

The classic sporadic outbreak occurs in areas where anthrax is enzootic. These outbreaks are sporadic, and usually involve initially only 1–3 animals. They originate in the soil, causing animals to become infected by grazing in contaminated pastures. Contamination arises from buried infected carcasses or when areas are irrigated with effluents from tanneries, or wool or hair mills. These outbreaks usually occur during the summer and tend to be more frequent during dry summers following brief rain showers, and are limited to alkaline calciferous soils, e.g. black steppe soils. The sporadic outbreaks are the most widespread, and although they represent a serious health problem, they seem to carry a low risk, while in reality maintaining soil recontamination with spores. In fact, in areas where anthrax is enzootic, breeders and veterinarians are usually aware of the disease and it is considered whenever there is an unexpected death. Proper management of an outbreak involves:

- avoiding the dispersion of biological fluids during sample collection
- correct handling of carcasses
- checking the temperatures of all animals and quickly vaccinating animals with normal temperatures that are at risk of infection
- delaying the vaccination of animals with suspected illness and initiating antibiotic treatment
- vaccinating these latter animals 10 days after suspension of antibiotic treatment
- performing a genotypic analysis of the isolated strain(s) to verify the origin of infection
- suspending the sale of milk and meat from animals on the infected farm for 10 days after vaccination or the last known death.

To prevent this type of outbreak, measures to reduce environmental contamination must be taken. These include:

- implementing programs of annual herd vaccination, especially of known affected herds and animals on adjoining farms
- identification of areas at risk through environmental analysis
- avoiding producing forage on soils with high levels of contamination
- compensating farmers who report illness and do not slaughter sick animals
- sensitizing stakeholders: farmers, butchers, veterinarians, and physicians
- training and information, with particular reference to school students and rural populations living in high-risk areas.

The atypical outbreak is associated with the use of forages (e.g. hay, silage) produced on contaminated land and with products of animal origin such as inadequately sterilized meat and bone meals derived from the infected carcasses. These products are very dangerous because they can cause unexpected anthrax outbreaks in conditions and situations epidemiologically very different from the classic episodes of telluric origin. The risk factors associated with atypical anthrax outbreaks can be identified as follows:

- they may occur in areas where the disease is unknown, or has disappeared, or has been eradicated for many years
- they can occur at any time of the year and in epidemiological situations very different from the classic form
- typically they involve animals that are not on pasture but are housed and receiving supplemental feeds, e.g. pigs, and dairy cows in winter or monsoon seasons
- simultaneous outbreaks may occur on several nonadjoining farms in the same area, or on distant farms sharing the same contaminated feed source.

Atypical anthrax outbreaks are the most dangerous to humans, especially when they develop in areas considered free of risk and where the disease is forgotten. The worst risk is an incorrect animal diagnosis that can result in humans becoming infected due to mismanagement of the carcasses, e.g. skinning. Another aspect that should not be underestimated is that physicians, not knowing the disease, may give a wrong diagnosis, with serious consequences for the patient's health. The management of this kind of outbreak is even more difficult in areas where the disease is unknown, because a correct diagnosis nearly always comes with a certain delay. The following steps must be taken:

- avoiding the dispersion of biological fluids during sample collection
- correct handling of carcasses, such as incineration, hollowing and site boundaries
- immediately ceasing the use of suspect feeds
- carrying out laboratory tests on samples of suspect feeds
- informing the sanitary authorities, which will prohibit the sale of the suspect feed until certified sterilization can be instituted in relation to meat and bone meals
- checking the temperatures of all animals and quickly vaccinating all animals at risk of infection with normal temperatures
- delaying the vaccination of animals with suspected illness and initiating antibiotic treatment
- vaccinating these latter animals 10 days after suspension of antibiotic treatment
- performing a genotypic analysis of the isolated strain and verifying its correspondence with the strains isolated at the origin of the forage
- suspending the sale of milk and meat from animals on the infected farm for 10 days after vaccination or the last known death.

This form of the disease is very difficult to predict and prevent but when the potential is recognized, farmers and ranchers can be quickly warned of the risk, and when it involves contaminated feedstuffs, a program for overseeing and certified sterilization can be put in place. Regular monitoring of meat and bone meals is more cost-effective than reactive livestock vaccination. A proper epidemiological investigation is needed in order to verify that animals have not been fed with fodder from areas at risk or with supplemental bone meal. The hallmark is when the outbreak occurs at a time or place where the disease is not usually seen outside the known surveillance areas.

Epidemic outbreaks are an evolution of the classic sporadic form due to the activities of hemophagic flies. Tabanids feeding on moribund animals, especially during the bacteremic phase, are able to transfer the pathogen to healthy animals in the same or neighboring herds, causing a disease characterized by extensive edema. However, under the right circumstances it can result in isolated cases stretching up to 10–15 km from the source outbreak. However, the danger for humans comes from bites by disease-carrying insects. A cutaneous case of human anthrax due to the bite of a horse fly has been reported (Fasanella et al. 2013a).

The features of epidemic anthrax outbreaks are:

- it develops in areas where the disease is enzootic and where vaccination programs may have been suspended or have never been implemented
- characteristically, they follow heavier than usual winter or spring rains, resulting in a markedly increased fly hatch, and a triggering sporadic outbreak but with some 4–6 or more animals sick or dead before veterinary help is sought by the owner
- it occurs at the end of summer, erratically as a result of a coincidental hatch of flies, and is characterized by many outbreaks involving an extensive area and a large number of animals.

The management of these outbreaks is not easy because it requires measures to block the spread of bacteria:

- avoid the dispersion of biological fluids during sample collection
- correct handling of carcasses, such as incineration, and hollowing site boundaries

- mass vaccination of animals in at least a 15 km radius of the index outbreak
- quarantine in insect-proof buildings for animals with suspected septicemia to avoid contact with the blood-sucking insects or, if not possible, sprinkle the body of animals with insect repellent
- antibiotic treatment of animals with suspected illness
- vaccination of animals after verifying that body temperature is normal
- a second vaccination 2 weeks after the first
- suspend handling of animals to minimize stress
- greater attention by physicians to possible increases of skin lesions in the exposed population.

To prevent this type of outbreak it is necessary to adopt the measures used to prevent the classic anthrax outbreaks.

27.8 Anthrax Vaccines for Wildlife

When outbreaks occur in wildlife, circumstances are likely to be very different, and a description of all eventualities is beyond the scope of this chapter. Sporadic cases in large wildlife conservation areas are likely to be seen as being of consequence only if livestock are at risk. Even with bigger outbreaks, in those large wildlife national parks from which livestock are excluded and which have "hands off" management policies for all but emergency situations, control actions may be regarded as interference with natural processes. Each area that encounters anthrax, or knows it is at risk of encountering anthrax, should have an action plan in place in line with its management policies and particular needs (Clegg 2006). In these areas, managing anthrax outbreaks is challenging because of either the unavailability of vaccine licensed for wildlife or the impossibility of vaccinating free-ranging animals. In natural parks, the management of anthrax cases should prevent transmission of the infection from dead animals to live ones.

Vaccines are not specifically produced for use in wild animals, but regional wildlife veterinarians and staff use some of the available vaccines in order to vaccinate wild animals. India and Myanmar include elephants in their schedules, albeit referring to domesticated representatives of the species. Although the prescribed method of administration of the vaccine in livestock is, with rare exceptions, the subcutaneous route, frequently wildlife vaccination is carried out using darts, thereby administering the vaccine intramuscularly. Seemingly, this is both effective and not dangerous for the animals (de Vos 1990; de Vos and Scheepers 1996; Turnbull et al. 2004).

27.9 Monitoring and Vaccine Effectiveness

27.9.1 Postvaccination Monitoring

Serological tests, which do not have a great diagnostic value, proved to be very useful epidemiological and research tools to evaluate the seroconversion following vaccination or naturally acquired infection (Turnbull et al. 1992; Quinn et al. 2004). ELISA and CFTs on livestock are useful to obtain epidemiological information in areas where the disease is endemic and to evaluate the efficacy of vaccination (Adone et al. 2016). However, there is still a general paucity of information related to the onset, kinetics, and magnitude of antibody response induced by vaccination in humans and animals. Effective serological tests should be satisfactory in terms of sensitivity and specificity, not expensive, and easy to standardize. The availability of diagnostic methods alternative to experimental infection could avoid the need for containment equipment and facilities that are required to reduce the risks for personnel exposed to biosafety level 3 agents (Little et al. 2004b).

Recently, Adone et al. (2016) conducted a study which evaluated the suitability of a Sterne-based CFT for the detection of specific antibodies in laboratory and target animals vaccinated with Sterne 34F2. They evaluated its specificity and sensitivity by testing unvaccinated and vaccinated animals, respectively, at different sampling times. The CFT results indicated that specific antibodies induced by vaccination with Sterne 34F2 did not persist over a long period of time (150 days after the first vaccination) in cattle (Adone et al. 2016). In many studies, conducted in cattle and goats, the antibody response following vaccination against anthrax was monitored using a PA-based ELISA, currently accepted as the best serological procedure, and different antibody kinetics were observed (Dipti et al. 2013; Roy et al. 2013; Hassan et al. 2015). The test utilizes purified toxin antigens PA and LF whose preparation is expensive and poorly standardized for purity, composition of antigens, and preparation procedure. Moreover, reference standard serum is not available. Furthermore, the comparison of serological data is very difficult since many factors affect the immune response of animals, such as the vaccine type, the age of vaccination, and, mostly, the health status of animals (Iowa Beef Center 2015).

27.9.2 Outbreaks in Vaccinated Animals

Questions arise from time to time regarding cases of anthrax that occur in herds which have been vaccinated, or about continuing cases after vaccination to control outbreaks. Kaufmann et al. (1973) investigated an outbreak involving more than 4000 cattle, and found that 0.1% died 8–14 days after vaccination and another 0.1% more than 15 days after vaccination. In the outbreak of 1987 described by Salmon and Ferrier (1992), five out of 10 deaths occurred 3, 5, 11, 68, and 126 days after vaccination and, in another case, 37 days after revaccination. In Africa, livestock owners know that some of their animals may still die after vaccination and this may lead to distrust of vaccination and resistance to it being done. Usually, it is not possible to identify the specific reasons for these vaccine failures. A possible reason that should be considered in the event of vaccine failures is that the potency of the vaccine itself has fallen for reasons beyond the control of the person or team carrying out the vaccination (WHO 2008).

27.10 Vaccine Adverse Reactions

The vaccine is widely used and adverse reactions have never been reported, except some rare reporting in horses, goats, and llamas. The vaccine appears to be safe in pregnant animals (Berrier & Hugh-Jones, personal communication, 2006).

27.11 Availability and List of Manufacturers

A complete list of manufacturers of livestock anthrax vaccine is in Annex 5, Table 18 of *Anthrax in Humans and Animals*, 4th edition. Geneva: World Health Organization, 2008.

27.12 Summary

The bioterrorist attack of 2001 heightened interest in the development of new vaccines against anthrax. It must not be forgotten, however, that anthrax is, first and foremost, a dangerous zoonosis. Having almost disappeared in most industrialized countries, sporadic anthrax outbreaks tend to occur where, in the past, infected animals had been buried, or associated with leather industry waste. Anthrax still represents a health problem in several nonindustrialized countries. A massive outbreak occurred in Zimbabwe between 1978 and 1980 (Davies 1982). In Bangladesh, between July and September 2010, there were 107 animal cases and 607 associated human cases (Fasanella et al. 2013b).

The Sterne vaccine is less expensive than recombinant vaccines and represents the best vaccine for routine anthrax control programs, especially if it is administered between April and May, to ensure the presence of protective immunity between August and October, when most anthrax outbreaks occur.

New vaccines should aim to improve mass vaccination programs in poor regions of the world. Research on the stability of anthrax vaccines is crucial, due to the long distances between the places where vaccines are produced and the remote areas where they are often needed. In the past, very little attention was paid to the improvement of anthrax vaccines for veterinary use. The effective control of animal anthrax requires the use of thoroughly protective vaccines, an objective which has so far not been attained. The Sterne vaccine still represents the best vaccine for routine anthrax control programs but not for emergency situations, where the recombinant PA vaccine seems more efficacious (Santra et al. 2005).

One of the advantages of recombinant vaccines is that they can be given simultaneously with antibiotics during anthrax outbreaks. Antibiotics given with Sterne, on the other hand, promptly kill the live vaccine. However, at the time of writing the recombinant vaccine for veterinary use is not publicly available, making the latter practice impracticable.

Finally, veterinary science should not refrain from exploring new biotechnologies, even those that were not originally developed for veterinary use. As new vaccination technologies become available and increasingly affordable, these should be applied to livestock for validation, so that they can be approved for widespread use. Another field of research on vaccines which needs to be developed is the standardization of a serological test able to identify the "protection parameter" induced by anthrax vaccine. The protective activity of anthrax vaccines mainly depends on their ability to elicit antibodies directed to toxin components (Little et al. 1997; Beedham et al. 2001; Reuveny et al. 2001; Kobiler et al. 2002). However, little is known on the effective duration of immunity, even if many studies have demonstrated the decline of the specific antibody response and the need for different vaccination schedules to ensure protection. New, improved livestock vaccines should be developed that induce a high level of protective antibodies in a very short time and which could be administered with long-acting antibiotics in the face of anthrax outbreaks and emergencies (Welkos et al. 2001; Fasanella et al. 2008; WHO 2008).

References

Adone, R., Sali, M., Francia, M. et al. (2016). Development of a Sterne-based complement fixation test to monitor the Humoral response induced by anthrax vaccines. *Front. Microbiol.* 7: 19.

Beall, F.A. and Dalldorf, F.G. (1966). The pathogenesis of the lethal effect of anthrax toxin in the rat. *J. Infect. Dis.* 116 (3): 377–389.

Beedham, R.J., Turnbull, P.C.B., and Williamson, E.D. (2001). Passive transfer of protection against *Bacillus anthracis* infection in a murine model. *Vaccine* 19: 4409–4416.

Berger, T., Kassirer, M., and Aran, A. (2014). Injectional anthrax – new presentation of an old disease. *Eurosurveillance* 19: 1–11.

Bradley, K.A., Mogridge, J., Mourez, M. et al. (2001). Identification of the cellular receptor for anthrax toxin. *Nature* 414 (6860): 225–229.

Brodzik, R., Bandurska, K., Deka, D. et al. (2005). Advances in alfalfa mosaic virus-mediated expression of anthrax antigen in planta. *Biochem. Biophys. Res. Commun.* 338: 717–722.

Brown, K.K., Parizek, R.E., and Stewart, R.C. (1976). Prevention of clostridial disease in cattle and sheep by vaccination with a multivalent bacterin-toxoid. *Vet. Med. Small Anim. Clin.* 71 (12): 1717–1722.

Cilli, V. (1951). Rassegna delle attività svolte dall'istituto vaccinogeno zooprofilattico di Asmara. In: *Archivio di scienze mediche tropicali e di parassitologia*, vol. XXXII, 135–138. Rome: Alto Commissariato per l'igiene e la sanità pubblica.

Clegg, S.B. (2006). Wildlife anthrax epizootic workshop working group. Preparedness for anthrax epizootics in wildlife areas [conference summary]. *Emerg. Infect. Dis.* https://doi.org/10.3201/eid1207.060458.

Cote, C.K., Rossi, C.A., Kang, A.S. et al. (2005). The detection of protective antigen (PA) associated with spores of *Bacillus anthracis* and the effects of anti-PA antibodies on spore germination and macrophage interactions. *Microb. Pathog.* 38 (5-6): 209–225.

Davies, J.C. (1982). A major epidemic of anthrax in Zimbabwe. *Cent. Afr. J. Med.* 28 (12): 291–298.

De Vos, V. (1990). The ecology of anthrax in the Kruger National Park, South Africa. *Salisbury Med. Bull.* 68S: 19–23.

De Vos, V. and Scheepers, G.J. (1996). Remote mass vaccination of large free-ranging wild animals for anthrax using Sterne spore vaccine. *Salisbury Med. Bull.* 87S: 116–121.

Dipti, M., Rashid, M.M., Ferdoush, M.J. et al. (2013). Morphological and immunological characterization of anthrax vaccine in cattle. *Bangladesh J. Vet. Med.* 11: 43–49.

European Pharmacopoeia. (2017). Anthrax spore vaccine (live) for veterinary use. No. 0441.

Fasanella, A., Losito, S., Trotta, T. et al. (2001). Detection of anthrax vaccine virulence factors by polymerase chain reaction. *Vaccine* 19: 4214–4218.

Fasanella, A., Tonello, F., Garofolo, G. et al. (2008). Protective activity and immunogenicity of two recombinant anthrax vaccines for veterinary use. *Vaccine* 26: 5684–5688.

Fasanella, A., Galante, D., Garofolo, G., and Jones, M.H. (2010). Anthrax undervalued zoonosis. *Vet. Microbiol.* 140 (3-4): 318–331.

Fasanella, A., Garofolo, G., Galella, M. et al. (2013a). Suspect vector transmission of human cutaneous anthrax during an animal outbreak in southern Italy. *Vector Borne Zoonotic Dis.* 13 (10): 769–771.

Fasanella, A., Garofolo, G., Hossain, M.J. et al. (2013b). Bangladesh anthrax outbreaks are probably caused by contaminated livestock feed. *Epidemiol. Infect.* 141 (5): 1021–1028.

Fasanella, A., Adone, R., and Hugh-Jones, M.E. (2014). Classification and management of animal anthrax outbreaks based on the source of infection. *Ann. Ist. Super. Sanità* 50 (2): 192–195.

Food and Agriculture Organization (FAO). (1991). Manual for the production of anthrax and blackleg vaccines. www.fao.org/docrep/004/T0278E/T0278E00.HTM

Friedlander, A.M. (1986). Macrophages are sensitive to anthrax lethal toxin through an acid-dependent process. *J. Biolumin. Chemilumin.* 261 (16): 7123–7126.

Garofolo, G., Fasanella, A., Chiocco, D. et al. (2007). Il vaccino vivo "Sterne" nella profilassi del carbonchio ematico in Italia. www.ordiniveterinaripiemonte.it/rivista/07n09/pdf/04.pdf

Glomski, I.J., Corre, J.P., Mock, M., and Goossens, P.L. (2007). Cutting edge: IFN-gamma-producing CD4 T lymphocytes mediate spore-induced immunity to capsulated *Bacillus anthracis*. *J. Immunol.* 178 (5): 2646–2650.

Gorantala, J., Grover, S., Goel, D. et al. (2011). A plant based protective antigen [PA(dIV)] vaccine expressed in chloroplasts demonstrates protective immunity in mice against anthrax. *Vaccine* 29 (27): 4521–4533.

Griazin, V.I., Sal'nikov, F.E., Pankratov, L.D. et al. (1970). Combined vaccines against brucellosis and anthrax in sheep. *Veterinariia* 7: 38–40.

Gwinn, W.M., Kirwan, S.M., Wang, S.H. et al. (2010). Effective induction of protective systemic immunity with nasally administered vaccines adjuvanted with IL-1. *Vaccine* 28 (42): 6901–6914.

Hambleton, P., Carman, J.A., and Melling, J. (1984). Anthrax: the disease in relation to vaccines. *Vaccine* 2: 125–132.

Hassan, J., Rahman, M.B., Chowdhury, S.M.Z.H. et al. (2015). ELISA based anthrax antibody titer in cattle induced by locally prepared anthrax vaccine originated from sterne F-24 strain in Bangladesh. *Microbes Health* 4: 36–38.

Hudson, M.J., Beyer, W., Böhm, R. et al. (2008). *Bacillus anthracis*: balancing innocent research with dual-use potential. *Int. J. Med. Microbiol.* 298 (5-6): 345–364.

Iowa Beef Center. (2015). Beef Cattle Handbook. www.iowabeefcenter.org/bch/TraceMineralsImmunology.pdf

Ivins, B.E., Welkos, S.L., Knudson, G.B., and Little, S.F. (1990). Immunization against anthrax with aromatic compound-dependent (Aro-) mutants of *Bacillus anthracis* and with recombinant strains of *Bacillus subtilis* that produce anthrax protective antigen. *Infect. Immun.* 58 (2): 303–308.

Ivins, B.E., Welkos, S.L., Little, S.F. et al. (1992). Immunization against anthrax with *Bacillus anthracis* protective antigen combined with adjuvants. *Infect. Immun.* 60 (2): 662–668.

Ivins, B.E., Fellows, P.F., and Nelson, G.O. (1994). Efficacy of a standard human anthrax vaccine against *Bacillus anthracis* spore challenge in Guinea-pigs. *Vaccine* 12 (10): 872–874.

Ivins, B.E., Pitt, M.L., Fellows, P.F. et al. (1998). Comparative efficacy of experimental anthrax vaccine candidates against inhalation anthrax in rhesus macaques. *Vaccine* 16 (11-12): 1141–1148.

Jackson, P.J., Hugh-Jones, M.E., Adair, D.M. et al. (1998). PCR analysis of tissue samples from the 1979 Sverdlovsk anthrax victims: the presence of multiple *Bacillus anthracis* strains in different victims. *Proc. Natl. Acad. Sci. U.S.A.* 95 (3): 1224–1229.

Jernigan, D.B., Raghunathan, P.L., Bell, B.P. et al. (2002). Investigation of bioterrorism-related anthrax, United States, 2001: epidemiologic findings. National Anthrax Epidemiologic Investigation Team. *Emerg. Infect. Dis.* 8 (10): 1019–1028.

Kaufmann, A.F., Fox, M.D., and Kolb, R.C. (1973). Anthrax in Louisiana, 1971: an evaluation of the Sterne strain anthrax vaccine. *J. Am. Vet. Med. Assoc.* 163 (5): 442–445.

Klimpel, K.R., Molloy, S.S., Thomas, G., and Leppla, S.H. (1992). Anthrax toxin protective antigen is activated by a cell surface protease with the sequence specificity and catalytic properties of furin. *Proc. Natl. Acad. Sci. U.S.A.* 89 (21): 10277–10281.

Kobiler, D., Gozes, Y., Rosenberg, H. et al. (2002). Efficiency of protection of Guinea pigs against infection with *Bacillus anthracis* spores by passive immunization. *Infect. Immunol.* 70: 544–550.

Little, S.F., Ivins, B.E., Fellows, P.F., and Friedlander, A.M. (1997). Passive protection by polyclonal antibodies against *Bacillus anthracis* infection in Guinea pigs. *Infect. Immun.* 65: 5171–5175.

Little, S.F., Webster, W.M., Ivins, B.E. et al. (2004a). Development of an in vitro-based potency assay for anthrax vaccine. *Vaccine* 22: 2843–2852.

Little, S.F., Ivins, B.E., Fellows, P.F. et al. (2004b). Defining a serological correlate of protection in rabbits for a recombinant anthrax vaccine. *Vaccine* 22 (3-4): 422–430.

Meselson, M., Guillemin, J., Hugh-Jones, M. et al. (1994). The Sverdlovsk anthrax outbreak of 1979. *Science* 266 (5188): 1202–1208.

Mikesell, P., Ivins, B.E., Ristroph, J.D., and Dreier, T.M. (1983). Evidence for plasmid-mediated toxin production in *Bacillus anthracis*. *Infect. Immun.* 39: 371–376.

Milne, J.C., Furlong, D., Hanna, P.C. et al. (1994). Anthrax protective antigen forms oligomers during intoxication of mammalian cells. *J. Biolumin. Chemilumin.* 269 (32): 20607–20612.

O'Brien, J., Friedlander, A., Dreier, T. et al. (1985). Effects of anthrax toxin components on human neutrophils. *Infect. Immun.* 47 (1): 306–310.

Odarenko, K.I., Zhanuzakov, K.I., Zadorozhnyi, K.I. et al. (1978). Associated vaccine against anthrax and blackleg. *Veterinariia* 7: 49–51.

OIE. (2017). Manual of Diagnostic Tests and Vaccines for Terrestrial Animals. www.oie.int/en/international-standard-setting/terrestrial-manual/access-online

Okinaka, R.T., Cloud, K., Hampton, O. et al. (1999). Sequence and organization of pXO1, the large *Bacillus anthracis* plasmid harboring the anthrax toxin genes. *J. Bacteriol.* 181 (20): 6509–6515.

Pankratov, L.D., Oreshkin, A.S., and Gorelov, I.M. (1977). Testing of an associated vaccine against anthrax and infectious ovine enterotoxemia. *Veterinaria* 2: 38–39.

Pasteur, L., Chamberland, C., and Roux, E. (2002). Summary report of the experiments conducted at Pouilly-le-fort, near Melun, on the anthrax vaccination, 1881. *Yale J. Biol. Med.* 75 (1): 59–62.

Quinn, C.P., Dull, P.M., Semenova, V. et al. (2004). Immune responses to *Bacillus anthracis* protective antigen in individuals with bioterrorism-associated cutaneous and inhalation anthrax. *J. Infect. Dis.* 190: 1228–1236.

Reuveny, S., White, M.D., Adar, Y.Y. et al. (2001). Search of correlates of protective immunity conferred by anthrax vaccine. *Infect. Immunol.* 69: 2888–2893.

Roy, P., Rashid, M.M., Ferdoush, M.J. et al. (2013). Biochemical and immunological characterization of anthrax spore vaccine in goat. *Bangladesh J. Vet. Med.* 11: 151–157.

Salmon, D.D. and Ferrier, G.R. (1992). Post-vaccination occurrence of anthrax in cattle. *Vet. Rec.* 130: 140–141.

Santra, S., Seaman, M.S., Xu, L. et al. (2005). Replication-defective adenovirus serotype 5 vectors elicit durable cellular and humoral immune responses in nonhuman primates. *J. Virol.* 79: 6512–6522.

Shlyakhov, E., Blancou, J., and Rubinstein, E. (1996). Vaccines against anthrax in animals, from Louis Pasteur to our day. *Rev. Sci. Tech.* 15: 853–862.

Smith, H., Keppie, J., and Stanley, J.l. (1955). The chemical basis of the virulence of *Bacillus anthracis*. V. The specific toxin produced by B. anthracis in vivo. *Br. J. Exp. Pathol.* 36 (5): 460–472.

Stanley, J.l. and Smith, H. (1961). Purification of factor I and recognition of a third factor of the anthrax toxin. *J. Gen. Microbiol.* 26: 49–63.

Stepanov, A.V., Marinin, L.I., Pomerantsev, A.P., and Staritsin, N.A. (1996). Development of novel vaccines against anthrax in man. *J. Biotechnol.* 44 (1-3): 155–160.

Sterne, M. (1937). The effects of different carbon dioxide concentration on the growth of virulent anthrax strains. Pathogenicity and immunity tests on Guinea pigs and sheep with anthrax variants derived from virulent strains Onderstepoort. *J. Vet. Sci. An. Ind.* 9: 49–67.

Tross, D. and Klinman, D.M. (2008). Effect of CpG oligonucleotides on vaccine-induced B cell memory. *J. Immunol.* 181 (8): 5785–5790.

Turnbull, P.C. (1991). Anthrax vaccines: past, present and future. *Vaccine* 9: 533–539.

Turnbull, P.C., Doganay, M., Lindeque, P.M. et al. (1992). Serology and anthrax in humans, livestock and Etosha National Park wildlife. *Epidemiol. Infect.* 108: 299–313.

Turnbull, P.C., Tindall, B.W., Coetzee, J.D. et al. (2004). Vaccine-induced protection against anthrax in cheetah (*Acinonyx jubatus*) and black rhinoceros (*Diceros bicornis*). *Vaccine* 22: 3340–3347.

Uchida, I., Sou-ichi, M., Tsutomu, S., and Nobuyuki, T. (1997). Cross-talk to the genes for *Bacillus anthracis* capsule synthesis by atxA, the gene encoding the frans-activator of anthrax toxin synthesis. *Mol. Microbiol.* 23 (6): 1229–1240.

Walberg, K., Baron, S., Poast, J. et al. (2008). Interferon protects mice against inhalation anthrax. *J. Interferon Cytokine Res.* 28 (10): 597–601.

Watson, J., Koya, V., Leppla, S.H., and Daniell, H. (2004). Expression of *Bacillus anthracis* protective antigen in transgenic chloroplasts of tobacco, a non-food/feed crop. *Vaccine* 22: 4374–4384.

Welkos, S., Little, S., Friedlander, A. et al. (2001). The role of antibodies to *Bacillus anthracis* and anthrax toxin components in inhibiting the early stages of infection by anthrax spores. *Microbiology* 147 (6): 1677–1685.

Welkos, S., Friedlander, A., Weeks, S. et al. (2002). In-vitro characterisation of the phagocytosis and fate of anthrax spores in macrophages and the effects of anti-PA antibody. *J. Med. Microbiol.* 51 (10): 821–831.

World Health Organization (WHO). (1967). Requirements for anthrax spore vaccine (live for veterinary use) (requirements for biological substances 13). Geneva: World Health Organization.

World Health Organization (WHO). (2008). *Anthrax in Humans and Animals*, 4e. Geneva: World Health Organization www.who.int/csr/resources/publications/AnthraxGuidelines2008/en

28

Capripox (Lumpy Skin Disease, Sheep Pox, and Goat Pox)

Eeva Tuppurainen[1], Charles Lamien[2], and Adama Diallo[3]

[1] *Friedrich-Loeffler-Institut, Greifswald, Germany*
[2] *Animal Health, Animal Production and Health Laboratory, Joint FAO/IAEA Division of Nuclear Techniques in Food and Agriculture, Department of Nuclear Sciences and Applications, International Atomic Energy Agency, Vienna, Austria*
[3] *ISRA/LNERV, Dakar Hann, Senegal*

28.1 Introduction

Lumpy skin disease (LSD), sheep pox (SPP), and goat pox (GTP) are economically important pox diseases of domestic ruminants caused by lumpy skin disease virus (LSDV), sheep pox virus (SPPV), and goat pox virus (GTPV). These three viruses compose the genus *Capripoxvirus* within the family Poxviridae. Due to the direct and indirect economic losses caused by capripoxvirus (CaPV) outbreaks, these are categorized as notifiable diseases by the World Organization for Animal Health (OIE) which provides recommendations for international trade standards in the LSD chapter (11.9) and SPP/GTP chapter (14.9) of the *Terrestrial Animal Health Code* (OIE 2018a) and for diagnostic assays and vaccines in the LSD chapter (3.4.12) and SPP/GTP chapter (3.7.12) of the *Manual of Diagnostic Tests and Vaccines for Terrestrial Animals* (OIE 2018b).

Currently, LSD is widespread throughout the African continent, excluding Morocco, Algeria, Tunisia, and Libya. Between 2012 and 2015, the disease spread across the Middle East and was reported by Israel, the Palestinian Autonomous Territories, Jordan, Lebanon, Kuwait, Saudi Arabia, Oman, Bahrain, Iran, and Iraq. Turkey was affected in 2013 and in late 2014, and the first cases were detected in the northern part of Cyprus from where it was swiftly eradicated by vaccination. In 2014, LSD spread to the Caucasus region, first to Azerbaijan, then to Georgia, south-western parts of the Russian Federation, Armenia, and Kazakhstan. Within south-east Europe, Greece was affected first in 2015, followed by Bulgaria, the Republic of North Macedonia, Kosovo region, Montenegro, Serbia, and Albania in 2016. In 2019, LSD outbreaks were reported in China, Bangladesh, and India.

In Africa, SPP and GTP occur from North Africa to Tanzania and the Democratic Republic of Congo. Their endemic zone is across the Middle East and the Indian subcontinent, Iran, Iraq, southern Russia, Kazakhstan, Kyrgyzstan, Afghanistan, Pakistan, Nepal, Mongolia, China, Bangladesh, Vietnam, and Chinese Taipei. SPP and GTP are widespread in Turkey and between 2013 and 2015, four outbreaks of SPP occurred in Bulgaria and several outbreaks were reported in Greece in 2014, and again in 2017.

28.1.1 Characteristic Clinical Signs

The incubation period of LSDV varies from 4 days to 5 weeks (Haig 1957) and is defined for official purposes as 28 days (OIE 2018a). About a week after infection, animals start to show ocular and nasal discharges and high fever. Highly characteristic skin lesions of 10–50 mm in diameter start to appear. The number of nodules varies from a few in mild cases to multiple nodules, covering the entire body, in severely affected animals. Enlarged subscapular and precrural lymph nodes can be detected at the onset of fever.

The incubation period for SPPV and GTPV is between 4 days and 2 weeks. Infection starts with nasal and ocular discharges and pyrexia (40–42 °C). Affected animals show laborious breathing, depression, and loss of appetite. Skin lesions develop first on the face, around the lips, nares, and on the eyelids. Skin nodules progress until a scab forms on top of the lesion. In severe cases, pox lesions may cover the whole body, but are more easily detected under the tail, on the belly, and on the mammary glands, where the hairless parts are.

Veterinary Vaccines: Principles and Applications, First Edition. Edited by Samia Metwally, Gerrit Viljoen, and Ahmed El Idrissi.

Typically, for all CaPV diseases, small necrotic plaques appear on the tongue and oral and nasal mucous membranes. Nasal discharges and saliva contain infectious virus. Lesions may also be found throughout the digestive and respiratory tracts and on the surface of almost any internal organ. LSDV may cause very painful ulcerative lesions in the cornea of one or both eyes, leading in some severe cases to blindness.

Pneumonia, caused by the virus itself or by secondary bacterial infection(s), is a common complication in severely affected cattle, sheep, and goats. Deep necrotic skin lesions in the legs and on top of the joints may become complicated with secondary bacterial infections, leading to lameness. Infected females often show mastitis and abortions. Fly strike may occur in skin ulcers.

28.1.2 Virulence and Host Specificity

For LSD, the morbidity rate varies between 5% and 45% and the mortality rate usually remains below 10%. However, both rates can be considerably higher (morbidity up to 100%) when an outbreak occurs for the first time in naïve European cattle breeds (Coetzer 2004). Highly infectious SPPV and GTPV may cause very high morbidity of 70–90% and mortality up to 50%. Young lambs and kids are especially susceptible and mortality among young animals may sometimes rise to 100% (Rao and Bandyopadhyay 2000). The virulence of different strains may vary to some extent, but the severity of the clinical disease depends more often on the host species, breed, age, immune status, and stage of production. European high-producing dairy cattle and sheep breeds, as well as animals in the peak of production, are often more severely affected.

In general, CaPVs are relatively host specific, causing clinical disease in either sheep, goats, or cattle. However, exceptions exist and some SPPV and GTPV strains can affect both sheep and goats. Interestingly, in a recent molecular study, GTPV was found to be solely responsible for all investigated outbreaks in both sheep and goats in Ethiopia (Gelaye et al. 2015). Recently, GTPV infection in wild ruminants, red serow (*Capricornis rubidus*), has been reported in Mizoram, India (Dutta et al. 2019).

Lumpy skin disease virus infects domestic cattle and Asian water buffalo (El-Nahas et al. 2011) while some strains may replicate in sheep and goats. The role of wildlife in the epidemiology of LSD is not well understood. Springbok (Lamien et al. 2011), impala, and giraffe (Young et al. 1970) are known to be susceptible and African buffaloes have been found to be seropositive (Davies 1982; Fagbo et al. 2014). In addition, antibodies have been detected in various wild ruminants, such as blue wildebeest, eland, giraffe, impala, and greater kudu (Barnard 1997).

28.1.3 Epidemiology

Transmission of LSDV is believed to occur mainly mechanically by blood-sucking insect and tick vectors, feeding frequently on cattle. The most important arthropod vector is likely to vary between affected regions, depending on the climate, season, environmental temperature, humidity, and vegetation, favorable for the biology of different insect and tick species.

The common stable fly (*Stomoxys calcitrans*) or other biting flies, mosquitoes, or midges have been the suspected vectors for spreading LSDV, although actual experimental evidence on the potential role of different blood-feeding insect species is still lacking. To date, only transmission of the virus by female *Aedes aegypti* mosquitoes has been experimentally demonstrated (Chihota et al. 2001). New studies are ongoing to investigate the vector capacity of different insects and more research data are expected to become available soon.

Tick vectors are likely to be of more importance in African environments than, for example, in the Middle East. Experimental evidence has been obtained on the role of the African brown ear tick (*Rhipicephalus appendiculatus*) (Tuppurainen et al. 2013a) and African bont tick (*Amblyomma hebraeum*) males (Tuppurainen et al. 2011; Lubinga et al. 2013) as well as African blue tick (*R.* [*Boophilus*] *decoloratus*) females (Tuppurainen et al. 2013b). Further proof on the transovarial mode of LSDV transmission by *R. annulatus* ticks has been reported by an Egyptian research group that collected engorged females from LSD-infected cattle, allowed females to oviposit, and were then able to isolate a live LSDV from subsequent larvae using chorioallantoic membranes of embryonated chicken eggs (Rouby et al. 2017). To date, no evidence on the actual multiplication of LSDV either in insect or tick vectors exists.

The efficiency of LSDV transmission by direct contact is believed to be relatively low. Infection can be transmitted through contaminated feed or water. LSDV is known to persist in semen of infected bulls and, therefore, natural mating or artificial insemination may be a source of infection for cows (Annandale et al. 2013). In the field, infected cows are known to give birth to calves with skin nodules (Rouby and Aboulsoud 2016). Iatrogenic transmission may happen when already infected herds are vaccinated or veterinary treatments are administrated without changing needles between animals.

Due to vector transmission, LSD spreads more easily during hot and humid seasons, although sporadic cases or outbreaks have also been reported during the vector-free season, such as during the most recent outbreaks in Georgia, Greece, and Albania. Typically, in endemic regions, LSD outbreaks occur in epidemics, with several years between the outbreaks (Davies 1991). Reemergence of the disease is likely to be associated with uncontrolled animal movements, accumulation of sufficient numbers of naïve animals, and abundance of blood-feeding vectors, generating favorable conditions for viral spread. It is not known precisely if and where in the environment the infectious virus can survive between outbreaks. Recently, the potential role of air currents in long-distance transport of LSDV-contaminated insects was investigated by Israeli scientists (Klausner et al. 2015).

Sheep pox and GTP are highly contagious diseases and direct contact between infected and naïve animals is the main mode of transmission. Outbreaks of these diseases occur throughout the year. SPPV and GTPV spread via contaminated aerosols following inhalation, oral absorption, or through skin abrasions. They can also spread indirectly via fomites originating from infected premises and carried by personnel, equipment, or vehicles. Experimentally, stomoxys flies have been demonstrated to transmit the virus in sheep and goats (Kitching and Mellor 1986).

In all CaPV diseases, high titers of virus are known to persist in skin lesions and in scabs that develop on top of the lesion. Virus-containing dried scabs are shed by infected animals, contaminating the environment.

In cattle, natural resistance to LSDV is believed to occur and asymptomatic LSDV infections are common in the field (Weiss 1968). In addition, approximately one-third of experimentally infected animals show no clinical signs at all, although all became viremic (Tuppurainen et al. 2005; Osuagwuh et al. 2007; Annandale et al. 2013). Viremic animals without skin lesions may be capable of transmitting the virus via arthropod vectors, which complicates the control and eradication of LSDV in those countries where slaughter of all infected and in-contact animals is not feasible. Thus, killing only those animals showing LSD skin lesions is unlikely to limit the spread of the virus if a modified stamping-out method is used without vaccination.

28.1.4 Currently Available Diagnostic Tests

Capripoxviruses are large, enveloped, double-stranded DNA viruses. The size of the genome is approximately 151 kb, comprising at least 147 putative genes in the SPPV/GTPV and 156 in LSDV genomes. In general, they are closely related but phylogenetically distinct viruses. Comparison of the full genome sequences of several CaPV isolates showed 96% of similarity between LSDV, SPPV, and GTPV compared with over 99% for intraspecies similarity (Tulman et al. 2001, 2002).

Several conventional and real-time polymerase chain reaction (RT-PCR) methods have been developed and are widely used for the detection of CaPVs. PCR kits for all CaPVs are also commercially available.

Species-specific molecular assays utilizing the G-protein-coupled chemokine receptor (GPCR) or 30 kDa RNA polymerase subunit (RPO30) genes have been described (Le Goff et al. 2005, 2009; Lamien et al. 2011a,b). Molecular assays for the differentiation of virulent and vaccine strains are needed for epidemiological field investigations. The first assay based on the detection of a 27-nucleotide difference, in the gene for an extracellular enveloped virion protein, between virulent and attenuated LSDV has been published (Menasherow et al. 2014), followed by gel-based and RT-PCR methods for SPPV (Haegeman et al. 2016; Chibssa et al. 2018). Alternative methods have been developed by Serbian (Vidanovich et al. 2016) and Greek (Agianniotaki et al. 2017) scientists. Sequencing of the GPCR-gene provides an alternative means to differentiate between field and vaccine viruses (Gelaye et al. 2015).

There are no pen-side tests commercially available for the detection of CaPV in the field. Two loop-mediated isothermal amplification (LAMP) assays for the specific identification of CaPV have been developed (Das et al. 2012; Zhao et al. 2014). Such assays, with the possibility of naked-eye reading, have great potential for use in diagnostic laboratories with limited resources and even in the field. PCR methods suitable for portable thermocyclers (Armson et al. 2017) and other simple molecular methods for pen-side testing (Shalaby et al. 2016) have been described, and more assays are expected to become available in the near future.

All serological tests in use (serum/virus neutralization, enzyme-linked immunosorbent assay [ELISA], fluorescent antibody, indirect fluorescent antibody, and agar gel immunodiffusion tests) are for CaPV group diagnosis. Except ELISA, none of them is suitable for testing large numbers of samples. Indirect ELISAs based on killed whole virus, recombinant antigens, or synthetic peptides have been developed (Babiuk et al. 2009; Bhanot et al. 2009; Bowden et al. 2009; Tian et al. 2010). In 2017, the first ELISA kit (ID Screen® Capripox Double Antigen Multi-species, IDvet, France) became commercially available for the detection of antibodies against CaPV, enabling serological surveillance for CaPV.

28.1.5 Disinfection

In general, purified LSDV is sensitive to many commonly used disinfectants when used at appropriate concentrations. CaPV is stable between pH 6.6 and 8.6 but due to the lipid-containing surface structure, the virus can be inactivated by most common detergents. Phenol (2%), sodium hypochlorite (2–3%), strong iodine compounds (1:33

dilution), Virkon® (2%), and quaternary ammonium compounds (0.5%) can be used for the disinfection of equipment, facilities, and vehicles. The virus is chloroform and ether (20%) sensitive and can be inactivated at 56 °C in 2 hours or at 65 °C in 30 minutes (www.oie.int/fileadmin/Home/eng/Animal_Health_in_the_World/docs/pdf/Disease_cards/LUMPY_SKIN_DISEASE_FINAL.pdf). More detailed practical recommendations for proper decontamination of premises, equipment, and environment are provided by the Food and Agriculture Organization (FAO) in the *Animal Health Manual* (FAO 2001).

28.2 Types of Vaccines

To date, only live attenuated CaPV vaccines are commercially available and all of them require an authorization prior to use in nonendemic countries. In the Balkan countries, affected with LSD between 2015 and 2017, use of live attenuated LSDV vaccines was authorized if the specific conditions set by the European Commission and national competent authorities were fulfilled. The superiority of live attenuated vaccines compared with the killed ones is well known. It is believed that in order for a vaccine to provide a solid protective immunity against CaPV *in vivo*, replication of the agent is required to mimic the natural infection. However, in specific circumstances, inactivated vaccines against CaPVs would be advantageous, and these products are likely to enter the markets in the near future.

28.2.1 Vaccines Against Lumpy Skin Disease

Homologous live vaccines against LSDV are derived either from the South African LSDV Neethling strain or alternatively from an attenuated LSDV field strain. Both vaccine types were widely used during the LSD outbreaks in south-eastern Europe. The efficacy of these vaccines against field LSDV is very good and when combined with high vaccination coverage, total or partial stamping-out policy, and movement restrictions, the spread of the disease can be effectively stopped within a short period of time. For example, in Bulgaria the vaccination effectiveness was 96% (EFSA 2018).

So-called "Kenyan sheep and goat pox virus" (KSGP) O-240 (also named KS1) and O-180 strains have been used in cattle against LSDV with varying success, for example in Egypt and Oman. As both these Kenyan strains were originally isolated from sheep (Davies 1976; Davies and Atema 1978; Davies and Mbugwa 1985; Kitching et al. 1987), they were consequently named according to the host as SPPV. However, after molecular techniques became available, these isolates were shown to be in fact LSDV strains (Black et al. 1986; Tulman et al. 2001; Lamien et al. 2011; Tuppurainen et al. 2014).

The efficacy of the different SPPV vaccine strains against LSDV is known to vary and final selection of the vaccine should always be based only on demonstrated efficacy. SPPV-derived vaccines have been used against LSDV in countries where SPP is endemic. For example, the Yugoslavian RM65 SPPV, at a 10 times stronger dose than used for sheep, has been used for cattle against LSDV in Israel and Jordan (Abutarbush et al. 2015; Ben-Gera et al. 2015). Since 2006, Romanian SPPV vaccine has been used for cattle in Egypt and Oman (Davies 1991; Brenner et al. 2009; Somasundaram 2011). In Turkey and the northern Caucasus region, the Bakirköy SPPV vaccine has been used in cattle at both three and 10 times the dose used for sheep.

Several studies have shown the efficacy of GTPV vaccines for protecting cattle from challenge by LSDV. The Kedong and Isiolo strains were isolated from sheep in Kenya during the 1950s but were later shown to be actually GTPV (Tuppurainen et al. 2014). In studies by Coackley and Capstick (1961), both strains were shown to protect cattle from LSDV challenge. Recently, in a study conducted in Ethiopia, an attenuated Gorgan GTPV-containing vaccine was demonstrated to provide good protection for cattle against a highly virulent LSD field strain (Gari et al. 2015). Currently, there is one GTPV-based vaccine commercially available against LSDV in cattle, from a Jordanian manufacturer (Table 28.1).

The price of SPPV and GTPV vaccines is considerably lower than that of homologous LSDV vaccines, which makes them attractive alternatives in countries with a large cattle population and limited financial resources available for disease control.

28.2.2 Vaccines against Sheep Pox and Goat Pox

KSGPV O-240, O-180, and RM65 vaccines are used against SPPV in the Middle East and Africa and the Bakirköy SPPV vaccine is used in Turkey. The Gorgan and Mysore GTPV strains are used in vaccines against GTPV (Kitching 1986b). Several local attenuated SPPV and GTPV strains are used in the Indian subcontinent.

28.2.3 Inactivated Vaccines

Killed vaccines are currently being developed against SPPV (Boumart et al. 2016) and LSDV and the field trials are ongoing. The availability of a safe, nonreplicating but effective vaccine with fewer side effects would assist both endemic and nonendemic countries to protect themselves against incursion of CaPV. As an inactivated vaccine causes fewer severe

Table 28.1 List of lumpy skin disease (LSD), sheep pox (SPP), and goat pox (GTP) vaccine manufacturers.

Manufacturer	Contact information	Product(s)[a]
Abic Biological Laboratories Ltd. (Phibro)	Abic Veterinary, Veterinary Products, 3 Hamelacha Street, P.O.B. 489, Beit Shemesh 99100, Israel Phone: +972 2 9906916 Fax: +972 2 9906900	RM65 SPPV
Agrovet	23 Academic Skryabin Street, 109472 Moscow, Russia Phone: +7 495 377 69.97 Fax: +7 495 377 69 87 Email: info@agrovet.ru www.agrovet.ru/index.eng.htm	Sheep Pox™ (Live SPPV Nishi)
Biopharma	Avenue Hassan II, km 2 route de Casablanca, Rabat-Akkari, Morocco Phone: +212 6 74 90 67 17/ +212 6 74 90 66 19 Fax:+ 212 5 37 69 36 32 Email: biopharma_ma@yahoo.fr	Romanian SPPV
Deltamune (Pty) Ltd.	PO Box 14167, Lyttleton 0140, South Africa Phone: +27 12 664 5730 Fax: +27 12 664 5149	Herbivac LS™ (Modified Neethling type)
Dollvet	Organize Sanayi Bölgesi 8, No: 3 Cadde Merkez Sanliurfa, Turkey Phone: +90 414 3691133 Fax: +90 414 3691662 Email: dollvet@dollvet.com.tr www.dollvet.com.tr	Poxdoll™ (Live SPPV Bakirköy strain) LSD-NDOLL (Neethling)
Federal Center for Animal Health (FGBI)	600901, Vladimir, Tur'evets, FGBI ARRIAH, Russia Phone: +7 4922 26 06 14 Fax: +7 4922 26 38 77 Email: mail@arriah.ru www.arriah.ru	Sheep pox Cultyral Dry™
Hester Biosciences Ltd.	1st Floor, Pushpak, Panchvati Circle, Motilal Hirabhai Road, Ahmedabad-380006, Gujarat, India Phone: +91 79 2644 5106, +91 79 2644 5107 Fax: +91 79 2644 5105 Email: mail@hester.in www.hesterbiosciences.co.in	Goat Pox Vaccine™ (Uttarkashi strain)
Indian Immunologicals Ltd	Road 44, Jubilee Hills, Hyderabad 500033, A.P., Telangana, India Phone: +91 40 23544585 Fax: +91 40 23544007 Email: info@indimmune.com www.indimmune.com	Raksha SP™
Institut Pasteur d'Algérie	Route du Petit Staouéli, Dély-Brahim, Alger Phone: +213 21 372674/ 363588 Fax: +213 21361748 Email: contact@pasteur.dz www.pasteur.dz	Sheep and goat pox (RM65 SPPV)

(Continued)

Table 28.1 (Continued)

Manufacturer	Contact information	Product(s)[a]
Intervac Pvt Ltd.	113/3 Allama Iqbal Road, Ghari Shahu, Lahore 54 141, Pakistan Phone: +92 42 36306957, +92 42 6364411 Fax: +92 42 6374378 Email: info@intervacpvtltd.com www.intervacpvtltd.com	Intervac sheep pox vaccine (RM65 SPPV)
Jordan Bio-Industries Center (JOVAC)	PO Box 43, Amman 11 941, Jordan Phone: +962 6 523 2162 Fax: +962 6 523 2210 Email: sales@jovaccenter.com www.jovaccenter.com	Jovivac™ (SPPV RM65) Caprivac (GTPV Gorgan strain) Kenyavac™ (KSGP O-240) Lumpyshield™ (GTPV Gorgan strain)
Intervet (Pty) South Africa/MSD Animal Health	20 Spartan Road, Spartan Ext 20, Kempton Park, 1619 South Africa Phone: +27 11 923 9300 Fax: +27 11 974 9320 www.msd-animal-health.co.za	Lumpyvax™ (attenuated LSDV field strain)
National Veterinary Institute	PO Box 19, Debre Zeit, Ethiopia Phone: +251 114 33 84 11/16 or 33 21 18 Fax: +251 114 33 93 00 Email: nvi-rt@ethionet.et	Sheep and goat pox vaccine (KSGP O-180) Lumpy skin disease vaccine (Neethling strain)
MCI Santé Animale	Lot 157, Zone Industrielle Sud-Ouest (ERAC) B.P.: 278 Mohammedia 28810, Morocco Phone: +212 523 30 31 32 Email: contact@mci-santeanimale.com	Bovivax LSD™ Ovivax ™ (SPP Perego strain) Lyopox™ (SPP and PPR)
Onderstepoort Biological Products	100 Old Soutpan Road, Onderstepoort 0110, Private Bag X07, South Africa Phone: +27 12 522 1500 Fax: +27 12 522 1591 Email: renah@obpvaccines.co.za, info@obpvaccines.co.za www.obpvaccines.co.za	Lumpy skin disease vaccine for cattle (Neethling strain)
Pendik Veterinary Control Institute/ Ministry of Agriculture	Batı Mah., Ankara Cad. No:1, 34890 Istanbul, Turkey Tel: +90 216 390 12 80-156 Fax: +90 216 354 76 92	Penpox-M™ Live SPPV (Bakirköy SPPV strain)
Razi Vaccine & Serum Research Institute	PO Box 31975/148 Hessarak, Karaj, Alborz, Iran Phone: +98 26 34554658 Fax: +98 26 34552194 Email: int@rvsri.ac.ir, www.rvsri.ac.ir	Sheep pox vaccine (RM65 SPPV) Goat pox vaccine (Gorgan GTPV)
Vetal Company	Gölbasi Yolu Uzeri 7 km, Adiyaman, Turkey Phone: +90 416 223 20 30 or +90 531 272 32 68 Fax: +90 416 223 1456 Email: vetal@vetal.com.tr www.vetal.com.tr	Poxvac™ Lumpyvac™
Veterinary Research Institute	59, Jalan Sultan Azlan Shah, 31400 Ipoh, Perak, Malaysia Phone: +605 5457166 or 187 Fax: +605 5463368 Email: admin@jphvri.gov.my	Sheep and goat pox

Table 28.1 (Continued)

Manufacturer	Contact information	Product(s)[a]
Veterinary Serum and Vaccine Research Institute	131 02 El-Sekka El-Bida St, Abbassia, Cairo, PO Box 131, 11381, Egypt Phone: + 02 23421866 or +02 23421406 Fax: +02 2342821 Email: svri@idsc.gov.eg http://vsvri-eg.com	Tissue culture sheep pox vaccine (KSGP O-240 or O-180)
Kenya Veterinary Vaccines Production Institute (KEVEVAPI)	P.O. Box 53260 00200, Head Office, Embakasi off Enterprise Road, Road A, Nairobi, Kenya www.kevevapi.org	S&G Vax™ Lumpivax™
China Animal Husbandry Group	Building 18-19, Block 8, 188 West Road, South 4th Ring Road, Beijing, P. R. China 100070 Fax: +86-10-5226-0088	Live goat pox vaccine
Laboratoire Central Vétérinaire	Km 8, Route de Koulikoro, BP 2295, Bamako, Mali Phone: +223 224 33 44/224 23 04/224 23 05 Fax: +223 224 98 09	Dermapox™
Institut Sénégalais de Recherches Agricoles (ISRA)	Route des Hydrocarbures, Bel-Air, BP 3120 Dakar, Sénégal Tel: +221 33 859 17 25 Fax: +221 33 832 24 27 www.isra.sn	Clavesec™

[a] This list of vaccines does not represent any authentication of the quality or efficacy of the products.

Disclaimer: It was the authors' intention to list all vaccine producers and are not responsible for the safety, quality, and effectiveness of the vaccines listed in the table.

side effects in fully susceptible animals than a live one, they could be ideal for use in preventive vaccination campaigns, for example in buffer zones created between affected and nonaffected countries. Inactivated vaccines could also be used to protect fully susceptible animals prior to importation from disease-free to recently affected regions. On arrival, the protection provided by the killed vaccine could be strengthened by giving a live attenuated booster vaccine. In some cases, the use of inactivated vaccines could also be considered as a short-term solution in an emergency (Tuppurainen and Oura 2014). However, protection provided by inactivated vaccines is shorter than that provided by live vaccines and booster vaccinations given twice per year are usually recommended (Kitching 1986b). Meanwhile, there is no difference in the current OIE or European Union (EU) trade regulations for live animals and their products whether the vaccine used by the exporting country is a live or inactivated one.

To date, no marker vaccines are commercially available against CaPV, making development of a differentiation between infected and vaccinated animals (DIVA) vaccine a major goal for vaccine research in coming years.

It should be underlined that vaccination with any type of vaccine should always be combined with other control and eradication measures, such as strict movement restrictions, a robust database for animal identification and health records, as well as stamping out where feasible.

28.3 Immune Response and Duration of Immunity

As for all poxviruses, immunity against CaPVs is both cell mediated and humoral. After vaccination or natural infection, antibodies appear within 15 days and reach a peak 21–30 days postinfection. The protective role of antibodies against CaPV has been demonstrated in sheep by passive transfer of sera from infected to naïve sheep (Kitching 1986a). However, locally, in the skin, the virus may spread from cell to cell without release of virus particles into the extracellular space. Therefore, a humoral response may not be sufficient to eliminate the infection completely (Kitching 1986b; Carn 1993).

Animals recovered from a natural infection with one member of the genus are believed to be protected from infection by another (Coackley and Capstick 1961; Kitching et al. 1987; Kitching 2003). However, this protection is likely to vary between different CaPV strains. Field studies in Israel and elsewhere have clearly demonstrated the superiority of homologous vaccines against LSDV (Ben-Gera et al. 2015). Calves, lambs, and kids born to immunized or naturally infected mothers have passive immunity that persists for approximately 3–6 months (Weiss 1968). New data on the persistence of the maternal antibodies in calves born to vaccinated dams have been published demonstrating that a significant number of calves were not protected by maternal antibodies after the age of 3 months and probably even after the age of 2 months (Agianniotaki et al. 2018).

Affected animals will clear the infection and no carrier stage is known to occur.

Duration of immunity provided by vaccination is likely to depend on the vaccine virus strain and host factors. It is estimated to vary between 12 and 23 months (Kitching 2003) and, therefore, an annual vaccination regimen is currently recommended by vaccine manufacturers. More studies are required to investigate the duration of antibody responses, using different serological methods. According to the validation report published by the manufacturer, the commercially available ELISA kit (ID Screen Capripox Double Antigen Multi-species) detected CaPV antibodies up to 7 months postvaccination.

28.4 Vaccine Quality Assurance and Control Testing

In commercially available CaPV vaccines, the origin of the vaccine virus should be clearly indicated. An even more essential part of vaccine quality control is to confirm the identity of the vaccine seed virus, using molecular methods, as there have been cases when molecular investigations revealed that the true identity of the vaccine virus was not what was believed. As an example, the KSGP O-240 strain vaccine was actually LSDV vaccine, being underattenuated and causing clinical signs for cattle but working well in sheep and goats (Tuppurainen et al. 2014). Failure to accurately identify the vaccine seed virus may lead to a situation where less effective or unsafe vaccines are used, or of accidentally using a vaccine containing a live CaPV otherwise absent in the country.

The titer of the virus in the CaPV vaccine product should exceed $10^{2.5}$–$10^{3.5}$ $TCID_{50}$, as recommended by the OIE *Manual of Diagnostic Tests and Vaccines* (OIE 2018b). As some vaccines against CaPV are propagated in primary lamb testis cell cultures, each vaccine batch should be tested for freedom from viruses that affect sheep, such as pestiviruses, different strains of bluetongue (BT), foot and mouth disease, and rabies viruses. In a recent study, LSD and SPP vaccines were shown to be contaminated by a BT serotype 26 virus (Bumbarov et al. 2016).

In addition, the product must be shown to be free of cross-contamination by other viruses handled in the same facilities, such as Aujeszky's disease (pseudorabies) virus. Freedom from *Mycoplasma* spp. and other adventitious bacterial and fungal organisms should be certified for each batch.

Animal species, breed, and numbers used for the safety and efficacy testing should be clearly indicated and potential adverse reactions described. A challenge model for LSD vaccine testing has been developed by researchers at Coda-Cerva, Belgium (Kris de Clercq, personal communication). The correct storage temperature and need for a cold chain during transport, as well as the shelf-life of the product, should be clearly indicated.

28.5 Vaccine Application for Disease Control

In general, live attenuated vaccines against CaPV provide good protection for cattle, sheep, and goats, so long as a homologous vaccine is used in combination with sufficient vaccination coverage. However, the available live vaccines may not provide each individual animal with complete protection against the disease. For a long time, it was believed that a single CaPV vaccine would protect against all members of the genus (Kitching et al. 1987) as more than 96% homology exists between the genomes of SPPV, GTPV, and LSDV (Black et al. 1986; Tulman et al. 2001; 2002; Balinski et al. 2007). However, recent experience obtained from the Middle East and the Horn of Africa indicates that the cross-protection provided by nonhomologue vaccines can be only partial (Khalafalla et al. 1993; Yeruham et al. 1994; Brenner et al. 2009; Somasundaram 2011; Ayelet et al. 2013; Tageldin et al. 2014). The experience obtained from LSDV outbreaks in Israel in 2012–2013 indicated the superiority of LSDV vaccines compared with SPPV vaccines for protecting cattle against LSDV (Ben-Gera et al. 2015). SPPV and GTPV containing vaccines can be used in countries where these CaPV diseases overlap.

Although a homologous vaccine is recommended against LSDV, the price of LSD vaccines is considerably higher than SPPV- and GTPV-containing vaccines. In countries with limited financial resources and a vast number of cattle, SPP or GTP vaccines may be a more affordable option. In these cases, selection of the vaccine should be based strictly on vaccine challenge trials to confirm that the vaccine is effective in cattle. Using heterologous vaccines, it is also possible to create sufficient herd immunity to stop the spread of the disease. In these cases, other supportive disease control and eradication measures, such as stamping out accompanied by an appropriate compensation policy, cattle movement controls, and a proper cattle ID, vaccination, and movement register should also be fully implemented. It should be underlined that in addition to full characterization of the vaccine seed virus, the safety and efficacy of any vaccine used for cattle against LSDV needs to be known prior to vaccine selection. For example, because of its residual pathogenicity for cattle, the KSGP O-240 (LSDV vaccine) caused serious adverse reactions in dairy cattle (Yeruham et al. 1994).

If homologous vaccines are not available or affordable, attenuated GTPV vaccine seems to be a good alternative for those regions where both LSD and GTP occur. Interestingly, in a recent vaccine challenge study in Ethiopia, a commercially available Gorgan GTPV vaccine (Caprivac™, Jordan Bio-Industries Center, Amman, Jordan) provided good protection for cattle against a highly virulent LSDV field strain (Gari et al. 2015).

More data on the safety and efficacy of a Gorgan GTPV-containing vaccine against LSDV in cattle are expected to be published soon by other research groups. Wider field studies need to be carried out to evaluate the safety and efficacy of other GTP virus vaccines against LSD.

28.5.1 Vaccination Strategy

In response to an outbreak, large-scale vaccination should be started without delay. All susceptible animals within and around the infected zone should be immunized, creating more than 80% vaccination coverage. Regional vaccinations are currently preferred and recommended instead of ring vaccinations. However, if a ring vaccination policy is adopted, the radius of the ring should be at least 25–50 km, covering the flying distance of blood-feeding insects and estimated animal movements to pasture, slaughterhouses, or for trade. The herd immunity should be maintained by an annual vaccination program.

Vaccination is recommended also around temporary slaughter plants or slaughterhouses and animal market places, because it is highly likely that during an outbreak, despite the ban on animal movements, some already affected or subclinically infected animals will be sent to slaughter or markets. Also, naïve pregnant animals should be vaccinated. Calves, lambs, and kids from vaccinated mothers should be immunized at the age of 3–6 months and from nonvaccinated mothers as soon as possible. Animals that are not healthy should be vaccinated without delay once recovered.

Ideally, animals showing characteristic clinical signs of CaPV diseases should be culled, but unfortunately, this is not affordable or feasible in all endemic countries. In these cases, vaccination of animals showing fever, skin lesions, or other typical clinical signs of LSD, SPP, or GTP is not recommended, as vaccination is likely to worsen the clinical disease of infected animals and after recovery affected animals will be protected from reinfection without vaccination. However, in these animals, CaPV infection should be confirmed by laboratory testing, in order to avoid a situation in which clinical signs were actually caused by some other conditions and these animals are left without protection. If animals are moved to seasonal grazing, they need to be vaccinated 28 days before the start of the event.

Correct handling of the live attenuated CaPV vaccines requires maintenance of a cold chain. Live pox vaccine must be protected from direct sunlight and opened bottles must be used within 2–6 hours and then discarded. Needles should be changed between animals, particularly if there is any doubt that the herd could be already incubating the disease.

28.6 Vaccines Against CaPV and Other Diseases

In Africa, the Middle East, and Asia, the geographic distribution of LSD, SPP, and GTP overlaps with the distribution of other, highly infectious, economically important or zoonotic diseases, such as peste des petits ruminants (PPR), contagious caprine pleuropneumonia, foot and mouth disease, and Rift Valley fever (RVF) against which vaccines are available.

The major cost of a vaccination campaign is delivery of the vaccine which is nearly the same whether animals are inoculated with one or more compatible vaccines. A significant cost–benefit improvement could be achieved by vaccination concurrently against several ruminant diseases (www.fao.org/3/a-i4460e.pdf), such as PPR, SPP, and GTP (Hosamani et al. 2006; Chaudhary et al. 2009). Alternatively, vaccination costs can be cut by using a single recombinant multivalent vaccine with a CaPV genome backbone and taking advantage of the following characteristics of the CaPV:

- the relative thermotolerance of a freeze-dried CaPV
- the large size and packaging flexibility of the CaPV genome, which contains genes that can be deleted and replaced by foreign genes without affecting the replication and performance of the resultant virus
- the limited host range of CaPV
- the lack of persistence of the virus in the host and the lack of integration of the virus genome in the host genome, facilitating the acceptance of CaPV-based recombinant vaccines.

The following recombinant capripox vaccines have been developed: CaPV/PPR virus (Diallo et al. 2002; Berhe et al. 2003; Chen et al. 2010; Caufour et al. 2014), CaPV/rinderpest (Romero et al. 1993, 1994; Ngichabe et al. 1997), CaPV/BT (Wade-Evans et al. 1996; Perrin et al. 2007), CaPV/rabies (Aspden et al. 2002), and CaPV/RVF virus (Wallace et al. 2006).

28.7 Vaccine Effectiveness and Postvaccination Monitoring

Due to various factors originating from either the host's immune response or varying efficacy of different vaccine products, not all animals will develop full protective immunity against LSDV. Incomplete protection by CaPV vaccines has been reported, for example, in Egypt (2006) (Salib and Osman 2011), Israel (2006) (Brenner et al. 2009), and Ethiopia (Ayelet et al. 2013; Gelaye et al. 2015). These cases were linked to both incomplete protection by the vaccine against the local LSDV strain and the use of SPP vaccine in cattle at the same dose as used for sheep.

The most common factor contributing to real or apparent vaccine breakdown is vaccination of an already infected herd or flock. During hectic mass vaccination campaigns, some animals may be accidentally missed. Sometimes catching free-ranging beef cattle for vaccination can be technically challenging and time-consuming, leaving small pockets of unvaccinated animals within otherwise fully vaccinated regions. Earlier, using the same needle for many animals for vaccine administration was a common practice but nowadays, due to better awareness, it rarely occurs. In cattle which are not used to handling, a subcutaneous administration of a vaccine can easily fail, or animals may receive only part of the vaccine dosage. Inappropriate storage of vaccine or failure in the maintenance of the cold chain can happen during hot summer months. Vaccine may also be inactivated due to exposure to direct sunlight in the field. Maternally derived antibodies may cause interference with the development of active immunity in calves less than 3–6 months of age (Carn 1993; Kitching 2003).

Postvaccination monitoring is based on passive or active clinical surveillance in vaccinated herds. Retrospective serological surveys are complicated by the fact that some vaccinated animals and those individuals showing mild disease may develop only low levels of neutralizing antibodies although these animals would be fully protected (Weiss 1968; Kitching 1986b). Current availability of a sensitive CaPV ELISA suitable for large-scale testing allows better monitoring of seroconversion and duration of humoral responses in vaccinated herds.

28.8 Vaccine Adverse Reactions

Mild adverse reactions may occur when using live attenuated LSDV vaccines. Small local reactions at the vaccination site are acceptable, showing that the vaccine virus is replicating and producing a good immune response. It is expected that the live vaccine virus can be isolated in skin samples collected from the vaccination site. Temporary fever and drop in milk yield have been reported in vaccinated animals. In a study investigating the adverse reactions caused by LSDV-containing vaccines in a cattle herd in Greece, the decrease in milk yield lasted for 12 days (Katsoulos et al. 2017). More data on the side effects caused by LSD vaccines have been obtained from Croatia which was the first country practising preventive vaccination in 2016. In a small number of cattle, vaccination caused a short low-level viremia and the presence of vaccine viral DNA was detected in nasal and skin samples (Beděković et al. 2017). It is also known that after vaccination, some animals may show mild generalized disease, the so-called "Neethling disease" (Ben-Gera et al. 2015; Abutarbush et al. 2016). However, the generalized skin lesions caused by an attenuated virus are smaller and clearly different from those caused by fully virulent field strains.

To date, there is no evidence of LSD vaccine viruses regaining their virulence. This may be the result of the laborious and lengthy attenuation process required to remove the virulence of LSDV viruses. For full attenuation, LSD prototype Neethling strain virus required 60 serial passages on lamb kidney cells, followed by 20 serial passages in the chorioallantoic membranes of 8-day-old embryonated chicken eggs (Weiss 1968). The whole attenuation process takes more than a year. During the preventive vaccination campaign in Croatia (2017), 421 720 cattle were vaccinated against LSD (with 85% vaccination coverage). Despite the large number of vaccinated cattle, no spread of the vaccine virus to fully susceptible animals, either within Croatia or in neighboring countries, has been reported. Understandably, farmers complained about the skin reactions and decrease in milk yield in vaccinated herds.

Adverse reactions due to residual pathogenicity have been reported in cattle in Israel (Yeruham et al. 1994) after use of the so-called KSGP O-240 strain for which the attenuation process was less than 20 passages (Tuppurainen et al. 2014). In many cases, generalized reactions were linked to utilization of the KS1 strain which is in fact an LSDV, as indicated earlier.

Sheep pox virus and GTPV vaccines rarely cause adverse reactions in cattle, although it has been reported (Aburtabush and Tuppurainen 2018). If cattle are vaccinated first with SPPV or GTP vaccine and then a booster vaccination is given using a LSDV vaccine, animals have shown fewer adverse reactions postvaccination with LSDV vaccine. Based on the field experience, adverse reactions are typically detected only after the first vaccination and the number of side effects reduces dramatically after the second round of vaccination. Farmers should be informed in advance about potential adverse reactions caused by live vaccines. In addition, if vaccines are purchased from black markets, cattle owners should be advised that these vaccines may not be safe, nor provide robust protection. Effective inactivated vaccines would offer a safer alternative for use in those countries practicing preventive vaccination.

28.9 Availability and a List of Manufacturers

Table 28.1 lists manufacturers of vaccines for lumpy skin disease, sheep pox, and goat pox.

28.10 Summary

In countries where CaPVs are endemic, where animal movement restrictions cannot be effectively implemented, and where active vector populations are abundant, large-scale immunization using effective vaccines is the only way to successfully control CaPVs. In general, live homologous vaccines provide excellent protection for cattle, sheep, and goats, if the vaccination coverage exceeds 80% and herd/flock immunity is maintained using annual vaccination. Vaccination campaigns should always be combined with other control and eradication measures. A homologous vaccine is preferred. The most recent study indicates that GTPV vaccines could provide a promising alternative for vaccinating cattle against LSD. Also, SPPV vaccines can be used for cattle if the dosage is adjusted accordingly. Importantly, if a heterologous vaccine is used, the efficacy and safety of the vaccine need to be confirmed by a challenge experiment. Effective, inactivated CaPV vaccines are being developed and are likely to become commercially available soon. Killed vaccines could be used in those countries not able to authorize live CaPV vaccines.

None of the vaccines provides all individuals with complete protection although sufficient herd immunity prevents further spread of the virus. The efficacy of CaPV vaccines may vary due to the capacity of the vaccine virus to replicate in nonhomologous host species. The finding that some vaccine strains were actually not what they were supposed to be underlines the importance of the molecular characterization of all commercially available vaccines.

Future vaccine research needs to focus on development of safer and more effective marker vaccines. Affordability of a vaccine is of major importance because the CaPV diseases mainly affect countries with limited financial resources and an outbreak has the most devastating effect on the livelihood of poor small-scale farmers. In particular, the currently available homologous LSDV vaccines are expensive. For example, in Africa, vaccines are used only by large commercial cattle farms. During 2015–2018, highly successful large-scale LSD vaccination campaigns in south-east Europe were co-financed by local governments and the European Commission. SPP and GTP vaccines are considerably cheaper although the actual manufacturing process does not differ between the LSD and SPP/GTP vaccines. An ideal single CaPV vaccine should be able to replicate well in cattle, sheep, and goats and it should have lost many of its pathogenic genes.

Along with the growing amount of genome sequence data, novel information is being accumulated on the pathogenesis of poxviruses. Expression of pathogenic or virulence proteins by the virus will influence the severity of disease. Poxviruses have developed a variety of strategies to divert the host immune response, such as by encoding proteins capable of masking signals associated with the virus infection, mimicking the host cytokines and receptors, and by blocking the host innate defense cell death mechanism (Johnston and McFadden 2003; Stanford et al. 2007). The attenuated vaccinia virus, NYVAC vaccine strain, was developed by disruption or deletion of most of those genes (Tartaglia et al. 1992; Paoletti 1994). Similar genes have been identified in the CaPV genome (Tulman et al. 2001, 2002; Balinsky et al. 2007; Lamien and Diallo, unpublished data) and are potential targets for studies to improve CaPV vaccines, such as deletion of the virus immunomodulatory genes (Tartaglia et al. 1992; Perdiguero et al. 2013; Filali-Mouhim et al. 2015). In order to improve the replication of the virus, the viral genes enabling replication in different host species could be combined in a single CaPV genome, as described for NYVAC vaccine (Kibler et al. 2011; Quakkelaar et al. 2011).

Alternatively, selected cytokine genes could be inserted in the CaPV genome, leading to their expression by the vector in the host. The delivery of the IL-12 and IL-18 genes by recombinant vaccinia virus improved the clearance of infection in mice (Gherardi et al. 2003). However, before an ideal CaPV vaccine will be developed, it is fundamental for the successful control and eradication of capripox diseases that the safety and efficacy of the currently used vaccines against LSD, SPP, and GTP are thoroughly evaluated by challenge experiments, using sufficient numbers of fully susceptible animals under controlled conditions and in the field.

References

Abutarbush, S.M. and Tuppurainen, E.S.M. (2018). Serological and clinical evaluation of the Yugoslavian RM65 sheep pox strain vaccine use in cattle against lumpy skin disease. *Transbound. Emerg. Dis.* 65 (6): 1657–1663.

Abutarbush, S.M., Ababneh, M.M., Al Zoubi, I.G. et al. (2015). Lumpy skin disease in Jordan: disease emergence, clinical signs, complications and preliminary-associated economic losses. *Transbound. Emerg. Dis.* 62 (5): 549–554.

Abutarbush, S.M., Hananeh, W.M., Ramadan, W. et al. (2016). Adverse reactions to field vaccination against lumpy skin disease in Jordan. *Transbound. Emerg. Dis.* 63 (2): 213–219.

Agianniotaki, E.I., Tasioudi, K.E., Chaintoutis, S.C. et al. (2017). Lumpy skin disease outbreaks in Greece during 2015-16, implementation of emergency immunization and genetic differentiation between field isolates and vaccine virus strains. *Vet. Microbiol.* 201: 78–84.

Agianniotaki, E.I., Babiuk, S., Katsoulos, P.D. et al. (2018). Colostrum transfer of neutralizing antibodies against lumpy skin disease virus from vaccinated cows to their calves. *Transbound. Emerg. Dis.* 65 (6): 2043–2048.

Annandale, C.H., Holm, D.E., Ebersohn, K., and Venter, E.H. (2013). Seminal transmission of lumpy skin disease virus in heifers. *Transbound. Emerg. Dis.* 61 (5): 443–448.

Armson, B., Fowler, V.L., Tuppurainen, E.S.M. et al. (2017). Detection of capripoxvirus DNA using a field-ready nucleic acid extraction and real-time PCR platform. *Transbound. Emerg. Dis.* 64: 994–997.

Aspden, K., van Dijk, A.A., Bingham, J. et al. (2002). Immunogenicity of a recombinant lumpy skin disease virus (Neethling vaccine strain) expressing the rabies virus glycoprotein in cattle. *Vaccine* 20 (21–22): 2693–2701.

Ayelet, G., Abate, Y., Sisay, T. et al. (2013). Lumpy skin disease: preliminary vaccine efficacy assessment and overview on outbreak impact in dairy cattle at Debre Zeit, Central Ethiopia. *Antivir. Res.* 98: 261–265.

Babiuk, S., Wallace, D.B., Smith, S.J. et al. (2009). Detection of antibodies against capripoxviruses using an inactivated sheeppox virus ELISA. *Transbound. Emerg. Dis.* 56: 132–141.

Balinsky, C.A., Delhon, G., Afonso, C.L. et al. (2007). Sheeppox virus kelch-like gene SPPV-019 affects virus virulence. *J. Virol.* 81: 11392–11401.

Barnard, B.J.H. (1997). Antibodies against some viruses of domestic animals in South African wild animals. *Onderstepoort J. Vet. Res.* 64: 95–110.

Bedeković, T., Šimić, I., Kresić, N., and Lojkić, I. (2017). Detection of lumpy skin disease virus in skin lesions, blood, nasal swabs and milk following preventive vaccination. *Transbound. Emerg. Dis.* 65 (2): 491–496.

Ben-Gera, J., Klement, E., Khinich, E. et al. (2015). Comparison of the efficacy of Neethling lumpy skin disease virus and ×10RM65 sheep-pox live attenuated vaccines for the prevention of lumpy skin disease – the results of a randomized controlled field study. *Vaccine* 33 (38): 4837–4842.

Berhe, G., Minet, C., Le Goff, C. et al. (2003). Development of a dual recombinant vaccine to protect small ruminants against peste-des-petits-ruminants virus and capripoxvirus infections. *J. Virol.* 77 (2): 1571–1577.

Bhanot, V., Balamurugan, V., Bhanuprakash, V. et al. (2009). Expression of P32 protein of goatpox virus in *Pichia pastoris* and its potential use as a diagnostic antigen in ELISA. *J. Virol. Methods* 162 (1–2): 251–257.

Black, D.N., Hammond, J.M., and Kitching, R.P. (1986). Genomic relationship between capripoxviruses. *Virus Res.* 5: 277–292.

Boumart, Z., Daouam, S., Belkourati, I. et al. (2016). Comparative innocuity and efficacy of live and inactivated sheeppox vaccines. *BMC Vet. Res.* 12 (1): 133.

Bowden, T.R., Coupar, B.E., Babiuk, S.L. et al. (2009). Detection of antibodies specific for sheeppox and goatpox viruses using recombinant capripoxvirus antigens in an indirect enzyme-linked immunosorbent assay. *J. Virol. Methods* 161: 19–29.

Brenner, J., Bellaiche, M., Gross, E. et al. (2009). Appearance of skin lesions in cattle populations vaccinated against lumpy skin disease: statutory challenge. *Vaccine* 27 (10): 1500–1503.

Bumbarov, V., Golender, N., Erster, O., and Khinich, Y. (2016). Detection and isolation of Bluetongue virus from commercial vaccine batches. *Vaccine* 34 (28): 3317–3323.

Carn, V.M. (1993). Control of capripoxvirus infections. *Vaccine* 11 (13): 1275–1279.

Caufour, P., Rufael, T., Lamien, C.E. et al. (2014). Protective efficacy of a single immunization with capripoxvirus-vectored recombinant peste des petits ruminants vaccines in presence of pre-existing immunity. *Vaccine* 32 (30): 3772–3779.

Chaudhary, S.S., Pandey, K.D., Singh, R.P. et al. (2009). A vero cell derived combined vaccine against sheep pox and Peste des Petits ruminants for sheep. *Vaccine* 27: 2548–2553.

Chen, W., Hu, S., Qu, L. et al. (2010). A goat poxvirus-vectored peste-des-petits-ruminants vaccine induces long-lasting neutralization antibody to high levels in goats and sheep. *Vaccine* 28: 4742–4750.

Chibssa, T.R., Grabherr, R., Loitsch, A. et al. (2018). A gel-based PCR method to differentiate sheeppox virus field isolates from vaccine strains. *Virol. J.* 15: 59.

Chihota, C.M., Rennie, L.F., Kitching, R.P., and Mellor, P.S. (2001). Mechanical transmission of lumpy skin disease virus by *Aedes aegypti* (Diptera:Culicidae). *Epidemiol. Infect.* 126 (2): 317–321.

Coackley, W. and Capstick, P.B. (1961). Protection of cattle against lumpy skin disease. I. Trials with a vaccine against Neethling type infection. *Res. Vet. Sci.* 2: 362–368.

Coetzer, J.A.W. (2004). Lumpy skin disease. In: *Infectious Diseases of Livestock* (eds. J.A.W. Coetzer and R.C. Tustin), 1268–1276. Oxford: University Press of Southern Africa.

Das, A., Babiuk, S., and McIntosh, M.T. (2012). Development of a loop-mediated isothermal amplification assay for rapid detection of capripoxviruses. *J. Clin. Microbiol.* 50 (5): 1613–1620.

Davies, F.G. (1976). Characteristics of a pox virus causing a pox disease of sheep and goats in Kenya with observations on the epidemiology and control. *J. Hyg.* 76: 163–171.

Davies, F.G. (1982). Observations on the epidemiology of lumpy skin disease in Kenya. *J. Hyg.* 88 (1): 95–102.

Davies, F.G. (1991). Lumpy skin disease of cattle: a growing problem in Africa and the Near East. *World Anim. Rev.* 68 (3): 37–48.

Davies, F.G. and Atema, C. (1978). The antibody response in sheep to infection with a Kenyan sheep and goat pox virus. *J. Comp. Pathol.* 88: 205–210.

Davies, F.G. and Mbugwa, G. (1985). The alterations in pathogenicity and immunogenicity of a Kenya sheep and goat pox virus on serial passage in bovine foetal muscle cell cultures. *J. Comp. Pathol.* 95: 565–572.

Diallo, A., Minet, C., Berhe, G. et al. (2002). Goat immune response to capripox vaccine expressing the hemagglutinin protein of peste des petits ruminants. *Ann. N.Y. Acad. Sci.* 969: 88–91.

Dutta, T.K., Roychoudhury, P., Kawlni, L. et al. (2019). An outbreak of goatpox virus infection in Wild Red Serow (*Capricornis rubidus*) in Mizoram, India. *Transbound Emerg Dis.* 66: 181–185. https://doi.org/10.1111/tbed.12997

EFSA (European Food Safety Authority) (2018). Scientific report on lumpy skin disease II. Data collection and analysis. *EFSA J.* 16 (2): 5176.

El-Nahas, E.M., El-Habbaa, A.S., El-Bagoury, G.F., and Radwan, M.E.I. (2011). Isolation and identification of lumpy skin disease virus from naturally infected buffaloes at Kaluobia, Egypt. *Glob. Vet.* 7 (3): 234–237.

Fagbo, S., Coetzer, J.A.W., and Venter, E.H. (2014). Seroprevalence of Rift Valley fever and lumpy skin disease in African buffalo (*Syncerus caffer*) in the Kruger National Park and Hluhluwe-iMfolozi Park, South Africa. *J. S. Afr. Vet. Assoc.* 85 (1): 1075.

FAO (2001). Manual on procedures for disease eradication by stamping out. In: *FAO Animal Health Manual*, vol. 12. www.fao.org/docrep/004/Y0660E/Y0660E00.HTM

Filali-Mouhim, A., Haddad, E.K., Harari, A. et al. (2015). Interleukin-1- and type I interferon-dependent enhanced immunogenicity of an NYVAC-HIV-1 Env-Gag-Pol-Nef vaccine vector with dual deletions of type I and type II interferon-binding proteins. *J. Virol.* 89: 3819–3832.

Gari, G., Abie, G., Gizaw, D. et al. (2015). Evaluation of the safety, immunogenicity and efficacy of three capripoxvirus vaccine strains against lumpy skin disease virus. *Vaccine* 33: 3256–3261.

Gelaye, E., Belay, A., Ayelet, G. et al. (2015). Capripox disease in Ethiopia: genetic differences between field isolates and vaccine strain, and implications for vaccination failure. *Antivir. Res.* 119: 28–35.

Gherardi, M.M., Ramírez, J.C., and Esteban, M. (2003). IL-12 and IL-18 act in synergy to clear vaccinia virus infection: involvement of innate and adaptive components of the immune system. *J. Gen. Virol.* 84: 1961–1972.

Haegeman, A., Zro, K., Sammin, D. et al. (2016). Investigation of a possible link between vaccination and the 2010 sheep pox epizootic in Morocco. *Transbound. Emerg. Dis.* 63 (6): 278–287.

Haig, D.A. (1957). Lumpy skin disease. *Bull. Epizoot. Dis. Africa* 5: 421–430.

Hosamani, M., Singh, S.K., Mondal, B. et al. (2006). A bivalent vaccine against goat pox and Peste des Petits ruminants induces protective immune response in goats. *Vaccine* 24 (35–36): 6058–6064.

Johnston, J.B. and McFadden, G. (2003). Poxvirus immunomodulatory strategies: current perspectives. *J. Virol.* 77: 6093–6100.

Katsoulos, P.-D., Chaintoutis, S.C., Dovas, C.I. et al. (2017). Investigation on the incidence of adverse reactions, viraemia and haematological changes following field immunization of cattle using a live attenuated vaccine against lumpy skin disease. *Transbound. Emerg. Dis.* 65 (1): 174–185.

Khalafalla, A.I., Gaffar Elamin, M.A., and Abbas, Z. (1993). Lumpy skin disease: observations on the recent outbreaks of the disease in the Sudan. *Rev. Elev. Med. Vet. Trop.* 46: 548–550.

Kibler, K.V., Gomez, C.E., Perdiguero, B. et al. (2011). Improved NYVAC-based vaccine vectors. *PLoS One* 6 (11): e25674.

Kitching, R.P. (1986a). Passive protection of sheep against capripoxvirus. *Res. Vet. Sci.* 41 (2): 247–250.

Kitching, R.P. (1986b). The control of sheep and goat pox. *Rev. Sci. Tech OIE* 5 (2): 503–511.

Kitching, R.P. (2003).Vaccines for lumpy skin disease, sheep pox and goat pox. Vaccines for OIE list A and emerging animal diseases, 16–18 September, 2002. Ames, Iowa, USA, pp. 161–167.

Kitching, R.P. and Mellor, P.S. (1986). Insect transmission of capripoxvirus. *Res. Vet. Sci.* 40 (2): 255–258.

Kitching, R.P., Hammond, J.M., and Taylor, W.P. (1987). A single vaccine for the control of capripox infection in sheep and goats. *Res. Vet. Sci.* 42: 53–60.

Klausner, Z., Fattal, E., and Klement, E. (2015). Using synoptic systems' typical wind trajectories for the analysis of potential atmospheric long-distance dispersal of lumpy skin disease virus. *Transbound. Emerg. Dis.* 64 (2): 398–410.

Lamien, C.E., Le Goff, C., Silber, R. et al. (2011a). Use of the capripoxvirus homologue of vaccinia virus 30 kDa RNA polymerase subunit (RPO30) gene as a novel diagnostic and genotyping target: development of a classical PCR method to differentiate goat poxvirus from sheep poxvirus. *Vet. Microbiol.* 149 (1–2): 30–39.

Lamien, C.E., Lelenta, M., Goger, W. et al. (2011b). Real time PCR method for simultaneous detection, quantitation and differentiation of capripoxviruses. *J. Virol. Methods* 171 (1): 134–140.

Le Goff, C., Fakhfakh, E., Chadeyras, A. et al. (2005). Host-range phylogenetic grouping of capripoxviruses: genetic typing of CaPVs. In: *Applications of Gene-Based Technologies for Improving Animal Production and Health in Developing Countries* (eds. H.P.S. Makkar and G.J. Viljoen), 727–733. The Netherlands: International Atomic Energy Association.

Le Goff, C., Lamien, C.E., Fakhfakh, E. et al. (2009). Capripoxvirus G-protein-coupled chemokine receptor: a host-range gene suitable for virus animal origin discrimination. *J. Gen. Virol.* 90: 1967–1977.

Lubinga, J.C., Tuppurainen, E.S.M., Stoltsz, W.H. et al. (2013). Detection of lumpy skin disease virus in saliva of ticks fed on lumpy skin disease virus-infected cattle. *Exp. Appl. Acarol.* 69 (1): 129–138.

Menasherow, S., Rubinstein-Giuni, M., Kovtunenko, A. et al. (2014). Development of an assay to differentiate between virulent and vaccine strains of lumpy skin disease virus (LSDV). *J. Virol. Methods* 199: 95–101.

Ngichabe, C.K., Wamwayi, H.M., Barrett, T. et al. (1997). Trial of a capripoxvirus-rinderpest recombinant vaccine in African cattle. *Epidemiol. Infect.* 118: 63–70.

OIE (2018a). *Terrestrial Animal Health Code*. Paris: Office International des Epizooties www.oie.int/international-standard-setting/terrestrial-code/access-online

OIE (2018b). Sheep and goat pox. Chapter 14.9. In: *Manual of Diagnostic Tests and Vaccines for Terrestrial Animals*. Paris: Office International des Epizooties https://www.oie.int/standard-setting/terrestrial-manual/access-online/

Osuagwuh, U.I., Bagla, V., Venter, E.H. et al. (2007). Absence of lumpy skin disease virus in semen of vaccinated bulls following vaccination and subsequent experimental infection. *Vaccine* 25 (12): 2238–2243.

Paoletti, E., Tartaglia, J., and Taylor, J. (1994). Safe and effective poxvirus vectors – NYVAC and ALVAC. *Dev. Biol. Stand.* 82: 65–69.

Perdiguero, B., Gómez, C.E., di Pilato, M. et al. (2013). Deletion of the vaccinia virus gene A46R, encoding for an inhibitor of TLR signalling, is an effective approach to enhance the immunogenicity in mice of the HIV/AIDS vaccine candidate NYVAC-C. *PLoS One* 8 (9): e74831.

Perrin, A., Albina, E., Bréard, E. et al. (2007). Recombinant capripoxviruses expressing proteins of bluetongue virus: evaluation of immune responses and protection in small ruminants. *Vaccine* 25: 6774–6783.

Quakkelaar, E.D., Redeker, A., Haddad, E.K. et al. (2011). Improved innate and adaptive immunostimulation by genetically modified HIV-1 protein expressing NYVAC vectors. *PLoS One* 6: e16819.

Rao, T.V. and Bandyopadhyay, S.K. (2000). A comprehensive review of goat pox and sheep pox and their diagnosis. *Anim. Health Res. Rev.* 1 (2): 127–136.

Romero, C.H., Barrett, T., Evans, S.A. et al. (1993). Single capripoxvirus recombinant vaccine for the protection of cattle against rinderpest and lumpy skin disease. *Vaccine* 11 (7): 737–742.

Romero, C.H., Barrett, T., Kitching, R.P. et al. (1994). Protection of cattle against rinderpest and lumpy skin disease with a recombinant capripoxvirus expressing the fusion protein gene of rinderpest virus. *Vet. Rec.* 135: 152–154.

Rouby, S. and Aboulsoud, E. (2016). Evidence of intrauterine transmission of lumpy skin disease virus. *Vet. J.* 209: 193–195.

Rouby, S.R., Hussein, K.H., Aboelhadid, S.M., and El-Sherif, A.M. (2017). Role of *Rhipicephalus annulatus* tick in transmission of lumpy skin disease virus in naturally infected cattle in Egypt. *Adv. Anim. Vet. Sci.* 5 (4): 185–191.

Salib, F.A. and Osman, A.H. (2011). Incidence of lumpy skin disease among Egyptian cattle in Giza Governorate, Egypt. *Vet. World* 4 (4): 162–167.

Shalaby, M.A., El-Deeb, A., El-Tholoth, M. et al. (2016). Recombinase polymerase amplification assay for rapid detection of lumpy skin disease virus. *BMC Vet. Res.* 12 (1): 10–15.

Somasundaram, M.K. (2011). An outbreak of lumpy skin disease in a Holstein dairy herd in Oman: a clinical report. *Asian J. Anim. Vet. Adv.* 6 (8): 851–859.

Stanford, M.M., McFadden, G., Karupiah, G., and Chaudhri, G. (2007). Immunopathogenesis of poxvirus infections: forecasting the impending storm. *Immunol. Cell. Biol.* 85: 93–102.

Tageldin, M.H., Wallace, D.B., Gerdes, G.H. et al. (2014). Lumpy skin disease of cattle: an emerging problem in the Sultanate of Oman. *Trop. Anim. Health Prod.* 46: 241–246.

Tartaglia, J., Perkus, E., Taylor, J. et al. (1992). NYVAC: a highly attenuated strain of vaccinia virus. *Virology* 188: 217–232.

Tian, H., Chen, Y., Wu, J. et al. (2010). Serodiagnosis of sheeppox and goatpox using an indirect ELISA based on synthetic peptide targeting for the major antigen P32. *Virol. J.* 7: 245.

Tulman, E.R., Afonso, C.L., Lu, Z. et al. (2001). Genome of lumpy skin disease virus. *J. Virol.* 75 (15): 7122–7130.

Tulman, E.R., Afonso, C.L., Lu, Z. et al. (2002). The genomes of sheeppox and goatpox viruses. *J. Virol.* 76 (12): 6054–6061.

Tuppurainen, E. and Oura, C. (2014). Lumpy skin disease: an African cattle disease getting closer to the EU. *Vet. Rec.* 175 (12): 300–301.

Tuppurainen, E.S.M., Venter, E.H., and Coetzer, J.A.W. (2005). The detection of lumpy skin disease virus in samples of experimentally infected cattle using different diagnostic techniques. *Onderstepoort J. Vet. Res.* 72 (2): 153–164.

Tuppurainen, E.S.M., Stoltsz, W.H., Troskie, M. et al. (2011). A potential role for ixodid (hard) tick vectors in the transmission of lumpy skin disease virus in cattle. *Transbound. Emerg. Dis.* 58 (2): 93–104.

Tuppurainen, E.S.M., Lubinga, J.C., Stoltsz, W.H. et al. (2013a). Mechanical transmission of lumpy skin disease virus by *Rhipicephalus appendiculatus* male ticks. *Epidemiol. Infect.* 141 (2): 425–430.

Tuppurainen, E.S.M., Lubinga, J.C., Stoltsz, W.H. et al. (2013b). Evidence of vertical transmission of lumpy skin disease virus in *Rhipicephalus decoloratus* ticks. *Ticks Tick-borne Dis.* 4 (4): 329–333.

Tuppurainen, E.S., Pearson, C.R., Bachanek-Bankowska, K. et al. (2014). Characterization of sheep pox virus vaccine for cattle against lumpy skin disease virus. *Antivir. Res.* 109: 1–6.

Vidanovic, D., Sekler, M., Petrovic, T. et al. (2016). Real-time PCR assays for the specific detection of field Balkan strains of lumpy skin disease virus. *Acta Vet-Beograd.* 66: 444–454.

Wade-Evans, A.M., Romero, C.H., Mellor, P. et al. (1996). Expression of the major core structural protein (VP7) of bluetongue virus, by a recombinant capripox virus, provides partial protection of sheep against a virulent heterotypic bluetongue virus challenge. *Virology* 220: 227–231.

Wallace, D.B., Ellis, C.E., Espach, A. et al. (2006). Protective immune responses induced by different recombinant vaccine regimes to Rift Valley fever. *Vaccine* 24: 7181–7189.

Weiss, K.E. (1968). Lumpy skin disease. *Virol. Monogr.* 3: 111–131.

Yeruham, I., Perl, S., Nyska, A. et al. (1994). Adverse reactions in cattle to a capripox vaccine. *Vet. Rec.* 135: 330–332.

Young, E., Basson, P.A., and Weiss, K.E. (1970). Experimental infection of game animals with lumpy skin disease virus prototype strain Neethling. *Onderstepoort J. Vet. Res.* 37 (2): 79–87.

Zhao, Z., Fan, B., Wu, G. et al. (2014). Development of loop-mediated isothermal amplification assay for specific and rapid detection of differential goat pox virus and sheep pox virus. *BMC Microbiol.* 14: 10.

29

Rabies

Charles Rupprecht[1] and Donna Gatewood[2]

[1] LYSSA LLC, Atlanta, Georgia, USA
[2] EDGE Veterinary Vaccines Consulting Group, LLC, Ames, Iowa, USA

29.1 Introduction

Rabies is a neglected viral zoonosis, with a substantial agricultural and public health burden (Hampson et al. 2015). Although one of the oldest described infectious diseases, with highly effective vaccines available for over a century, rabies remains enzootic throughout Africa, the Americas, and Eurasia. Despite significant technical progress and the highest associated case fatality of common infectious diseases, rabies appears to lack the same cachet for prioritization and political will for action among national veterinary authorities, in contrast to other viral diseases, for a variety of complex biological, economic, and social reasons (Meltzer and Rupprecht 1998; Rupprecht and Burgess 2015). Beyond agriculture officials and commercial producers, primary motivation for additional improvements to current vaccines may need to arise directly from the private sector, such as the farmer, pet owner, biomedical professional, environmental enthusiast, and conservationist, which will require more focused education on the applied epidemiology, prevention, and control of this disease as a public good.

29.1.1 Etiology

The etiological agents belong to the family Rhabdoviridae, genus *Lyssavirus*. All lyssaviruses are highly neurotropic and cause rabies. The most important and widely distributed member is the type species, rabies virus – the only lyssavirus perpetuated in the New World (Rupprecht et al. 2011). New lyssavirus species have been detected increasingly since the 1950s, due in part to renewed interests in pathogen discovery and technical improvements in diagnosis and characterization (https://talk.ictvonline.org/ictv-reports/ictv_online_report/negative-sense-rna-viruses/mononegavirales/w/rhabdoviridae/795/genus-lyssavirus). No human or veterinary biologics have an adequate panreactive spectrum to protect against all lyssaviruses, given the considerable antigenic variation. Even experimental recombinant vaccines have limitations in spanning the breadth of the genus (Weyer et al. 2008). However, modern potent rabies virus vaccines should protect against all phylogroup I lyssaviruses throughout the world, including rabies virus (Brookes et al. 2005; Malerczyk et al. 2009). Considering genetic diversity across the genus, the prospect for any substantial improvements to cross-reactivity from new biologics remains a challenge (Rupprecht et al. 2017).

29.1.2 Hosts

All warm-blooded vertebrates are believed to be susceptible to rabies (Rupprecht and Kuzmin 2015). Reservoirs include mammalian carnivores (e.g. dogs, foxes, mongoose, raccoons, skunks, etc.) and bats, which are responsible for disease maintenance, predominantly via bite transmission. In general, livestock are essentially victims of spillover from infected carnivores and bats, and are usually a dead end for transmission (Figure 29.1). Bats are major global lyssavirus reservoirs on all inhabited continents, with spillover infections to humans, domestic animals, and wildlife. Because of this, variant-specific prevention, control, and selective elimination are possible for some wildlife species, but not the vast majority, so the viruses are perpetuated, despite effective vaccines for domestic animals (Rupprecht et al. 2017).

Primary vaccination with licensed products would remove the risk of infection for most domestic animals, but would need to occur on a routine and regular basis, without the actual prospect of fundamental eradication because of disease maintenance among wildlife, such as bats (Rupprecht et al. 2017).

Veterinary Vaccines: Principles and Applications, First Edition. Edited by Samia Metwally, Gerrit Viljoen, and Ahmed El Idrissi.

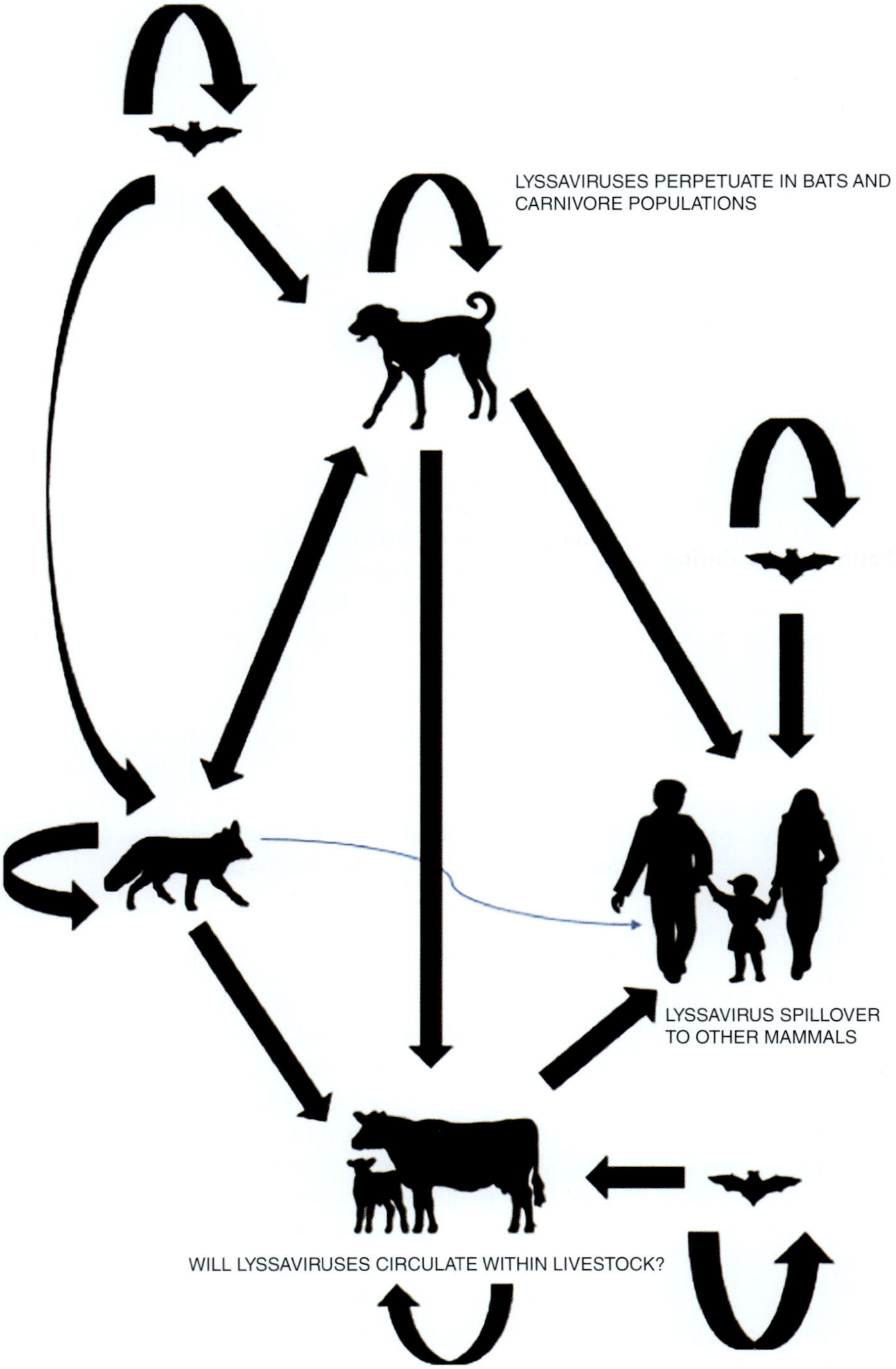

Figure 29.1 Generalized depiction of intraspecific transmission pathways of lyssaviruses perpetuated within principal reservoirs in the Carnivora (e.g. domestic dogs and wildlife such as foxes, raccoons, skunks, etc.) and Chiroptera (e.g. hematophagous, insectivorous, frugivorous bats, etc.), with interspecific spillover infections to other mammals (e.g. livestock, humans, etc.), typically resulting in dead-end rabies cases.

29.2 Types of Vaccines

Over the past century, developments in animal vaccines have largely mirrored similar progress in human rabies biologics (Rupprecht et al. 2016). The gradual evolution of rabies vaccines and the history of production methods covered the same gamut of diversity as other veterinary biologics, from animal passages, to primary organ propagation, through the use of tissue culture and recombinant technology (Wu et al. 2011).

29.2.1 First-Generation Vaccines

At the end of the nineteenth century, the first vaccines were produced in adult animal brains (e.g. rabbits, sheep, etc.), by methods very much akin to those originally used by Pasteur (Rappuoli 2014). As such, Pasteur coined the term "street" viruses, defined as wild-type rabies viruses perpetuated in nature, in contrast to "fixed" rabies viruses whose characteristics were altered in the laboratory by continuous passages, originally in adult animal brains. Such nerve tissue-based products contained residual, infectious "fixed" rabies virus, which was not completely inactivated by drying. The later addition of chemicals, such as ether, phenol, chloroform, or formalin, was an attempt to stabilize the substrate and reduce any adverse events from laboratory rabies viruses, to maintain potency, and minimize the risk of possible vaccine-associated rabies cases. As an example, one rabies virus biologic in Latin America during the early twentieth century was produced by passage in the brain of calves or horses, after which a phenolized emulsion of 20% brain tissue in glycerol and water was used as the vaccine.

Unfortunately, these early vaccines were labor intensive and expensive to produce, and also of fairly low potency, requiring large volumes and multiple doses. Decades later, to avoid concerns related to myelin sensitization and adverse events from vaccines produced within adult animal nervous tissue, rabies virus was propagated successfully in suckling mouse brains, which, when supplemented with an adjuvant, appeared to provide immunity for at least 1 year (Fuenzalida et al. 1978).

29.2.2 Second-Generation Vaccines

By the mid-twentieth century, production using primary cells from fetal or newborn animals, avian embryos, and mammalian tissue cultures (e.g. hamster, canine or porcine kidney cells) sparked a second generation of animal rabies virus vaccines (Koprowski and Cox 1947; Abelseth 1964; Reculard 1996). The agents were isolated as street viruses, which formed the origin of common seed viruses used in attenuated virus vaccines, some still in use for livestock today. While control was often focused upon vaccination of the primary vector, such as dogs, the first widespread use of modified live vaccines in livestock began throughout Latin America, due to the associated burden with vampire bat rabies (Pawan 1959). Thereafter, because of the possibility of vaccine-induced rabies cases, use of some live virus strains was no longer recommended, in favor of other, safer vaccines (Sikes 1970; Lawson et al. 1987).

After the 1970s, animal rabies vaccines progressed gradually from modified live viruses to products produced in high concentrations and inactivated with irradiation (such as ultraviolet light) or chemicals (such as β-Propiolactone). Most animal rabies vaccines available today are inactivated and adjuvanted, although several attenuated viral vaccines persist on the market. Over time, with technology transfer, individuals in several developed countries shared seed viruses, cell cultures, protocols, and production methods to assist rabies vaccine production in developing countries (Devleesschauwer et al. 2016). Nevertheless, there is an underrepresentation of production in both Africa and Asia, where the rabies burden appears to be highest.

29.2.3 Third-Generation Vaccines

The transition to a third generation of animal rabies vaccines began near the end of the twentieth century, with the development of recombinant technology. Several recombinant vaccines have been constructed, based upon adeno-, pox-, or rabies viruses (Pastoret and Vanderplasschen 2003; Gomme et al. 2011; Fry et al. 2013; Martins et al. 2017). These recombinant vaccines have been tested in a variety of domestic animals for safety and some have been licensed, eventually, for other species, such as companion animals or wildlife. However, none thus far has included licensed products with livestock as the target. Similarly, the use of nucleic acid-based vaccines has been suggested in veterinary medicine for decades, but without licensure in livestock (Biswas et al. 2001; Yang et al. 2013). Newer technology, based upon mRNA, may provide alternatives for livestock vaccination, as shown experimentally in swine (Schnee et al. 2016). Production of rabies virus-like particles (VLPs) may also have application as future vaccines (Fontana et al. 2016).

Undoubtedly, rabies biologics for humans, domestic animals, and wildlife have evolved for the better over the past century. Hopefully, novelty and innovation will not be hampered by fears of liability or overzealous regulatory concerns in the design and use of the next generation of rabies vaccines particularly for the *in situ* delivery of multiple antigens (Petricciani et al. 1989; Aspden et al. 2002).

29.2.4 Related Applications

Historically, most inactivated vaccines have contained adjuvants. The majority have been limited to alum and its derivatives, although a few have considered incorporation of plant-based compounds, such as saponins (Yendo et al. 2016). Besides such historical use of aluminum hydroxide, in the future, the use of novel adjuvants is anticipated (Asgary et al. 2016).

Concerning application, to date, all livestock vaccines have been applied by the parenteral route, either intramsucularly

(IM) or subcutaneously (SC). However, other applications may also be relevant. For example, oral vaccines have been successful for the control of rabies among wild carnivores (Slate et al. 2009; Müller et al. 2015). Experimentally, sheep were fed a plant-based vaccine and were protected against rabies virus challenge (Loza-Rubio et al. 2012). Other scenarios exist where similar approaches might be extended to domestic livestock more broadly, including swine or free-ranging, managed hoofed stock, such as kudu (Scott et al. 2012; Yang et al. 2016). Other applications may include development of a single-dose vaccine with a longer duration of immunity, with or without adjuvant, minimizing the need for frequent boosters.

29.3 Immune Response

29.3.1 Virions

Lyssaviruses are composed of a single strand of nonsegmented, negative-sense RNA. The virions consist of five structural proteins and have a bullet-shaped morphology (Figure 29.2).

Biochemical and structural details of these proteins provide insight into viral pathobiology and vaccine-provoked immunity. The outer glycoprotein (G) is embedded in the viral envelope, with peplomer spikes involved in host cellular receptor binding (Fernando et al. 2016). In addition, the viral G protein is the external antigen responsible for the induction of virus-neutralizing antibodies (VNA). As such, the virion-associated G protein is the most critical component of livestock rabies vaccines (Piza et al. 2002). Internally, a helical nucleocapsid includes several structural proteins and the viral RNA. The matrix protein (M) forms a scaffold between the G protein and the nucleocapsid. The inner nucleoprotein (N) is bound tightly to the RNA, to form a ribonucleoprotein (RNP) complex, which protects from destruction by cellular nucleases. Among lyssaviruses, the RNP is the group-specific component and more conserved, whereas the G protein is the major antigen determining serotype, with considerable antigenic diversity. Although much less important than the G protein, administration of the viral RNP has also been documented to confer protective immunity (Dietzschold et al. 1987).

Besides its role as a structural component of the viral nucleocapsid, the N protein is also responsible for the formation of intracytoplasmic inclusions in neurons, which when stained appropriately can be identified by light microscopy as Negri bodies, virion-producing factories (Nikolic et al. 2017) that are a diagnostic hallmark of rabies. The RNA-dependent RNA polymerase (L) protein transcribes and replicates the viral genome (Ogino et al. 2016). The N, P, and L proteins are also involved in viral pathogenicity, through suppression of the host interferon response (Tian et al. 2015).

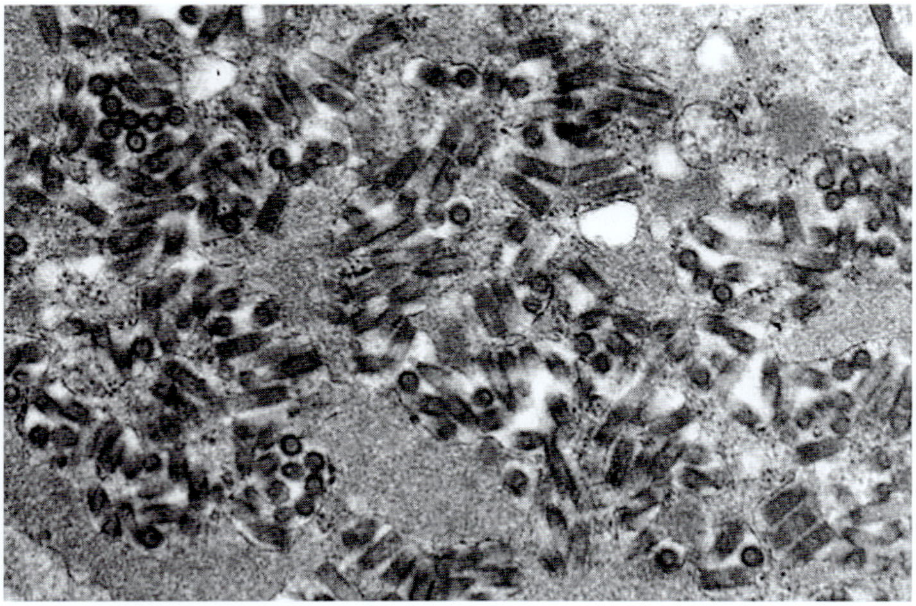

Figure 29.2 A representative lyssavirus virion with a typical bullet-shaped particle, the helical nucleocapsid and the outer glycoprotein envelope, as well as a cross-section of a virion. Source: Adaptation of an electron micrograph courtesy of the US Public Health Image Library within the public domain.

29.3.2 Herd Immunity

Although documented in some wildlife reservoirs such as bats, natural or acquired immunity to rabies in the naïve host is otherwise uncommon. Evidence of prior exposure to rabies virus may be suggested under certain circumstances in unvaccinated animals, but such findings, based upon serology, are essentially irrelevant to the development of effective herd immunity in livestock and should not be used as evidence to avoid primary immunization of animals at risk of viral infection (Gilbert et al. 2015).

29.3.3 Pathobiology

Nonspecific anatomical barriers to pathogen invasion, in part, may provide a shield or buffer and include layered fur, as in musk oxen, bison or camelids, or thickened, intact skin, such as in buffalo, as lyssaviruses cannot penetrate an undamaged epidermis. However, once a transdermal or mucosal exposure has occurred, lyssaviruses avoid local removal efforts by a dual combination of stealth and suppression, as quintessential neurotropic agents (Dietzschold et al. 2008). After virion deposition and reception in the peripheral nerves, viral tropism occurs in retrograde fashion to the spinal cord and brain. The predominance of viral replication occurs in the central nervous system as an immunologically privileged site, largely free from immunological surveillance.

During replication, viral products induce upregulation of host cellular processes to evade primary immune responses, which increases success for productive generation of viral progeny. Concomitantly, viral proteins inhibit specific immune responses, resulting in the dampening of downstream opportunities for the host to clear active viral infection. Once clinical signs and encephalitis manifest, death ensues within a relatively short morbidity period.

29.3.4 Acquired Immunity

In theory, limited immunity against a productive lyssavirus infection in the naïve animal is provided by a combination of both innate and adaptive responses. Innate responses are triggered by the interaction between pathogen-associated molecular patterns and host reciprocal pattern recognition receptors, leading to secretion of proinflammatory cytokines (Li et al. 2011). However, this innate response alone does not promote total viral clearance. Adaptive immune responses develop more slowly in the unvaccinated animal. Typically, antibodies in naïve livestock infected with rabies virus only become detectable, if at all, several days after onset of neurological illness. In general, such antibodies, once induced, are only found in serum, but not, or only at lower titers, within the cerebrospinal fluid (CSF) of animals who succumb, as opposed to the rarity of survivors with sequelae (Bell and Moore 1979; Gnanadurai et al. 2013). This late and commonly weaker antibody response may suggest that the dose of the infecting viral inoculum is inadequate to trigger effective T and B cell activation at the site of infection.

An intact blood–brain barrier minimizes the effectiveness of penetration of any antibodies that may develop in the periphery. Humoral responses are also limited by the inhibition of interferon signaling, which may prevent B cell maturation.

29.3.5 Humoral Responses

Long-lasting immunity after rabies vaccination is complex, but seems provided primarily via VNA. The basic definition of a successful rabies vaccination outcome is the measurement of an international standard of VNA at a level of 0.5 IU mL^{-1}. Although this arbitrary value is not considered as "sero-protective" *per se*, it can be taken as an indicator of an appropriate response in the individual immune-competent animal. In reality, the true measure of the efficacy of rabies vaccination is protection against a virulent viral challenge in the surviving animal.

Development of rabies VNA requires assistance from $CD4^+$ cells, which are induced by inactivated rabies vaccines. Responses occur via T helper cell-independent, shorter-lived plasma cells, developing outside germinal centers and producing IgM. Longer-lived plasma cells develop in germinal centers and produce switched, affinity-matured IgG antibodies. Nearly all healthy animals which receive a dose of rabies vaccine will respond with detectable VNA within 7–14 days, peaking at around day 30, then beginning a gradual decline by around day 90 and finally starting to drop below 0.5 IU/mL by about 12–15 months (Côrtes et al. 1993; Sihvonen et al. 1994; Filho et al. 2012). Rabies vaccines also induce memory B cells that may persist for life, considering they can be recalled years later, as observed in vaccinated humans (Malerczyk et al. 2007). Upon booster immunization at 12–36 months, rather than a more typical, shorter interval between doses, VNA appear more sustained. In properly vaccinated animals, an anamnestic response may result in a favorable outcome, regardless of the absolute VNA level at the time of viral exposure (Rupprecht and Dietzschold 1987).

Not all animals develop VNA to the same level or duration. In any population of livestock, both low and high responders to rabies vaccination are detected (Thompson et al. 2016). Response may be influenced by genetics, nutrition, and overall health. Somewhat surprisingly, parasite load did not appear to significantly affect vaccine efficacy

(Charlier et al. 2013). Regardless, with respect to overall response, a normal distribution of immunological response is expected in a herd over time. In contrast to $CD4^{+}$cells, $CD8^{+}$ cells do not appear to contribute substantially to protective immunity and are not induced by conventional inactivated animal rabies vaccines.

29.4 Presentation, Indications, and Dosage

Rabies vaccines for veterinary use are unique in a One Health context, considering that their use in domestic animals and wildlife provides an important public health benefit by creating a barrier between rabies virus reservoirs and human populations. In addition, they provide direct utility in agriculture and conservation biology. As a result of these factors, regulatory authorities have a keen interest in ensuring that rabies vaccines meet stringent requirements for safety, purity, potency, and efficacy. Safety considerations involve not only the intended species but also nontarget species, such as humans.

29.4.1 Potency, Efficacy, and Duration of Immunity

Relative estimates of the test vaccine potency are compared with a reference standard using the United States National Institutes of Health (NIH) test. The NIH test has been used for several decades and involves large numbers of mice. Alternatives are being sought to minimize the use of animals for potency determination (Lewis et al. 2012). All reference vaccines are based on the International Standard for Rabies Vaccine provided by the World Health Organization (WHO) and should be carefully calibrated to ensure that a potency of at least 1 IU mL^{-1} is met (Hermann et al. 2012).

Efficacy involves testing the effectiveness of rabies vaccine in species for which the product is intended, using animals of appropriate age and gender. For example, a canine vaccine might use puppies of both sexes at 3 months of age. Most authorities require vaccination/challenge studies to demonstrate product efficacy.

True duration of immunity is the length of time during which vaccine recipients are resistant to virulent viral challenge. For ethical and practical reasons, such studies are rarely conducted for veterinary vaccines. Rather, a revaccination interval is established for new products by demonstrating protection against a virulent challenge at a defined period of time, typically 1–3 years postvaccination.

29.4.2 Access

Many authorities require that rabies vaccines be administered by or under the supervision of a veterinarian, so they are often not available for sale directly to animal owners or the general public. Especially because of the important public health implications, rabies vaccine should only be obtained from manufacturers operating under the oversight of a robust and competent regulatory authority.

29.4.3 Specifications

Desired specifications when ordering rabies vaccines are necessarily closely linked to their intended use. Most manufacturers offer single-dose and multiple-dose vials for use in domestic animals, including dogs, cats, cattle, horses, sheep, ferrets, and wildlife. Products for use in wildlife are typically prepared as single doses in individual baits. Vaccination of wildlife is generally conducted only under the auspices of a government agency, and the products are not usually available to nongovernmental entities or individuals.

When ordering vaccine for livestock operations or for use in kennels, catteries, animal shelters, or mass vaccination clinics, multiple-dose vials are likely to provide the most economical option. When using multiple-dose vials, once opened, any unused portion of the vial should be discarded and not stored for future use. For vaccination of individual companion animals or "pet" livestock, single-dose vials may be the best option to ensure that product sterility or potency is not compromised.

29.4.4 Boosters

The revaccination interval is an important consideration. Most rabies vaccines have 1–3-year revaccination recommendations. Some veterinarians object to the use of 3-year interval vaccines, for several reasons. Some believe client compliance is better when annual revaccination is the standard practice, because it may be easier for clients to remember to schedule an annual visit. Others assume that the 3-year vaccines have substantially more antigen and are therefore potentially more reactive. There are no data to support either of these beliefs, so the revaccination interval specification should be based on local conditions and intended use. When conducting mass vaccination campaigns in rabies-endemic areas, a 3-year product is generally the preferred option, as it offers the longest demonstrated efficacy.

29.4.5 Stability

Product shelf-life and stability are other important parameters to consider when selecting rabies vaccines. Pricing is often based on quantity purchased, so buying large quantities may be an economical choice, but care should be taken to ensure that the amount purchased will be used prior to the product expiry date for the particular batch or lot being purchased. Most rabies vaccines have a shelf-life of 1–3 years, so if large quantities are being ordered, it is advisable to request a batch or lot that was recently produced, to maximize the length of time for which it can be used.

29.4.6 Wildlife

Rabies vaccines for use in wildlife are available with efficacy claims for several wildlife species, such as foxes, raccoon dogs, coyotes, and raccoons (Slate et al. 2009; Müller et al. 2015). When ordering vaccine for use in a wildlife vaccination campaign, several factors must be considered. Ideally, the vaccine selected should have proven laboratory and field efficacy for the species being targeted. However, there are situations where it is reasonable to begin a campaign on an experimental basis, if there are data to suggest that the product will be effective in the target species.

With regard to wildlife vaccines, stability of the product in the field after distribution is a critical consideration (Hermann et al. 2011). Manufacturers should have data to demonstrate field stability of their products, and this information should be evaluated in the context of the planned bait distribution density, target species population density, foraging behavior of the target species, and climatic conditions.

29.4.7 Public Health Issues

All veterinarians and others at occupational risk of exposure to animals with suspected rabies should be vaccinated against the disease. For the naïve person exposed to a rabid animal, measures consist of local wound care, infiltration of rabies immune globulin, and administration of multiple doses of vaccine (Rupprecht et al. 2016). Modern human rabies vaccines are inactivated tissue culture-derived products. Detailed specifications and recommendations for pre- and postexposure use are available at several national or international sources (ACIP 2008; WHO 2018).

29.5 Regulations and Quality Assurance

When purchasing rabies vaccines for veterinary use that are licensed in Canada or the USA, or are registered in the European Union (EU), or Japan, end-users can be confident that the products meet the standards established by those regulatory authorities. Vaccines produced in accordance with the Canadian Food Inspection Agency's (CFIA) requirements, the United States Title 9 of the Code of Federal Regulations (9CFR), or under European Pharmacopoeia Good Manufacturing Processes (EP GMP) requirements have undergone extensive evaluations for safety, purity, potency, efficacy, and postmarketing surveillance. Such vaccines should not require control testing by the end-user or the importer.

While the EP, CFIA, and 9CFR regulatory approaches are slightly different, all achieve the same results of assurance for safe, pure, potent, and effective products. These approaches require preauthorization characterization and testing of the master seeds, master cells, and ingredients of animal origin to ensure purity of the end-product. Batch testing includes controlled sterility, safety, and potency testing. Further, these authorities require that facilities meet stringent requirements to prevent the possibility of product contamination. Certificates accompanying a vaccine order from the EU, Canada, or USA should include evidence that the product was made in approved facilities, as well as evidence that it is approved for distribution and sale, and is labeled for use in the species of interest.

When considering products manufactured under the purview of other regulatory authorities, the Certificate of Analysis should describe the final product testing. At a minimum, final product should be tested for purity, safety, and potency. For conventional inactivated rabies vaccines, the assays used should be at least equivalent to either the EP monograph entitled Rabies Vaccine (Inactivated) for Veterinary Use, or the United States 9CFR Part 113.209.

Historically, the trend in developed countries has been to move from modified live to inactivated rabies vaccines for use in domestic animals. Such inactivated rabies vaccines have been tested for potency using the mouse potency test (or some modification thereof) developed by the US NIH. As mentioned previously, this assay is problematic for a number of reasons, and several groups are investing substantially in efforts toward the development of an *in vitro* assay or a battery of assays to replace the NIH test (Schiffelers et al. 2014). In the near future, ELISA-based techniques may be preferred to *in vivo* testing (Sigoillot-Claude et al. 2015). However, until a replacement assay is validated and adopted by the requisite regulatory authorities, potency should be conducted using the NIH test or an equivalent assay.

Besides classic inactivated products, there are several approved, modified live, biotechnology-derived vaccines, which utilize a vector virus expressing the rabies virus G protein (Hicks et al. 2012). These are typically evaluated for potency by conducting a simple titration of the vector virus coupled with an expression assay to confirm expression of the G protein. The batch release requirements for these products are based on performance of the efficacy batch when tested in the approved test system. Besides overcoming potency and efficacy concerns, technical improvements and next-generation sequencing methods will provide greater ease in the identification of viral seed strains used for production as well as genetic stability, particularly in the use of biologics intended for the vaccination of free-ranging wildlife (Höper et al. 2015).

In summary, most manufacturers conduct adequate testing prior to the release of vaccine batches. However, it is advisable to request proof of country of origin as well as a list or reference to the testing conducted for each batch release.

29.6 Vaccine Application for Disease Prevention in Livestock and Other Animals

Applications of rabies vaccination to livestock will vary, dependent in part upon life history stage, immunological status, and exposure circumstances. Modern veterinary vaccines are highly efficacious, especially when used in a preexposure strategy. Rabies is quite rare in properly vaccinated animals. Most reported cases of rabies in livestock occur in naïve animals. Vaccination of animals with clinical suspicion of rabies has no proven utility and is not recommended, based upon a lack of evidence, wasted economic outlay, and the public health risk of viral exposure.

29.6.1 Livestock

Unlike domestic carnivore rabies vaccination, which should be mandatory starting with puppies and kittens in enzootic areas, global practices for livestock vaccination vary greatly from country to country and region to region, based in part on risk perceptions. Regardless of species and rabies epidemiological conditions, the majority of livestock are not vaccinated anywhere in the world. Historically, livestock vaccination was considered prohibitive in cost, recognizing the primary source in dogs or wildlife, while management preferences centered upon insurance and indemnification (Korns and Zeissig 1948; Miguens 2007; Swai et al. 2010). Education of owners, producers, and veterinarians is needed to change this perception (Hundal et al. 2016).

At a minimum, because of the zoonotic aspect of the disease, in enzootic regions rabies vaccination should occur for all animals in close contact with the public, such as at livestock fairs, petting zoos, etc., or those used in international competition (Brown et al. 2016). Vaccination is not needed in "rabies-free" areas, provided that such countries meet the criteria for such self-declarations. Even a continent considered historically free of rabies, such as Australia, has enzootic lyssaviruses, with reservoirs in bats. Similarly, Taiwan was considered free of rabies, until surveillance was expanded to wildlife and the recognition of reservoirs among ferret badgers and bats (Hu et al. 2018).

Rabies vaccines are usually formulated as monovalent products. On occasion, the vaccine has been combined with others, such as with foot and mouth disease virus (FMDV) vaccines in ruminants (Palanisamy et al. 1992). In general, immunogenicity of the monovalent or combined vaccines appeared equivalent. Another example, in horses, includes the combination of rabies and Potomac fever vaccines (Brown et al. 2016).

29.6.2 Frequency

The frequency of boosters is an issue of economics and practicality, especially for animals on range, not readily available for multiple rounds of parenteral immunization. Most vaccine labels call for annual boosters, but this may not be necessary for all products and species. For example, based upon VNA serological comparisons, a booster interval greater than 1 year may be appropriate for previously vaccinated horses, but not for naïve animals, after receiving their first dose (Harvey et al. 2016). Similarly, in cattle, priming at ~6 months of age gave an acceptable anamnestic response when boosted up to 3 years later (Yakobson et al. 2015). Other investigators also reported the utility of booster vaccinations in previously vaccinated livestock, to maintain rabies VNA in excess of 0.5 IU mL^{-1} (Albas et al. 1998; Monaco et al. 2006).

29.6.3 Epizootic Application

If vaccines are to be used in the face of an outbreak, efficacy will vary if animals are already exposed and incubating. Postexposure prophylaxis, using vaccine only, has been used in naïve animals (Blancou et al. 1991; Basheer et al. 1997; Wilson and Clark 2001). One schedule for buffalo suggests using vaccine within 24 hours of the exposure, followed by boosters on days 3, 7, 14, 28, and 90 (www.buffalopedia.cirb.res.in/index.php?option=com_content&view=article&id=209&Itemid=117&lang=en). In Nepal, the annual reports of ~100 fatal cases of rabies in livestock and more than 1000 cases of rabies prophylaxis administered to livestock per year were felt to be gross underestimates (Devleesschauwer et al. 2016). However, the efficacy of postexposure prophylaxis in unvaccinated livestock is questionable, especially for severe exposures. Ideally, in a One Health context, it is better to strive toward complete protection in such postexposure settings, and a source of immune globulin should be available for use in addition to vaccine, as recommended by the WHO for exposed persons (Mitmoonpitak et al. 2002).

29.6.4 Related Concerns

Because cases of rabies in livestock originate from either other domestic animals or wildlife, attention must also be given to reducing their exposure from these sources. In less developed countries, most cases of rabies in livestock are due to transmission from dogs. Clearly, the single most important element for the prevention of livestock cases in canine rabies enzootic areas is the mass vaccination of dogs (Gibson et al. 2016). Plans have been created for elimination of canine rabies globally (http://caninerabiesblueprint.org). Where canine rabies has been controlled and other carnivores, such as foxes or raccoons, are the major source of infection, oral wildlife vaccination and related management strategies should be considered (Slate et al. 2009; Müller et al. 2015).

Regardless of other benefits, neither canine rabies elimination nor oral vaccination of wild carnivores will provide benefit to livestock under all scenarios. With a distribution from Mexico to Argentina, rabies virus transmitted by vampire bats has a major impact upon the livestock industry, with multiple attempts aimed at control. Historically, before the development of effective vaccines, rabies control was nonspecific, such as by destroying suspected vampire bat roosts (and many beneficial species). In the mid-to-late twentieth century, anticoagulants were used as a more specific method of vampire bat control. Vampire bats were captured, spread with anticoagulant pastes and allowed to return to their roosts, where grooming by conspecific roost mates resulted in multiple deaths. Such methods allowed targeting to the species of interest and multiplication of effect from treated individuals, but was labor intensive, requiring staying late throughout the evening to capture vampires at affected ranches. Alternatively, livestock were injected with anticoagulants directly, which vampire bats would ingest during a blood meal. This technique allowed veterinarians to treat multiple farms during the day, but was more expensive and required a bat bite upon a treated animal for effectiveness. Both techniques suffered the limitation of toxic environmental contamination with potential impacts to other fauna, as well as the opportunity of vampire bat population disruption, roost switching, and colony dispersal, exacerbating the infectious disease threat. Neither was effective without concomitant vaccination of the herd at risk (Benavides et al. 2017). Inconsistent use of anticoagulants throughout the region as a whole, combined with decreasing availability of products and increasing costs, has lessened the utility of vampire bat population reduction as a principal long-term or widespread solution to control this highly adaptive and unique vertebrate reservoir, requiring novel, more integrated solutions (Stoner-Duncan et al. 2014).

As an example of one small country in Central America that has successfully controlled canine rabies but has vampire bats, Costa Rica reported more than 75 outbreaks in livestock over a 30-year period, with more than 780 fatal cases diagnosed in cattle (Hutter et al. 2016). Recent reports suggest that bovine paralytic rabies is spreading into areas that were previously unaffected (Bárcenas-Reyes et al. 2015). If climate change trends continue, vampire bat-transmitted rabies is expected to increase over widespread cattle-rearing regions, such as Mexico, Central America, Brazil, Paraguay, and perhaps the USA (Hayes and Piaggio 2018). Although livestock vaccination appears quite beneficial, the cost–benefit of vampire bat control may not always be high (Anderson et al. 2014).

29.7 Monitoring and Vaccine Effectiveness

The measure of any rabies vaccine and vaccination program should be the protection of vaccinated subjects from a productive lyssavirus infection. Postvaccination monitoring and a vaccine adverse event reporting system (VAERS) are essential parts of an effective prevention and control program and a major indicator of success. All suspected rabies cases should be reported, confirmed, and thoroughly investigated, including collection and analysis of spatiotemporal data, species demographics, clinical signs, history of human and animal exposures, vaccination status, etc. True vaccine failures should be rare. To minimize this risk, and for a variety of ethical, regulatory, and public health reasons, all rabies vaccination should be conducted by, or under the supervision of, a licensed veterinarian (Rollin 1995; Brown et al 2016).

In addition to the basic laboratory diagnosis of rabies, molecular methods should be utilized to characterize the various lyssaviruses present and differentiate indigenous from any introduced cases. In some regions, only a single lyssavirus species will predominate (e.g. rabies virus, Australian bat lyssavirus, etc.). Viral characterization may indicate the emergence or translocation of a new pathogen that could impact vaccine efficacy. Similarly, if modified live rabies vaccines (e.g. LEP, SAD, etc.) are used, such methods will readily differentiate seed viruses used for production (and the possibility of vaccine-associated rabies) from native street viruses (Höper et al. 2015).

Serological monitoring for VNA is possible. It should not be necessary as a routine measure for all applications, but may provide some insight in the management of exposed livestock. For example, after viral exposure, all vaccinated animals should be boosted. Unvaccinated animals may be euthanized or quarantined. Although all records of vaccination should be readily available, if such documentation is lacking, prospective serological monitoring might be considered, as suggested for dogs and cats (Moore et al. 2015; Brown et al. 2016). Depending upon the product and its immunogenicity, rabies VNA may be detected or an anamnestic response can be measured within ~5–7 days of a booster vaccination, indicating the vaccination status of the animal in question. Moreover, if multiple vaccines from different producers are used concomitantly, postmarketing surveillance may be useful to differentiate the utility of multiple products, not only on the basis of cost but other factors, such as basic VNA response and duration of immunity under field conditions (Gilbert et al. 2015).

Analysis of the occurrence of livestock cases in space and time, viral characterization, and subsequent ecological modeling may provide long-term information on any species-specific or geographic patterns or seasonality. For example, regardless of vaccination status, introduction of livestock into new areas may have unexpected consequences. Recent observations of vampire bat foraging activity in Amazonia are consistent with the idea that introducing alternative prey could affect the numbers of human rabies cases in local high-risk communities (Streicker and Allgeier 2016).

29.7.1 Vaccine Adverse Reactions

In general, modern rabies vaccines are quite safe, compared with older, nerve tissue-derived products. Local reactions may include pain, swelling, redness, alopecia, pruritus, or other signs of mild inflammation. Granulomas may occur, particularly with vaccines containing adjuvants. Systemic signs may include fever, multifocal vasculitis, transient lameness or, rarely, anaphylaxis (Quirozr et al. 1964). Epinephrine should be readily available in case the latter occurs. Among domestic animals, vaccine injection site sarcomas have been reported (Hartmann et al. 2015; Jacobs et al. 2017). Nonviral components of vaccines may sensitize animals for future adverse responses (Gershwin et al. 2012).

The most serious adverse events are vaccine-associated rabies and vaccine failure. Vaccine-associated rabies cases were uncommon, even after first-generation vaccines were used more widely, especially when compared with the millions of doses of modified live vaccines applied globally. The advent of characterization by monoclonal antibodies and later by genetic sequencing enabled proper differentiation of fixed laboratory strains from street viruses (Hostnik et al. 2014; Robardet et al. 2016). Very rare cases in livestock have been reported in association with rabies virus vaccines used for the oral vaccination of wildlife (Fehlner-Gardiner et al. 2008; Vuta et al. 2016). Reports of rabies cases in animals with a history of vaccination must differentiate among variables related to the vaccine, the vaccinated subject, and the vaccinator. True vaccine failures are quite rare. Vaccinated animals may have a compromised immune system and fail to respond appropriately. Interference from maternal immunity may also occur. Breaks in the cold chain may lead to vaccine instability. Similarly, choice of an improper product, diluent, route, age, boosters, etc. are also variables that may be associated with rabies in an exposed animal with a documentation of prior vaccination.

Creation of a national VAERS program related to veterinary vaccines and a searchable database for such licensed biologics would complement existing surveillance systems for the detection of acute or chronic reactions by product, species, and circumstances.

29.8 Availability

A comprehensive list of all manufacturers of livestock rabies vaccines is not possible. The pharmaceutical field is quite dynamic and lists may become obsolete quickly. Companies may merge and minimize product duplication. New start-up facilities are created with novel products based upon regulatory approval and others may be recalled based on the occurrence of adverse events following postmarketing surveillance. Annual reviews are needed on a national and regional basis to remain current (Brown et al. 2016). One apparent trend is that older, less potent nerve tissue biologics are being replaced gradually by tissue culture vaccines and the prior monopoly of products requiring routine annual boosters is being supplemented gradually by vaccines having a minimum duration of immunity of several years.

Historically, rabies vaccines were produced primarily in the Americas and Eurasia, but slowly are becoming more available on a global basis. By comparison, during 2016, based upon incomplete, self-reported data provided to the OIE by region (www.oie.int/wahis_2/public/wahid.php/Countryinformation/Vaccines), more than 150 million doses were produced by countries in the Americas, compared with fewer than 50 000 doses produced in Africa and Asia (excluding China and India). Based upon current vaccines and their distributional use, no major shortages are forecast in the Americas or Europe. In the future, emerging markets in Asia, such as India, are expected to contribute more to the overall diversity and dose numbers for the subcontinent and surrounding region, even while concerns elsewhere abound (McLaughlin 2016). In particular, within China, canine rabies is widespread and outbreaks involving other domestic species appear to be on the increase. Problematically, specific rabies vaccines for large animals are not readily available, particularly in rural provinces. Under such limitations and emergency settings, in one study, a single injection of a "double dose" canine vaccine was economical and convenient for local veterinarians and induced adequate levels of VNA for at least 1 year in cattle and camels, underscoring the opportunities and challenges throughout rural Asia (Liu et al. 2016).

Considering the needs for canine rabies elimination, additional production capacity is required, predicated in part upon a more accurate assessment of the populations at risk, the required number of doses to accomplish this objective, better engagement with industry, and a sound business plan for completion (Rupprecht et al. 2017).

In general, vaccines are available for all the major mammalian species that may be considered at risk. However, some gaps exist. Where a need for vaccination in a particular species is not apparent geographically, a product with the greatest taxonomic cross-reactivity and the longest duration of immunity may be considered. For example, in conservation medicine, parenteral inactivated vaccines are often used off-label to protect valuable zoo stock in rabies enzootic regions (Miller and Fowler 2012). While such use does not preclude proper public health measures, if human exposure occurs to a suspect or documented rabid animal, such vaccination would lessen the relative risk of a case in a vaccinated animal, and lessen the impact of occupational exposures to staff on a routine basis (Brown et al. 2016).

Obviously, it would be unreasonable to expect a unique product licensed for every possible species, on economic grounds alone. For example, if a national authority is interested in a rabies vaccine for a new species, but in which no prior application is documented, review of the recent comparative literature and current vaccine product insert lists may be relevant for importation or technology transfer, rather than embarking upon *de novo* indigenous production for every possible application. Given the potency and safety of modern animal rabies vaccines today, a relatively broad margin of cross-reactivity would be expected, based upon inference alone and comparative serological testing (Wallace et al. 2016). By extension, one broadly applicable vaccine already proven to be efficacious in dogs, cats, cows, sheep, horses, ferrets, etc. would also be expected to be useful, *ad hoc*, in elephants, guinea pigs, llamas, musk oxen, reindeer, yaks, etc., especially in an emergency. Such off-label or investigational use of other marketed vaccines might have utility during an outbreak, protect valuable animals, and help prevent additional disease spread, but caution is advisable if livestock need to be translocated and these animals should not be assumed to be protected for the purposes of international trade.

29.9 Summary

Vaccination is a critical part of the prevention and control of rabies, as a neglected viral zoonosis, with the highest case fatality of any conventional infectious disease. This acute, progressive encephalitis is global in distribution, with rare exceptions. The etiological agents are single-stranded, negative-sense RNA viruses in the family Rhabdoviridae, genus *Lyssavirus*. All mammals are believed to be susceptible. Major reservoirs include domestic and wild carnivores and bats. In general, livestock are victims and dead-end hosts, although they can serve as vectors to humans and in very rare cases result in animal-to-animal transmission. Most livestock are infected either by bite exposure via rabid domestic dogs or wild carnivores, particularly in Africa and Asia, or hematophagus bats throughout Latin America.

Biologics have progressed over the past century from nerve tissue-based products to modified live viruses to cell culture vaccines and in the near future many newer derivatives may be based upon recombinant technology. The viral G protein is the most important antigen for the induction of VNA and protective immunity. Pure, potent, safe, and efficacious vaccines for preexposure vaccination are widely available for most common species, but with some limitations in supply.

All livestock should be considered for vaccination in rabies enzootic areas. Priority should be given to particularly valuable animals and those in frequent contact with humans in public settings. Primary vaccination of juveniles, followed by a booster dose around a year later, leads to a long-lasting duration of immunity. Postexposure prophylaxis of the naïve individual is possible, if conducted in a timely and appropriate manner, but is much more complicated and expensive. Therapy of animals after the advent of clinical signs is futile. Rabies should be a notifiable disease and enhanced, local, laboratory-based surveillance is necessary to determine the burden of livestock rabies, generate economic impacts in rural areas, and document the need for medical investigation of those persons exposed to suspect animals.

Future research should entail: development of biologics with a broader spectrum of activity across the antigenic diversity of the *Lyssavirus* genus; additional robust and safer adjuvants; methods to maximize thermostability under tropical conditions; relevant, humane techniques to manage bovine paralytic rabies associated with vampire bats; and simpler vaccination regimens that may entail a single dose, or at most a prime-boost administration, for maximal duration of immunity for free-ranging animals, without the need for routine annual boosters.

As espoused by the FAO, OIE, and PAHO/WHO, in a One Health context, the single overriding strategy to minimize the risk of rabies in many livestock is the mass vaccination of dogs, to eliminate the perpetuation of canine rabies as a common public good from the joint perspectives of agriculture, human health, and conservation medicine (Rupprecht et al. 2019).

References

Abelseth, M.K. (1964). An attenuated rabies vaccine for domestic animals produced in tissue culture. *Can. Vet. J.* 5 (11): 279–286.

Advisory Committee on Immunization Practices (ACIP) (2008). Human rabies prevention – United States, 2008: recommendations of the Advisory Committee on Immunization Practices. *MMWR Recomm. Rep.* 57 (RR-3): 1–28. www.cdc.gov/mmwr/preview/mmwrhtml/rr5703a1.htm.

Albas, A., Pardo, P.E., Gomes, A.A. et al. (1998). Effect of a booster-dose of rabies vaccine on the duration of virus neutralizing antibody titers in bovines. *Rev. Soc. Bras. Med. Trop.* 31 (4): 367–371.

Anderson, A., Shwiff, S., Gebhardt, K. et al. (2014). Economic evaluation of vampire bat (*Desmodus rotundus*) rabies prevention in Mexico. *Transbound. Emerg. Dis.* 61 (2): 140–146.

Asgary, V., Shoari, A., Baghbani-Arani, F. et al. (2016). Green synthesis and evaluation of silver nanoparticles as adjuvant in rabies veterinary vaccine. *Int. J. Nanomed.* 11: 3597–3605.

Aspden, K., van Dijk, A.A., Bingham, J. et al. (2002). Immunogenicity of a recombinant lumpy skin disease virus (neethling vaccine strain) expressing the rabies virus glycoprotein in cattle. *Vaccine* 20 (21–22): 2693–2701.

Bárcenas-Reyes, I., Loza-Rubio, E., Zendejas-Martínez, H. et al. (2015). Epidemiological trends in bovine paralytic rabies in Central Mexico, 2001–2013. *Rev. Panam. Salud Publica* 38 (5): 396–402.

Basheer, A.M., Ramakrishna, J., and Manickam, R. (1997). Evaluation of post-exposure vaccination against rabies in cattle. *New Microbiol.* 20 (3): 289–294.

Bell, J.F. and Moore, G.J. (1979). Allergic encephalitis, rabies antibodies, and the blood/brain barrier. *J. Lab. Clin. Med.* 94 (1): 5–11.

Benavides, J.A., Rojas Paniagua, E., Hampson, K. et al. (2017). Quantifying the burden of vampire bat rabies in Peruvian livestock. *PLoS Negl.Trop. Dis.* 11 (12): e0006105.

Biswas, S., Reddy, G.S., Srinivasan, V.A., and Rangarajan, P.N. (2001). Preexposure efficacy of a novel combination DNA and inactivated rabies virus vaccine. *Hum. Gene Ther.* 12 (15): 1917–1922.

Blancou, J., Baltazar, R.S., Molli, I., and Stoltz, J.F. (1991). Effective postexposure treatment of rabies-infected sheep with rabies immune globulin and vaccine. *Vaccine* 9 (6): 432–437.

Brookes, S.M., Parsons, G., Johnson, N. et al. (2005). Rabies human diploid cell vaccine elicits cross-neutralising and cross-protecting immune responses against European and Australian bat lyssaviruses. *Vaccine* 23 (32): 4101–4109.

Brown, C.M., Slavinski, S., Ettestad, P. et al. (2016). National Association of State Public Health Veterinarians (NASPHV); compendium of animal rabies prevention and control committee, compendium of animal rabies prevention and control. *J. Am. Vet. Med. Assoc.* 248 (5): 505–517.

Charlier, J., Forbes, A., van Gucht, S. et al. (2013). Serological evidence of *Ostertagia ostertagi* infection in dairy cows does not impact the efficacy of rabies vaccination during the housing period. *Res. Vet. Sci.* 95 (3): 1055–1058.

Côrtes, J.A., Rweyemamu, M.M., Ito, F.H. et al. (1993). Immune response in cattle induced by inactivated rabies vaccine adjuvanted with aluminium hydroxide either alone or in combination with avridine. *Rev. Sci. Tech.* 12 (3): 941–955.

Devleesschauwer, B., Aryal, A., Sharma, B.K. et al. (2016). Epidemiology, impact and control of rabies in Nepal: a systematic review. *PLoS Negl. Trop. Dis.* 10 (2): e0004461.

Dietzschold, B., Wang, H.H., Rupprecht, C.E. et al. (1987). Induction of protective immunity against rabies by immunization with rabies virus ribonucleoprotein. *Proc. Natl. Acad. Sci. U.S.A.* 84 (24): 9165–9169.

Dietzschold, B., Li, J., Faber, M., and Schnell, M. (2008). Concepts in the pathogenesis of rabies. *Future Virol.* 3 (5): 481–490.

Fehlner-Gardiner, C., Nadin-Davis, S., Armstrong, J. et al. (2008). Era vaccine-derived cases of rabies in wildlife and domestic animals in Ontario, Canada, 1989–2004. *J. Wildl. Dis.* 44 (1): 71–85.

Fernando, B.G., Yersin, C.T., José, C.B., and Paola, Z.S. (2016). Predicted 3D model of the rabies virus glycoprotein trimer. *Biomed. Res. Int.* 2016: 1674580.

Filho, O.A., Megid, J., Geronutti, L. et al. (2012). Vaccine immune response and interference of colostral antibodies in calves vaccinated against rabies at 2, 4 and 6 months of age born from antirabies revaccinated females. *Res. Vet. Sci.* 92 (3): 396–400.

Fontana, D., Etcheverrigaray, M., Kratje, R., and Prieto, C. (2016). Development of rabies virus-like particles for vaccine applications: production, characterization, and protection studies. *Methods Mol. Biol.* 1403: 155–166.

Fry, T.L., Vandalen, K.K., Duncan, C., and Vercauteren, K. (2013). The safety of ONRAB® in select non-target wildlife. *Vaccine* 31 (37): 3839–3842.

Fuenzalida, E., Díaz, A.M., and Rivenson, S. (1978). Suckling mouse brain rabies vaccine supplemented with an adjuvant. Its use in cattle. *Rev. Asoc. Argent. Microbiol.* 10 (2): 47–53.

Gershwin, L.J., Netherwood, K.A., Norris, M.S. et al. (2012). Equine IgE responses to non-viral vaccine components. *Vaccine* 30 (52): 7615–7620.

Gibson, A.D., Handel, I.G., Shervell, K. et al. (2016). The vaccination of 35,000 dogs in 20 working days using combined static point and door-to-door methods in Blantyre, Malawi. *PLoS Negl. Trop. Dis.* 10 (7): e0004824.

Gilbert, A., Greenberg, L., Moran, D. et al. (2015). Antibody response of cattle to vaccination with commercial modified live rabies vaccines in Guatemala. *Prev. Vet. Med.* 118 (1): 36–44.

Gnanadurai, C.W., Zhou, M., He, W. et al. (2013). Presence of virus neutralizing antibodies in cerebral spinal fluid correlates with non-lethal rabies in dogs. *PLoS Negl. Trop. Dis.* 7 (9): e2375.

Gomme, E.A., Wanjalla, C.N., Wirblich, C., and Schnell, M.J. (2011). Rabies virus as a research tool and viral vaccine vector. *Adv. Virus Res.* 79: 139–164.

Hampson, K., Coudeville, L., Lembo, T. et al. (2015). Global alliance for rabies control partners for rabies prevention. Estimating the global burden of endemic canine rabies. *PLoS Negl. Trop. Dis.* 9 (4): e0003709.

Hartmann, K., Day, M.J., Thiry, E. et al., European Advisory Board on Cat Diseases. (2015). Feline injection-site sarcoma: ABCD guidelines on prevention and management. *J. Feline Med. Surg.* 17 (7): 606–613.

Harvey, A.M., Watson, J.L., Brault, S.A. et al. (2016). Duration of serum antibody response to rabies vaccination in horses. *J. Am. Vet. Med. Assoc.* 249 (4): 411–418.

Hayes, M.A. and Piaggio, A.J. (2018). Assessing the potential impacts of a changing climate on the distribution of a rabies virus vector. *PLoS One* 13 (2): e0192887.

Hermann, J.R., Fry, A.M., Siev, D. et al. (2011). Stability of vaccinia-vectored recombinant oral rabies vaccine under field conditions: a 3-year study. *Can. J. Vet. Res.* 75 (4): 278–284.

Hermann, J., Fry, A., Reising, M. et al. (2012). Rabies vaccine standards: comparison of the 5th and 6th WHO international reference standards to the USDA veterinary reference standard. *Vaccine* 30 (48): 6892–6896.

Hicks, D.J., Fooks, A.R., and Johnson, N. (2012). Developments in rabies vaccines. *Clin. Exp. Immunol.* 169 (3): 199–204.

Höper, D., Freuling, C.M., Müller, T. et al. (2015). High definition viral vaccine strain identity and stability testing using full-genome population data – the next generation of vaccine quality control. *Vaccine* 33 (43): 5829–5837.

Hostnik, P., Picard-Meyer, E., Rihtarič, D. et al. (2014). Vaccine-induced rabies in a red fox (*Vulpes vulpes*): isolation of vaccine virus in brain tissue and salivary glands. *J. Wildl. Dis.* 50 (2): 397–401.

Hu, S.C., Hsu, C.L., Lee, M.S. et al. (2018). Lyssavirus in Japanese Pipistrelle, Taiwan. *Emerg. Infect. Dis.* 24 (4): 782–785.

Hundal, J.S., Sodhi, S.S., Gupta, A. et al. (2016). Awareness, knowledge, and risks of zoonotic diseases among livestock farmers in Punjab. *Vet. World* 9 (2): 186–191.

Hutter, S.E., Brugger, K., Sancho Vargas, V.H. et al. (2016). Rabies in Costa Rica: documentation of the surveillance program and the endemic situation from 1985 to 2014. *Vector Borne Zoonotic Dis.* 16 (5): 334–341.

Jacobs, T.M., Poehlmann, C.E., and Kiupel, M. (2017). Injection-site sarcoma in a dog: clinical and pathological findings. *Case Rep. Vet. Med.* 2017: 6952634.

Koprowski, H. and Cox, H.R. (1947). Studies on rabies infection in developing chick embryos. *J. Bacteriol.* 54 (1): 74.

Korns, R.F. and Zeissig, A. (1948). Dog, fox, and cattle rabies in New York state; evaluation of vaccination in dogs. *Am. J. Public Health Nations Health* 38 (1 Pt1): 50–65.

Lawson, K.F., Black, J.G., Charlton, K.M. et al. (1987). Safety and immunogenicity of a vaccine bait containing ERA strain of attenuated rabies virus. *Can. J. Vet. Res.* 51 (4): 460–464.

Lewis, C.E., Fry, A.M., Hermann, J.R. et al. (2012). Potency testing of veterinary rabies vaccines: replacement of challenge by in vitro testing: considerations for development of alternative assays. *Dev. Biol. (Basel)* 134: 29–33.

Li, J., Faber, M., Dietzschold, B., and Hooper, D.C. (2011). The role of toll-like receptors in the induction of immune responses during rabies virus infection. *Adv. Virus Res.* 79: 115–126.

Liu, Y., Zhang, H.P., Zhang, S.F. et al. (2016). Rabies outbreaks and vaccination in domestic camels and cattle in Northwest China. *PLoS Negl. Trop. Dis.* 10 (9): e0004890.

Loza-Rubio, E., Rojas-Anaya, E., López, J. et al. (2012). Induction of a protective immune response to rabies virus in sheep after oral immunization with transgenic maize, expressing the rabies virus glycoprotein. *Vaccine* 30 (37): 5551–5556.

Malerczyk, C., Briggs, D.J., Dreesen, D.W., and Banzhoff, A. (2007). Duration of immunity: an anamnestic response 14 years after rabies vaccination with purified chick embryo cell rabies vaccine. *J. Travel Med.* 14 (1): 63–64.

Malerczyk, C., Selhorst, T., Tordo, N. et al. (2009). Antibodies induced by vaccination with purified chick embryo cell culture vaccine (PCECV) cross-neutralize non-classical bat lyssavirus strains. *Vaccine* 27 (39): 5320–5325.

Martins, M., Joshi, L.R., Rodrigues, F.S. et al. (2017). Immunogenicity of ORFV-based vectors expressing the rabies virus glycoprotein in livestock species. *Virology* 511: 229–239.

McLaughlin, K. (2016). Scandal clouds China's global vaccine ambitions. *Science* 352 (6285): 506.

Meltzer, M.I. and Rupprecht, C.E. (1998). A review of the economics of the prevention and control of rabies. Part 2: rabies in dogs, livestock and wildlife. *Pharmacoeconomics* 14 (5): 481–498.

Miguens, L. (2007). The opinion of the production sector on the role of vaccines in the control and eradication of livestock diseases in Argentina. *Rev. Sci. Tech.* 26 (2): 479–483. 485–8.

Miller, R.E. and Fowler, M. (2012). *Zoo and Wild Animal Medicine: Current Therapy*, vol. 7. St Louis: Elsevier.

Mitmoonpitak, C., Limusanno, S., Khawplod, P. et al. (2002). Post-exposure rabies treatment in pigs. *Vaccine* 20 (16): 2019–2021.

Monaco, F., Franchi, P.M., and Lelli, R. (2006). Studies on an inactivated vaccine against rabies virus in domestic animals. *Dev. Biol. (Basel)* 125: 233–239.

Moore, M.C., Davis, R.D., Kang, Q. et al. (2015). Comparison of anamnestic responses to rabies vaccination in dogs and cats with current and out-of-date vaccination status. *J. Am. Vet. Med. Assoc.* 246 (2): 205–211.

Müller, T., Freuling, C.M., Wysocki, P. et al. (2015). Terrestrial rabies control in the European Union: historical achievements and challenges ahead. *Vet. J.* 203 (1): 10–17.

Nikolic, J., Le Bars, R., Lama, Z. et al. (2017). Negri bodies are viral factories with properties of liquid organelles. *Nat. Commun.* 8 (1): 58.

Ogino, M., Ito, N., Sugiyama, M., and Ogino, T. (2016). The rabies virus L protein catalyzes mRNA capping with GDP polyribonucleotidyltransferase activity. *Viruses* 8 (5): 144.

Palanisamy, R., Ramanna, B.C., Ananda Rao, K., and Srinivasan, V.A. (1992). Combined vaccination of cattle against FMD and rabies. *Microbiologica* 15 (1): 45–49.

Pastoret, P.P. and Vanderplasschen, A. (2003). Poxviruses as vaccine vectors. *Comp. Immunol. Microbiol. Infect. Dis.* 26 (5–6): 343–355.

Pawan, J.L. (1959). The transmission of paralytic rabies in Trinidad by the vampire bat (*Desmodus rotundus murinus* Wagner). *Caribb. Med.* J21: 110–136.

Petricciani, J.C., Grachev, V.P., Sizaret, P.P., and Regan, P.J. (1989). Vaccines: obstacles and opportunities from discovery to use. *Rev. Infect. Dis.* 11 (Suppl 3): S524–S529.

Piza, A.T., Pieri, K.M., Lusa, G.M. et al. (2002). Effect of the contents and form of rabies glycoprotein on the potency of rabies vaccination in cattle. *Mem. Inst. Oswaldo Cruz* 97 (2): 265–268.

Quirozr, D.E., Sutmoeller, P., and Barroeta, M. (1964). Factors associated with anaphylactic reactions to chicken embryo foot-and-mouth disease vaccine and Flury rabies vaccine in cattle of Venezuela. *Am. J. Vet. Res.* 25: 1627–1634.

Rappuoli, R. (2014). Inner workings: 1885, the first rabies vaccination in humans. *Proc. Natl. Acad. Sci. U.S.A.* 111 (34): 12273.

Reculard, R. (1996). Cell-culture vaccines for veterinary use. In: *Laboratory Techniques in Rabies*, 4e (eds. F.X. Meslin, M.M. Kaplan and H. Koprowski), 314–323. Geneva: WHO.

Robardet, E., Picard-Meyer, E., Dobroštana, M. et al. (2016). Rabies in the Baltic States: decoding a process of control and elimination. *PLoS Negl. Trop. Dis.* 10 (2): e0004432.

Rollin, B.E. (1995). An ethicist's commentary on whether rabies vaccine for livestock should be sold over the counter. *Can. Vet. J.* 36 (3): 178.

Rupprecht, C.E. and Burgess, G.W. (2015). Viral and vector zoonotic exploitation of a homo-sociome memetic complex. *Clin. Microbiol. Infect.* 21 (5): 394–403.

Rupprecht, C.E. and Dietzschold, B. (1987). Perspectives on rabies virus pathogenesis. *Lab. Invest.* 57 (6): 603–606.

Rupprecht, C.E. and Kuzmin, I.V. (2015). Why we can prevent, control and possibly treat – but will not eradicate rabies. *Future Virol.* 10 (5): 517–535.

Rupprecht, C.E., Turmelle, A., and Kuzmin, I.V. (2011). A perspective on lyssavirus emergence and perpetuation. *Curr. Opin. Virol.* 1 (6): 662–670.

Rupprecht, C.E., Nagarajan, T., and Ertl, H. (2016). Current status and development of vaccines and other biologics for human rabies prevention. *Expert Rev. Vaccines* 15 (6): 731–749.

Rupprecht, C., Kuzmin, I., and Meslin, F. (2017). Lyssaviruses and rabies: current conundrums, concerns, contradictions and controversies. *F1000Res.* 6: 184.

Rupprecht, C.E., Kuzmin, I.V., Yale, G. et al. (2019). Priorities in applied research to ensure programmatic success in the global elimination of canine rabies. *Vaccine* 37: A77–A84.

Schiffelers, M.J., Blaauboer, B., Bakker, W., and Hendriksen, C. (2014). Replacing the NIH test for rabies vaccine potency testing: a synopsis of drivers and barriers. *Biologicals* 42 (4): 205–217.

Schnee, M., Vogel, A.B., Voss, D. et al. (2016). An mRNA vaccine encoding rabies virus glycoprotein induces protection against lethal infection in mice and correlates of protection in adult and newborn pigs. *PLoS Negl.Trop. Dis.* 10 (6): e0004746.

Scott, T., Hasse, R., and Nel, L. (2012). Rabies in kudu (*Tragelaphus strepsiceros*). *Berl. Munch. Tierarztl. Wochenschr.* 125 (5–6): 236–241.

Sigoillot-Claude, C., Battaglio, M., Fiorucci, M. et al. (2015). A versatile *in vitro* ELISA test for quantification and quality testing of infectious, inactivated and formulated rabies virus used in veterinary monovalent or combination vaccine. *Vaccine* 33 (32): 3843–3849.

Sihvonen, L., Kulonen, K., and Neuvonen, E. (1994). Immunization of cattle against rabies using inactivated cell culture vaccines. *Acta Vet. Scand.* 35 (4): 371–376.

Sikes, R.K. (1970). Guidelines for the control of rabies. *Am. J. Public Health Nations Health* 60 (6): 1133–1138.

Slate, D., Algeo, T.P., Nelson, K.M. et al. (2009). Oral rabies vaccination in North America: opportunities, complexities, and challenges. *PLoS Negl.Trop. Dis.* 3 (12): e549.

Stoner-Duncan, B., Streicker, D.G., and Tedeschi, C.M. (2014). Vampire bats and rabies: toward an ecological solution to a public health problem. *PLoS Negl.Trop. Dis.* 8 (6): e2867.

Streicker, D.G. and Allgeier, J.E. (2016). Foraging choices of vampire bats in diverse landscapes: potential implications for land-use change and disease transmission. *J. Appl. Ecol.* 53 (4): 1280–1288.

Swai, E.S., Schoonman, L., and Daborn, C.J. (2010). Knowledge and attitude toward zoonoses among animal health workers and livestock keepers in Arusha and Tanga, Tanzania. *Tanzan. J. Health Res.* 12 (4): 280–286.

Thompson, M.K., Fridy, P.C., Keegan, S. et al. (2016). Optimizing selection of large animals for antibody production by screening immune response to standard vaccines. *J. Immunol. Methods* 430: 56–60.

Tian, D., Luo, Z., Zhou, M. et al. (2015). Critical role of K1685 and K1829 in the large protein of rabies virus in viral pathogenicity and immune evasion. *J. Virol.* 90 (1): 232–244.

Vuta, V., Picard-Meyer, E., Robardet, E. et al. (2016). Vaccine-induced rabies case in a cow (*Bos taurus):* molecular characterisation of vaccine strain in brain tissue. *Vaccine* 34 (41): 5021–5025.

Wallace, R.M., Niezgoda, M., Waggoner, E.A. et al. (2016). Serologic response in eight alpacas vaccinated by extralabel use of a large animal rabies vaccine during a public health response to a rabid alpaca in South Carolina. *J. Am. Vet. Med. Assoc.* 249 (6): 678–681.

Weyer, J., Kuzmin, I.V., Rupprecht, C.E., and Nel, L.H. (2008). Cross-protective and cross-reactive immune responses to recombinant vaccinia viruses expressing full-length lyssavirus glycoprotein genes. *Epidemiol. Infect.* 136 (5): 670–678.

Wilson, P.J. and Clark, K.A. (2001). Postexposure rabies prophylaxis protocol for domestic animals and epidemiologic characteristics of rabies vaccination failures in Texas: 1995–1999. *J. Am. Vet. Med. Assoc.* 218 (4): 522–525.

World Health Organization (2018). WHO expert consultation on rabies. Third report. *World Health Organ. Tech. Rep. Ser.* 1012: 1–183.

Wu, X., Smith, T.G., and Rupprecht, C.E. (2011). From brain passage to cell adaptation: the road of human rabies vaccine development. *Expert Rev. Vaccines* 10 (11): 1597–1608.

Yakobson, B., Taylor, N., Dveres, N. et al. (2015). Cattle rabies vaccination – a longitudinal study of rabies antibody titres in an Israeli dairy herd. *Prev. Vet. Med.* 121 (1–2): 170–175.

Yang, D.K., Kim, H.H., Lee, K.W., and Song, J.Y. (2013). The present and future of rabies vaccine in animals. *Clin. Exp. Vaccine Res.* 2 (1): 19–25.

Yang, D.K., Kim, H.H., Choi, S.S. et al. (2016). A recombinant rabies virus (ERAGS) for use in a bait vaccine for swine. *Clin. Exp. Vaccine Res.* 5 (2): 169–174.

Yendo, A.C., de Costa, F., Cibulski, S.P. et al. (2016). A rabies vaccine adjuvanted with saponins from leaves of the soap tree (*Quillaja brasiliensis*) induces specific immune responses and protects against lethal challenge. *Vaccine* 34 (20): 2305–2311.

Index

Veterinary Vaccines: Principles and Applications, First Edition. Edited by Samia Metwally, Gerrit Viljoen, and Ahmed El Idrissi.